Neurosurgical
Pain
Management

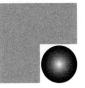

Neurosurgical Pain Management

KENNETH A. FOLLETT, MD, PhD
Department of Neurosurgery
University of Iowa Hospitals and Clinics
Iowa City, Iowa

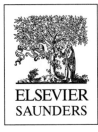

ELSEVIER
SAUNDERS

ELSEVIER
SAUNDERS

The Curtis Center
170 S. Independence Mall W 300 E
Philadelphia, Pennsylvania 19106

NEUROSURGICAL PAIN MANAGEMENT   ISBN 0-7216-9241-9

Notice

Medicine is an ever-changing field. Standard safety precautions must be followed, but as new research and
clinical experience broaden our knowledge, changes in treatment and drug therapy may become necessary
or appropriate. Readers are advised to check the most current product information provided by the
manufactuer of each drug to be administered to verify the recommended dose, the method and duration of
administration, and contraindications. It is the responsibility of the licensed prescriber or health care
provider, relying on experience and knowledge of the patient, to determine dosages and the best treatment
for each individual patient. Neither the publisher nor the author assumes any liability for any injury and/or
damage to persons or property arising from this publication.

The Publisher

Library of Congress Cataloging-in-Publication Data
Neurosurgical pain management/[edited by] Kenneth A. Follett — 1st ed.
    p.   ; cm.
    Includes bibliographical references.
    ISBN 0-7216-9241-9
  1. Pain—Surgery.   2. Chronic pain—Surgery.   3. Nervous system—Surgery.   4. Neuralgia.
    I. Follett, Kenneth A.
    [DNLM: 1. Neuralgia—rehabilitation.   2. Neuralgia—surgery.   3. Neurosurgical
    Procedures—methods.   4. Treatment Outcome. WL 544 N4948 2004]
RD595.5.N483 2004
616′.0472—dc22

                                                                    2004042740

Acquisitions Editor: *Rebecca Schmidt Gaertner*
Editorial Assistant: *Suzanne Flint*
Project Manager: *Dan Clipner*

Printed in the United States of America

Last digit is the print number: 9   8   7   6   5   4   3   2   1

_____

To Karen, Daniel, and Matthew,
with love and appreciation.

_____

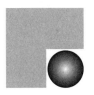

Contributors

Nicholas M. Barbaro, MD
Professor of Neurological Surgery, University of California
at San Francisco, San Francisco, CA
Cordotomy

Devin K. Binder, MD, PhD
Resident, Department of Neurological Surgery, University of
California at San Francisco, San Francisco, CA
Cordotomy

Amy Bleyer, MD
Clinical Instructor of Medicine, New York University School
of Medicine, New York; Murray Hill Medical Center,
New York, NY
Outcome Assessment

Jeffrey A. Brown, MD
Professor, Department of Neurological Surgery, Wayne State
University School of Medicine, Detroit, MI
*Motor Cortex Stimulation for the Treatment of
Neuropathic Pain Syndromes; Trigeminal Neuralgia—
Percutaneous Trigeminal Nerve Compression*

Daniel M. Doleys, PhD
Director, Pain and Rehabilitation Institute, Birmingham, AL
Psychological Considerations in Spine Surgery

Kenneth A. Follett, MD, PhD
Professor, Neurosurgery, University of Iowa Hospitals and
Clinics, Iowa City, IA
*Failed Back Surgery Syndrome; Spinal Ablative Therapies:
Myelotomy*

John P. Gorecki, FRCS(C), FACS, MD
Clinical Assistant Professor, University of Kansas School of
Medicine; Active Staff, Via Christi Regional Medical
Center; Active Staff, Wesley Medical Center,
Wichita, KS
Brainstem Ablative Procedures

J. David Haddox, DDS, MD, DABPM, MRO
University of Connecticut School of Medicine, Farmington,
CT; Vice President, Health Policy, Purdue Pharma L.P.,
Stamford, CT
Pharmacologic Therapies for Pain

Naeem Haider, MD, MBBS
Assistant Professor, University of Iowa College of Medicine;
Assistant Professor, University of Iowa Hospitals and
Clinics, Iowa City, IA
Complex Regional Pain Syndrome

Samuel J. Hassenbusch, MD, PhD
Professor, Department of Neurosurgery, MD Anderson
Cancer Center, Houston, TX
Peripheral Nerve Stimulation

Michael Horowitz, MD
Associate Professor of Neurosurgery, University of
Pittsburgh Medical Center, Pittsburgh, PA
*Posterior Fossa Procedures for Cranial
Neuralgias*

Amin Kassam, MD
Associate Professor of Neurosurgery, University of
Pittsburgh Medical Center, Pittsburgh, PA
Posterior Fossa Procedures for Cranial Neuralgias

Robert M. Levy, MD, PhD
Professor, Departments of Neurological Surgery and
Physiology, Northwestern University Medical School;
Northwestern Memorial Hospital, Chicago, IL
*Building (and Surviving) a Neurosurgical
Pain Practice*

Kenneth M. Little, MD
Chief Resident, Division of Neurosurgery, Duke University
Medical Center, Durham, NC
Brainstem Ablative Procedures

L. Dade Lunsford, MD
Professor and Chairman, Department of Neurological
Surgery, University of Pittsburgh Medical Center,
Pittsburgh, PA
*Trigeminal Neuralgia—Percutaneous Glycerol
Rhizotomy*

Norman Marcus, MD
Associate Professor of Psychology, New York University
School of Medicine; Senior Attending in Psychiatry and
Medicine, Lenox Hill Hospital; Director, Norman Marcus
Pain Institute, New York, NY
Outcome Assessment

Patrick Mertens, MD, PhD
Professor of Anatomy, University of Lyon, Lyon, France
Dorsal Root Entry Zone Lesions

John C. Oakley, MD
Director of Pain Management, Northern Rockies Pain
Rehabilitation Center, St. Vincent's Healthcare,
Billings, MT
Spinal Cord Stimulation for the Treatment of Chronic Pain

Richard K. Osenbach, MD
Assistant Professor, Division of Neurological Surgery, Duke University Medical Center, Durham, NC
Nontrigeminal Craniofacial Pain Syndromes; Peripheral Ablative Techniques

Ronald P. Pawl, MD
Associate Professor, Neurosurgery, University of Illinois, Chicago, IL; Medical Director, Lake Forest Hospital, Lake Forest, IL
The Multidisciplinary Pain Treatment Program

Richard D. Penn, MD
Professor, University of Chicago, Chicago, IL
Neuraxial Analgesic Administration

Donald E. Richardson, MD
Chairman and Program Director, Professor, Tulane University Health Sciences Center, School of Medicine; Chairman of Neurosurgery, Tulane University Hospital and Clinic; Chief of Neurosurgery, Medical Center of Louisiana at New Orleans; Consulting Physician, Veterans Medical Center, New Orleans, LA
Intracranial Stimulation Therapies: Deep-Brain Stimulation

Richard W. Rosenquist, MD
Associate Professor of Anesthesia; Director, Pain Medicine Division, University of Iowa; Medical Director, Center for Pain Medicine and Regional Anesthesia, University of Iowa Hospitals and Clinics, Iowa City, IA
Complex Regional Pain Syndrome

Hubert L. Rosomoff, MD, D Med Sci, FAAPM
Professor and Chairman Emeritus, Department of Neurological Surgery, University of Miami School of Medicine, Miami, FL; Medical Director, The Rosomoff Comprehensive Pain and Rehabilitation Center, Miami Beach, FL
Myofascial Pain Syndromes

Oren Sagher, MD
Associate Professor, Department of Neurosurgery, University of Michigan Health System, Ann Arobor, MI
Trigeminal, Geniculate, and Glossopharyngeal Neuralgia

Joel L. Seres, MD
Clinical Professor, Department of Neurosurgery, Oregon Health and Science University, Portland, OR
Approach to the Patient with Pain

Richard K. Simpson, Jr, MD, PhD, FACS
Professor, Department of Neurosurgery, Anesthesiology, and Physical Medicine and Rehabilitation, Baylor College of Medicine; Chief, Neurosurgical Section, Houston VA Medical Center, Houston, TX
Central and Deafferentation Pain Syndromes

Marc P. Sindou, MD, DSc
Professor of Neurosurgery, University of Lyon; Chairman, Department of Neurosurgery, Hôpital Neurologique Pierre Wertheimer, Lyon, France
Dorsal Root Entry Zone Lesions

Renee Steele-Rosomoff, BSN, MBA
Adjunct Associate Professor, University of Miami School of Medicine; Rosomoff Comprehensive Pain and Rehabilitation Center, Miami, FL
Myofascial Pain Syndromes

Richard L. Stieg, MD, MHS
Associate Clinical Professor of Neurology, University of Colorado Health Sciences Center, Denver, CO
Disability and Impairment in the Patient with Pain

Jamal M. Taha, MD
Director, Office of Neuroscience Technology Development, Kettering Medical Center, Dayton, OH
Trigeminal Neuralgia—Percutaneous Radiofrequency Rhizotomy

R.R. Tasker, MD, FRCSC
Professor Emeritus, Division of Neurosurgery, Toronto Western Hospital; Honorary Neurosurgeon, Toronto Western Division, University Hospital Network, Toronto, Canada
Intracranial Ablative Procedures

Bradley K. Taylor, PhD
Department of Pharmacology, Tulane University Health Sciences Center, New Orleans, LA
The Pathophysiology of Neuropathic Pain

Todd P. Thompson, MD
Peachtree Neurosurgery, Atlanta, GA
Trigeminal Neuralgia—Percutaneous Glycerol Rhizotomy

Richard J. Traub, PhD
Associate Professor, Department of Biomedical Sciences-Dental School, Program in Neuroscience Research Center for Neuroendocrine Influences on Pain, University of Maryland, Baltimore, MD
The Neuroanatomic and Neurophysiologic Basis of Pain

Sridhar V. Vasudevan, MD
Clinical Professor, Medical College of Wisconsin, Madison, WI; Medical Director, Center for Pain and Work Rehabilitation, St. Nicholas Hospital, Sheboygan, WI
Physical Medicine and Rehabilitation in Pain Management

Marc Y. Wasserman, MD
Senior Resident, Neurology, Rush University Medical Center, Chicago, IL
Physical Medicine and Rehabilitation in Pain Management

Richard L. Weiner, MD, FACS
Clinical Associate Professor, Department of Neurosurgery, University of Texas Southeastern Medical School; Chair, Department of Neuroscience, Presbyterian Hospital of Dallas, Dallas, TX
Treatment of Occipital Neuralgia and Related Posterior Headache Syndromes

Harold A. Wilkinson, MD, PhD
Clinical Affiliate in Neurosurgery, Massachusetts General Hospital, Boston, MA
Trigeminal Neuralgia—Peripheral Neurectomy

Andrew S. Youkilis, MD
Staff Neurosurgeon, Neurological Associates Inc., St. Louis, MO
Trigeminal, Geniculate, and Glossopharyngeal Neuralgia

Ronald F. Young, MD
Medical Director, Northwest Hospital Gamma Knife Center, Seattle, WA
Radiosurgery for Pain Management

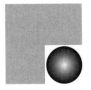

Introduction

The past two decades have seen evolutionary changes in the practice of pain management. Many of the changes have come about as a result of a growing understanding of pain pathophysiology, including recognition of chronic pain as a biopsychosocial disease, and increasing awareness on the part of patients, physicians, payors, and regulatory agencies that pain can and should be treated. Within neurosurgery, as in other pain management specialties that offer primarily interventional techniques, historically important (and sometimes still clinically important) ablative procedures have by-and-large given way to augmentative neuromodulation therapies. Against this backdrop of change, neurosurgeons have maintained their role in the field of pain medicine as practitioners and as contributors to the development and refinement of innovative pain therapies.

Management of chronic pain frequently requires comprehensive patient evaluation and multidisciplinary treatment, with specific therapy tailored to meet the needs of each individual patient. To accomplish this, pain management specialists, regardless of background medical specialty, must remain knowledgeable about mechanisms of nociception and pain pathophysiology, psychosocial factors that contribute to or cause pain and influence responses to treatment, and the indications and relative advantages and disadvantages of the variety of interventional and non-interventional pain therapies currently available. Most physicians engaged in pain management, including neurosurgeons, typically understand and provide the pain therapies they were taught during training in their parent specialty. This approach to pain care tends to restrict treatment options to those offered personally by the treating physician, places the burden of finding the appropriate physician with the appropriate therapies on the shoulders of the patients, and leads to uncoordinated, fragmented pain care. In contrast, pain management physicians who have a broad understanding of pain disorders and therapies can facilitate the delivery of more comprehensive, better coordinated care because they can recommend treatments selected from the full range of pain management options, not just those they provide personally. Even surgeons who believe their role in pain care should be limited to that of "technician," performing whatever interventional treatment (e.g., spinal cord stimulator implant, intrathecal drug infusion system implant) is requested by the patient's primary pain management physician, need to understand basic principles of pain care because the surgeon is responsible ultimately for deciding the proper type and timing of the surgical procedures he or she performs.

Within the realm of interventional procedures, it is important for practitioners to be familiar with ablative and non-ablative techniques. Contemporary surgical therapies for pain treatment are primarily neuroaugmentative techniques such as spinal cord stimulation and intrathecal analgesic administration. Pain management practitioners should be familiar with these non-ablative surgeries because they are useful, increasingly common procedures for pain management. On the other hand, ablative therapies (e.g., cordotomy, myelotomy, DREZ) that are considered classically to lie within the neurosurgical domain may be more appropriate than neuroaugmentative therapies for certain patients. These ablative procedures must remain part of the pain medicine armamentarium if patients are to receive the best care possible. Neurosurgeons are uniquely suited to offer these ablative procedures and should remain knowledgeable about them. Pain management physicians from other parent specialties should be familiar with these techniques as well in order to know when to refer patients for these procedures.

This book is intended to serve as a practical reference to facilitate the continued participation of neurosurgeons in the field of pain medicine and to provide physicians in non-neurosurgical disciplines a concise source of information about neurosurgically-relevant pain disorders and therapies. A broad range of topics of fundamental importance to the general practice of pain management is presented, reflecting the interdisciplinary nature of basic pain care. Pain disorders encountered frequently by neurosurgeons are described in detail, including craniofacial pain syndromes, pain associated with the "failed back surgery syndrome," and myofascial pain. Pain therapies provided typically by neurosurgeons are reviewed, including classical ablative therapies as well as contemporary and innovative treatments.

This textbook could not have been completed without the help of many individuals. I am indebted greatly to the authors, each of whom took precious time from their professional activities, medical practices, and families to contribute. I extend special thanks to Rebecca Schmidt Gaertner and her colleagues at Elsevier and to Ellen Sklar at P. M. Gordon Associates for their efforts in bringing this book to completion.

I offer my thanks also to the many patients I have encountered in my day-to-day activities as a pain medicine physician. Every patient has something to teach his or her physicians and I have learned much from my patients. Each day brings new patients, new lessons, new challenges, and new opportunities for a better understanding of pain and its treatment.

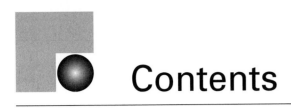

Contents

Contributors / vii

Introduction / xi

SECTION I
Fundamental Considerations in Pain Treatment / 1

CHAPTER 1
Approach to the Patient with Pain / 3

CHAPTER 2
The Neuroanatomic and Neurophysiologic Basis of Pain / 17

CHAPTER 3
The Pathophysiology of Neuropathic Pain / 29

CHAPTER 4
Psychological Considerations in Spine Surgery / 38

CHAPTER 5
Pharmacologic Therapies for Pain / 46

SECTION II
Pain Syndromes of Neurosurgical Importance / 55

CHAPTER 6
Myofascial Pain Syndromes / 57

CHAPTER 7
Failed Back Surgery Syndrome / 73

CHAPTER 8
Nontrigeminal Craniofacial Pain Syndromes / 84

CHAPTER 9
Treatment of Occipital Neuralgia and Related Posterior Headache Syndromes / 99

CHAPTER 10
Trigeminal, Geniculate, and Glossopharyngeal Neuralgia / 102

CHAPTER 11
Central and Deafferentation Pain Syndromes / 110

CHAPTER 12
Complex Regional Pain Syndrome / 119

SECTION III
Neurosurgical Pain Therapies / 129

CHAPTER 13
Spinal Cord Stimulation for the Treatment of Chronic Pain / 131

CHAPTER 14
Peripheral Nerve Stimulation / 144

CHAPTER 15
Neuraxial Analgesic Administration / 150

CHAPTER 16
Intracranial Stimulation Therapies: Deep-Brain Stimulation / 156

CHAPTER 17
Motor Cortex Stimulation for the Treatment of Neuropathic Pain Syndromes / 160

CHAPTER 18
Cordotomy / 165

CHAPTER 19
Spinal Ablative Therapies: Myelotomy / 172

CHAPTER 20
Dorsal Root Entry Zone Lesions / 176

CHAPTER 21
Brainstem Ablative Procedures / 189

CHAPTER 22
Intracranial Ablative Procedures / 194

CHAPTER 23
Peripheral Ablative Techniques 200

CHAPTER 24
Trigeminal Neuralgia—Peripheral Neurectomy / 210

CHAPTER 25
Trigeminal Neuralgia—Percutaneous Trigeminal Nerve Compression / 214

CHAPTER 26
Trigeminal Neuralgia—Percutaneous Glycerol Rhizotomy / 219

CHAPTER 27
Trigeminal Neuralgia—Percutaneous Radiofrequency Rhizotomy / 227

CHAPTER 28
Posterior Fossa Procedures for Cranial Neuralgias / 232

CHAPTER 29
Radiosurgery for Pain Management / 237

SECTION IV
Miscellaneous Topics / 245

CHAPTER 30
Physical Medicine and Rehabilitation in Pain Management / 247

CHAPTER 31
The Multidisciplinary Pain Treatment Program / 255

CHAPTER 32
Disability and Impairment in the Patient with Pain / 262

CHAPTER 33
Outcome Assessment / 265

CHAPTER 34
Building (and Surviving) a Neurosurgical Pain Practice / 271

Index / 275

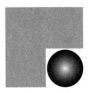

Fundamental Considerations in Pain Treatment

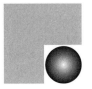

C H A P T E R 1

Approach to the Patient with Pain

JOEL L. SERES, MD

People respond to pain in vastly differing ways.[1–6] So do the surgeons they consult.[7–11] Patients see pain as something they want to get rid of; the surgeon often sees significant palliation as the goal. Some patients respond positively to palliation, others continue to seek a complete "cure." Sometimes the cure as envisioned by the patient is not realistic; sometimes neither is the result envisioned by the surgeon.[12] This chapter explores the importance of understanding your patients, their concept of their pain, and its resulting impairments in planning any pain-relieving operation.

Chronic pain is different. It is not the same as acute pain, or postoperative pain, or pains that we can explained by physical examination, imaging studies, or findings at surgery.[13] Some tolerate chronic pain without medical care.[14] Others tax the ingenuity of the most brilliant among us to find a way to make the pain tolerable enough to justify continued life.[15] Most patients are somewhere between these extremes.[16] Those who come for surgical help represent a separate division by themselves. And those who fail to benefit despite all our machinations document the limit of our knowledge and force us to face the reality of our inadequacies in providing relief.[17]

Historically, the surgical management of pain has gone through a variety of informative epochs.[18,19] This means that while each has added to our understanding of the patient in pain, none have provided the ultimate treatment.[20] Our current approaches are the extension of these efforts and should be viewed as additional stepping-stones. Common among our past efforts has been enthusiasm for newer therapies later diminished by the reality of outcomes.[21–23] Until we know more, our present treatments must be viewed with the skepticism justified by experience. All too often, however, some of the efficacies that have resulted are ignored as new procedures stimulate the enthusiastic vigor of the next generation of surgeons.[24–26]

Opioids defined the first modern era of effective pain control.[27] Eventually, it was found that opioids failed in some patients to provide enough continued relief to justify their use. Others seemingly did well. We have never been able to explain these differences except through the expression of such vague concepts as "individual differences," "different thresholds of pain," or because of some mysterious and even now unexplained psychological or cerebral mechanisms.[28] The eventual identification of opioid inadequacies renewed the search for more direct attacks on the perceived source of pain, the "pain generator."[29] Repeated back surgery, wider decompressions, and attempts to reduce the rate of fusion failures all failed to deliver expected outcomes in many patients.[30] Initially, the enthusiastic developers of new tools and techniques led us to expect remarkable results.[31] After the blush of impressive outcomes, more practical data became available. This information, now not as influenced by some of the funding sources of the earlier studies, gave a better taste of reality.[32,33] Still, newer and more technically elaborate procedures have resulted. Each bears the promise of solving the pain and the way it impacts our patients.

Direct ablative surgery on parts of the peripheral nervous system initially seemed to solve some difficult pain problems.[34] But there were those whose pain seemed to recur later despite the degree of initial efficacy.[35] Ablation procedures on the spinal cord seemingly worked well for the cancer patient but offered little long-term benefit for most with longer survivals. Newer techniques of percutaneous cord ablative procedures promised to avoid previous problems[36]; in fact, they created their own.[37] Brain ablative procedures eventually targeted so many cerebral and brainstem structures that it seemed that almost any central nervous system lesion could affect pain perception at least for a while. The review of outcomes of ablative surgery for pain control seemed to parallel the same fate of other less exotic procedures.[38–40] Most recently, neuroaugmentative procedures have held new promise but only in "appropriately selected patients."[41] Despite a remarkable array of psychological and psychosocial preoperative testing, we still cannot outline clearly what we mean by an "appropriate patient."[42,43] When failures result from newer procedures, we tend to malign those mysterious psychosocial issues that we had defined were not present with preoperative testing.[44] Doesn't this challenge the validity of the kind of testing we are doing? Yet little has seemingly been done to focus our tests more accurately. Because the tests do not predict outcomes, we understand our failures here no more completely than we comprehend the failures experienced in previous epochs of pain treatment. Even now when all fails, we revert yet again back to the use of narcotics by a variety of delivery means.[45] Again some of this works in some people some of the time.

3

In our literature we extol our successes. Yet a global view of the management of pain must include our failures and the messages that they teach. If the intervertebral disk is opined as the cause of the patient's pain, why do some still hurt after its removal, its fusion, or its obliteration through electrical coagulation or enzymatic digestion? If the patient responds positively to a trial of spinal stimulation or spinal opioids, why do some fail to benefit later with a permanent implant? The operational answer is quite simple, but difficult to accept. We just do not have all the answers for all patients who come to us for aid. And this means that we do not understand well enough the mechanisms of pain and their meaning. It also infers that we do not yet understood enough about people and their pain responses to truly understand the phenomenon of chronic pain. What we do know we can use. What we do not know becomes visible every time a patient seeks our help for the first time. That new patient who you are seeing represents the failure of the last treatment. And that treatment was provided with very best of intentions . . . and supposedly with a good chance for aid. In the final analysis, it is not physicians' intentions that count in treating the chronic pain patient, it is the result that is paramount and decisive. And it is not the result for a short temporal quantum that is important. Cessation of pain and a future without recurrence is.

WHY CHRONIC PAIN IS DIFFERENT

Chronic pain is different than acute pain problems because it infers the failure of medical care. After all, if previous treatments had been successful, the patient would not be experiencing chronic pain. Chronic pain requires an understanding of the mechanisms behind previous failures before it is reasonable to proceed with something new.

The failure of medical or surgical care to relieve pain may be due to the failure of the treatment itself, but it might also be related to a variety of underlying psychosocial issues. Pain relief that is judged as adequate by a previous physician may not have been helpful enough for the patient. This means that the level of improvement that the patient envisions must be explored and understood before proceeding. Even relieving a substantial portion of residual pain that might seem like an adequate result by the surgeon might again be viewed as less than satisfactory by the patient who needs more.

The presence of chronic pain despite previous treatment places a special burden on any new physician trying to help. There exists now a special requirement that no new treatment should be considered unless it stands a good chance for success. It is not appropriate just to do something else and see what happens. Success must be assured first. Repeated failures of adequate relief only further add to the frustrations of the patient, and demoralization and depression. These problems make it more difficult for the patient to cope with their predicament. Consider this when prescribing repeated nerve blocks, epidural steroids, trigger point injections, and the variety of treatments that predictably produce only short-term effects at best.

It appears at times that we create a new dependency relationship with the patient who enters our practice with previous failures. The patient depends on our ability to make things right. In some this augments the already existing passivity of the patient. That preexisting passivity may be the only visible sign of serious underlying emotional, motivational, and personal problems.

WHY HAVING A NEUROSURGEON SEE THE PATIENT IS DIFFERENT

Neurosurgeons are usually seen as the last of "last resorts." In reality, neurosurgical efforts often become part of the on-going history as the patient searches for relief. From the moment of consultation with the neurosurgeon the patient expects the ultimate of care. It is important that the physician understands the impact of such expectations. Sadly, we often see that when patients do not do well after pain treatment surgeons commonly lose interest in the patient and her or his care. Because patients presenting for pain treatment usually represent the failures of previous care, it is important that someone must be willing to remain as their advocate. If the surgeon is not able to do this, it is important that someone else assumes this position before proceeding with care. Psychologists often see patients before a pain-relieving operation. But they are often not consulted when patients fail later. We should encourage psychologists to expand their role in judging the prognosis of the proposed treatment and in offering a post-treatment plan that includes the management of failure if it should occur. As we will discuss subsequently, if psychosocial issues are impugned as explanations for the failure of adequate pain relief it is likely that they were present, and thus identifiable, before the procedure. Again, failure to identify their importance beforehand is a common scenario in patients who later do not do well.

OBLIGATIONS OF CHRONIC PAIN CARE

The implication that the chronic pain syndrome infers the failure of previous treatments creates a special obligation on the pain-treating physician. The patient who has failed to gain enough benefit from previous care is commonly in the midst of a life crisis. Not only has chronic pain resulted in marked lifestyle changes but also it has wrested away the controls of the patient's life. Reliance on medical practitioners who now imply, if not overtly promise, benefit augments the patient's passivity. Most do not understand much of what they are told regarding the reasons for their continued pain, its impact, or proposed treatments. Just test this out by asking your patient to repeat what their last practitioner had said or what you had discussed at your last meeting with him or her.[46]

Undertaking the care of the patient in chronic pain requires an understanding of the patient's predicament in terms that must include its meaning to the patient. It is unfair to consider relief of just some of the pain (say a 50% reduction) as an adequate goal unless that goal provides the impact needed by the patient. The implication of all this is that the surgeon must be willing to envision his or her ultimate role in the care of the patient and to define it beforehand.

Sadly, funding issues determine what happens to many of our patients. While there might be funding for a pain-relieving operation, there might not be money available for rehabilitation or for long-term follow-up. This follow-up might be more important to the support of our patient's well being than the degree of surgical benefit. Because a significant number of patients undergoing pain operations fail to improve this issue must become part of overall care planning.

OUTCOMES VERSUS OUTCOMES

The literature on pain relieving surgical procedures seems to present a picture of outcome that transcends reality. In most pain surgical practices there are many patients who, seemingly improved with surgery continue to augment their pain relief with narcotics; and display impaired levels of function, continued emotional difficulties, and the search for yet more improvement. In literature reports, outcomes statements are often exaggerated and stress positive results. Little is often made of the relatively large groups of failed patients. Unfortunately, once printed such outcomes are the major points quoted to patients seeking help.

One study, starting with 40 pre-screened candidates for morphine pump instillation, documented that only eight patients claimed a 50% pain reduction at 2 years. The paper concludes that ". . . intrathecal morphine can be a safe, effective therapy for the management of severe, nonmalignant pain among a carefully selected patient population . . . "[43] Quoting this outcome to a needy or desperate pain patient belies the more likely result. It is more likely than not that the patient will achieve less than a 50% relief of pain based upon this study. This study documents that it is probably more realistic to wait at least 2 years after treatment to define efficacy. Think for a moment what our outcome literature would look like if 2-year follow-up were a requirement of every journal editorial staff. Unfortunately, much of our literature looks at much shorter outcomes. Further research that never seems to get done is suggested.

A listing of the patient's expectations should be part of preoperative planning. A simple checklist might be helpful (Fig. 1-1). Such a list can provide a reasonable source of reality discussion. The major point is that outcomes assessment must start with preoperative expectations. Outcomes that the patient finds valuable are more important than percentages of pain improvement. And what the patient plans to do with the improvement has more to do with the meaning of results than any other measure.

PAIN CONCEPTS AND TREATMENT

William Sweet who has spent a creative and fruitful life treating chronic pain tells us in the twilight of his career that . . . "It has become steadily more obvious that, not only does persistent pain involve mysterious cerebral mechanisms, but also that we do not understand them."[28] Ever-evolving concepts of pain theory provide insights into the complexity of pain and its perception. The newly proposed neuromatrix theory implies the importance of neural mechanisms within the brain that are normally activated and modulated by inputs from the body but they can also act in the absence of any inputs.[47] The origins of these lie in neural networks within the brain that are genetically determined and involve neural-hormonal mechanisms of stress response and sensory transmission.[48] More and more the complexity of pain and its impact is exposed by the progressive complexity of our pain theories. The full elucidation of pain mechanisms of both reception and impact will require yet the works of another generation of scientists. Until then our concepts of pain and its management remained based more directly on the observed effects of our surgical and chemical machinations because each patient is impacted differently. These differences demand a level of humility as we approach our patients and promise outcomes. Often we still do not have enough information to be smug about what we promise.

To help provide a reasoned approach given the inadequate nature of our current comprehension of pain, its mechanisms, and its impact, we have classically described pain in a variety of subtypes. These lists are the results of observed clinical differences in the expression of pain and its response to treatment. In an introductory chapter such as this, it is reasonable to discuss each type of pain and its meaning briefly. Continue to remember, however, that if we really fully understood the mechanisms of pain physiology at a molecular and at a global level, we might speak in entirely different ways. What we write here no doubt will be discarded with the same antipathy that we express for earlier theories once we understand more.

For now a simple classification can be a starting point (Table 1-1).

Acute Pain

Acute pain is often separated from chronic pain syndromes because of the way the patient reports their pain and the way they respond to treatment. Acute pain is the result of tissue damage or the threat of tissue damage. It should be clear that this definition is more of a crutch upon which to build discussions than a clue to the mechanisms involved. Acute pain is often self-limited, short-lived, and effectively responsive to opioids.

There are, however, some acute pain syndromes that are similar to chronic states. These are the recurring acute pain syndromes that result in psychosocial impairments similar to those seen in chronic states. These syndromes often create the same type of existential impairments that are present in the persistent states of pain. Such syndromes include the recurring pain of sickle cell disease, the inflammatory arthritides, and a variety of episodic neuropathic pain syndromes including tic douloureux, neuroma pain, and the pain associated with some brain disorders.

Sisters to the acute pain syndromes are those that might be described as subacute. These syndromes carry a degree of two more of the psychosocial concomitants seen in the chronic pain syndromes. These syndromes provide the interface between the acute and more responsive pain problems and those that are classified as chronic and therefore less responsive. This subacute phase is often missed when treating acute pain. Its presence often portends of poor outcomes

---

Patient Expectations

1. Pain relief

   ☐ 25% ☐ 50% ☐ 75% ☐ 100%

2. Return to Work

   ☐ Same job at time of injury
   ☐ Different job. Specify _____
      Will you need training for this job? ☐ Yes ☐ No
      Have you arranged for this yet? ☐ Yes ☐ No
   ☐ Am retired. Do not plan to return to work

3. What family activities can you not engage in now?_____
   _____
   _____
   _____

4. Which of these do you plan to resume if your operation is successful?
   _____
   _____
   _____

5. If you get significant pain relief, what physical activities do you plan to resume?
   _____
   _____
   _____

6. Do you have an attorney regarding your disability?

   ☐ Yes ☐ No
   If your answer is "yes," what is it that your attorney is doing at this time on your behalf?
   _____
   _____
   _____
   _____

7. Do you have an open compensation claim or lawsuit at this time regarding your disability?

   ☐ Yes ☐ No
   If your answer is "yes," what are your plans regarding it if your operation is successful?
   _____
   _____
   _____
   _____

8. Do you know what is the cause of your pain?

   ☐ Yes ☐ No
   If your answer is "yes," what is your understanding for its cause?
   _____
   _____
   _____
   _____

9. What do you plan to do if this operation or treatment is not successful in relieving a substantial part of your pain?
   _____
   _____
   _____
   _____

10. Please share with us your opinion of the medical care you have received to date for your pain.
   _____
   _____
   _____
   _____

FIGURE 1-1 These are just some of the questions about your patient's expectations that can help you plan treatment in a more realistic way. It is not necessary to give the patient this form. Consider using it as a guide and having the answers available before you decide to proceed with an operation for pain management.

● **T A B L E 1 - 1** • A Simple Classification of Pain

I. Pain based on its temporal presentation

- Acute and postoperative pain
- Subacute pain
- Chronic pain
- Recurring pain

II. Pain defined by its physiology

- Nociceptive pain
- Neuropathic pain

III. Pain associated with complicating factors

- Failed pain syndrome
- Pain in the workplace
- Pain associated with psychological complicating issues
- Pain and societal expectations

for acute pain treatment after the pain has later become chronic.

Chronic Pain

Chronic pain syndromes are really a mixed variety of pain syndromes that have similar aspects. They are long-lived and are associated with a variety of psychological responses and societal influences. They do not respond as well to opioids and their response to pain-relieving treatments are variable and tend to be inconsistent. Chronic pain patients improve as a group for a time after surgical, behavior/cognitive, and other psychological and social interventions.[14,16,17] They document short-term improvement after a variety of physical therapies that include manipulative therapy. They seemingly respond for a time to a myriad of alternative medical treatments. Regression of apparent initial benefit is common. Exaggerated negative responses to pain and minimal positive response to its improvement are characteristic. Yet within this group there are those who respond dramatically, just as those in acute pain respond to surgery, narcotics, to simple counseling, and to a vast array of approaches. The chronic pain patient represents the largest group of outcome failures and the most difficult of treatment groups. They define the deficiencies of our current comprehension of pain mechanisms.

Nociceptive Pain

Nociceptive pain is often included in the acute pain syndromes because it infers a more linear cause-and-effect relationship. Such is not always the case. There are patients who clearly have a "pain generator" whose presence is defined by the response to local anesthetics yet which continue to cause pain despite their removal. Diskogenic pain that seemingly can be relieved by coagulation of the disk, by radio frequency lesions of the facets, and by local blocks often does not respond to diskectomy or to a variety of fusion techniques,[49] or by permanent denervation by dorsal root ganglionectomy.[50] Patients with nociceptive pain may have the same psychosocial impairments seen in patients with each of the other pain syndromes.

Many of these patients cease to suffer after becoming actively involved in their care.[3] Despite the persistence of a definable pain generator, suffering behaviors stop. The response of the patient with nociceptive pain therefore teaches volumes about what we do not understand about the pain response.

Neuropathic Pain

This special form of chronic pain is related to peripheral nerve or central nervous system (CNS) damage. This form of pain does not respond as well to opioids and is associated with a variety of peripheral responses whose nature still remains controversial.[51] On the other hand, there are some forms of neuropathic pain that respond just as well as acute syndromes to opioids and to surgery. Some patients with tic douloureux, postlaminectomy nerve damage, postcordotomy pain, and the variety of complex regional pain syndromes sometimes respond in very gratifying ways. Some have most of the emotional complications of those in chronic pain and some of these respond poorly to any treatment. Yet even in this group some make dramatic improvements. While we can make some generalizations regarding patients with neuropathic pain, this syndrome defines more than most our lack of understanding.

Failed Pain Syndrome

The failed pain syndrome results from the failure of a variety of treatments that have not provided adequate improvement. As we suggest above, this group requires a much more comprehensive approach before proceeding with yet another attempt. Some of these patients respond well to specific surgical treatment, others do not. Some respond well to opioids, others do not. Some respond to neuroaugmentative procedures, others do not. Some exhibit marked and refractory psychological responses that others do not. Some are depressed and discouraged while others are seemingly impassive. The failed pain syndrome patient presents our greatest challenge. Before proceeding with care for this group, we must first define the reasons for the prior failures.

Were the Failures Due to the Failure of the Treatment Itself?

Treatment for acute pain syndromes is usually directed at removal of the source of the pain. Sometimes diagnostic studies inappropriately direct us. For example, not all patients with concordant diskographic pain will respond positively to the radical excision of the disk.[23,49] Degenerative changes at one level may not explain the cause for backache or neckache.[52] Effectively eradicating the pain with a directed localized nerve block may not predict any long-term benefit from denervation.[50] Indeed, we may view the trial of spinal stimulation or spinal opioids in the same way when the patient who initially responds loses the efficacy of the implanted device within a short time. Early failure suggests that the procedure did not eradicate the cause of the pain.

Were the Failures Due to Inherent Personality or Genetic Factors?

There exists within the comprehension of the lay public and in the minds of some physicians that there is a lower pain threshold in some patients. From a neurophysiologic viewpoint, this is not true. Within narrow limits of variability, our peripheral receptors and nociceptive fibers all act similarly.[53] There does appear to be a difference in the way that individuals respond to pain.[54,55] This may be the result of some earlier conditioning,[56] responses to certain behaviors, or perhaps to as-yet not understood genetic factors. The point is that because reception at the lowest level of our nociceptive anatomy functions similarly, attacking only that level when planning pain relief is less likely to be helpful in the over-responsive person. Moreover, it appears that over-responsivity is variable across time and wide array of variables.

Were the Failures Due to Motivational Issues?

People have to have something to do with an improvement of their pain state. While there are probably very few people who actively choose pain as a coping mechanism, it is also true that there are many who do not know what to do with improvement in their pain. It is interesting to talk to prospective patients about how their lives might be better if their pain improved. Often we hear that they plan to return to work. Yet when we question them about the type of work they might want to do, there are no plans in place. Commonly, such people will indicate that the only job they know how to do was the job they had been doing. But now they haven't done that job in years, have not kept up with its advancements, and despite total cessation of their pain would not be able physically to do that job. Statistics regarding return-to-work potential speak volumes.[57–61] When return to work is not likely, many patients will make no plans for future activities. Think about this for a moment. If a person is not working because of their pain and their pain is made better, what reason will they give for not working? In our experience, it is the residual pain that then becomes the reason. Thus, the patient tells us of dramatic improvement, and complains to others about the limitations imposed by the persisting pain.

The point of this all is simply that the motivational issues are available for study before the next attempt.[62] Know that they exist, know what they are, and know how they will influence your outcome before you proceed. The motivational factors may represent the most important of prognostic matters.

Were the Failures Related to Compensation Factors?

Behavioral theory suggests that it is the responses to behaviors that help to extinguish or to augment them. In chronic pain, certain behaviors result in at least a degree of financial security. While most patients who have been out of work for long periods will indicate their desire to return to work, few seemingly make any definitive plans.[63] Alternative employment possibilities are commonly not explored in our experience even with the forceful aid of a professional vocational counselor.[15]

Compensation factors may be a cause for motivational issues. Many workers' compensation plaintiffs' attorneys seem to be more interested in financial compensation than what really might be best for the client. I once raised the ire of a group of attorneys attending the annual meeting of the Oregon Trial Lawyers Association when I asked the group when they had last called a client 6 months or longer after the settlement to see how they were doing. Some quite vociferously pleaded that was not their job. Their job was to get them money and that was all! On the other hand, how many pain surgeons are really interested enough to contact their patients afterward, except perhaps for research purposes?

Unfortunately, for many some form of compensation is their only realistic option. If the compensation is not adequate, the residual pain then becomes more important in order to justify more compensation. These statements are not meant in a pejorative sense; it just seems that this is the way things seem to be.

Complicating the compensation issues are the remarkable array of compensation systems that exist in our country. Each state has its own workers' compensation system, each with its own way of assessing impairment and disability. There is a different system for federal employees, for railroad workers, and for long shore employees. There is Social Security (SS), Supplemental Security Income (SSI), Social Security Disability Insurance (SSDI), and an array of differing jury awards that sometimes transcend reason or logic. Each of these exerts its own and commonly different nefarious influence on the patient who also must cope with pain. In simple discussions with pain surgeons, many do not understand the differences in these systems and how the doctors' reports may impact their patient. Indeed, saying something in one system might be helpful while the same statement in another system might have negative influences. Someone who helps you in assessing the patient for surgery must be able to explain this to you about each patient if you do not have the knowledge yourself.

Did Domestic Relation Issues Influence the Failures?

After the remarkable success in mobilizing a chronic back patient, I was taken aback by the attack of the patient's wife. "Do you realize what you have done!!!," she screamed after storming into my office. "He needed me before . . . I always knew where he would be . . . now he spends all his time down at the tavern . . . and I don't know who he is with!" While this was a rare and extreme response, it did alert our staff to the powers inherent in domestic relations. We see such a remarkable variety of responses. We define many of these behaviors as red flags:

- The significant other who answers for the patient. This may be a benign form of response. It might indicate anxiety. It might also indicate an excessive level of involvement by the significant other who discusses "our pain."
- The significant other who directs you. This direction may come during your examination . . . "be sure to check such and such." It may occur during your treatment planning. It may occur at the end of the visit when the significant other tells you what to prescribe, what studies to order, or what operation to perform.
- The significant other who controls the patient's drug consumption. "I only give him medication when he 'needs' it, doc." This might be a clue to other "enabling behaviors." As in any behavioral situation, the presence of an enabler limits the efficacy of treatment. It suggests a level of dependency on the significant other. When this is too great a factor, it is likely that negative influences will result.
- The significant other who is angry. That anger may be at another physician, or at you. It might be transposed anger at the patient that can be expressed in no other way.
- The impassive significant other. Seemingly uninterested in the proceedings leading to a new treatment might suggest a variety of issues. Some of these are depression. Many significant others become withdrawn as they find their own avenues for communication closed. I have often suggested to such people that there might be something worse than the pain the patient is suffering while I look directly at the patient. I then turn to the significant other and suggest, "living with you, might just be worse than having the pain itself . . . what do you think?" Sometimes the response of the patient is dramatic. A very passive person often becomes animated and angry, really angry. Sometimes this will break the ice, but other times it does little. Often, the significant other will start to cry with tears pent up representing years of distress. This can sometimes be an important breakthrough.
- The significant other who has enthusiastic plans that are not shared by the patient.
- The significant other who seems to have developed a maternal role for the childlike patient. "Well, here he is, doc . . . just fix him up!" While improvement may be expressed as the goal by the significant other when it occurs it might be a threat to the integrity (meaning control pattern) of the relationship. Emancipated patients, just as adolescents, often rebel against forces that they might interpret as tyrannical once they assume control of their lives.

Some of the best relationships we have had with significant others have been when we paid attention to their needs, their concerns, and their lack of knowledge about the realities of their mates' predicaments. The hostile significant other poses special problems for the physician and may interfere with the outcome. Clues regarding this problem usually come first from your staff. Listen to them carefully and find some way to deal with the issues before you proceed to discuss or to provide treatment. Some hostility might be justified based on previous difficulties. But it cannot be accepted if it is severe enough to be a negative factor in your relationship with your patient. It is worthwhile to remember that hostility against previous providers of care is likely to be a repetitious scenario. You might be the next source of hostility and anger regardless of how effectively you work with your patient.

Were the Failures Related to Workplace Environmental Problems?

Attitude, aptitude, potential for advancement, and job satisfaction are issues that can influence pain management outcomes.[64–66] Patients who have no job to return to must consider starting at the lowest rung of a new occupation. Most patients who find this option distasteful will announce their dilemma by considering only return to their old job. Such excuses as, "I won't work at anything that will pay me less than my old job," while perhaps reasonable at one level often precludes any possibility of work return. Such patients may have been out of work for long periods without any effort on their part to search for job opportunities or to gain new skills or to obtain a graduate equivalency certification (GED). Because there are many such clues, this malevolent group of forces is usually easy to spot. However, it is too commonly ignored before proffering a surgical attempt at pain relief. Afterward, it becomes obvious how influential this issue is. In our experience, it has been present usually for some time and probably influenced the outcomes of previous treatments. Can you see then how important it is to document the reasons for previous failures?

There are several specific workplace-related issues that deserve comment.

- Wage replacement ratio. Studies by economists have documented that incentives regarding return to work are predicated to a remarkable degree on how much a person might earn at a new job entry position in comparison to the compensation (and to the lack of responsibility in many cases) while being disabled.[67,68] While most in the working years of life express the goal of work return, the percentages tell another story.
- Seniority issues. Just 1 year before his back injury, a 45-year-old machinist had been offered a supervisory position. Because he had been employed the longest he had been offered the job when his former supervisor had retired. Our patient realized that he would really rather be "one of the guys" than act as supervisor to his peer group. Besides, he wasn't sure he could handle the job. And he was fearful that that his boss would detect his inadequacies. When a junior worker who had some business education was made the supervisor, working lost much of its sparkle for our patient. He now realized that he was in a dead-end job. He could no longer dream about how he would work if he were the supervisor; he could no longer complain to his peers about what the supervisor did that he felt was wrong. He had given up the chance, hadn't he? Finally, and probably even worse, he now had to take orders from the younger worker who really didn't know as much about the business as he did. The back injury

and time away from work, away from the responsibilities and the pressures seemed to solve many problems. It is easy to see how factors such as these influence the thinking of patients and their behavior in response to pain treatment. Our machinist had very few options about work that he felt were reasonable.

- New technology. At a plant making a popular national brand of cookies, electricians were given the opportunity to learn the electronics of a new assembly line control system. They were permitted to match up to 4 hours weekly that they were paid for learning on a self-guided computer program. Obviously, their advancement would be based on their comprehension of the newer system. This posed a real threat to many of the workers who lacked the necessary computer and learning skills. Our clinic became involved when we noted that three electricians who worked there were our patients with a variety of vague and difficult-to-diagnose back and neck pain problems. Coincidence? Perhaps, but the connection was easy to make once the facts were known.

Workplace issues should be an important part of any pain surgery preoperative assessment. While it is sometimes difficult to get the facts, the patient's affect while discussing work often provides an important clue. This is where the psychologist's assessment can be of real help. Sadly, these issues are often ignored in favor of scores on paper-and-pencil tests. Again, understanding some of the factors that influenced previous outcomes may help you prevent their repetition.

Were Previous Failures Related to Attitude Issues?

The attitude of patients is tempered by their expectations.[69] Unfortunately, a sense of entitlement is becoming more common in our workplace it seems. Such attitudes as "Fix me or pay me," "I never had a backache before . . . I don't care if you can't find a cause," "Am I retired, doc?" or "I want to be trained for any job you think I can do!" are just some of the attitudinal issues we see in patients who have failed to prosper despite the initial effects of treatment. Patients in chronic pain are often in the midst of a major existential crisis. Their lives cannot continue on their previous course. Sadly, the addition of the adversarial influences in our legal and compensation systems add to the patient's predicament.[70]

In our experience it seems that there are many plaintiffs' attorneys who seem to be more interested in higher financial awards than in pain relief, proper medical care, or return to work. In all fairness, there are some lawyers who are more global in their representation and can be helpful to your efforts. A major question therefore to ask your patient is, "What is your attorney trying to get for you?" An answer that we commonly get is that the patient doesn't know. In fact, one does not hire an attorney and not know what they are trying to do. When patients indicate to us that they do not know what the attorney is expecting, we often find that the lawyer's goal is more than the patient feels they themselves are entitled to. Sometimes it is necessary to communicate with the attorney to get the facts. Certainly, if retirement is the goal and you think that you can support it, you and the attorney can work synergistically. On the other hand, if you and the patient think

that return to work is possible, it is important to be sure that the attorney is on your team. We have had attorneys tell their clients to "go through" with any treatment the doctor suggests. The implication is for minimal enough compliance to keep the doctor involved without any expectations for improvement.

It is important to reflect on your patients' attitudes regarding their previous medical care. Attitudes regarding initially good results we will discuss subsequently. The patient's and the patient's family's attitudes about previous care as we have noted may presage their feelings eventually about you. Understanding this principle can provide some interesting tools for your use to minimize their influence. Again, this is the kind of information you should expect from preoperative psychological assessment.

Did a Dichotomous Lack of Comprehension Regarding Outcome Issues Compound the Problem?

A colleague recently quipped, "Where in the world do all these chronic pain patients come from when the results of treatment look so good in the articles I read?" Often, at the end of a treatment adventure, the physician might feel satisfied with the reduction in pain the patient admits to. And this might solve the problems for the patient.[71,72] But too often the patient merely moves on to yet another physician, another treatment adventure, and another "excellent" or "good" result. There appears to be a serious dichotomy between outcomes as viewed by the physician and the outcome as seen by the patient. This is not altogether only in a negative direction. There appear many patients who felt they had a good result whose physicians judged the outcome otherwise![73]

This discussion suggests the importance of understanding the meaning of the outcome to the patient, not just the percent of improvement, the change in analogue scale measures, or changes the patient describes in usual activities. Improvement in pain may not be enough for the patient as we have already noted. Some patients describe remarkable improvement in pain level, activities, sense of well-being, improved function, and the like, and yet seek continued narcotics, doctor contacts, and even "cures" from others.

Fifty percent pain relief is seemingly an accepted industry standard.[74] But it might mean little in practical terms. It is not the pain measure that is important. No longer requiring the presence of medical practitioners in the patient's life is a more important issue. We see patients who continue narcotics and their level of impairment at the same levels as preoperatively who indicate remarkable improvement from pain surgery to their surgeons.

Unfortunately, some of our own literature adds to the dichotomies of expectations. Outcomes, especially when funded by instrument or drug manufacturers, must be viewed circumspectly. The remarkable results originally published from studies on a variety of spinal fusions,[31] deep brain stimulation,[75] cordotomy,[76] disk coagulation, and digestion[77] did not withstand more objective review. Yet, each seemed to have helped some patients whose selection criteria seem to be repeatedly suggested as fodder for future research that never seems to get done. Why indeed have our surgical indications not become more objectively selective and predictive?

How Did Previous Initial Improvement Impact the Patient?

We generally expect that people in pain desire improvement. That being the case, it is reasonable to expect a level of elation when improvement occurs. Unfortunately, in many patients with chronic pain, such is not the case. They improve but remain emotionally flat, even those who are not especially depressed. We have observed this repeatedly through the years and can draw some conclusions from it. Improvement might mean a variety of things. It might mean loss of the degree of support that had been there during the suffering phase. It might mean that the patient now has to become more responsible for the family's activities, including its support. It might mean more demands from an overwhelmed significant other. It might mean developing a realistic plan for the future. Such plans had been on hold during the severity of the pain. It might mean a new self-appraisal that might not be pleasant. It might mean that any pain relief less than complete is deemed inadequate by the patient. Or it might mean that the patient is skeptical of the duration of improvement.

A lack of positive response to improvement is strongly suggestive in our view of serious motivational, personal, emotional, or environmental factors. It is often not easy to obtain information of this kind from the patient. Interviews with family members, however, can be quite informative. Because of the complexity of the patient with chronic pain, we think that it is worth the effort to understand this principle in each patient.

There is a further consideration along these same lines that can help your understanding of your potential surgical patient. How your patient responds to your discussions about your expectations of your proposed treatment can provide an important clue. When you see no enthusiasm, consider asking the patient to explain the reason. Ask the psychologist with whom you work to provide some help here.

What Effect Did Previous Regression of Initial Benefit Have on the Patient's Emotional Response? On the Response of Significant Others?

The patient you are seeing for a pain-relieving operation is one who has not benefited from a previous effort. A characteristic of many patients is some initial improvement followed by regression of benefit. There are a variety of explanations for this. It is likely that whatever was done only resulted in partial eradication of the cause for the pain. Another explanation is that whatever the process there has been a progression of the underlying disorder. Obviously, movement of electrodes and catheters and the variety of mechanical factors all need to be considered also.

Equally important, however, is the commonality that seems to exist between initial surgical and initial behavioral and cognitive outcomes. Many patients seem to do better initially, then later regress with a variety of treatments. From a psychological standpoint, the initial improvement might be viewed as a form of cognitive dissonance.[78] The patient has put so much effort into having an operation, being involved in therapy or exercise, making decisions about the future, and the like that they must have a feeling of improvement to justify the efforts. Later, as reality descends, the real effect of treatment and the meaning that it implies become evident.

Whatever the reasons behind initial improvement, the patient's response to regression of benefit deserves careful scrutiny. Patients who desire improvement should become chagrined and upset about regression. One would anticipate the patient requesting restoration to the previous level of benefit. Instead, one often sees apathy. In many there is no response that one can interpret as being upset by the regression of benefit.

In sum, if patient improvement is the goal, was the patient happy about initially doing better and was there a negative emotional response to regression? If not, why not? Answer this question before you proceed and you will save yourself a longer list of less than ideal outcomes. You will also help your patient to face reality and what can truly be accomplished earlier enough to make a difference.

To maximize outcome be sure that these questions are adequately explored before you proceed. They should be at minimum the kind of information you obtain from pretreatment psychological evaluation.

The point is that, given the wisdom of several generations of pain surgeons, it is important to accept and to understand those factors that seem to predict outcome far more accurately than the patient's admitted degree of pain relief.

PSYCHOSOCIAL FACTORS

It has been generally agreed that the chronic pain phenomenon is a biopsychosocial disorder.[79] That is, the psychology of the patient and societal factors play a role in the patient's exhibition of suffering. The important lesson that our experience teaches is that there are elements of all these factors in all the patients we treat for chronic pain disorders. The difficult part is to understand the meaning of this fact in the way that influences the way that pain impacts our patients. Most surgeons leave this to the psychologist to unravel. Unfortunately, pretreatment psychological testing and interviews have apparently failed to provide enough prediction of outcome to move us to the next level of understanding the pain phenomenon.[47] It is not enough to recognize the presence of psychosocial influences. Their impact on the patient and means of reducing their influence on outcomes must become a key element in understanding who should be a candidate for more care. It is this principle that will provide better results for our patients. It is much more important than which area of the nervous system to target for pain relief.

It is important to note how often we impugn psychosocial issues later as the cause for the patient's failure to improve after treatment. In every case these same factors were present before our treatment. It is just that we did not understand them, did not recognize their importance, or chose to ignore their presence. It is clearly not reasonable to look at the global patient who has failed when we focus only on the patient's pain biology before we treat. A comprehensive and global view of the patient is necessary beforehand.

PREOPERATIVE EVALUATION

While many pain physicians espouse a preoperative global assessment of the patient with chronic pain, in many quarters little is actually done. It seems that some see the patient briefly, verify the presence of pain, discuss the procedure, and do a clinical trial to see if it might work. If the patient then agrees to a 50% pain reduction during the trial, a more permanent procedure is done. Preoperative assessments of this variety do not provide the higher levels of outcomes reported in our literature. In my experience, however, such physicians commonly quote to the prospective patient the literature-documented outcomes.

The validity of the preoperative assessment is impeached each time a patient fails to benefit from treatment. The failure of significant benefit means that the indications for the procedure missed something big. The physician who truly cares about the patient learns from the failure and adds that information to a more mature preoperative assessment of the next patient.

Some surgeons view the time and difficulty involved in the selection of patients as an unreasonable burden. Probably, such physicians should not be performing the evaluations themselves. Each of us possesses unique skills that limit the scope of our practices. We tend to do those things that we enjoy the most. If our skills do not include the appropriate selection of patients for pain treatment, then others should be given this function. Many surgeons object to the epithet of "mechanic," yet many seem to function in that way. This can further limit the patient's options for help after failure to benefit occurs. Surgeons who limit their comprehension of the overall problem really provide a disservice to the needy patient if they function without a proper support team. Because there are so many failures from each of our current treatments of chronic pain, the impact of this is tremendous.

Some important issues seemingly have a major impact on patient selection and outcome. If the surgeon's expressed goal is a moderate (50%) pain reduction during the clinical trial, the patient may concur that such has occurred. If the promised level of relief occurs, the surgeon often feels validated. The patient, on the other hand, might be left with still unmet expectations.

Because regression of pain benefit is common after any form of pain treatment, a goal of only 50% reduction during the clinical trial may condemn the patient to a less than satisfactory result. Review of many series suggests that a 50% relief during the trial does not guarantee a substantial benefit in many patients later.[74]

Patients need to be assessed for the changes in their life that pain improvement might have. Even in behavioral programs the expectations that many patients have transcends available efficacy.[80] Some see the pain as their only impairment. If it is fixed everything in their lives would be fine. When we question patients we find that they often actually expect to be able to relive a significant part of their lives once the pain is fixed. Patients who preoperatively are not willing to deal with the impact of their predicament and the effects of those issues other than the pain affecting their lives are not likely to do so afterward.

Vocational adjustment is an important determinant of outcome. For many in chronic pain there really is no realistic vocational goal.[79] Yet, often they see return to their former job as the major goal of treatment. Often such patients will consider no other work options. This attitude should be a "red flag" that requires further investigation before proceeding with treatment. Certainly for many, retirement is the only reasonable option. In these people, acceptance of this and their avocational activity planning become of equal importance. Not dealing with these issues can have major nefarious effects after treatment.

The needs and goals of the significant other must be considered before offering surgery for pain relief. Support and encouragement add to outcome while enabling and controlling behaviors often do not.

It is important to understand that frequently many of these issues act in synergy producing effects that compound one another. The patient who has no real goal or understanding of what she or he will do with the relief promised is not likely to continue to prosper after treatment.

Intraoperative Management

Commonly, the patient is asked to do little during the perioperative period. There are some important considerations during this time for the physician to consider. It is known that the time the patient is inactive or out of work can play an important role in outcome.[81,82] It is reasonable therefore to plan for your patient's activities and work-related decisions early. When surgery enters the picture it is easy to wait for the results before requiring any action from the patient. However, because most pain-relieving procedures are elective, there is time to plan for the patient's activities before and during convalescence. All too often we wait to see how the patient does before suggesting increased involvement in future planning, return to work efforts, or increased physical activities. When the patient doesn't do well (as occurs in up to 80% in some studies),[42] we start over again. This tends to add to the delay in dealing with psychosocial issues that so significantly impact outcome.

It is more productive to get patients to deal with vocational issues, activity schedules, physical restoration, and increased involvement in household functions before an elective procedure. This planning takes the time and effort of ancillary personnel. A report of these efforts should be part of preoperative planning for your patient. While financial resources might limit the amount of this that is done, it should not stop it entirely. Failures are too often influenced by the lack of this kind of planning.

Postoperative Issues

Patients seemingly respond better when they have an idea of what to expect in the postoperative stage. How long can they consider to be disabled? How long on oral pain relievers for the effects of the operations? How long before restorative activities are possible? All of these issues can become part of the preoperative planning. Then, even if the patient doesn't do as well as we had hoped, some therapeutic effect could still result. In the chronic pain patient it is really not appropriate to wait to see how the patient does after a procedure before deciding what might be next. There are still too many patients who continue to have problems for that to be an acceptable approach.

MAXIMIZING OUTCOMES BY UNDERSTANDING THE MEANING OF A MULTIDISCIPLINARY APPROACH

Typically, patients are sent from one physician or therapist to another to provide the best efforts of each. This model works best in the acute pain situation. Patients usually respond appropriately to surgery, a variety of physical and vocational therapies, and go on with their lives. Even sending a depressed patient to a psychologist works well in this context.

Things are different in the patient with chronic pain. Here integration of efforts is paramount. While the psychologist might help the patient's depression, the pain is in the way. While the physical therapist can increase the patient's physical abilities, the pain, the lack of vocational planning, and attitude issues get in the way. While a vocational counselor tries to help the patient to explore work options, the pain, the depression, and the motivation get in the way. Often patients will discuss more limitation due to residual pain to the physical therapist, vocational counselor, or to the psychologist than to the physician. The surgeon feeling that all is well due to improvement reported by the patient is often unaware of the rest of the problems. The gist of all this is that in the patient with chronic pain, all clinicians who are involved in the care must work synergistically. This requires a level of communication not usually required of the medical team. Too frequently we have seen patients whose surgeon was satisfied with the 60% or 70% pain relief that the patient reports. The others involved with the patient remain stymied by the residual problems that remain unknown to the surgical team.

A multidisciplinary approach requires some form of team meeting. We now understand the impact of too many of the variables to ignore them. Pain relief is meaningful to a patient who is able to do something with it. It is usually not possible for each practitioner to spend enough time to understand the meaning this has to each patient. A multidisciplinary approach is therefore a necessity. A multidisciplinary team that truly works together could be described as interdisciplinary. However much of this you can achieve will add to the ultimate benefit that you are able to provide to your patient.

Multidisciplinary or interdisciplinary are not the same as "serial consultations." Merely having all the pieces together for the patient doesn't work as well as communication and integration between the members of the treatment team.

PUTTING IT INTO CONTEXT

Understanding basic principles is really not enough. How those principles influence what we do is the major point. The justification for what we do must be based on how well we help the patient in terms that are meaningful to the patient.

For the Busy Surgeon

The patient usually considers that the surgeon or one he or she designates is in charge of their care. It is not common in our experience for patients to consider that the psychologist, counselor or therapist, or even a physiatrist is really in charge. This belief is commonly reinforced by the variety of disability and insurance forms the surgeon is asked to complete. Unfortunately, there are many of us and many of our brethren in anesthesiology who perform pain-relieving surgeries who function only superficially in the patient's overall care. It is certainly reasonable for a busy practitioner to want to avoid the ancillary issues. However, because of their importance, it is not appropriate to ignore them. Appropriately, it is important to appoint others to flesh-out the treatment package you provide. Regular meetings with other members of the team is one option. Another is to withdraw from the team's functions. However, this should be done as an active decision not as passive disregard. For this to work the surgeon must no longer then make the decisions regarding the patient's continued care, return to work, impairment assessments, and continued pain management. The other team members can make these decisions while the surgeon functions as the person who performs the procedures the whole unit has decided on.

We have treated a patient who truly felt ready to return to work. The patient suddenly decided on having an operation that the surgeon had just brought back from a national meeting. The promise of greater pain relief influenced the patient. The whole program was put on hold until the new procedure was done. With really no greater relief (the psychologist had predicted this beforehand), the entire team approach fell apart. The patient's apathy and disinterest made it impossible to get him ready for work again. In this case it would have been best if the surgeon had communicated with the team before even discussing the possible value of a new treatment for the patient. The surgeon must not function in a vacuum in this regard.

For the Psychologist

Because the psychologist does not usually make surgical decisions, her or his role is not usually well defined. Indeed, while some tests are in common use, there really is no standard for what consists an adequate preoperative patient assessment. Indeed, the lack of predictive value of most of the techniques that we now use suggests the need for a new hard look at the role of the psychologist. Psychosocial issues influence outcome and explain many failures. But which issues and how do they specifically and in chorus actually affect outcome? And what are the current tools that can avert their influence?

The psychologist can be more accurate in predicting outcome than the surgeon. Given the high rate of less-than-ideal results with pain surgery and the rate of regression of benefit, the psychologist must be more selective in "passing" patients for surgery. But this might extract too high a price for some. If the psychological assessment is honed to an accuracy that is closer to the actual outcome data, then many more patients will be denied operations for pain. While there are some among us who feel this might be appropriate, there are those who do not. Indeed, there are many who do not even use preoperative psychological assessment. We hear commonly that the operator is just as accurate as the psychologist in making predictions. If this is really so, the psychological consultant is probably not doing the job that needs to be done.

Outcomes assessment also positions the psychologist to more effectively pick up clues regarding the emergence of some negative influences. The psychologist is then positioned well to help abort them or their influences. A psychologist who can be assertive when appropriate and function as a predictor of outcome can help the avoidance of many unsuccessful surgical odysseys.

For the Next "Expert"

It is truly interesting to read the records of patients who have passed through the hands of many, each offering something special in the way of relief. For the new expert it is not so much whether or not a procedure exists that can be tried. The real responsibility is to avoid adding her or his name to the list of those who promised a lot, but delivered little. Commonly, we find in the review of files that the same psychosocial issues are impugned as the cause for repeated failures. The next "expert" who has "the cure" commonly ignores them. For the patient with chronic pain, anything offered will be seen as even more of a panacea than is promised. The disappointment that attends the regression of benefit adds to the problem.

The point is that the next one who offers hope to the patient must consider several important points.

1. Is there a distinct likelihood that the procedure now offered will do better than the last? Why?
2. What will the patient be able to do with the improvement?
3. What factors are likely to influence the outcome in this patient?
4. What will I do if the procedure really does little? Whose responsibility will the patient be?

Generally speaking, justify your right to become involved with a patient who has failed to benefit from the attempts of others. The only reasonable justification is that you can offer more, and the more that you offer has meaning for the patient. Another false hope is not justified now that we know some of the results.

For the Patient

Patients want you to "fix" them. Their concept of "fix" may not be realistic. The patient's understanding of both what is causing the pain and what it is you are planning influences expectations. As we discussed previously, many patients really do not understand the cause of their pain. Unfortunately, neither do we in many situations. Especially in these circumstances, it is important that the patient understand the problem as well as you can explain it.

We evaluated one patient who had done rather well after a pain-relieving operation for failed back surgery pain. The patient arrived in a mechanized wheelchair, yet he stood and walked normally. He had no limp or expression of discomfort. When we asked about the wheelchair, he explained that he had a "deteriorating spine." His first surgeon had told him that unless he had an operation he would end up in a wheelchair. Since he still had the deteriorating spinal condition even though his pain had been improved, he indicated that he still envisioned a wheelchair in his future. When a neighbor who had used the mechanized wheelchair died, he bought the appliance from the widow. He told us that he wanted to learn

how to use it before he really needed it thus making the transition to its use easier. This patient still spoke of returning to work as a truck driver as his goal.

Obviously, this is an extreme example. It does, however, illustrate a common problem. Most patients do not understand their problem or what our treatment really might mean for them. In the patient with chronic pain, education is important. Ask your patient to repeat the information you or others give. Someone must understand how the patient interprets this before any additional treatment is offered.

In addition, patients must understand the role they must play. When physical therapy will start, how drugs will be used, when work issues will be resolved. They must understand how to handle residual pain. And they must understand its meaning. Until we can eradicate pain entirely, the patient must understand the active role they must play. Apathy and passivity are not as helpful as activity, future planning, and active participation in the emancipation from the effects of pain. The patient must understand that it is the impact of the pain and not its severity that is most important. The impact of pain is personal, individual, and variable across a broad range of time and space.

A FINAL PHILOSOPHICAL POINT

Because of our need to do something for everybody who comes to us suffering from chronic pain, there is a tendency to offer one treatment after another. An inappropriate philosophical point that we hear in pain management circles is that since a certain percentage seem to do well after each procedure, we are justified in offering more and more procedures if the current one does not work well. This philosophy suggests a progressively decreasing pool of failures. However, this attitude seems to negate the efforts of those pain scientists and practitioners of the past who tried to understand pain more scientifically. Just because there is something else that we can always find to offer a patient in need is not justification to do that. Since we know that psychosocial factors are so important, we cannot just continue to offer pain relief with surgery unless it can cure enough. Only then do the other negative factors lose their importance. A practical understanding of the true meaning of our outcome should help to focus our indications and to improve our results. If our results are not improving we must ask, "why not?" Could it be that we are not narrowing our approach to those for whom we truly can offer help? Ask yourself the question each time you approach a new chronic pain patient, "when and what will be the very last of the 'last resorts' for this patient?"

CONCLUSIONS

Chronic pain sufferers offer one of the most difficult of challenges to the pain physician. It is possible to understand the meanings that the chronic pain state has to the patient. In understanding these we can become more selective in our approach to our patient. We must understand the meanings of our proposed outcomes. We must understand that chronic pain patients will most likely require continued support and care. Before proceeding we must define how this will work operationally.

Finally, the approach to the patient with chronic pain must be more than just offering a pain treatment option and letting them decide whether or not to proceed. We must factor in the education that the past several decades of pain surgery have provided. We must guide our patients in making their decisions about treatment. To do less ignores the lessons we have learned. It is no longer appropriate to start with each patient as though we were at the beginning of surgical pain treatment again by offering something to see if it will work. We just have garnered too much information for us to approach our patients in that manner. Our approach to the patient must include an honest appraisal of what it is that we can actually accomplish for them. It is seductive to offer simply a mechanical treatment for the pain. However, we must also include an understanding of our patients and their needs. The suffering patient deserves nothing less.

REFERENCES

1. Hazard RG, Haugh LD, Green PA, et al. Chronic low back pain: the relationship between patient satisfaction and pain, impairment and disability outcomes. Spine 19:881–887, 1994.
2. de Schepper AM, Francke AL, Abu-Saad HH. Feelings of powerlessness in relation to pain: ascribed causes and reported strategies. Cancer Nurs 20:422–429, 1997.
3. Arnstein P, Caudill M, Mandle CL, et al. Self efficacy as a mediator of the relationship between pain intensity, disability and depression in chronic pain patients. Pain 80:483–491, 1999.
4. Tan V, Cheatle MD, Macken S, et al. Goal setting as a predictor of return to work in a population of chronic musculoskeletal pain patients. Int J Neurosci 92:161–170, 1997.
5. Mancuso C, Salvati EA, Johanson NA. Patient's expectations and satisfaction with total hip arthroplasty. J Arthroplasty 12:387–396, 1997.
6. Schmitz U, Saile H, Nilges P. Coping with chronic pain: flexible goal adjustment as an interactive buffer against pain-related distress. Pain 67:41–51, 1996.
7. White AA. Compassionate patient care and personal survival in orthopaedics. A 35-year perspective. Clin Orthop 361:250–260, 1999.
8. Boden SD, Dreyer SJ, Levy HI. Management of low back pain. Current assessment and formulation of a blueprint for the health care delivery system of the future. Phys Med Rehabil Clin North Am 9:419–433, 1998.
9. Owens DK. Spine update. Patient preferences and the development of practice guidelines. Spine 23:1073–1079, 1998.
10. Deyo RA. Promises and limitations of the Patient Outcome Research Teams: the low-back pain example. Proc Assoc Am Physicians 107:324–328, 1995.
11. Loeser JD, Melzack R. Pain. An overview. Lancet 353:1607–1609, 1999.
12. Epstein NE, Hood DC, Bender JF. A comparison of surgeon's assessment to patient's analysis (Short form 36) after far lateral lumbar disc surgery. Spine 22:2422–2428, 1997.
13. Zaza C, Stolee P, Prkachin K. The application of goal attainment scaling in chronic pain settings. J Pain Symptom Manage 17:55–64, 1999.
14. Vendrig AA. Prognostic factors and treatment-related changes associated with return to work in the multimodal treatment of chronic back pain. J Behav Med 22:217–232, 1999.
15. Jordan KD, Mayer TG, Gatchel RJ. Should extended disability be an exclusion criterion for tertiary rehabilitation? Socioeconomic outcomes of early versus late functional restoration in compensation spinal disorders. Spine 23:2110–2116, 1998.
16. Long DM, BenDebba M, Torgerson WS, et al. Persistent back pain and sciatica in the United States: patient characteristics. J Spinal Disord 9:40–58, 1996.
17. Cutler RB, Fishbain DA, Lu Y, et al. Prediction of pain center treatment outcome for geriatric chronic pain patients. Clin J Pain 10:10–17, 1994.
18. Bonica JJ. History of pain concepts and pain therapy. Mt Sinai J Med 58:191–202, 1991.
19. Seres JL. The neurosurgical management of pain: a critical review. Clin J Pain 9:284–290, 1993.
20. Menges LJ. Pain: still an intriguing puzzle. Soc Sci Med 19:1257–1260, 1984.
21. Agazzi S, Reverdin A, May D. Posterior lumbar interbody fusion with cages: an independent review of 71 cases. J Neurosurg 91:186–192, 1999.
22. France JC, Yaszemshi MJ, Lauerman WC, et al. A randomized prospective study of posterolateral lumbar fusion. Outcomes with and without pedicle screw instrumentation. Spine 24:553–560, 1999.
23. Wetzel FT, LaRocca SH, Lowery GL, et al. The treatment of lumbar spinal pain syndromes diagnosed by discography. Lumbar arthrodesis. Spine 19:792–800, 1994.
24. McDonald GJ, Lord SM, Bogduk N. Long-term follow-up of patients treated with cervical radiofrequency neurotomy for chronic neck pain. Neurosurgery 45:61–68, 1999.
25. Seres JL. Long-term follow-up of patients treated with cervical radiofrequency neurotomy for chronic neck pain [letter]. Neurosurgery 45:1499–1450, 1999.
26. Bogduk N. Response. Neurosurgery 45:1499–1500, 1999.
27. Jaffe JH, Martin WR. Chapter 22: Opioid analgesics and antagonists. In Gilman AG, Goodman LS, Gilman A (eds). The Pharmacological Basis of Therapeutics (6th ed). New York, Macmillan, 1980, pp 494–534.
28. Sweet WH. An analysis of opinions considered adverse to the thesis of the main communication. Pain Forum 5:118–120, 1996.
29. Cho J, Park YG, Chung SS. Percutaneous radiofrequency lumbar facet rhizotomy in mechanical low back pain syndrome. Stereotact Funct Neurosurg 68(1–4 Pt 1):212–217, 1997.
30. Nachemson A, Zdeblick TA, O'Brien JP. Lumbar disc disease with discogenic pain. What surgical treatment is most effective? Spine 21(15):1835–1838, 1996.
31. Hinkley BS, Jaremko ME. Effects of 360-degree lumbar fusion in a workers' compensation population. Spine 22(3):312–322, 1997.
32. Paice JA, Penn RD, Shott S. Intraspinal morphine for chronic pain: a retrospective, multicenter study. J Pain Symptom Manage 11:71–80, 1996.
33. Agazzi S, Reverdin A, May D. Posterior lumbar interbody fusion with cages: an independent review of 71 cases. J Neurosurg 91(Suppl 2):186–192, 1999.
34. Nathan PW. Results of antero-lateral cordotomy for pain in cancer. J Neurol Neurosurg Psychiatry 26:353–362, 1963.
35. White JC. Anterolateral cordotomy—its effectiveness in relieving pain of non-malignant disease. Neurochirurgia (Stuttg) 15:83–102, 1963.
36. Sano K. Neurosurgical treatments of pain—a general survey. Acta Neurochir Suppl (Wein) 38:86–96, 1987.
37. Polatty RC, Cooper KR. Respiratory failure after percutaneous cordotomy. South Med J 79:897–899, 1986.
38. Spiegel EA, Wycis HT, Szekely EG, Gildenberg P, et al. Combined dorsomedial, intralaminar and basal thalamotomy for relief of so-called intractable pain. J Int Coll Surg 42:160–168, 1964.
39. Mark VH, Ervin FR, Yakovlev PI. Correlation of pain relief, sensory loss, and anatomical lesion sites in pain patients treated with stereotactic thalamotomy. Trans Amer Neurol Ass 86:86–90, 1961.
40. Mark VH, Ervin FR, Hackett TP. Clinical aspects of stereotactic thalamotomy in the human. Part I. The treatment of chronic severe pain. AMA Arch Neurol 3:351–367, 1960.
41. Valentino L, Pillay KV, Walker J. Managing chronic nonmalignant pain with continuous intrathecal morphine. J Neurosci Nurs 30:233–239, 243–244, 1998.
42. North RB, Kidd DH, Wimberly RL, et al. Prognostic value of psychological testing in patients undergoing spinal cord stimulation: a prospective study. Neurosurgery 39:301–311, 1996.
43. Anderson VC, Burchiel KJ. A prospective study of long-term intrathecal morphine in the management of chronic nonmalignant pain. Neurosurgery 44:289–301, 1999.
44. Robbins RA, Moody DS, Hahn MB, et al. Psychological testing variables as predictors of return to work by chronic pain patients. Percept Mot Skills 83:1317–1318, 1996.
45. Bannwarth B. Risk-benefit assessment of opioids in chronic noncancer pain. Drug Saf 21(4):283–296, 1999.
46. Epstein NE, Hood DC, Bender JF. A comparison of surgeon's assessment to patient's analysis (short form 36) after far lateral lumbar disc surgery. Spine 22:2422–2428, 1997.
47. Dubner R, Ren K. Endogenous mechanisms of sensory modulation. Pain (Suppl 6):S45–S53, 1999.

48. Melzack R. From the gate to the neuromatrix. Pain (Suppl 6): S121–S126, 1999.
49. Knox BD, Chapman TM. Anterior lumbar interbody fusion for discogram concordant pain. J Spinal Disord 6(3):242–244, 1993.
50. North RB, Kidd DH, Campbell JN, et al. Dorsal root ganglionectomy for failed back surgery syndrome: a 5-year follow-up study. J Neurosurg 74:236–242, 1991.
51. Boas RA. Sympathetic nerve blocks: in search of a role. Reg Anesth Pain Med 23:292–305, 1998.
52. Wood KB, Schellhas KP, Garvey TA, et al. Thoracic discography in healthy individuals. A controlled prospective study of magnetic resonance imaging and discography in asymptomatic and symptomatic individuals. Spine 24:1548–1555, 1999.
53. Yamaski H, Kakigi R, Watanabe S, et al. Effects of distraction on pain perception: magneto- and electro-encephalographic studies. Brain Res Cogn Brain Res 8:73–76, 1999.
54. Vlaeyen JW, Crombez G. Fear of movement/(re)injury, avoidance and pain disability in chronic low back pain patients. Man Ther 4:187–195, 1999.
55. Nelson BW, O'Reilly E, Miller M, et al. The clinical effects of intensive, specific exercise on chronic low back pain: a controlled study of 895 consecutive patients with 1-year follow up. Orthopedics 18:971–981, 1995.
56. Walker EA, Katon WJ, Hansom J, et al. Psychiatric diagnoses and sexual victimization in women with chronic pelvic pain. Psychosomatics 36:531–540, 1995.
57. Fishbain DA, Cutler RB, Rosomoff HL, et al. Impact of chronic pain patients' job perception variables on actual return to work. Clin J Pain 13:197–206, 1997.
58. Tan V, Cheatle MD, Mackin S, et al. Goal setting as a predictor of return to work in a population of chronic musculoskeletal pain patients. Int J Neurosci 92:161–170, 1997.
59. Fishbain DA, Cutler RB, Rosomoff HL, et al. Prediction of "intent," "discrepancy with intent," and " discrepancy with nonintent" for the patient with chronic pain to return to work after treatment at a pain facility. Clin J Pain 15:141–150, 1999.
60. Lofvander M. Attitudes towards pain and return to work in young immigrants on long-term sick leave. Scand J Prim Health Care 17:164–169, 1999.
61. Hubbard JE, Tracy J, Morgan SF, et al. Outcome measures of a chronic pain program: a prospective statistical study. Clin J Pain 12:330–337, 1996.
62. Burns JW, Sherman ML, Devine J, et al. Association between workers' compensation and outcome following multidisciplinary treatment for chronic pain: roles of mediators and moderators. Clin J Pain 11:94–102, 1995.
63. Keith RA. Patient satisfaction and rehabilitation services. Arch Phys Med Rehabil 79:1122–1128, 1998.
64. Lowdermilk A, Panus PC, Kalbfleisch JH. Correlates of low back pain outcomes in a community clinic. Tenn Med 92:301–305, 1999.
65. Donceel P, DuBois M, Lahaye D. Return to work after surgery for lumbar disc herniation. A rehabilitation-oriented approach in insurance medicine. Spine 24:9, 872–876, 1999.
66. Seitz FC. The evaluation and understanding of pain: clinical and legal/forensic perspectives. Psychol Rep 72:643–657, 1993.
67. Krause N, Asinger LK, Deegan LJ, et al. Alternative approaches for measuring duration of work disability after low back injury based on administrative workers' compensation data. Am J Ind Med 35:604–618, 1999.
68. Dasinger LK, Krause N, Deegan LJ, et al. Duration of work disability after low back injury: a comparison o administrative and self-reported outcomes. Am J Ind Med 35:619–631, 1999.
69. Andersson GB. Epidemiological features of chronic low-back pain. Lancet 354:581–585, 1999.
70. Bigos SJ, Andary MT. Practitioner's guide to industrial back problems. Neurosurg Clin North Am 2:863–875, 1991.
71. Tandon V, Campbell F, Ross ER. Posterior lumbar interbody fusion. Association between disability and psychological disturbance in non-compensation patients. Spine 24:1833–1838, 1999.
72. van Kleef M, Barendse GA, Kessels A, et al. Randomized trial of radiofrequency lumbar facet denervation for chronic low back pain. Spine 24:1937–1942, 1999.
73. Epstein NE, Hood DC, Bender JF. A comparison of surgeon's assessment to patient's analysis (short form 36) after far lateral lumbar disc surgery. Spine 22:2422–2428, 1997.
74. Seres JL. The fallacy of using 50% pain relief as the standard for satisfactory pain treatment outcome. Pain Forum 8:183–188, 1999.
75. Levy RM, Lamb S, Adams JE. Treatment of chronic pain by deep brain stimulation: long term follow-up and review of the literature. Neurosurgery 21:885–893, 1987.
76. White JC. Anterlateral cordotomy—its effectiveness in relieving pain of non-malignant disease. Neurochurgia (Stuttg) 15:83–102, 1963.
77. Javid MJ. Postchemonucleolysis diskcectomy versus repeat discectomy: a prospective 1- to 13- year comparison. J Neurosurg 85:231–238, 1996.
78. Painter JR, Seres JL, Newman RI. Assessing benefits of the pain center: why some patients regress. Pain 8:101–113, 1980.
79. Main CJ, Watson PJ. Psychological aspects of pain. Man Ther 4:203–215, 1999.
80. Seres JL, Painter JR, Newman RI. Multidisciplinary treatment at the Northwest Pain Center. NIDA Res Monogr 36:41–65, 1981.
81. Allen C, Glaziou P, Del Mar C. Bed rest: a potentially harmful treatment needing more careful evaluation. Lancet 354:1229–1233, 1999.
82. Gallagher RM, Rauh V, Haugh LD, et al. Determinants of return-to-work among low back pain patients. Pain 39:55–67, 1989.

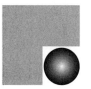

C H A P T E R   2

The Neuroanatomic and Neurophysiologic Basis of Pain

RICHARD J. TRAUB, PhD

The perception of pain depends on the integration and modulation of activity in the spinal cord and brain. Activity in multiple components of the nervous system affects our perception of external (or internal) stimuli. Pain processing is not static and hard-wired, but rather a dynamic process reflecting the complex integration of many components of the nervous system. Changing activity or function in one component affects the function of other components. This functional modulation, or plasticity, underlies the expression of three pain states: acute, inflammatory (also called persistent or subchronic), and chronic (i.e., neuropathic). The perception of pain to a given stimulus (e.g., pinprick) will differ depending on the state of the nervous system, the spinal cord in particular (Fig. 2-1).

Under "normal" conditions, noxious stimuli excite nociceptive afferent fibers, which transduce the external energy into action potentials that encode the location, intensity, quality, and duration of the external stimulus. This information is transmitted centrally and processed in the spinal cord and brain, evoking a reflex withdrawal from the stimulus and the perception of acute pain. If the stimulus produces tissue damage, chemical substances are released at the site of injury from primary afferent fibers and surrounding tissue. This is the first site where modulation of function is reflected as an alteration in pain perception. The injured tissue becomes inflamed and the released substances sensitize and/or activate nociceptive afferents (*peripheral sensitization*). The sensitized afferent fibers discharge at a higher rate in response to noxious stimuli, have a decreased threshold for discharge initiation, and discharge spontaneously producing a greater sensation of pain than otherwise expected in the injured area (*primary hyperalgesia*). The resulting increased afferent barrage into the spinal cord initiates changes in the response of dorsal horn neurons, increasing excitability, reducing threshold, and increasing spontaneous activity (*central sensitization*). The dorsal horn then, is another site where plasticity results in an alteration of pain perception. One consequence of central sensitization is increased pain sensitivity in normal tissue adjacent to the injured tissue, that is, hyperalgesia in noninjured tissue (*secondary hyperalgesia*). The primary and secondary hyperalgesia persist for the duration of the tissue damage and are reduced as the tissue heals.

Both acute and inflammatory pain serve protective functions. Withdrawal reflexes away from the noxious stimulus reduce the amount of time the skin is in contact with the stimulus reducing the chance for further tissue damage. Inflammation and hyperalgesia limit the range of motion or use of the injured tissue facilitating healing and recovery. Under certain circumstances, however, pain does not subside as the injury heals. This may result from direct injury or damage to a peripheral nerve or the central nervous system (CNS), changing the structure and function of the circuitry within the nervous system. This produces neuropathic pain, which is usually chronic and serves no useful purpose, becoming a disease itself.

We are only beginning to understand the complex interactions that occur in the spinal cord and brain that lead to the perception of pain. In this chapter, the anatomy, physiology, and pharmacology of the spinal mechanisms involved in acute, inflammatory, and chronic pain are reviewed. Emphasis is on mechanisms that contribute to inflammatory and to a lesser extent, chronic pain, because these conditions are most likely to prompt an individual to seek medical attention. Acute pain is discussed as a means to understand mechanisms of persistent and chronic pain. Most of our knowledge of pain mechanisms derives from experimental manipulation of the skin of animals because it is readily accessible. However, from what has already been ascertained, most concepts apply to humans. When appropriate, parallels to deep somatic and visceral pain are pointed out. This review is not meant to be comprehensive (cancer pain is not addressed), but provide an overview of spinal cord function that is intrinsic to the perception of pain. The reader is referred to several reviews and book chapters that discuss these concepts in more depth.[1–24]

PERIPHERAL MECHANISMS OF SOMATIC PAIN

It is generally accepted that the signaling of peripheral events into the spinal cord and CNS occurs over primary afferent fibers that are specific to the adequate stimuli that excite them. Sherrington in the early 1900s described nociceptors as

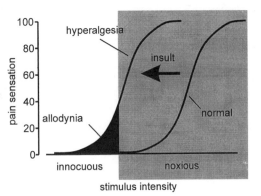

FIGURE 2-1 The relationship between stimulus intensity and pain sensation evoked from normal and injured tissue. Pain is normally perceived following stimulation of nociceptive afferents (*curve on right*). As the stimulus intensity increases in the noxious range, the pain sensation increases. Innocuous stimuli do not produce pain. Following tissue injury, there is a leftward shift in the curve. Innocuous stimuli evoke pain sensations (i.e., allodynia) and noxious stimuli evoke greater pain sensations than normal (i.e., hyperalgesia). (From Cervero F, Laird JMA. Mechanisms of touch-evoked pain (allodynia): a new model. Pain 68(1):14, 1996, with permission.)

sensory afferent fibers that respond to tissue damage or the threat of tissue damage. Tissue damage is not necessary to evoke the sensation of pain and many nociceptors have thresholds below the pain threshold. However, the discharge rate of these afferent fibers increases with stimulus intensity. On the other hand, low threshold afferent fibers encode nonnoxious stimuli and the response either plateaus or the afferent fibers cease firing when the stimulus intensity becomes painful.

Cutaneous Afferent Fibers

Primary afferent fibers are divided into three classes based on size and conduction velocity (size and conduction velocity are positively correlated). Large myelinated or Aβ fibers (>40 m/sec conduction velocity), smaller myelinated Aδ fibers (2–40 m/sec conduction velocity), and small, unmyelinated C fibers (<2 m/sec conduction velocity). In normal tissue, Aβ and some Aδ and C fibers transmit nonnoxious mechanical (e.g., brush, touch, hair movement, vibration) and thermal (cool and warm) stimuli. Aβ fibers normally do not transmit noxious stimuli, but do contribute to allodynia in some inflammatory and chronic pain states. However, the majority of Aδ and C fibers transmit noxious stimuli (painful mechanical, thermal, and chemical stimuli) and are nociceptors.

The receptive field of primary afferent fibers differs with location on the body. Afferent fibers innervating the trunk or proximal limbs have larger receptive fields (several square centimeters) than afferent fibers innervating the hands and fingers (<1 cm^2). Smaller receptive fields provide more accurate localization of the stimulus and better discrimination. Typically, the receptive field of nociceptive afferent fibers is composed of discrete spots of high sensitivity surrounded by regions of lesser sensitivity. Receptive fields of afferent fibers overlap, so an area of lesser sensitivity for one afferent may be highly sensitive for another.

Aδ and C fibers are broadly categorized into several classes of nociceptive afferent fibers based on response properties to varying thermal and mechanical stimuli. Aδ type II nociceptors, C mechanoheat, and C polymodal nociceptors signal the initial pain from noxious heat while Aδ type I fibers, initially unresponsive to heat, become sensitized signaling the prolonged burning sensation. Both Aδ and C fibers signal noxious mechanical stimuli.

Silent Nociceptors

An important group of nociceptive afferent fibers are referred to as silent afferents or sleeping nociceptors. These fibers innervate skin, joints, and the viscera. They are mostly unmyelinated fibers and are unresponsive to intensely noxious mechanical or thermal stimuli. Following injury and inflammation, these fibers become sensitized and subsequently respond to thermal and mechanical stimulation. Estimates of the number of silent afferent fibers in various tissues range from 20% to 30% to as high as 80% of all unmyelinated fibers. Activation or recruitment of these fibers following tissue damage increases the total afferent input to the spinal cord thereby contributing to central sensitization. Because these afferent fibers become sensitized during inflammation, they are chemosensitive, but whether one or many inflammatory mediators are necessary to "awaken" them is unknown.

Deep Somatic Nociceptive Afferent Fibers (Muscle and Joint)

Most muscle afferent fibers are larger myelinated fibers (group I and II) and signal proprioceptive information about the muscle. Group III (thinly myelinated) and group IV (unmyelinated) nociceptive muscle afferent fibers (analogous to Aδ and C fibers, respectively) generally respond to tissue damaging and chemical stimuli (decreased pH from lactic acid formation). Correspondingly, muscle pain results from direct trauma and inflammation, strenuous exercise, and sustained muscular contraction (lactic acid accumulation). These fibers can be excited by histamine, serotonin, bradykinin, and potassium that would accumulate in muscle tissue following injury.

Similar to muscle, most joint afferent fibers are proprioceptive, signaling the position and movement of the joint. Joint nociceptors also fall into the smaller fiber range. Some group III and group IV joint afferent fibers signal movement beyond the normal range or intense pressure on the joint. A third group of joint afferent fibers are silent nociceptors and only start to respond following joint injury and inflammation.

Visceral Afferent Fibers

The spinal afferent innervation of the viscera differs from somatic tissue in several ways. First, visceral afferents are Aδ and C fibers. There are few Aβ fibers innervating the viscera. Second is the degree of specificity of visceral afferent fibers to noxious and non-noxious stimuli. Most visceral afferent fibers do not respond to cutting, crushing, or burning of viscera, stimuli that are highly noxious to somatic tissue. Spinal visceral afferent fibers do, however, depending on the tissue, respond to hollow organ distention, ischemia, inflammation, smooth muscle spasm, and traction on the mesentery. Third are the response properties of visceral afferent fibers. In tissue where humans report no conscious sensation except pain (e.g., solid organs, ureter), most spinal afferent fibers respond to stimuli that are tissue damaging or potentially tissue damaging (e.g., tumors stretching the visceral peritoneum, calculus deposits distending the ureter or bile duct). These afferent fibers are considered nociceptive visceral afferent fibers. On the other hand, spinal afferent fibers that innervate hollow organs (e.g., colon, bladder) have thresholds well below the threshold for pain, and these fibers have increasing stimulus-response functions that extend into the noxious range. Most spinal afferent fibers to these organs convey both noxious and non-noxious stimuli and therefore do not fit into the somatic tissue definition of a nociceptive afferent.

Neurochemistry of Nociceptive Afferent Fibers

Under normal conditions, most nociceptive afferent fibers use several neurotransmitters and modulators. These excitatory amino acids and neuropeptides colocalize in different combinations and to date it has not been possible to assign a particular combination of transmitters with a specific type of nociceptive afferent. However, most nociceptive afferent fibers contain glutamate and some combination of neuropeptides.

Immunocytochemical labeling studies have shown dorsal root ganglion neurons contain excitatory amino acids, although their presence in cell bodies makes it difficult to ascribe a transmitter function because they are components of most proteins. However, primary afferent terminals in the spinal cord label for these amino acids suggesting a transmitter function. Furthermore, several physiologic effects firmly establish a role for excitatory amino acids as neurotransmitters in low threshold and nociceptive afferents. First, intrathecal administration of glutamate produces biting and scratching behaviors in rats and mice that is interpreted as pain-related behavior. Second, application of glutamate to spinal neurons *in vivo* and *in vitro* evokes neuronal activity, which is blocked by specific excitatory amino acid receptor antagonists. Finally, inflammation-induced pain behavior and spinal neuron activity is attenuated by excitatory amino acid receptor antagonists.

Most nociceptive afferents also contain one or more neuropeptides and/or other substances (e.g., adenosine triphosphate [ATP], nitric oxide, neurotrophins) that are expressed constitutively or are induced and modulate synaptic activity. Calcitonin gene–related peptide (CGRP) and substance P (SP) are the most common neuropeptides and are colocalized in 50% to 60% of nociceptive afferent fibers. Most notably, SP has documented functions in nociceptive transmission in the generation of central sensitization and hyperalgesia in persistent pain states. Intrathecal administration of SP receptor (NK-1 receptor) antagonists attenuate the generation of inflammatory hyperalgesia. More recently, SP conjugated to the neurotoxin saporin is reported to prevent persistent pain by killing the pain-signaling neurons in the spinal cord that express the NK-1 (substance P) receptor.

Inflammation and nerve injury induce changes in peptide levels in nociceptive afferent fibers. Substance P and CGRP levels decrease in primary afferents during the first few days following tissue injury and inflammation. The increase in afferent activity increases the release of peptides in the spinal cord depleting the cellular stores. During this time, the neuron increases transcription of peptide message so following the initial decrease in peptide levels, the cell increases translation of the message into protein. By 48 to 72 hours, the peptide level returns to normal and then increases to maintain enough peptide for use as a transmitter for the duration of the peripheral inflammation. In contrast, following nerve damage, substance P and CGRP levels decrease in nociceptive afferent fibers and remain decreased. However, substance P is induced in large diameter, low threshold afferent fibers that normally do not express substance P. In the nociceptive afferent fibers, other peptides that are rarely found in primary afferent fibers are induced and increase to substantial levels. These changes in the primary afferent phenotype contribute to alterations in sensory processing contributing to hyperalgesia and allodynia.

Efferent Function of Sensory Afferent Fibers

In addition to the classical role as neurotransmitters between primary afferents and dorsal horn neurons, SP and other neuropeptides, excitatory amino acids, ATP, nitric oxide, and prostaglandins also act peripherally. They cause vasodilatation, plasma extravasation, degranulation of mast cells, and excitation/sensitization of primary afferents. They are released from primary afferent fibers by action potentials that invade the afferent terminal. This can be evoked by an axon reflex (activity in one branch of an afferent propagating into other branches of the same fiber evoking release of peptides) or dorsal root reflex (activity originating in the spinal cord propagating out to the peripheral terminal). These peripherally propagating action potentials produce neurogenic inflammation, which contributes to the wheal and flare following tissue damage creating the zone of primary hyperalgesia.

Inflammation and Nociceptor Sensitization

Tissue-damaging stimuli release chemicals from damaged tissue, immunocompetent cells, vasculature, and primary afferent and sympathetic efferent terminals. The capacity of primary afferents to respond to these perturbations in their environment depends on the chemical receptors in the membrane of the afferent terminal. Activation of the afferent terminal through these receptors can directly excite the fiber, sensitize the fiber to other stimuli, or change the phenotype of the receptor altering its function in the periphery and in the spinal cord.

The chemical receptors located in the afferent terminal membrane belong to two broad families of receptors: those associated with an ion channel (ligand-gated channels) and those associated with G-proteins/second messenger systems (Fig. 2-2).

The ligand-gated channels increase inward cationic currents, which depolarize the afferent terminal generating action potentials. Several inflammatory mediators (ligands) and receptors belong to this group. Serotonin, ATP, glutamate, and

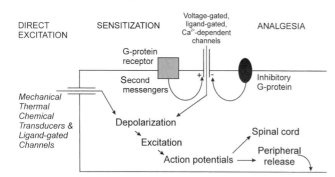

DIRECT EXCITATION SENSITIZATION ANALGESIA

FIGURE 2-2 A simplified scheme illustrating three outcomes of primary afferent stimulation in the periphery. Excitatory substances (e.g., ACh, ATP, glutamate, H$^+$, serotonin) bind receptors or stimulate a transducer to directly open the ligand-gated channels depolarizing the afferent to discharge action potentials. The action potentials are transmitted to the central terminal in the spinal cord evoking transmitter release. Action potentials also evoke release of neurotransmitters in the periphery via axon reflexes. Sensitizing substances (e.g., adenosine, bradykinin, histamine, prostaglandins, substance P) bind G-protein–coupled receptors that activate second messenger pathways within the afferent terminal. Second messengers sensitize neurons by modulating activity at voltage-gated, ligand-gated, and Ca^{2+}-dependent ion channels. Increasing sodium and calcium currents and decreasing potassium currents increases the excitability of the afferent terminal so subsequent stimuli will elicit a greater discharge. Analgesic substances (opioids) bind inhibitory G-protein–coupled receptors that inhibit second messengers and negatively modulate voltage-gated, ligand-gated, and Ca^{2+}-dependent ion channels reducing excitability of the afferent terminal.

acetylcholine, as well as acidic pH (protons, H$^+$), capsaicin, and noxious heat directly excite afferent terminals evoking the centripetal propagation of action potentials. When these substances are applied to healthy tissue (topically or injected into the skin), they produce pain.

G-protein–coupled receptors are not directly associated with ion channels. Activity at these receptors activates second messenger pathways that modulate activity at voltage-gated, ligand-gated, and Ca^{2+}-dependent ion channels. Changing the kinetics of the voltage- and ligand-gated channels increases or decreases ionic conductances, altering the excitability of the afferent terminal, but usually does not produce sufficient depolarization to initiate action potential activity. Rather, the afferent is sensitized to other modes of stimulation so many action potentials will be generated instead of a few. Potent sensitizing agents include bradykinin (BK), serotonin, histamine, and prostaglandins.

Several of these inflammatory mediators act at both ligand-gated channels and G-protein–coupled receptors. The effect of the ligand will depend on the receptor subtype that it binds. Through multiple receptor subtypes, some substances can be both algogenic and analgesic. For example, adenosine sensitizes afferents to produce hyperalgesia via A$_{2A}$ receptors, but antihyperalgesia via A$_1$ receptors.

A third group of ligands, neurotrophins or growth factors, especially nerve growth factor (NGF), are increased in inflamed or nerve-injured tissue and bind to tyrosine kinase (Trk) receptors on primary afferent terminals. Binding to these receptors does not excite or initially sensitize the afferent. These receptors initiate genetic activity increasing the production of membrane ion channels and upregulating or inducing new transmitter synthesis altering the phenotype of the afferent fiber.

Attenuation of Inflammatory Pain

Nonsteroidal anti-inflammatory drugs (NSAIDs) are potent drugs for attenuating inflammatory pain. They primarily inhibit prostaglandin synthesis by blocking the cyclooxygenase enzymes COX-1 and COX-2. COX-1 is constitutively active in the nervous system and in other organ systems. Chronic use of COX-1 inhibitors can have detrimental side effects such as generation of gastric ulcers because prostaglandins stimulate mucus secretion that protects the gastric lining from gastric acid. On the other hand, COX-2 is induced by inflammation. Inhibitors that are specific for COX-2 are effective anti-inflammatory drugs with decreased risk of side effects.

Opioids have some clinical use as peripheral analgesics. Opioids do not affect the nociceptive threshold of normal tissue, but inflammation activates opioid receptors in primary afferents. Opioids bind the receptors in inflamed tissue producing antinociception by inhibiting second messenger systems decreasing afferent terminal excitability.

DORSAL HORN OF THE SPINAL CORD

Primary afferent fibers provide the first site of active integration in pain processing. The second site is in the dorsal horn (Fig. 2-3). The spinal gray matter is a layered structure; laminae I–V and VI–VII comprise the dorsal horn and intermediate gray, respectively. Laminae VIII and IX (motoneuron pools) comprise the ventral horn and lamina X surrounds the central canal (central gray). Primary afferent fibers enter the spinal cord through the dorsal roots and send collateral projections over several segments (two to three for somatic afferent fibers, five to ten for visceral afferent fibers) to form synaptic connections in the gray matter. Nociceptive afferents (Aδ and C fibers) terminate in the superficial dorsal horn (laminae I and II) and lamina V, while Aβ afferents terminate deep to lamina II. Primary afferent projections form a somatotopic map of the body along the rostrocaudal and mediolateral axes of the spinal cord, so primary afferent fibers with adjacent receptive fields terminate closely in the spinal cord.

Three types of neurons based on responses to cutaneous stimuli are located in the dorsal horn. Nociceptive specific (NS) neurons that only respond to noxious stimuli are located in the superficial dorsal horn and to a lesser extent in the deep dorsal horn. Low threshold cells that respond to non-noxious stimuli (low threshold) are mainly located in laminae III and IV. Wide dynamic range (WDR) cells that encode noxious and non-noxious stimuli are in the deeper laminae (V–VII, X), but also in lamina I. Most NS and WDR neurons in the superficial dorsal horn, deep dorsal horn, and lamina X also respond to visceral stimuli. An exception are cells in the cervical (brachial) and lumbar enlargements that receive innervation from the limbs where few cells respond to visceral stimuli. Dorsal horn neurons are also classified as projection or interneurons. Projection neurons send axons to distal spinal segments (propriospinal) or higher brain areas (supraspinal projection). Interneurons are excitatory (e.g., glutamate, SP) or inhibitory (e.g., GABA, glycine, opioids) depending on their transmitters and their postsynaptic effects.

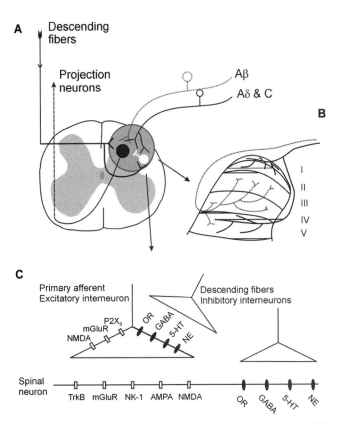

FIGURE 2-3 The organization of the spinal dorsal horn. *A,* Large (Aβ) and small (Aδ, C) diameter primary afferent fibers and descending fibers provide input onto interneurons and projection neurons. *B,* Generalized projection pattern of Aβ (*dashed line*) low threshold mechanoreceptors and Aδ and C (*solid line*) nociceptive afferent fibers into the spinal dorsal horn. The laminar designation is on the right. Aβ fibers terminate in laminae III and IV. Nociceptive afferents terminate in the superficial dorsal horn (laminae I, II) and lamina V–VI. Some nociceptive afferent fibers and visceral afferent fibers also project to lamina X (not shown). *C,* Schematic illustrating the synaptic organization in the spinal cord. A primary afferent or excitatory interneuron synapses onto a spinal neuron producing postsynaptic excitation. Descending fibers and inhibitory interneurons inhibit transmitter release from presynaptic terminals or inhibit postsynaptic spinal neurons decreasing excitability. The *open rectangles* are receptors that produce excitatory effects and the *closed ovals* are receptors that produce inhibitory effects. Not every cell has every receptor. 5-HT, serotonin; AMPA, α-amino-3-hydroxy-5-methyl-4-isoxazole propionic acid; GABA, gamma-aminobutyric acid; mGluR, metabotropic glutamate receptor; NE, norepinephrine; NMDA, N-methyl-D-aspartate; NK-1, neurokinin-1 (substance P receptor); OR, μ, δ, κ opioid receptor; P2X₃, purinoreceptor type 2X3; TrkB, tyrosine kinase B.

The synaptic interactions in the dorsal horn are quite complex. The state of processing in the spinal cord and the activity in supraspinal projection neurons depends on the magnitude of synaptic activity produced by primary afferent fibers, and modulation of activity by descending fibers and interneurons. A dorsal horn neuron will receive hundreds if not thousands of synaptic contacts from primary afferents, descending fibers, and interneurons. The presynaptic terminals of these fibers are subject to modulation (Fig. 2-3C). Autoreceptors on nociceptive afferent terminals augment transmitter release while descending fibers and spinal interneurons inhibit transmitter release. The postsynaptic neuron is excited by mono- and polysynaptic primary afferent input, but is also inhibited by descending fibers

and spinal interneurons. It is the dynamic modulation of this circuitry in the spinal cord that determines the pain state, the output of the spinal cord to the brain, and the quality and magnitude of pain perception to a noxious stimulus.

Spinal Mechanisms of Acute Pain

Glutamate, the most prevalent excitatory neurotransmitter, binds to two classes of ionotropic receptors termed *NMDA* (N-methyl-D-aspartate) and *non-NMDA* (AMPA and kainate) on the basis of their specificity to selective agonists. When the spinal cord is in its normal state in the absence of tissue damage, there is a voltage-dependent Mg^{2+} block of the NMDA receptor ion channel. When nociceptive afferent fibers are excited by a noxious stimulus (e.g., pinprick; Fig. 2-4), glutamate is released from the central terminals exciting postsynaptic neurons via AMPA receptors. Sodium flows through the AMPA receptor ion channel eliciting fast excitatory postsynaptic potentials (EPSPs) that are measured in milliseconds. The EPSPs evoked by afferent fibers that form the excitatory receptive field of the dorsal horn neuron summate (temporal and spatial) to sufficiently depolarize the neuron to fire a few action potentials. EPSPs in the neurons evoked by other afferent fibers are not strong enough to generate action potentials. These form subthreshold or silent synapses. The receptive fields of these afferent fibers form a subthreshold area that surrounds the excitatory receptive field of the dorsal horn neuron. Two pathways are thus excited by the pinprick: one evokes a reflex withdrawal from the stimulus and the other sends the information to the cortex evoking a brief sensation of pain. Even though the dorsal horn neuron fires action potentials, there is not sufficient depolarization to alleviate the voltage-dependent Mg^{2+} block of the NMDA receptor. In the absence of further noxious stimulation, the spinal cord remains in this normal state and acute pain has been experienced.

Spinal Mechanisms of Inflammatory Pain

When an organism is presented with a tissue-damaging stimulus, the injured area becomes inflamed and nociceptive afferents become sensitized. The persistent activity of the primary afferents from direct stimulation by the noxious stimulus in addition to spontaneous activity produced by afferent sensitization produces a continual barrage of action potentials into the spinal cord. Several events then occur. The constant activity increases excitability of the primary afferent terminals increasing transmitter (glutamate) release. Glutamate binds to presynaptic autoreceptors (Fig. 2-3C) further increasing excitability of the presynaptic terminal in a feed-forward cycle that evokes additional transmitter release. Glutamate also binds to postsynaptic AMPA receptors as well as a third class of non-NMDA receptor, the metabotropic glutamate receptor. This receptor is not associated with an ion channel, but is a G-protein–coupled receptor that initiates a second messenger cascade increasing the intracellular Ca^{2+} concentration and phosphorylating the NMDA receptor. This phosphorylation is sufficient to change the tertiary conformation of the NMDA receptor reducing the voltage dependence of the Mg^{2+} block.

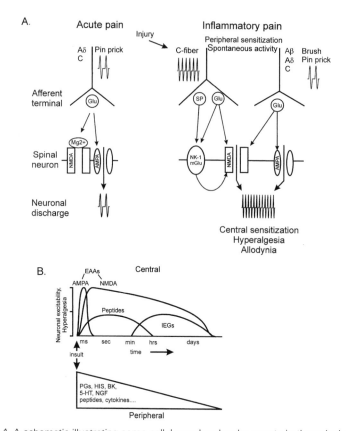

FIGURE 2-4 *A*, A schematic illustrating some cellular and molecular events in the spinal cord involved in changing from an acute pain state to an inflammatory pain state. Acute pain (*left*), caused by a pinprick produces a few action potentials (⊦⊦) in nociceptive afferents that are transmitted centrally to the spinal cord. Glutamate is released from the presynaptic terminals to bind to NMDA and AMPA receptors. The NMDA receptor is blocked by Mg^{2+} preventing current flow through the receptor channel. The AMPA receptor allows Na^+ to flow into the cell, briefly depolarizing the neuron to produce a few action potentials. A tissue damaging injury sensitizes and excites primary afferent fibers. They become hyperexcitable and discharge spontaneously (peripheral sensitization). The increased afferent activity releases substance P (SP) and glutamate from the afferent terminal in the dorsal horn. Substance P and glutamate bind G-protein–coupled receptors (NK-1 and mGlu, respectively) activating second messenger pathways that remove the Mg^{2+} block from the NMDA receptor. Now pinprick to the injured tissue increases primary afferent activity increasing the spinal release of glutamate, which binds to NMDA and AMPA receptors. The NMDA receptor, no longer blocked by Mg^{2+}, allows Ca^{2+} and Na^+ to enter the cell producing sufficient depolarization to fire multiple action potentials. Simultaneously, glutamate binds AMPA receptors producing additional neuronal discharges. This increase in cellular excitability (central sensitization) lowers the stimulation threshold so previously ineffective synapses produce action potentials expanding the receptive field of the neuron. The increase in neuronal discharge, the decrease in stimulation threshold, and the increase in the number of neurons excited due to expanded receptive fields will increase the output of the spinal cord producing primary hyperalgesia and allodynia from the injured tissue and secondary hyperalgesia from adjacent noninjured tissue. *B*, The time course of peripheral and central events during central sensitization and hyperalgesia. Acute pain, mediated by AMPA receptors, uses fast synaptic transmission on the order of milliseconds. Injury results in the release of inflammatory mediators in the periphery that sensitize/excite primary afferents. The quantity of inflammatory mediators decrease as the tissue heals. The process of central sensitization following injury takes place over seconds to minutes. The initial activity in dorsal horn neurons evoked by NMDA receptors lasts hundreds of milliseconds to seconds and ultimately lasts for days. The effects of peptides lasts seconds to minutes/hours. Immediate early genes (IEGs) increase protein synthesis and increase cellular activity. These processes take minutes to hours to produce effects that last for days.

In addition, the persistent activity in the primary afferent evokes the release of neuropeptides that colocalize with glutamate in the primary afferent terminal. The most well documented of these is substance P (SP), which binds to the NK-1 receptor. The NK-1 receptor is also a G-protein–coupled receptor that can evoke phosphorylation of the NMDA receptor via a second messenger cascade. In addition, SP produces a long-lasting depolarization of the dorsal horn neuron increasing the resting membrane potential further alleviating the Mg^{2+} block of the NMDA receptor. In contrast to the fast synaptic transmission through the AMPA receptor, these synaptic events last hundreds of milliseconds. Now glutamate binding to the NMDA receptor produces an inward cationic (Ca^{2+}, Na^+) conductance further increasing neuronal excitability and neuronal discharge that has a time course much longer than the AMPA receptor–mediated events. The increase in intracellular Ca^{2+} initiates a downstream cascade of events including activation of nitric oxide (NO) synthase forming NO and induction of immediate-early gene families such as *fos* and *jun*. NO is a retrograde messenger that diffuses out of the cell back into the presynaptic terminal where it can produce long-term changes in terminal excitability and transmitter release. Immediate-early genes such as *fos* and *jun* regulate the expression of proteins and enzymes in the postsynaptic cell that change the excitability of the neuron with a time course of hours to days. At this point, the dorsal horn neuron is sensitized; the neurons become spontaneously active, the threshold for excitation decreases, and a noxious stimulus (pinprick) evokes a greater response (the cell fires more action potentials). The increased excitability of the dorsal horn also allows the previously silent or ineffective synapses to reach threshold to generate action potentials. This expands the receptive field of the dorsal horn neuron so it is excited by stimulation over a larger area. Noxious stimulation to an area will now excite more dorsal horn neurons, which have overlapping receptive fields that have expanded into the stimulation site. It is likely that more supraspinal projection neurons are excited by a stimulus leading to hyperalgesia. This inflammatory pain continues over the duration of the injury and slowly subsides as the injury heals.

An understanding of the sequence of events that generates central sensitization and hyperalgesia led to the concept of pre-emptive analgesia. It was reasoned that inflammatory pain such as postoperative pain should be reduced if central sensitization was prevented. Animal studies have shown that spinal block of NMDA and NK-1 receptors attenuates inflammatory hyperalgesia. Both NMDA and NK-1 receptor antagonists work pre-emptively, but only NMDA antagonists are effective following injury.

Spinal Mechanisms of Chronic Pain

The plasticity associated with inflammatory pain changes the state of processing in the spinal cord increasing excitability of supraspinal projection neurons. With the resolution of inflammation, the spinal cord moves from this state of hyperexcitability back to the normal state. Inflammatory mediators decrease and the second messenger pathways in nociceptive afferents that were turned on by the inflammatory process slow down and return to normal. With the disappearance of primary sensitization, especially the decrease in spontaneous activity, the driving force for central sensitization is removed and dorsal horn neurons return to their normal state of activity. The plasticity in the spinal cord was functional and there was no change in the anatomic organization of the dorsal horn.

Chronic pain differs from inflammatory pain in that there often is a synaptic rearrangement within the dorsal horn. Two mechanisms will be discussed here. When a peripheral nerve is injured, several events take place. First, the damaged axon will signal the cell body about the damage. This can be through the loss of retrogradely transported trophic factors from the periphery or changes in membrane properties. The cell responds to the injury by becoming spontaneously active (ectopic activity). This increase in activity may originate at the site of injury, in the cell body, or at any point along the axon. One mechanism that contributes to this is an increase in sodium channels inserted into the membrane. This increase in excitability and spontaneous and evoked discharges can produce excitotoxicity in the spinal cord. Excessive excitation of dorsal horn neurons can increase intracellular Ca^{2+} to a point that it damages and eventually kills the cell. Inhibitory interneurons are particularly sensitive to neural excitotoxicity. The loss of inhibitory interneurons in the dorsal horn results in disinhibition of spinal projection neurons increasing their excitability (central sensitization). In contrast to inflammatory pain, resolution of the injury in the periphery would not reduce the central sensitization, and the hyperexcitability of spinal neurons persists into a chronic state.

A second consequence of a peripheral nerve injury is degeneration and cell death of the damaged cells, especially C fibers. The central terminals of damaged C fibers degenerate reducing the density of the neuropil in lamina II of the dorsal horn. This signals central terminals of larger myelinated fibers that terminate in lamina III to sprout into lamina II, producing a situation where low threshold afferents directly drive lamina II excitatory and inhibitory interneurons involved in nociceptive processing. Now, low threshold stimulation excites nociceptive projection neurons producing allodynia. This process takes place over days to weeks producing structural and functional rearrangement in the dorsal horn. Because these changes are not readily resolved, pain becomes chronic.

Ascending Pain Pathways

The state of activity in the spinal cord partly determines what information relating to location, intensity, quality, and duration of a noxious stimulus is sent to higher brain nuclei for further modulation and integration and ultimately to cortical areas to bring the pain to the level of conscious perception. When viewed in the context that pain is a multidimensional sense, separate ascending pathways appear to contribute to the sensory-discriminative and affective-motivational aspects of pain.

The identification of ascending pathways and the functional characteristics of each have been determined from human studies following spinal injury and from animal studies. An understanding of the effects of lesions to different white matter fiber tracts can be partially ascertained from reports of sensory loss following damage to ascending spinal pathways. Early studies using sensory testing following spinal injury tried to differentiate which sensory modalities were transmitted in different fiber tracts. However, clinical studies suffer from the inability to determine the extent of damage and to a lack of specificity of an injury to a single ascending pathway. On the other hand, animal studies, which are more reproducible, lack the verbal description of sensory deficits. Loss of sensory function can only be determined from behavioral changes of awake animals and loss of response properties of sensory neurons at several levels of the neuraxis above and/or below the lesion. Nevertheless, both clinical and experimental findings have contributed to our understanding of how information about our environment reaches consciousness.

An important consideration when using surgical methods to treat pain is that in many patients, pain returns within months to years following initially successful surgery. This suggests that new pathways take over the function of lesioned

Ascending Pain Pathways

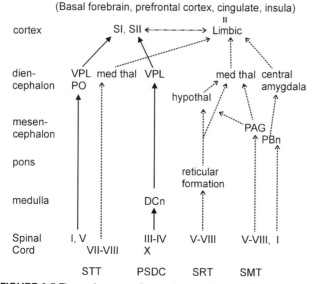

FIGURE 2-5 The major ascending pathways that contribute to the sensory-discriminative and affective-motivational aspects of pain. The spinothalamic tract (STT) and postsynaptic dorsal columns/medial lemniscus (PSDC) form the sensory-discriminative pathways (*solid lines*). Spinal projection neurons reach the lateral thalamic nuclei (ventral posterior lateral, VPL; and posterior complex: PO) directly or polysynaptically via the dorsal columns nuclei. Thalamic neurons project to the primary and secondary sensory cortices (SI, SII). The affective-motivational pathways (*dashed lines*): Neurons in the deep spinal laminae project in the spinoreticular tract (SRT) to the pontomedullary reticular formation and the spinomesenchephalic tract (SMT) to the mesencephalon including the periaqueductal gray (PAG) and parabrachial nuclei (PBn). Polysynaptic projections connect the brainstem to the limbic cortex. At the level of the cortex, limbic areas and somatosensory areas are interconnected.

pathways, but also that there is redundancy in the rostrad transmission of nociceptive information (Fig 2-5).

Sensory-Discriminative Pathways

The sensory-discriminative component of pain is processed through the ventral posterior lateral (VPL) nucleus and posterior complex of the thalamus which project to the primary and secondary sensory cortices. There are two main pathways for sensory information to reach the thalamus: the spinothalamic tract (STT) and the dorsal (posterior) columns/medial lemniscus.

Spinothalamic Tract

The spinothalamic tract is the main pathway for sensory discrimination of somatic pain. Disruption of the STT produces a loss of pain and thermal sensation contralateral to and below the site of the lesion. The STT is composed of fibers in the anterolateral (ventrolateral in animals) white matter. Cell bodies of the STT are located in the superficial dorsal horn, the deep dorsal horn, and the ventral horn. Most cells receive input from the ipsilateral side of the body. Receptive fields are relatively small, especially on the distal limbs. Most neurons respond to innocuous and/or noxious stimuli, WDR and NS

neurons. The axons of STT cells decussate in the anterior (ventral) commissure of the spinal cord within a few segments of the cell body and project to the contralateral thalamus (VPL and Po). Within the white matter, axons of STT cells are somatotopically organized. Axons from cervical cells are pushed medial as the axons from more caudal levels are added. Within the cervical spinal cord, STT axons from cervical levels are located close to the gray matter and axons from sacral segments are the most superficially located.

Dorsal Columns/Medial Lemniscus

The dorsal or posterior columns contain axons of spinal neurons (postsynaptic dorsal column neurons; PSDC) that project to the dorsal column nuclei as well as ascending branches of large diameter sensory afferent fibers. The dorsal columns/medial lemniscal pathway conveys information related to touch, vibratory sense, two-point discrimination, and proprioception. Cell bodies of PSDC neurons are mostly located in laminae III and IV. Receptive fields are small and most neurons respond exclusively to low threshold mechanical stimuli or innocuous and noxious stimuli (WDR neurons). The axons of PSDC neurons ascend in the ipsilateral dorsal columns with axons of lower thoracic, lumbar, and sacral cells located medially in the fasciculus gracilis and axons of rostral thoracic and cervical cells located more laterally in the fasciculus cuneatus. They synapse on neurons in the dorsal column nuclei (nucleus gracilis, nucleus cuneatus) neurons whose axons decussate in the caudal medulla forming the medial lemniscus, which terminates in the ventral posterior lateral nucleus and posterior complex of the thalamus.

Recently, the dorsal column has been studied as a pathway for transmitting visceral stimuli to the thalamus. Neurons in the dorsal column nuclei respond to noxious visceral stimulation and lesions to the dorsal columns significantly attenuate the response of dorsal column nuclei neurons and VPL thalamic neurons to visceral stimuli. Many of these visceroceptive PSDC neurons are located in lamina X around the central canal. Surgical intervention, a midline myelotomy, reduces chronic pelvic pain. However, this surgery also cuts axons conveying touch, vibratory sense, two-point discrimination, and proprioception, so it is a surgery of last resort.

Affective-Motivational Pathways

The affective-motivational component is the unpleasant nature of pain and provides the motivation to reduce pain as quickly as possible. Sensory pathways conveying the affective component project to the reticular formation and midbrain to access autonomic centers and to the limbic system to provide the emotional component of the pain. Several pathways contribute to the affective-motivational component as will be described. There are no direct projections into the limbic system proper with most pathways passing through the medial thalamus or hypothalamus.

Spinoreticular Tract

Cells of the spinoreticular tract (SRT) send axons through the anterolateral (ventrolateral) funiculus to synapse on neurons throughout the medullary and pontine reticular formation. The spinal neurons that form the SRT are mostly located in the deeper laminae, V–VIII. SRT neurons have large receptive fields that can encompass several limbs and the trunk on both sides of the body. With such large receptive fields, SRT neurons cannot provide accurate information about the location of a stimulus, they lose the somatotopic organization of the body. However, this makes these cells well suited to activate autonomic, visceromotor, and somatomotor systems when the body is injured. Axons of SRT neurons join with STT and SMT (see subsequent sections) neurons to form the ascending pathway in the anterolateral funiculus. However, it is not clear what percentage of SRT neurons project ipsilateral or contralateral to the cell body. Estimates range from all fibers projecting in the ipsilateral pathway to 80% contralateral. Upon reaching the brainstem, these fibers project the length of the reticular formation. Of interest are the strong projections to the nucleus raphe magnus and nucleus reticularis gigantocellularis where SRT neurons activate descending inhibitory and facilitatory systems. Neurons from several areas of the reticular formation also project to the medial thalamus (central lateral, dorsomedial, parafascicular nuclei). These nuclei have diffuse projections to the cerebral cortex and limbic system mediating the emotional aspect of pain perception.

Spinomesencephalic Tract

The spinomesencephalic tract (SMT) actually consists of two separate pathways. SMT cells in lamina I of the spinal cord project in the ipsilateral and contralateral dorsolateral fasciculi to synapse in the parabrachial and surrounding nuclei. Because they are in lamina I, most of these cells are nociceptive specific with small to medium size receptive fields. Some third order neurons in the parabrachial nuclei project to the amygdala accessing the limbic system with information pertaining to noxious stimuli.

SMT cells in lamina V and to a lesser extent VI to VII, form the larger SMT pathway. These cells send axons through the anterolateral funiculus (joining the STT and SRT) to synapse on neurons in the ventrolateral PAG, nucleus cuneiformis, the superior colliculus, nucleus Darkschewitsch, and nucleus Edinger-Westphal. Neurons in the PAG project back down to the rostroventral medulla activating descending systems, but also to the hypothalamus and medial thalamus accessing the limbic system.

Ventral Spinothalamic Tract

A smaller group of fibers ascends in the anterior (ventral) columns to synapse in the thalamus forming a ventral STT. The full extent and function of these fibers is unclear. Some project to the ventral posterior lateral thalamus and functionally appear no different than the larger STT. Others are thought to project to the medial thalamus making them part of the affective-motivational pathway.

Multisynaptic Ascending System

A system of intersegmentally projecting spinal neurons has been described in the spinal cord. Rather than a set of neurons with axons that project to supraspinal targets, this is a chain of neurons that ascend the spinal cord providing another pathway to access the reticular formation.

Descending Modulation of Pain

The modulation of activity in spinal projection neurons by descending pathways has been recognized for many years. Studies over the past 30 years have identified multisynaptic pathways originating in the ventrolateral PAG that descend into the spinal cord and inhibit or facilitate activity in supraspinal projection neurons. Studies demonstrating descending inhibitory influences in the spinal cord date back to the early 1900s, but Melzack and Wall first proposed a specific descending pain modulatory system as part of their Gate Control Theory.[11] Subsequently, electrical stimulation or microinjection of morphine into the PAG was demonstrated to attenuate responses of spinal nociceptive neurons and behavioral responses to noxious stimuli in animals and man. In addition, stress was found to be analgesic suggesting that attention and state of mind modulate pain perception. This led to recognition of a limbocortical–diencephalic–mesopontomedullary–spinal cord circuit for the control of nociceptive transmission in the spinal cord (Fig. 2-6). This circuit encompasses parallel descending pathways and multiple transmitters and receptors underscoring the complexity of spinal pain processing. Because spinal neurons project to the supraspinal sites involved in descending modulation of nociceptive transmission, this produces a feedback mechanism whereby the activity in the spinal projection neurons modulates the descending modulatory pathways. Therefore, the state of spinal processing will affect descending modulation. Recent studies have shown that changes in descending modulation of spinal neuronal activity are important to the generation and maintenance of hyperalgesia in noninjured tissue. It appears then, that several descending circuits exist that modulate spinal neuronal activity. Whether this modulation inhibits or facilitates nociceptive transmission depends on the state of the animal and the intensity and duration of the stimulus.

Descending Pathways

The ventrolateral PAG is critically involved in descending inhibition of spinal nociceptive transmission, but has few direct projections to the spinal cord. Rather, antinociceptive effects of PAG stimulation are mediated by two generalized regions of the brainstem. Neurons in the rostroventral medulla (RVM), which includes the nucleus raphe magnus and adjacent reticular formation (nucleus reticularis magnocellularis and nucleus reticularis paragigantocellularis) comprise the largest brainstem projection to the spinal cord. These projections descend in the dorsolateral funiculus (DLF) and anterior (ventral) columns as part of the reticulospinal tract. Reticulospinal spinal fibers in the DLF project to laminae I, II, V to VII, and X. Fibers in the ventral reticulospinal tract project to laminae VIII and IX to influence the motoneuron pools.

The RVM is the major source of serotonin (5-HT) to the spinal cord although 5-HT neurons only form a minor portion of the RVM spinal projection. Nevertheless, 5-HT is critically involved in descending modulation of nociceptive transmission. Stimulation in the NRM or DLF produces antinociception and inhibition of spinal neuronal responses to noxious stimuli,

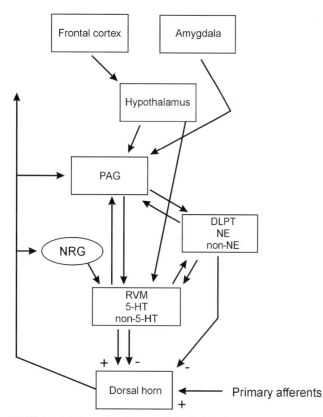

FIGURE 2-6 Schematic diagram of the limbic-diencephalic-mesopontomedullary-spinal descending pain modulatory system. Limbic structures directly and indirectly project to the PAG. These midbrain structures project to the RVM and DLPT. The RVM and DLPT project to the spinal cord to inhibit (−) nociceptive processing. The RVM also facilitates (+) nociceptive processing under certain circumstances. RVM, nucleus raphe magnus, nucleus reticularis magnocellularis, nucleus reticularis paragigantocellularis; DLPT, nucleus cuneiformis, locus coeruleus, A5, A7 cell groups; nRG, nucleus reticularis gigantocellularis. (Adapted from Fields HL, Basbaum AI. Central nervous system mechanisms of pain modulation. In Wall PD, Melzack R (eds). Textbook of Pain (4th ed). New York, Churchill Livingstone, 1999, p 312.)

which are attenuated by spinal 5-HT receptor antagonists. Likewise, destruction of 5-HT–containing neurons in the RVM partially blocks opioid-induced antinociception and spinal administration of 5-HT agonists produces antinociception.

Neurons in the dorsolateral pontine tegmentum (DLPT) including the nucleus cuneiformis, A5 and A7 cell groups, and the locus coeruleus form the other major brainstem projection to the spinal cord. Neurons in the locus coeruleus and A5 and A7 cell groups project through the dorsal and ventral parts of the lateral funiculus to all laminae of the spinal cord. These cell groups form the major source of norepinephrine (NE) to the spinal cord. Similar to 5-HT, NE produces inhibition of spinal responses and antinociception through α_2-adrenergic receptors. α_2-antagonists block antinociception induced by stimulation in the PAG or DPLT and stimulation in these areas evokes release of NE in the spinal cord.

In the spinal cord, descending inhibition of nociceptive processing occurs via pre- and postsynaptic mechanisms. Presynaptic inhibition decreases transmitter release from primary afferent terminals attenuating nociceptive transmission. This occurs monosynaptically via noradrenergic axons

originating in the DLPT (A5 and A7 cell groups) and polysynaptically via descending excitation of spinal GABAergic or enkephalinergic inhibitory interneurons, which inhibit primary afferent transmitter release. Inhibition is also postsynaptically mediated via mono- and polysynaptic projections from descending fibers. Descending serotonergic fibers from the RVM synapse on spinothalamic tract neurons inhibiting output of these cells. Descending fibers also synapse on inhibitory and excitatory interneurons in the superficial dorsal horn. Inhibition of excitatory interneurons or excitation of inhibitory interneurons that synapse upon spinal nociceptive projection neurons will decrease nociceptive transmission in these cells. It is clear from these connections that both excitatory and inhibitory modulation of spinal nociceptive processing is possible producing a very complex interaction between these systems.

Neurons in the RVM, PAG, and DLPT that modulate nociceptive transmission in the spinal cord are described as ON and OFF cells. ON cells are normally silent and begin to fire before initiation of a reflex movement evoked by a noxious stimulus. OFF cells have some degree of spontaneous activity and cease firing before the reflex movement. Therefore, ON cells appear to be pronociceptive as they facilitate spinal neuron activity to noxious stimuli while OFF cells are antinociceptive as they inhibit spinal neuronal activity. ON and OFF cells have spinal terminations in laminae I, II, V, and X, providing the anatomic specificity necessary for the proposed modulatory functions.

Pharmacology of Opioid Analgesia

Opioids are potent analgesics for relief of inflammatory and chronic pain that act by inhibiting spinal nociceptive processing. Morphine administered systemically or locally into the PAG, RVM, or amygdala produces antinociception and attenuation of spinal neuronal responses to noxious stimuli. Studies with receptor selective antagonists have shown that three subtypes of opioid receptor—μ, δ, and κ—contribute to the antinociception. These receptors are found throughout the neural circuitry involved in descending inhibition of pain processing along with several endogenous transmitters that are natural ligands for these receptors. Microinjection of μ, δ, or κ opioid receptor antagonists into these sites block the analgesic effects of systemic morphine.

There are several opioid peptides that likely are the endogenous ligands for the μ, δ, and κ opioid receptors. These endogenous opioids derive from several different precursor proteins that also form nonopioid hormones. Met- and Leuenkephalin derive from preproenkephalin. These opioid peptides have high affinity for μ and δ receptors and could be endogenous ligands for both. β-endorphin and the hormones adrenocorticotropic hormone and melanocyte stimulating hormone are derived from pro-opiomelanocortin. β-endorphin, which contains the N-terminal sequence of Metenkephalin also has high affinity for μ and δ receptors. Preprodynorphin gives rise to dynorphin peptides, which have the N-terminal sequence of Leuenkephalin and have high affinity for κ receptors, and α-neoendorphin. Endomorphins, which do not have the enkephalin sequence, have much higher affinity for μ receptors than δ or κ receptors. For the most part, these opioid peptides are localized in presynaptic terminals in close relation to the appropriate receptor, but this is not absolute.

Opioid-containing neurons in the descending inhibitory circuitry are inhibitory interneurons. They produce effects presynaptically by inhibiting a voltage-dependent calcium conductance decreasing transmitter release or postsynaptically by increasing a potassium conductance hyperpolarizing the neuron. Figure 2-7 diagrams a circuit for opioid-mediated ON and OFF cell modulation of nociceptive transmission in the spinal cord. In order for morphine to produce effects similar to electrical stimulation of the PAG, which is inhibition of spinal nociceptive transmission, opioid receptor–containing neurons must also be inhibitory interneurons. Opioids inhibit these inhibitory interneurons increasing activity in PAG neurons that project to the RVM and DPLT. This projection excites RVM neurons that are also opioid interneurons. They inhibit ON cells that are themselves inhibitory neurons. The decrease in activity of ON cells disinhibits OFF cells increasing RVM inhibition of spinal nociceptive transmission.

Nonopioid Inhibition of Nociception

Noxious stimulation to one area of the body can attenuate the perception of pain to another area of the body. This phenomenon is called diffuse noxious inhibitory controls (DNIC) or counterirritation. Experimental studies have shown that DNIC is mediated by a spino-bulbo-spinal loop involving the caudal medulla and the nucleus reticularis dorsalis, but not the RVM. Activation of this system seems to sharpen one noxious stimulus while producing inhibition throughout the rest of the body. Stimulation in the nucleus reticularis dorsalis can facilitate reflex responses to noxious stimuli suggesting that DNIC produces a balance of excitatory and inhibitory modulation within the nervous system.

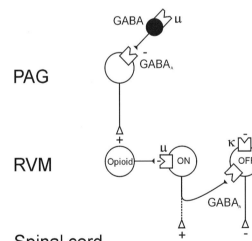

FIGURE 2-7 Diagram of intrinsic opioid–mediated brainstem connectivity. PAG neurons, disinhibited by opioids or GABA-A antagonists, activate an opioid (presumably enkephalinergic) interneuron in the RVM. This endogenous opioid inhibits mu (μ) opioid receptor–bearing ON cells. The inhibition of the ON cell disinhibits the OFF cell, which inhibits nociceptive transmission at the level of the dorsal horn. (From Fields HL, Basbaum AI. Central nervous system mechanisms of pain modulation. *In* Wall PD, Melzack R (eds). Textbook of Pain (4th ed). New York, Churchill Livingstone, 1999, p 316, with permission.)

Descending Modulation of Inflammatory Pain

Recent studies have also shown that the descending modulatory sites in the brainstem are necessary for the generation and maintenance of secondary hyperalgesia via a spinal-bulbo-spinal loop. Joint inflammation or topical application of mustard oil (a C-fiber excitant) produces secondary hyperalgesia away from the injured tissue. Lesions of the RVM or spinal cord DLF prevent or attenuate the secondary hyperalgesia without affecting primary hyperalgesia. This secondary hyperalgesia depends on an NMDA receptor–mediated excitation in the RVM since NMDA receptor antagonists or nitric oxide synthase inhibitors attenuate the secondary hyperalgesia. Interestingly, AMPA receptor antagonists in the RVM facilitate the hyperalgesia, suggesting there are dual descending modulatory effects; an NMDA receptor–mediated facilitation and an AMPA receptor–mediated inhibition. The expression of secondary hyperalgesia to persistent noxious input depends on a shift in the balance of these descending modulatory circuits.

SUMMARY AND CONCLUSIONS

The perception of painful stimuli is dependent on the interaction of multiple systems. Primary afferent fibers are modulated by the environment surrounding the afferent terminals. The interaction of multiple inflammatory mediators with the receptor composition of the afferent terminal will affect the excitability of the afferent to subsequent stimuli. This information is passed centrally to the spinal cord where the neurochemical composition of the afferent fiber interacts with the receptor composition of dorsal horn neurons. The intensity and persistence of afferent activity will contribute to the state of spinal nociceptive processing affecting the output of the dorsal horn. Information diverges from the dorsal horn over multiple ascending pathways. Some drive descending modulatory circuits that feedback onto dorsal horn neurons shaping the responses to subsequent stimuli. Other pathways bring information to different areas of higher processing that contribute to different aspects of the painful experience.

REFERENCES

1. Dubner R, Gold MS. Colloquium on the Neurobiology of Pain. Washington, DC, National Academy of Sciences, 1999.
2. Basbaum AI. Spinal mechanisms of acute and persistent pain. Reg Anesth Pain Med 24:59–67, 1999.
3. Besson JM. The neurobiology of pain. Lancet 353:1610–1615, 1999.
4. Bonica JJ. The Management of Pain. Philadelphia, Lea & Febiger, 1999.
5. Cervero F. Sensory innervation of the viscera: peripheral basis of visceral pain. Physiol Rev 74:95–138, 1994.
6. Coggeshall RE, Carlton SM. Receptor localization in the mammalian dorsal horn and primary afferent neurons. Brain Res Rev 24:28–66, 1997.
7. Dubner R, Ren K. Endogenous mechanisms of sensory modulation. Pain (Suppl 6):S45–S53, 1999.
8. Dubner R, Ruda MA. Activity-dependent neuronal plasticity following tissue injury and inflammation. TINS 15:96–103, 1992.
9. Furst S. Transmitters involved in antinociception in the spinal cord. Brain Res Bull 48:129–141, 1999.
10. Lewin GR, Mendell LM. Nerve growth factor and nociception. Trends Neurosci 16:353–359, 1993.

11. Melzack R, Wall PD. Pain mechanisms: a new theory. Science 150:971–979, 1965.
12. Millan MJ. The induction of pain: an integrative review. Prog Neurobiol 57:1–164, 1999.
13. Petersen-Zeitz KR, Basbaum AI. Second messengers, the substantia gelatinosa and injury-induced persistent pain. Pain S5–S12, 1999.
14. Ruda MA, Bennett GJ, Dubner R. Neurochemistry and neural circuitry in the dorsal horn. Prog Brain Res 66:219–268, 1986.
15. Stein C. Peripheral mechanisms of opioid analgesia. Anesth Analg 76:182–191, 1993.
16. Treede RD, Kenshalo DR, Gracely RH, Jones AK. The cortical representation of pain. Pain 79:105–111, 1999.
17. Treede RD, Meyer RA, Raja SN, Campbell JN. Peripheral and central mechanisms of cutaneous hyperalgesia. Prog Neurobiol 38:397–421, 1992.

18. Urban MO, Gebhart GF. Central mechanisms in pain. Med Clin North Am 83:585–596, 1999.
19. Wall PD, Melzack R. Textbook of Pain. Edinburgh, Churchill Livingstone, 1999.
20. Willis WD. Hyperalgesia and Allodynia. New York, Raven, 1992.
21. Willis WD Jr, Coggeshall RE. Sensory Mechanisms of the Spinal Cord. New York, Plenum, 1991.
22. Yaksh TL. Pharmacology and mechanisms of opioid analgesic activity. Acta Anaesthesiol Scand 41:94–111, 1997.
23. Yaksh TL. Spinal systems and pain processing: development of novel analgesic drugs with mechanistically defined models. Trends Pharmacol Sci 20:329–337, 1999.
24. Yaksh TL, Dirig DM, Malmberg AB. Mechanism of action of non-steroidal anti-inflammatory drugs. Cancer Invest 16:509–527, 1998.

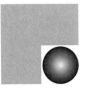

The Pathophysiology of Neuropathic Pain

BRADLEY K. TAYLOR, PhD

SCOPE OF NEUROPATHIC PAIN

Neuropathic pain represents a major neurologic complication associated with neuronal injury. Common clinical examples include pain resulting from diabetic neuropathy (~600,000 cases in the United States), postherpetic neuralgia (~500,000 cases), neuralgia associated with late-stage cancer (~200,000 cases), partial nerve injury (leading to causalgia), multiple sclerosis, amputation, and some forms of back pain. When these examples are taken together, neuropathic pain is conservatively estimated to affect 1.5% of the0 population.[1] Because neuropathic pain is often immutable and maladaptive in nature, it can reduce the patient's ability to work, walk, or sleep, as with other forms of chronic pain. Indeed, the societal and financial impact of chronic neuropathic pain is tremendous.

PHYSIOLOGICAL VERSUS NEUROPATHIC PAIN

With recent advances in our understanding of the pathophysiology and pharmacotherapy of pain, we can now distinguish neuropathic pain from other types of pain— transient pain and inflammatory pain.[2] A transient noxious stimulus, such as brief exposure to hot metal or a sharp object, causes what is termed *transient pain* (other use the synonymous terms *normal pain* or *reflexive pain*). Transient pain serves several protective functions. In particular, it acts as an early warning device that helps to prevent tissue damage by eliciting a coordinated, reflexive response constellation. Behavioral responses include withdrawal from the stimulus, autonomic responses include increases in blood pressure and heart rate, and other stress responses include activation of the hypothalamo-pituitary-adrenal axis.[3,4] Until the past decade or two, most laboratory studies were designed from this perspective.

If non-neural tissue damage does occur, as in the setting of inflammatory pain, a set of excitatory changes in the periphery and in the central nervous system establish a more persistent, but reversible, hypersensitivity in the inflamed and surrounding tissue. Inflammatory pain is associated with hyperalgesia and an expansion of receptive fields, typically of a *quantitative* nature.[5] The resulting immobilization and protective behaviors prevent further damage and thus assist in wound repair. As illustrated in Figure 3-1, transient and acute inflammatory pain represent adaptive responses to the external milieu, and on that basis can be collectively termed *physiologic pain*. The previous term, *nociceptive pain,* was originally used in basic science research and then spilled into the clinical arena many years ago; being an ambiguous term, it has outlived its usefulness as a descriptor of clinical pain.

In contrast to non-neural tissue damage, nerve injury can produce sensory/motor deficits and other paradoxical sensations of a *qualitative* nature. As might be expected, impaired conduction of afferent nerve activity leads to an area of sensory deficit, felt by patients as numbness, while impaired conduction of efferent nerve activity leads to muscle deficits, experienced by patients as weakness. These are termed *negative symptoms,* or *negative phenomena.* Many patients, however, also report enhanced sensations; these are termed *positive phenomena,* or *positive symptoms.* They range from paresthesias such as tingling and prickling sensations, to hyperesthesias (heightened but nonpainful appreciation of sensation), to dysesthesias (unpleasant or painful sensations).[6] Thus, the quality and pattern of altered sensitivity in neuropathic pain clearly differs from that of transient or inflammatory pain. For example, a cold stimulus such as ice may reduce inflammatory pain in the normal person, but produce excruciating pain in the patient with neuropathic pain. These qualitative differences in sensation suggest that nerve injury leads to a *reorganization* of sensory transmission pathways that persist long after the normal healing period. Such a reorganization in the nervous system would suggest that simple knowledge of pain pathways and neurotransmission is not enough to understand chronic neuropathic pain.

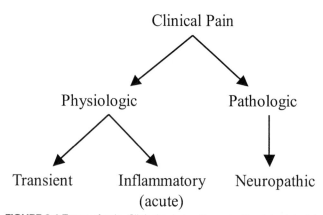

Clinical Pain

Physiologic   Pathologic

Transient   Inflammatory   Neuropathic
                  (acute)

FIGURE 3-1 Types of pain. Clinical pain is either adaptive (physiologic) or maladaptive (pathologic). Physiologic pain is either transient (e.g., exposure to a hotplate or a pinprick) or inflammatory (involving non-neural tissue damage). Pathologic pain occurs in the setting of neural tissue damage (neuropathic). In some cases (see Table 3-1), chronic inflammation will produce a neuropathic pain state.

CLINICAL SYMPTOMS FOLLOWING NERVE DAMAGE

The International Association for the Study of Pain (IASP) has brought order to the terminology used to define neuropathic pain[7]: "Pain initiated or caused by a primary lesion or dysfunction in the nervous system." The quality of neuropathic pain sensation can be further divided into overlapping categories: allodynia, hyperalgesia, spontaneous pain, and hyperpathia.[6] *Allodynia* refers to the pain evoked by a gentle tactile stimulus; it is usually found in the cutaneous territory innervated by the damaged nerves, the skin itself being otherwise healthy. The term *allodynia* is increasingly being used inappropriately to imply a distinct pathophysiologic mechanism, and should be avoided in that context. *Hyperalgesia* refers to an exaggerated pain that is disproportionately produced by a noxious stimulus. *Spontaneous* abnormal sensations reported by patients include tingling, prickling, electric,

burning, and lancinating. *Hyperpathia* is a delayed painful after-sensation to a stimulus, particularly when presented repetitively. This rare, paradoxical pain often occurs in an area that is normally hypoesthetic, but can become explosive after exposure to a noxious stimulus or a stimulus that normally produces another sensation.

Certain characteristics of reported abnormal sensations may suggest a diagnosis of neuropathic pain.[8] Of these sensations, tactile allodynia is the most striking. Even very mild somatosensory stimuli, such as slight bending of hairs, contact with bedcovers, or the wearing of clothes, can become excruciating. In addition, neuropathic pain commonly has a burning and/or shooting quality with unusual tingling, crawling, or electrical dysesthesias. A third suggestive feature is the progressive worsening of pain during slow repetitive stimulation with a mildly noxious stimulus, such as a pinprick. Fourth, if small-diameter fibers of a cutaneous nerve are damaged, then the area of skin reported as painful may be coextensive with or within a zone of hypoesthesia to noxious stimulation. In considering the diagnosis of neuropathic pain, it must be kept in mind that patients with peripheral nerve lesion or dysfunction can experience more than one type of abnormal sensation.

HETEROGENEITY OF NEUROPATHIC PAIN

Although most neuropathic pain patients experience one or more of the abnormal sensations described previously, numerous etiologies and anatomic sites of nerve lesions can produce a wide variety of neuropathic pain syndromes. Indeed, the most complex cases involve multiple nerves and/or multiple somatic and visceral structures. This diversity in cause and site is reflected by the numerous categories of neuropathic pain patients with peripheral nerve disease,[9,10] as depicted in the classification of neuropathic pain by etiology and anatomic distribution (Table 3-1).

This classification might be useful for diagnosis and treatment of the disease itself. However, because we know little of

● TABLE 3-1 • Classification of Neuropathic Pain by Etiology and Anatomy

Category	Type of Neuropathy	Specific Example
Focal or multifocal neuropathies	Neuralgias Entrapment	Trigeminal neuralgia Nerve compression
	Neuroma	Surgical nerve damage
	Diabetes	Diabetic neuropathy
	Malignancy	Nerve/plexus invasion
	Angiopathic	Nerve inflammation/ischemia
	Infectious	Postherpetic neuralgia, AIDS
Generalized polyneuropathies	Metabolic disorders Toxin exposure	Vitamin deficiency Anticancer drugs
	Immune-mediated	Multiple sclerosis
	Heredity	Inherited sensory neuropathies

the relationship between the disease state and chronic pain, this classification does not even allow us to predict which patient will develop neuropathic pain. And without an understanding of mechanism, we cannot reliably predict outcome of an intervention for the clinical management of pain. Thus, treatment of neuropathic pain remains largely empirical.[11] Apart from the strong response of trigeminal neuralgia to carbamazepine, and the recently demonstrated responsiveness of diabetic neuropathy[12,13] and postherpetic neuralgia[12,14] to gabapentin and tricyclic antidepressants, we cannot provide adequate treatment to a vast number of patients with established neuropathic pain.

RECENT ADVANCES

Over the past decade, we have experienced an explosion of research directed toward an understanding of the pathophysiologic neural changes associated with neuropathic pain. Most of this research stems from the development of new animal models of peripheral nerve injury,[15] and from experimental human studies of pain and sensory changes after dermal injection of capsaicin. In the capsaicin model, controlled clinical information usually comes in the form of neurophysiologic recordings and the results of pharmacologic treatment trials.[16]

As illustrated in Table 3-2, the new animal models involve partial injury of a peripheral nerve, or ligation of spinal nerves. In contrast to previous models involving complete section of the sciatic nerve, these newer models leave a large proportion of motor fibers intact, allowing behavioral measurement. Several important mechanisms common to various animal models of neuropathic pain likely contribute to the clinical features of neuropathic pain. Thus, nerve injury–induced painlike behavior in animals and neuropathic pain in humans share some key distinguishing characteristics, particularly tactile allodynia and cold hyperalgesia.[1] For example, the dermal application of thin von Frey hairs, normally felt at the threshold of detection, can produce allodynia in patients with neuropathic pain and withdrawal responses in nerve-injured rats. Also, both patients with complex regional pain syndrome (CRPS 2) and causalgia (burning pain after nerve injury) and neuropathic rats exhibit abnormal temperature abnormalities at the affected limb. Certainly, key differences exist between human clinical pain and animal behavioral allodynia/hyperalgesia, particularly with respect to specificity of neural damage and to temporal progression and decline of symptoms. But it is by understanding the similarities that we will make progress in our understanding and pharmacotherapy of neuropathic pain.

With these new basic science and clinical methods, recent and upcoming advances in pain research have provided, and will continue to provide, important clues toward a new understanding of the specific mechanisms that underlie the positive symptoms of neuropathic pain. Already, detailed studies of neuropathic pain in patients and animal models have converged to indicate that changes in both the peripheral and central nervous system cause and maintain signs of abnormal sensory function following nerve damage. These alterations include biochemical, anatomic, and physiologic changes in the somatosensory system at the level of the primary afferent neuron, spinal cord dorsal horn, and brain. Intense research is determining the relative contributions of these reactive changes to neuropathic pain.

PERIPHERAL MECHANISMS

As alluded to previously, the peripheral mechanisms generating physiologic pain are quite different from those generating neuropathic pain. In transient pain, events at the peripheral terminals of nociceptors initiate axonal impulses. Peripheral nociceptive terminals selectively express transducer proteins that respond to thermal, tactile, or chemical stimuli. If the current is sufficient, action potentials are initiated and conducted to the central terminals in the spinal cord, leading to the release of nociceptive transmitters such as glutamate. Glutamate activates alpha-amino-3-hydroxy-5-methyl-4-isoxazolepropionic acid (AMPA) and kainate ligand-gated ion channels on second-order neurons in the spinal cord, which then relay the nociceptive signals to a number of brainstem areas including the thalamus. It is these pathways that also mediate inflammatory pain; if the pain is severe and persistent, numerous changes may take place within the nervous system. Some of these are also characteristic of neuropathic pain, such as central sensitization, changes in neurochemical signature, and certain supraspinal mechanisms, as discussed below. However, injury to the nervous system produces additional long-term changes that contribute to neuropathic pain. We begin with a discussion of how primary afferent neurons acquire spontaneous and stimulus-evoked activity at loci other than peripheral terminals, namely the nociceptor axons and cell bodies, respectively.

● TABLE 3-2 • Prevalent Animal Models of Neuropathic Pain

Model	Year of Publication	Lesion Location	Key Modality of Hypersensitivity
Chronic constriction injury	1988	Sciatic nerve (4 loose ligatures)	Heat
Partial nerve lesion	1990	Sciatic nerve (partial ligation)	Heat
Spinal nerve ligation	1992	Spinal nerve (L5 ± L6)	Touch
Spared nerve injury	2000	Common peroneal and tibial nerves	Touch

The Neuroma and Ectopic Activity

Research in the area of neuropathic pain began with studies of experimental neuromas.[17] Nerve transection can produce an aberrant regenerative response at the site of injury. As illustrated in Figure 3-2, the result is a disorganized collection of regenerating axon tips ("sprouts"), small patches of demyelinated terminal endings of the cut parent axons, and a proliferation of other cellular neural components. The sprouts of the neuroma are often of small diameter and contain substance P, and thus may have originally been nociceptors. Wall and Gutnick found that spontaneous (stimulus-independent) activity and robust mechanical (stimulus-dependent) sensitivity develops in the afferent axonal sprouts innervating the neuroma (see Fig. 3-2).[17] The abnormal impulses arising from these sites are called *ectopic* because they do not originate from the normal transduction elements of peripheral terminals of the primary afferent nociceptor. Ectopic activity has been observed in the newer animal models of neuropathic pain (although in a small percentage of neurons[18]), and is now widely believed to contribute to the generation and maintenance of positive neuropathic symptoms.[19] Beyond this, the sensory disturbances and types of pain that may be associated with neuromas vary greatly among individuals, and are not well understood.

Stimulus-Dependent Activity of Neuromas

Healthy sensory nerve axons are normally insensitive to nonnoxious mechanical stimulation. In the setting of nerve injury, however, they develop extreme mechanical sensitivity, such that arterial pulsations may become painful. The mechanosensitivity of neuromas has been shown by manipulating them or probing their surface, which produces bursts of impulses, sometimes in long trains.[19] In humans, electrical discharges from neuromas have been recorded using microelectrodes placed within the nerves. Such microneurographic recordings from patients with traumatic or amputation neuromas have shown that tapping the neuroma evokes nerve discharges accompanied either by sensations of electric shocks (Tinel's sign) or pain.[20] These responses can often be blocked with local anesthetic injections directly at the neuroma, suggesting that stimulus-dependent pain arises from the neuroma itself. Unfortunately, surgical resection of a neuroma tends to have only short-lasting benefits, as a new painful neuroma invariably forms.

Stimulus-Independent Activity of Sensory Neurons

Normally, the spontaneous activity of primary afferent neurons is quite low. In patients with chronic peripheral neuropathy, however, direct microneurographic recordings demonstrated enhanced spontaneous firing of nociceptors innervating the painful region, indicating that abnormally active nociceptors contribute to neuropathic pain.[20] Also, animal models demonstrate that nerve transection produces a brief injury discharge lasting a few seconds, followed by electrical silence. Later, as a neuroma forms, other electrical discharges occur. These discharges reach a maximum by about 2 weeks. After 4 weeks, only a few of the axons proximal to the neuroma show evidence of spontaneous activity.[19,21]

Where does the spontaneous activity arise? Local anesthetic application, such as lidocaine infiltration of a peripheral neuroma, does not change spontaneous discharge and pain, indicating that spontaneous pain impulses arise away from the neuroma.[20] Damaged and regenerating distal axon terminals do not appear to be the source of generation of ectopic impulses. Rather, as illustrated in Figure 3-2, animal studies suggest that a region near the dorsal root ganglion becomes capable of generating spontaneous impulses after nerve injury.[19,22] These secondary changes may be at least as important as the neuroma itself in producing and maintaining sensory symptoms, especially spontaneous pain.

Mechanism of Ectopic Activity

Sodium channels mediate the initiation of the action potential and are thought to be a major contributor to stimulus-independent pathological pain states. Nerve injury triggers a redistribution of Na^+ channels at the neuroma site and along the axon.[23–25] The resulting accumulation of Na^+ channels may lower action potential threshold and cause spontaneous activity, leading to the appearance of loci of hyperexcitability and ectopic action potential discharge in injured nociceptors. Anticonvulsants, such as carbamazepine, and antiarrhythmics, such as mexiletine (both are used in the treatment of neuropathic pain), may block these sodium channels at these sites of spontaneous ectopic discharge and thus stabilize membranes at aberrantly active loci. Although the dose required for such actions is small relative

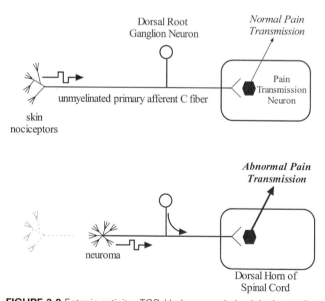

FIGURE 3-2 Ectopic activity. *TOP:* Under normal physiologic conditions, stimulation of nociceptor endings innervating the peripheral tissues triggers the action potential (*squiggly arrow*), leading to the release of neurotransmitters in the dorsal horn of the spinal cord, and subsequent stimulation of nociceptive pathways to the brain. *BOTTOM:* Under the pathologic conditions induced by nerve transection, a neuroma forms. Alterations in sodium channel gene expression and protein translocation then contribute to stimulus-dependent ectopic firing from the neuroma, or stimulus-independent ectopic firing from a site in or near the dorsal root ganglion (*curved arrow*), leading to abnormal pain transmission.

to effects on uninjured axons, it is still high enough to significantly inhibit Na^+ channels on cardiac myocytes. Therefore, certain types found only in dorsal root ganglion neurons (SNS/PNS, SNS2/NaN, and alpha-III) are particularly attractive targets.[26–28]

Unclear Contribution of the Sympathetic Nervous System

Evidence for Sensory-Sympathetic Coupling

Sensory-sympathetic coupling in the setting of nerve injury may contribute to some types of stimulus-independent neuropathic pain. Under physiologic conditions, primary afferent nerve endings are not sensitive to catecholamines and are functionally distinct from the efferent sympathetic nervous system. Thus, sympathetic activation does not produce pain. Nerve injury, however, can induce a noradrenergic supersensitivity to noxious stimulation. In humans, the application of norepinephrine at or near a neuroma increases electrical discharges and produces severe burning pain.[29] Furthermore, animal studies suggest that intraarterial injections of noradrenaline can activate or sensitize intact C nociceptors in the partially injured nerve.[30] Finally, electrical stimulation of the sympathetic chain, causing endogenous release of norepinephrine, increases the discharge of unmyelinated sprouts that have regenerated into a neuroma.[31] α_2-Adrenergic receptors contribute to the increased sensitivity to norepinephrine,[30] but the relative importance of the α_1 receptor (or a new type of adrenoceptor specific to nerve damage) remains controversial.[32]

Anatomic Evidence for Sensory-Sympathetic Coupling

After nerve damage in the rat, norepinephrine-containing sympathetic postganglionic fibers that normally innervate small blood vessels sprout, a process that is likely triggered by a neurotrophin such as nerve growth factor.[33] In addition to making nonsynaptic contacts with sensory endings, sympathetic sprouts can actually encircle large-diameter dorsal root ganglion (DRG) somata, forming "baskets."[34] The net result of this increased sympathetic innervation could be the creation of a new source of releasable norepinephrine. Whether or not this additional neurotransmitter is complemented by an increased expression of adrenergic receptor in DRG neurons, however, is not known.

Clinical Significance of the Sympathetic Nervous System

Several lines of clinical evidence implicate a sympathetic contribution to neuropathic pain.[33] First, surgical destruction or pharmacological blockade of sympathetic outflow to the affected region often produces pain relief. Second, neuropathic pain is worsened by stimuli that evoke a sympathetic discharge, including the startle response and emotional arousal. Third, patients with neuropathic pain often have accompanying signs possibly attributable to abnormal sympathetic activity, including skin vasomotor and sweating abnormalities and dystrophic changes in skin, hair, nails, and bone. Despite this and other evidence, however, adrenosensitivity does not contribute to as many cases as was once thought. For example, recent randomized, placebo-controlled trials of patients with CRPS have failed to demonstrate a large benefit of sympatholytic procedures.[35] Likewise, neuropathic pain in many animal models of neuropathic pain are resistant to sympathectomy.[36] And although sympathectomy reduces pain, paresthesias, and autonomic instability in some patients, these symptoms usually return after 6 months. Thus, despite intensive study over the past two decades, the contribution of the autonomic nervous system to neuropathic pain remains frustratingly uncertain.

Changes in Neurochemical Signature of DRG Neurons

Nerve injury elicits a complex pattern of neurochemical phenotype ("signature") changes in DRG neurons. Some of these changes are related to repair or regeneration, while others may contribute to the maintenance or inhibition of neuropathic pain. Under normal conditions, for example, unmyelinated C fiber, but not myelinated $A\beta$ fibers, contains the pronociceptive peptide substance P (SP). After nerve injury, however, $A\beta$ fibers begin to express SP and also the antinociceptive peptide, NPY.[37,38] The induction of a pronociceptive substance like SP in normally non-noxious large fibers may contribute to the tactile allodynia so characteristic of neuropathic pain. The induction of an antinociceptive substance like NPY may represent an attempt by the nervous system to counteract the actions of SP. The final balance between pronociceptive and antinociceptive changes in neurochemical signature in the DRG neuron may determine the degree of positive neuropathic pain symptoms following nerve injury.

Nerve Inflammation

As with damage to non-neural tissue, injury to nerves leads to an inflammatory response. At the site of nerve damage, macrophages and other immunocompetent cells have been found in injured nerves and in dorsal root ganglion.[39] Activated macrophages at the site of nerve inflammation produce numerous proinflammatory substances, such as tumor necrosis factor-α (TNF-α) and interleukin 1β. When injected subcutaneously, TNF-α induces ectopic activity in primary afferent nociceptors and produces pain behavior.[40,41] The target of inflammatory substances could be nociceptors along the trunk of the nerve itself, specifically in the nervi nervorum, which innervates the connective tissues of the nerves. As such, the nerve becomes a pain-sensitive structure similar to other somatic and visceral tissue.[42] The possible interaction between the immune system and the nervous system suggest that drugs modulating the immune system may be useful therapies in some neuropathic pain states.[43]

Pathologic Fiber Interactions

In the intact peripheral nervous system, each primary sensory neuron functions as an independent communication channel until it reaches the first central synapse. In the setting of nerve injury, however, the ensuing disruption of glial ensheathment allows adjacent denuded axons to make contact, permitting both electrical (ephaptic) and chemical (via a diffusible substance) cross-excitation. Furthermore, the activity of a group of neurons can alter the endogenous repetitive firing activity of their neighbors. Indeed, a key pathogenic mechanism of neuropathic pain involves the appearance of abnormal responses in primary afferent axons that travel in the damaged nerve. This "crossed afterdischarge" can occur between undamaged neurons of different types.[44] By these mechanisms, A fibers may directly activate C fibers so that a nonnoxious stimulus can produce pain. In this way, the peripheral nervous system itself can account for tactile allodynia. Mechanosensitive, low threshold, Aβ-fiber activity also drives tactile allodynia by several other mechanisms involving the spinal cord, as described subsequently.

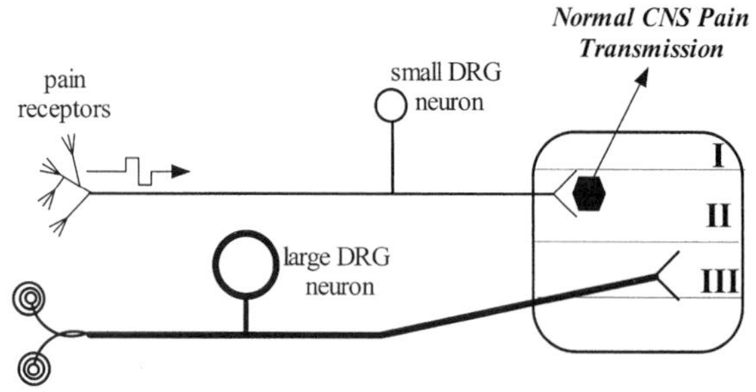

FIGURE 3-3 Under normal physiologic conditions, stimulation of unmyelinated C fibers activates pain transmission neurons of the spinal cord dorsal horn, including those in lamina II. These neurons then relay nociceptive information to the brain. In contrast, stimulation of myelinated Aβ fibers activates non-nociceptive somatosensory pathways, some of which travel through lamina III. Under the pathologic conditions induced by nerve injury, enhanced transmission of Aβ fiber input to neurons in the superficial dorsal horn may occur, possibly via excitatory interneurons.

SPINAL MECHANISMS

In addition to primary afferent mechanisms in the periphery, studies over the past 15 years strongly suggest that long-term changes in the spinal cord and brain contribute to the dysesthesias associated with neuropathic pain. Indeed, it is no longer surprising that neuropathic pain is often not suppressed by isolation of the damaged nerve from the central nervous system (CNS), whether by nerve block or surgical nerve/root transection. Even after these peripheral treatments, abnormal activities in the CNS may continue to drive neuropathic pain.

Anatomic Reorganization Following Injury

In the intact nervous system, as illustrated in Figure 3-3, many neurons in the superficial dorsal horn (lamina I and II) receive direct input from unmyelinated small-diameter primary afferent neurons (C fibers) and best transmit noxious sensations, while deeper neurons (lamina III and IV) receive afferent input from large-diameter primary afferent neurons (Aβ fibers) and best transmit innocuous sensations. The transection of peripheral nerves leads to a substantial degeneration and loss of the central terminals of C fibers in lamina II (see Fig. 3-3). This deafferentation deprives pain transmission neurons in the superficial dorsal horn of their normal nociceptive input and causes patients to lose normal transient pain in the affected areas, and experience negative symptoms.[45] In addition, however, a controversial speculation suggests that a switch to *regenerative* mechanisms can occur, leading to positive symptoms.[46] The effects of this organizational change are compounded by the phenotypic transformation of Aβ fibers to a SP-synthesizing mode,[38] and by the upregulation of SP (NK-1) receptors in the superficial dorsal horn.[47] After

such reorganization and phenotypic change, light mechanical stimulation of Aβ fibers (or their spontaneous ectopic firing) could aberrantly activate pain transmission neurons in the spinal cord, and be misinterpreted by the brain as noxious.

It is difficult to prove that this functional reorganization is a mechanism of allodynia in the clinical situation; however, it is intriguing that some patients with postherpetic neuralgia report intense allodynia along with the more expected loss of normal transient pain.[45] Presumably, the normal function of C fibers was destroyed by the virus, and had been replaced with allodynia mediated by A fibers. These patients have experienced a shift in the *quality* of pain, from physiologic to pathologic, as predicted by a shift in pain processing from C fibers to Aβ fibers.

Pathologic Central Sensitization

Any prolonged or massive input from C-nociceptors enhances the response of dorsal horn neurons to all subsequent afferent inputs.[48] In the setting of inflammation, for example, dorsal horn neuron threshold and pain threshold are reduced. In addition, the receptive field of the dorsal horn neuron grows.[49] This process, called central sensitization, involves the spinal release of neuropeptides and glutamate from nociceptors. These excitatory neurochemicals act at neurokinin, AMPA, and NMDA receptors on postsynaptic spinal neurons, leading to a depolarization-induced influx of calcium and the subsequent triggering of secondary events such as nitric oxide synthesis and protein phosphorylation. Central sensitization is a normal physiological response of the undamaged nervous system, and functions as a protective mechanism in the setting of inflammation. It is normally kept in check by a balance of inhibitory controls, such as an enhancement of GABA-mediated inhibition.[50]

Once established, central sensitization critically depends on persistent primary afferent input, and is normally reversible in the setting of acute inflammation.[3] In the absence of ectopic activity, central sensitization will subside as input declines during tissue healing. In the setting of abnormal ectopic activity and its associated afferent input to the spinal cord, however, established central sensitization may persist indefinitely. For example, partial peripheral nerve injury leads not only to ectopic activity but also to an increase in the activity of spinal cord neurons.[51] Thus, central sensitization may contribute to the pathologic positive symptoms associated with neuropathic pain.

In summary, it is now widely believed that the persistent ectopic activity associated with peripheral nerve injury leads to excessive glutamate and substance P release in the dorsal horn; a pathologic activation of NMDA and NK-1 receptors; a chronic sensitization of pain transmission neurons in the dorsal horn; and, possibly, allodynia and hyperalgesia associated with nerve damage. If true, then NK-1 receptor antagonists, in combination with pain-specific glutamate receptor antagonists (currently in development) could be extremely beneficial to some patients with neuropathic pain.

Loss of Endogenous Pain Inhibitory Controls

The normal nervous system has at its disposal several endogenous pain inhibitory systems. In the setting of nerve injury, however, loss of these inhibitory controls (disinhibition) may increase pain transmission, leading to spontaneous pain, hyperalgesia, and allodynia.

Loss of Presynaptic Inhibition

Melzack and Wall observed that selective blockade of large myelinated primary afferent axons increases pain, and thus proposed that Aβ-fiber activity normally excites interneurons that then inhibit pain transmission neurons in the spinal cord.[52] This gate control theory further proposed that selective damage to Aβ fibers could lead to neuropathic pain, and, conversely, that the selective activation of surviving Aβ fibers would decrease pain. In support of this hypothesis, transcutaneous electrical nerve stimulation (TENS) decreases pain in patients with painful traumatic mononeuropathies.[53] Furthermore, dorsal column stimulation selectively activates the central branches of large diameter primary afferents and is effective for some patients with neuropathic pain.[54] Thus, release of dorsal horn pain transmission cells from inhibition by myelinated axons may contribute to some cases of neuropathic pain; however, further research is necessary to support this hypothesis.

Loss of Spinal Cord Inhibitory Neurotransmission

Many interneurons in the spinal cord contain inhibitory neurotransmitters such as GABA, and may exert an inhibitory tone on pain transmission neurons in the dorsal horn or on central terminals of C fibers. In the setting of nerve injury, a loss of this inhibitory activity could release

the brake on central sensitization of dorsal horn neurons. Experimental nerve injury produces a decrease in spinal cord GABA concentrations and GABA receptor–binding sites,[55] and spinal administration of GABA decreases hypersensitivity in an animal model of nerve injury.[56] The loss of spinal GABA concentrations following sciatic nerve injury could be restored with spinal cord stimulation in rats.[57] This suggests that spinal cord stimulation may exert its analgesic actions by activating GABA-mediated inhibitory systems in the spinal cord.

SUPRASPINAL MECHANISMS

Increase in Supraspinal Facilitation

The brainstem rostral ventral medulla (RVM) exerts both inhibitory and excitatory influences on dorsal horn neurons.[58] Inhibitory bulbospinal pathways have long been known to contribute to the analgesic effects of opioids with regard to transient pain,[59] and a nerve injury–induced antagonism of this pathway could theoretically contribute to neuropathic pain. However, recent evidence suggests that it is an enhancement of the *facilitatory* pathways that contributes to neuropathic pain.[60,61] For example, inactivation of the RVM with lidocaine attenuates the tactile allodynia and thermal hyperalgesia that accompanies spinal nerve injury.[62,63] The persistent noxious input associated with inflammatory pain causes long-term changes in the activity of RVM neurons and the release of neurotransmitters in the RVM region,[64,65] and further RVM microinjection studies indicate that both glutamate and the neuropeptide cholecystokinin may drive this tonic descending facilitation to maintain neuropathic pain.[62,66] Thus, nerve injury shifts the overall influence of descending pain modulation away from an inhibitory influences that modulates physiologic pain, and toward a persistent enhancement of nociceptive transmission that maintains neuropathic pain. This raises an important consideration: such a mechanism may limit the usefulness of intracranial stimulation for the relief of neuropathic pain.

Changes in Thalamus and Cortex

As discussed elsewhere in this book, nociceptive signals are sent to the thalamus and cortex for higher levels of processing. Although data are limited, nerve injury may increase the excitability of and reorganize the connections of neurons in these supraspinal centers.[67] For example, patients with neuropathic pain demonstrate a dramatic reorganization of sensory modalities in the thalamus.[68] Also, the phantom limb pain following arm amputation is associated with a spatial reorganization of somatosensory cortical mapping.[69] In rats, sciatic ligation increased the responsiveness of thalamic and S1 neurons to tactile and cold thermal stimulation of the paw, and S1 displayed a reorganization of somatic input.[70] Thus, like the spinal cord dorsal horn, plasticity in supraspinal centers may contribute to the severity and quality of neuropathic pain. This may underlie reports that posterior thalamus lesions significantly reduce pain in patients with peripheral nervous system lesions.

THE TREATMENT OF NEUROPATHIC PAIN

Because neuropathic pain appears to involve long-lasting *qualitative* alterations of sensory transmission pathways, neuropathic pain must be studied and treated separately from inflammatory pain. Indeed, certain drugs that block inflammatory pain, such as nonsteroidal anti-inflammatory drugs, produce only small analgesic effects at best in neuropathic pain. Opioids, such as morphine, only work in a subset of neuropathic pain patients, and must be given in very high doses with high incidence of adverse effects. In contrast, certain drugs, such as the new generation of anti-epileptics, reduce neuropathic pain but not physiologic pain.

With improvements in our mechanistic understanding of the pathophysiology of neuropathic pain, a rational pharmacotherapy will likely develop. Of course, the cause of neuropathic pain should first be targeted. In certain situations, certain diagnoses call for the administration of specified treatments. For example, the neurosurgical management of neuropathic pain; in particular entrapment neuropathies, are best treated with neurolysis, transposition, or decompression.[71] But this is not possible in many neuropathic pain disorders. For example, the pain of postherpetic neuralgia persists even after healing has taken place. In such situations, pain control is the only therapy left.

In most cases, the treatment of neuropathic pain remains largely empirical. The complexities of chronic neuropathic pain require a comprehensive treatment regimen. One must consider not only pharmacologic therapies (administered with a sequential trial strategy), but also nonpharmacologic, psychological, and physical medicine therapies; local anesthetic block procedures; and neurostimulation techniques.

Further progress in neuropathic pain management is contingent upon further clinical and basic science research leading to a more detailed description of the symptoms and pathophysiologic mechanisms associated with neuropathic pain. Symptoms of inflammatory and neuropathic pain must be distinguished on the basis of pathophysiologic mechanism rather than etiology or anatomic location. Ideally, each stimulus-dependent and stimulus-independent symptom will correspond to a distinct mechanism, and thus respond to a specific treatment.[72] Such progress will lead to specific pharmacologic, surgical, or physical therapy interventions for each identified mechanism involved in a particular syndrome. Until that time, certain guidelines can be followed. For example, in patients with focal neuropathies, one can follow an algorithm of treatment involving the following sequence: sympathetic block, tricyclic antidepressants, gabapentin, mexiletine or carbamazepine, tramadol, opioids, then invasive treatment.[11]

The final choice, invasive treatment, includes a number of surgical procedures, some of which are described in later chapters of this book. Most surgical procedures were originally based on the concept that if the source of pain can be isolated from the central nervous system, then the pain can be abolished. As discussed in this chapter, however, our new understanding of the pathophysiology of neuropathic pain indicates that certain surgical procedures can actually be predicted not to reduce pain, but to *worsen* the quality of pain. Thus, following the reorganization produced by the nerve injury associated with some types of neurosurgery, hyperalgesia that was once mediated by C fibers might be replaced with allodynia mediated by Aβ fibers. Indeed, many believe that all invasive treatments fail to consistently provide long-term pain relief in patients who have not responded to noninvasive treatments.[22]

ACKNOWLEDGMENT

The author would like to thank Dr. M-M Backonja for helpful discussions regarding the clinical aspects of the manuscript.

REFERENCES

1. Bennett GJ. Neuropathic pain: new insights, new interventions. Hosp Pract (Off Ed) 33:95–110, 1998.
2. Woolf CJ, Salter MW. Neuronal plasticity: increasing the gain in pain. Science 288:1765–1769, 2000.
3. Taylor B, Peterson MA, Basbaum A. Persistent cardiovascular and behavioral nociceptive responses to subcutaneous formalin require peripheral nerve input. J Neurosci 15:7575–7584, 1995.
4. Taylor BK, Akana SF, Peterson MA, Dallman MF, Basbaum AI. Pituitary-adrenocortical responses to persistent noxious stimuli in the awake rat: endogenous corticosterone does not reduce nociception in the formalin test. Endocrinology 139:2407–2413, 1998.
5. Dubner R, Ruda MA. Activity-dependent neuronal plasticity following tissue injury and inflammation. TINS 15:96–103, 1992.
6. Stewart JD. Focal Peripheral Neuropathies (3rd ed). New York, Lippincott Williams & Wilkins, 2000.
7. Merskey H, Bogduk N. Pain terms. *In* Merskey H, Bogduk N (eds). Classification of Chronic Pain. Seattle, IASP Press, 1998, pp 207–213.
8. Backonja MM, Galer BS. Pain assessment and evaluation of patients who have neuropathic pain. Neurol Clin 16:775–790, 1998.
9. Koltzenburg M. Painful neuropathies. Curr Opin Neurol 11:515–521, 1998.
10. Scadding JW. Peripheral neuropathies. *In* Wall PD, Melzack R (eds). Textbook of Pain. Edinburgh, Churchill Livingstone, 1999, pp 815–834.
11. Fields HL, Baron R, Rowbotham MC. Peripheral neuropathic pain: an approach to management. *In* Wall PD, Melzack R (eds). Textbook of Pain. Edinburgh, Churchill Livingstone, 1999, pp 1523–1533.
12. Max MB. Treatment of post-herpetic neuralgia: antidepressants. Ann Neurol 35:S50–S53, 1994.
13. Rowbotham M, Harden N, Stacey B, Bernstein P, Magnus-Miller L. Gabapentin for the treatment of postherpetic neuralgia: a randomized controlled trial. JAMA 280:1837–1842, 1998.
14. Backonja M, Beydoun A, Edwards KR, et al. Gabapentin for the symptomatic treatment of painful neuropathy in patients with diabetes mellitus: a randomized controlled trial. JAMA 280:1831–1836, 1998.
15. Bennett GJ. New frontiers in mechanisms and therapy of painful peripheral neuropathies. Acta Anaesthesiol Sin 37:197–203, 1999.
16. Petersen KL, Fields HL, Brennum J, Sandroni P, Rowbotham MC. Capsaicin evoked pain and allodynia in post-herpetic neuralgia. Pain 88:125–133, 2000.
17. Wall PD, Gutnick M. Properties of afferent nerve impulses originating from a neuroma. Nature 248:740–743, 1974.
18. Liu X, Eschenfelder S, Blenk KH, Janig W, Habler H. Spontaneous activity of axotomized afferent neurons after L5 spinal nerve injury in rats. Pain 84:309–318, 2000.
19. Devor M, Seltzer Z. Pathophysiology of damaged nerves in relation to chronic pain. *In* Wall PD, Melzack R (eds). Textbook of Pain. Edinburgh, Churchill Livingstone, 1999, pp 129–164.
20. Nystrom B, Hagbarth KE. Microelectrode recordings from transected nerves in amputees with phantom limb pain. Neurosci Lett 27:211–216, 1981.
21. Govrin-Lippmann R, Devor M. Ongoing activity in severed nerves: source and variation with time. Brain Res 159:406–410, 1978.
22. Kajander KC, Wakisaka S, Bennett GJ. Spontaneous discharge originates in the dorsal root ganglion at the onset of a painful peripheral neuropathy in the rat. Neurosci Lett 138:225–228, 1992.

23. Devor M, Govrin-Lippmann R, Angelides K. Na + channel immunolo-calization in peripheral mammalian axons and changes following nerve injury and neuroma formation. J Neurosci 13:1976–1992, 1993.

24. England JD, Happel LT, Kline DG, et al. Sodium channel accumulation in humans with painful neuromas. Neurology 47:272–276, 1996.

25. Novakovic SD, Tzoumaka E, McGivern JG, et al. Distribution of the tetrodotoxin-resistant sodium channel PN3 in rat sensory neurons in nor-mal and neuropathic conditions. J Neurosci 18:2174–2187, 1998.

26. Akopian AN, Souslova V, England S, et al. The tetrodotoxin-resistant sodium channel SNS has a specialized function in pain pathways. Nat Neurosci 2:541–548, 1999.

27. Porreca F, Lai J, Bian D, et al. A comparison of the potential role of the tetrodotoxin-insensitive sodium channels, PN3/SNS and NaN/SNS2, in rat models of chronic pain. Proc Natl Acad Sci U S A 96:7640–7644, 1999.

28. Waxman SG, Kocsis JD, Black JA. Type III sodium channel mRNA is expressed in embryonic but not adult spinal sensory neurons, and is reex-pressed following axotomy. J Neurophysiol 72:466–470, 1994.

29. Chabal C, Jacobson L, Russell LC, Burchiel KJ. Pain response to peri-neuromal injection of normal saline, epinephrine, and lidocaine in humans. Pain 49:9–12, 1992.

30. Sato J, Perl ER. Adrenergic excitation of cutaneous pain receptors induced by peripheral nerve injury. Science 251:1608–1610, 1991.

31. Devor M, Janig W. Activation of myelinated afferents ending in a neu-roma by stimulation of the sympathetic supply in the rat. Neurosci Lett 24:43–47, 1981.

32. Lee DH, Liu X, Kim HT, Chung K, Chung JM. Receptor subtype medi-ating the adrenergic sensitivity of pain behavior and ectopic discharges in neuropathic Lewis rats. J Neurophysiol 81:2226–2233, 1991.

33. Janig W, Levine JD, Michaelis M. Interactions of sympathetic and pri-mary afferent neurons following nerve injury and tissue trauma. Prog Brain Res 113:161–184, 1996.

34. McLachlan EM, Janig W, Devor M, Michaelis M. Peripheral nerve injury triggers noradrenergic sprouting within dorsal root ganglia. Nature 363:543–546, 1993.

35. Kingery WS. A critical review of controlled clinical trials for peripheral neuropathic pain and complex regional pain syndromes. Pain 73:123–139, 1997.

36. Ringkamp M, Eschenfelder S, Grethel EJ, et al. Lumbar sympathectomy failed to reverse mechanical allodynia- and hyperalgesia-like behavior in rats with L5 spinal nerve injury. Pain 79:143–153, 1999.

37. Noguchi K, De Leon M, Nahin RL, Senba E, Ruda MA. Quantification of axotomy-induced alteration of neuropeptide mRNAs in dorsal root ganglion neurons with special reference to neuropeptide Y mRNA and the effects of neonatal capsaicin treatment. J Neurosci Res 35:54–66, 1993.

38. Noguchi K, Kawai Y, Fukuoka T, Senba E, Miki K. Substance P induced by peripheral nerve injury in primary afferent sensory neurons and its effect on dorsal column nucleus neurons. J Neurosci 15:7633–7643, 1995.

39. Wagner R, Janjigian M, Myers RR. Anti-inflammatory interleukin-10 therapy in CCI neuropathy decreases thermal hyperalgesia, macrophage recruitment, and endoneurial TNF-alpha expression. Pain 74:35–42, 1998.

40. Junger H, Sorkin LS. Nociceptive and inflammatory effects of subcuta-neous TNFalpha. Pain 85:145–151, 2000.

41. Sorkin LS, Xiao WH, Wagner R, Myers RR. Tumour necrosis factor-alpha induces ectopic activity in nociceptive primary afferent fibres. Neuroscience 81:255–262, 1997.

42. Asbury AK, Fields HL. Pain due to peripheral nerve damage: an hy-pothesis. Neurology 34:1587–1590, 1984.

43. Bennett GJ. A neuroimmune interaction in painful peripheral neuropathy [In Process Citation]. Clin J Pain 16:S139–S143, 2000.

44. Amir R, Devor M. Functional cross-excitation between afferent A- and C-neurons in dorsal root ganglia. Neuroscience 95:189–195, 2000.

45. Baron R, Saguer M. Postherpetic neuralgia. Are C-nociceptors involved in signalling and maintenance of tactile allodynia? Brain 116: 1477–1496, 1993.

46. Shortland P, Woolf CJ. Chronic peripheral nerve section results in a rearrangement of the central axonal arborizations of axotomized A beta primary afferent neurons in the rat spinal cord. J Comp Neurol 330:65–82, 1993.

47. Abbadie C, Brown JL, Mantyh PW, Basbaum AI. Spinal cord substance P receptor immunoreactivity increases in both inflammatory and nerve injury models of persistent pain. Neuroscience 70:201–209, 1996.

48. Woolf CJ, Wall PD. Relative effectiveness of C primary afferent fibers of different origins in evoking a prolonged facilitation of the flexor reflex in the rat. J Neurosci 6:1433–1442, 1986.

49. McMahon SB, Lewin GR, Wall PD. Central hyperexcitability triggered by noxious inputs. Curr Opin Neurobiol 3:602–610, 1993.

50. Dickenson AH. Balances between excitatory and inhibitory events in the spinal cord and chronic pain. Prog Brain Res 110:225–231, 1996.

51. Laird JM, Bennett GJ. An electrophysiological study of dorsal horn neurons in the spinal cord of rats with an experimental peripheral neuro-pathy. J Neurophysiol 69:2072–2085, 1993.

52. Melzack R, Wall PD. Pain mechanisms: a new theory. Science 150:971–979, 1965.

53. Meyer GA, Fields HL. Causalgia treated by selective large fibre stimula-tion of peripheral nerve. Brain 95:163–168, 1972.

54. Kumar K, Toth C, Nath RK. Spinal cord stimulation for chronic pain in peripheral neuropathy. Surg Neurol 46:363–369, 1996.

55. Castro-Lopes JM, Tavares I, Coimbra A. GABA decreases in the spinal cord dorsal horn after peripheral neurectomy. Brain Res 620:287–291, 1993.

56. Eaton MJ, Martinez MA, Karmally S. A single intrathecal injection of GABA permanently reverses neuropathic pain after nerve injury. Brain Res 835:334–339, 1999.

57. Stiller CO, Linderoth B, O'Connor WT, Franck J, Falkenberg T, Ungerstedt U, Brodin E. Repeated spinal cord stimulation decreases the extracellular level of gamma-aminobutyric acid in the periaqueductal gray matter of freely moving rats. Brain Res 699:231–241, 1995.

58. Zhuo M, Gebhart GF. Biphasic modulation of spinal nociceptive trans-mission from the medullary raphe nuclei in the rat. J Neurophysiol 78:746–758, 1997.

59. Basbaum AI, Fields HL. Endogenous pain control mechanisms: review and hypothesis. Ann Neurol 4:451–462, 1978.

60. Ossipov MH, Lai J, Malan TP Jr, Porreca F. Spinal and supraspinal mechanisms of neuropathic pain. Ann N Y Acad Sci 909:12–24, 2000.

61. Urban MO, Gebhart GF. Supraspinal contributions to hyperalgesia. Proc Natl Acad Sci U S A 96:7687–7692, 1999.

62. Kovelowski CJ, Ossipov MH, Sun H, Lai J, Malan TP, Porreca F. Supraspinal cholecystokinin may drive tonic descending facilitation mechanisms to maintain neuropathic pain in the rat. Pain 87:265–273, 2000.

63. Pertovaara A, Wei H, Hamalainen MM. Lidocaine in the rostroventrome-dial medulla and the periaqueductal gray attenuates allodynia in neuro-pathic rats. Neurosci Lett 218:127–130, 1996.

64. Taylor BK, Basbaum AI. Neurochemical characterization of extracellular serotonin in the rostral ventromedial medulla and its modulation by nox-ious stimuli. J Neurochem 65:578–589, 1995.

65. Terayama R, Guan Y, Dubner R, Ren K. Activity-induced plasticity in brain stem pain modulatory circuitry after inflammation. Neuroreport 11:1915–1919, 2000.

66. Wei H, Pertovaara A. MK-801, an NMDA receptor antagonist, in the ros-troventromedial medulla attenuates development of neuropathic symp-toms in the rat. Neuroreport 10:2933–2937, 1999.

67. Lenz FA, Lee JI, Garonzik IM, Rowland LH, Dougherty PM, Hua SE. Plasticity of pain-related neuronal activity in the human thalamus. Prog Brain Res 129:259–273, 2000.

68. Lenz FA, Gracely RH, Baker FH, Richardson RT, Dougherty PM. Reorganization of sensory modalities evoked by microstimulation in region of the thalamic principal sensory nucleus in patients with pain due to nervous system injury. J Comp Neurol 399:125–138, 1998.

69. Flor H, Elbert T, Knecht S, et al. Phantom-limb pain as a perceptual cor-relate of cortical reorganization following arm amputation. Nature 375:482–484, 1995.

70. Guilbaud G, Benoist JM, Levante A, Gautron M, Willer JC. Primary somatosensory cortex in rats with pain-related behaviours due to a peripheral mononeuropathy after moderate ligation of one sciatic nerve: neuronal responsivity to somatic stimulation. Exp Brain Res 92: 227–245, 1992.

71. Dawson D. Entrapment Neuropathies. Boston, Little, Brown, 1983.

72. Woolf CJ, Mannion RJ. Neuropathic pain: aetiology, symptoms, mecha-nisms, and management. Lancet 353:1959–1964, 1999.

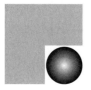

C H A P T E R 4

Psychological Considerations in Spine Surgery

DANIEL M. DOLEYS, PhD

"Never vague or tentative, surgery has its place in the narrow spectrum of cases with clearly established, well circumscribed, structural pathology unresponsive to non-surgical treatment and producing significant persistent disability. Identifying valid indications and options within the plethora of choices requires knowledge of what is available, what can actually be accomplished, and what limitations apply."[1]

Hall

It is estimated that 10% of patients suffering from lumbar pain account for more than 80% of total healthcare and social costs. The 1% of patients who undergo surgery comprise the most expensive group. Surgical procedures are responsible for approximately one third of healthcare costs.[2] Approximately 236,000 diskectomies were carried out in 1987 with an estimated failure rate of 8%; 59,000 spinal fusions were performed with a failure rate of 15%. The number of lumbar surgeries carried out in the United States approaches ten times the rate of lumbar surgeries performed in Great Britain. Surgery is performed nearly twice as often on the West Coast of the United States than the East Coast.[3] Cervical spine surgeries have increased by approximately 45% over the past decade; cervical fusion by 70%, lumbar diskectomy by 40%, and lumbar fusion by 33%.[4] The estimated lifetime incidence of spine surgery is 10% to 12% with an overall success rate of 40% to 90%.[5] Abnormal radiologic studies, such as contrast-enhanced magnetic resonance imaging (MRI), do not correlate on a one-to-one basis with outcome.[6] Indeed, some patients described as having a successful outcome may, in fact, evidence abnormal postoperative morphologic studies.[7]

Outcomes analyses of spine surgery, particularly lumbar spine surgery, continue to create controversy. As in most human endeavors in this area, the majority of published studies fail to meet rigorous experimental design characteristics. Nonetheless, several randomized controlled trials do exist and when evaluated have yielded fairly convincing conclusions.[8] While it appears clear that the majority of "well-selected" patients profit from surgical intervention, the debate over the most efficacious approach continues. For example, microdiskectomy, standard diskectomy, automated percutaneous diskectomy, laser surgery, anterior versus posterior fusion, and fusion with or without instrumentation each have

their own proponents. The reason(s) that all patients do not profit from surgical intervention is often unclear and varies from one study to another. Timing of the surgery, number and type of dependent variables evaluated, degree and type of structural abnormality, patient selection criteria, demographics, and psychological variables are the more commonly cited factors.[9]

Pain relief and functional restoration are common goals in spine surgery. Both, however, are very complex concepts and require consideration of more than just the identifiable physical pathology. Indeed, the outcome of spine surgery might best be approached by considering its purpose; that is, whether it was conducted to correct structural abnormalities/deformities, for the cessation or reversal of progressive neurologic symptoms, or for pain relief and functional restoration. Resolution of pain appears to be the most elusive and unpredictable of outcomes. This may be a consequence of the complexity of pain,[10] the manner in which it is measured, the influence of as yet identified physiologic or neurochemical processes, and/or patient variables. Efforts must continue to identify those factors that may enhance or interfere with a successful surgical outcome because the minority of patients who fail to respond to appropriately executed spine surgery constitute a large economic burden on society, not to mention the intangible "cost" of continued suffering. We must guard against an attitude of complacency justified by the fact that these apparent "failures" constitute a "statistical minority" of patients treated. Accepting a 10% to 30% failure rate as a "natural consequence" of surgical intervention may result in approaching the prospective surgical candidate with an unacceptable degree of indifference. It is important to remember that a portion of these "failures" may in fact be worse than presurgical position.[11] Spine surgery performed with a degree of impunity would seem contrary to the primary dictum of "first do no harm."

This chapter will focus on several psychological variables thought to be relevant in patient selection and outcome of spine surgery. It is not an attempt to present an exhaustive review but rather to summarize information in this area. It is not intended for the surgeon to take on the role of a mental health practitioner, but rather to become aware of the various factors that may play a role in surgical outcome and therefore require consideration in the decision-making process.

Hopefully, the discussion to follow will provide a foundation for determining when psychological consultation should be sought and the type of questions to pose the consultant.

There will also be a brief discussion of the hypothesized physiologic and neurochemical mechanisms by which some of the psychological factors are believed to exert their influence. This is an important matter because psychological issues are frequently thought to be a manifestation of the patient's "state of mind" and easily altered by the properly motivated patient. This somewhat parochial attitude ignores the rather significant and enduring effect(s) such factors can have on physiologic and neurochemical processes. This apparent reductionistic approach to psychological variables is not necessary to validate their importance, but placing them in this context may encourage a more general acceptance in much the same way as one would consider the role of diabetes mellitus or hypertension in determining the suitability of a patient to undergo spine surgery.

PSYCHOLOGICAL FACTORS RELATED TO SURGICAL OUTCOMES

The history of exploring psychological factors as they relate to surgical outcomes notes a tendency to identify patients as having a "functional" versus "organic" problem. This dichotomy was rejected many decades ago[12] in favor of an approach that views the setting in a biopsychosocial perspective. Consistent with this model Watkins and colleagues[13] noted that while the Minnesota Multiphasic Personality Inventory (MMPI) did not predict surgical outcomes, they thought that it was useful in describing and understanding the patient. This emphasis on "description versus prediction" has been reinforced by Doleys and Doherty.[14] Nonetheless, Moeller and Hedlund[15,16] used pain drawings to separate patients into "organic" and "nonorganic" groups. Postoperative improvement was defined as 50% reduction in pain as well as improvement in functional disability. At 1 year, 47% of the "organic" and only 11% of the non-organic group met these criteria, and at 2 years, 48% and 16%, respectively. This may not be unique to patients with low back pain because there are indications that personality traits and coping styles are similar in patients awaiting lumbar surgery versus other types of surgery.[17]

Return to work is often viewed as an important outcome measure under the general category of improved functioning. Reports in this area are quite discrepant. Berger, for example, reports that 71% of patients with a single lumbar surgery and 95% of those with multiple surgeries had not returned to work at 4 years after surgery.[18] Taylor noted that 82% of patients with one surgery and 59% of patients with multiple surgeries returned to work.[19] Hodges and colleagues estimated 55% of patients who underwent lumbar spine surgery returned to work, further indicating that 72% who underwent microdiskectomy returned, while only 43% of patients who underwent fusion surgery returned.[20] Factors that seem to be associated with return to work include preoperative anxiety and depression[21] and the psychological aspects of work such as occupational mental stress.[22]

The relationship between objective physiologic measures and psychological factors to outcomes is fairly complex. For example, Schade and colleagues reported that radiologic findings such as MRIs did predict postoperative improvement in activities of daily living, but that return to work appeared more correlated with depression, mental stress, job satisfaction, and social support.[22] Similarly, Trief and colleagues found return to work correlated with anxiety and depression, lack of change in pain with somatic anxiety and depression, and lack of change in function with somatic anxiety.[21] In this study, hostility did not correlate with any of the outcome measures. Junge and colleagues[23] and Tandon and colleagues[24] noted preoperative psychological factors, especially depression and pain behavior, to predict postoperative changes in pain but not frequency of physician visits or work status. These data are similar to those of Spengler and colleagues, noting that imaging studies, including MRI, correlate highly with operative findings but psychological factors were more predictive of overall outcomes.[25] It is, perhaps, this discrepancy that has encouraged many to explain their findings by noting "the operation was successful but the patient didn't respond."

Overall patient satisfaction is a frequently used outcome measure. In some cases, it exceeds what would be predicted based on the objective evaluation of surgical outcome.[26] Higher levels of depression, anxiety, and pain have been associated with patient dissatisfaction.[27] In this regard, it may be the degree to which the outcome matches the patient's expectation rather than the actual outcome that determines patient satisfaction.[28] Interactive videodiscs with and without an accompanying booklet have been shown to enhance patient knowledge and also influence their acceptance of surgery and a feeling of involvement in the clinical decision.[29] Patient expectations appear to correlate more highly with the level of disappointment as it relates to postoperative pain than to rate of recovery or return to work status. Indeed, Iversen and colleagues reported patients having more numerous expectations of pain relief to be associated with greater report of pain and decreased satisfaction with pain relief 6 months postoperatively.[30] Conversely, patients with more numerous expectations as to improved functioning did better than those with moderate or low expectations. In general, it would seem that outcomes and patient satisfaction can, therefore, be increased by treating significant levels of depression and anxiety preoperatively, and encouraging patients to have significant but realistic expectations for functional improvement but moderate expectations for change in pain.

The search for a single or limited number of factors that are associated with a positive outcome for spine surgery seems to have given way to identifying a constellation of variables whose individual importance may vary from patient to patient. Cashion and Lynch list patients that are stable psychologically, cautious, affectively defensive, self-confident, realistic regarding their illness, mildly depressed, generally optimistic, and able to cope with emergent situations without over-reaction as good surgical candidates.[31] Pearce identified several "risk factors" including wrong diagnosis, repeated disability certification, failed surgery, symptoms incongruous with signs and imaging, multiple surgical procedures, poor social support, poor motivation, psychological illness, clinical depression before or after injury or surgery, and pending litigation as associated with a negative outcome.[32] The role of childhood traumas including physical abuse, sexual assault, abandonment, and rearing by alcoholic or drug-abusing parents has been emphasized by Shofferman and colleagues.[33] Psychological factors also appear relevant in patients awaiting other forms of surgery,[17] diskography,[34] and radiofrequency cervical dorsal root ganglia.[35] The influence of preoperative psychological stress has been found as much as 7 years postoperatively.[36] Indeed, "normal" MMPI testing is not necessarily associated with a positive outcome at least in the treatment of pain via drug administration system.[37]

A consequence of inadequate attention to the role of psychological factors, particularly in considering surgical intervention for the treatment of pain, is an overemphasis and reliance on identifiable physical pathology as the "pain generator." In fact, as many as 30% to 40% of asymptomatic patients may have abnormal radiologic findings.[38] Positive diskography results, a frequently used criteria for lumbar fusion, can also be found in asymptomatic patients and influenced by psychological factors.[34,38] Epidural scarring, although present, may not be the single or even one of many contributing factors to pain.[39] There is a whole host of chemical mediators including enkephalins, norepinephrine, serotonin, and substance P as well as morphologic changes that may have been precipitated by injury, disease, or trauma, and whose deleterious effects may be independent of any identifiable structural abnormality.[40] This fact may help explain the persistence of "pain" following the surgical correction of physical pathology.

PSYCHOLOGICAL "RISK FACTORS"

Table 4-1 identifies a variety of psychological "risk factors" for poor surgical outcome.[41] These risk factors are not arranged in any specific order and may be found singularly or in combination. They appear to have general applicability to spine surgery and to date have not been differentially associ-

ated with type of surgery, that is, fusion versus diskectomy; laminectomy versus microdiskectomy. The appearance of these risk factors is not universal in the literature but each appears frequently enough to warrant inclusion. Each must be evaluated qualitatively and quantitatively. Their mere presence does not constitute a contraindication for surgical intervention but may suggest the advantage of greater preparation and/or planned follow-up.[42]

Depression is one of the more commonly cited mood disorders associated with outcomes from spine surgery. The incidence of major depressive disorder associated with low back pain has been estimated to be as high as 45% point prevalence, and 64% lifetime prevalence.[43] Whether the depression precedes the onset of spinal disorder and pain or comes about consequent to it is sometimes difficult to ascertain. Instruments such as the Beck Depression Inventory[44] and the Zung Depression Inventory[45] have been applied with a fair degree of regularity. These are easily administered and can provide a fairly accurate estimate of the degree of depression. Interview data can also be helpful. For example applying the pneumonic device, SIGECAPS, information can be sought regarding sleep disturbance (S), decreased interest (I), guilt (G), decreased energy (E), concentration (C), appetite (A), psychomotor retardation (P), and suicidality (S). The presence of five of these criteria correlates highly with the diagnosis of depression or major affective disorder.

The existence of progressive neurologic symptoms, remarkable spinal instability, and/or a severe compressive lesion may necessitate the spinal surgery despite the existence of major depression. In such cases, Rush and colleagues have suggested the following as a means of enhancing the outcome of surgery[42]: (1) reduce stressful environmental factors, such as job, legal, marital if possible; (2) involve the family and encourage them to provide a supportive network; (3) provide realistic estimates of benefits/risks; (4) manage any psy-

● TABLE 4-1 • Risk Factors for Poor Surgical Outcome Identified in the PPS Interview

Risk Factor	Risk Level
Pending legal actions related to injury	High risk
Workers' compensation	High risk
Job dissatisfaction 　　Moderate 　　Extreme	 Moderate risk High risk
Heavy job demands (frequent lifting >50 lb)	High risk
Substance abuse 　　Preinjury 　　Current/untreated	 Moderate risk High risk
Reinforcement of disability by family members	Moderate to high risk
Marital dissatisfaction	Moderate risk
Physical or sexual abuse 　　Preinjury 　　Current	 Moderate risk High risk
Preinjury psych problems 　　Outpatient treatment 　　Inpatient treatment	 Moderate risk High risk

From Block AR. Presurgical Psychological Screening in Chronic Pain Syndromes: A Guide for the Behavioral Health Practitioner. Mahwan, NJ, Erlbaum Press, 1996.

chopathology following surgery; and (5) if time allows, reduce psychopathology before surgery.

Perhaps more important than the mood disorders, referred to as axis I diagnoses in DSM-IV,[46] are the personality disorders or axis II diagnoses. A personality disorder represents a rather enduring pattern of behavior that deviates markedly from the expectations of the individual's culture. Furthermore, it is pervasive and inflexible having its onset in adolescence or early childhood and is stable over time leading to distress and impairment. The Diagnostic and Statistics Manual IV (DSM-IV) categories personality disorders into three main clusters. Cluster A includes those disorders exhibiting odd, eccentric, or inclusive traits such as paranoid or schizoid personalities. Cluster B disorders incorporate those that demonstrate dramatic emotional or manipulative traits, including the borderline and antisocial disorders. Finally, cluster C refers to anxious, fearful, and depressive patients such as the dependent or obsessive-compulsive personality disorder. In one study, more than 50% of patients with low back pain had at least one axis II diagnosis. The most common were paranoid, borderline, and avoidant personality.[43]

These personality disorders may not declare themselves immediately. Only after several visits may the practitioner or staff "get a funny feeling" about the patient. Such individuals are more often recognized by office staff and nurses because of increased frequency of contact. One advantage to tests such as the MMPI is its ability to help identify personality disorders.[47] Presence for the personality disorder can make patient treatment extremely difficult particularly in the case of the cluster B disorders.

Problems of addiction are frequently associated with personality disorders. Their prevalence among patients with spine-related pain has been estimated as high as 36%.[48] It is important to understand that the presence of tolerance and/or physical dependence, naturally occurring and expected pharmacologic consequences of certain types of medications especially opioids, does not define addiction.[49] Compulsive use of a substance, preoccupation with acquisition of the substance, use despite harm, and loss of control are more defining characteristics. Patients with a remote history of substance abuse as well as active involvement in a recovery program are at much less risk for a negative outcome than those actively using drugs. Urine drug screens at the time of an office visit or admission to the hospital may help in identifying the substance abuser. Asking certain questions such as those represented in the pneumonic CAGE ("C" represents an urge to "cut back"; "A" the report of being "annoyed" by comments from others; "G" a sense of "guilt" about substance use, especially alcohol; and "E" the need for a "eye opener") can be a rather easy way of identifying a potential alcoholic. One should not underestimate the willingness of an addict to undergo surgical procedures as a mechanism to obtain or justify the use of his or her substance of abuse.

Anxiety is another commonly identified negative state. In some instances, this can be a generalized pervasive anxiety or one more related to physical symptoms and frequently referred to as "somatic anxiety." Somatic anxiety may manifest itself in hypochondriasis.[50] While increased knowledge, support, and reassurance may help the generally anxious patient, it is likely to have little effect on the more pathologically anxious patient. The use of tranquilizing agents or antidepressants may likewise have little long-term effect.

The apparent absence of "normal anxiety" may reflect a type of somatization. Some patients exhibit a degree of indifference disproportionate to the demands of the situation. The presence of "pain" or at least their "pain behavior" may serve some adaptive function. This may be seen in cases where financial or personal gain is associated with the outcome. Some have hypothesized that the suppression or repression of emotional conflict may be functionally related to the patient's symptoms. If so, one would hardly expect the symptoms to improve by merely altering the physical pathology in the spine.

Issues of job satisfaction and workers' compensation are identified with great regularity. They perhaps go hand in hand as patients who find their jobs highly desirable and rewarding are less likely to remain on disability benefits and to allow their physical problems to interfere with return to work any longer than absolutely necessary. Others will find disability payments very rewarding and will undergo procedures to help validate their complaints. Clearly, one or more surgical scars with the possibility of postoperative epidural fibrosis can provide fertile ground for a stronger disability claim than a "virgin back." Nonetheless, it would be unfair to assume that every impaired worker is so motivated. Generalizations of this type can lead to inappropriate and untimely treatment or the lack thereof. Indeed, if disability payments were the sole source of the workers' compensation patient's complaints, it would be hard to reconcile with the fact that many of these patients continue to have disabling pain even after their claims are resolved. Many such patients often undergo irretrievable financial and personal losses. It may be more important to determine where the patient is in the "disability process." That is, the more eminent case resolution, deposition, or court, the more likely it will influence the overall outcome. It has been suggested that patients 2 or more years removed from their case settlement do not have outcomes different from non–workers' compensation patients.[22,51,52]

PSYCHOLOGICAL ASSESSMENT

A comprehensive psychological assessment can be a rather demanding task when done properly.[9,14] The outcome of the evaluation is likely to be more meaningful if the evaluator has some minimally acceptable comprehension of the type of surgery proposed. A background in pain assessment is essential for appropriate interpretations of interview and test data. The incorporation of the mental health practitioner, who is part of a "team" evaluating and working with the patient and surgeon, can pay dividends. Patients are less likely to resist psychological evaluation if it is appreciated as part of the overall process and done for their benefit rather than to question the authenticity of their complaints. All too often, psychological assessments are performed in an effort to justify not doing a procedure than to assist in improving the outcome of the procedure.

The MMPI-I and -II is perhaps the most recognizable of psychological tests.[47] It has found wide application and acceptance in the literature. Its value as a "predictor" of outcome remains unproven. Its use in identifying potentially troublesome patients is undeniable. The MMPI is only a tool and neither inherently good nor bad. It is recommended that the overall

MMPI profile analysis lead to a description of the patient and suspected psychological issues rather than an instrument to be used in a "go, no-go" fashion. Contrary to a past popular opinion, the MMPI cannot determine the existence or etiology, that is "organic versus nonorganic" nature of a patient's complaints.

Formal psychological or neuropsychological testing may be required of a minority of patients. There are many brief inventories and questionnaires that can be used as screening devices, including the already mentioned Beck Depression Inventory[41] in much the same way as one might obtain a routine chemistry profile or complete blood cell count to identify medical abnormalities that may require investigation. Table 4-2 gives examples of some of the more commonly used instruments for evaluating psychological states, coping mechanisms, level of functioning, and pain.

REQUESTING PSYCHOLOGICAL CONSULTATION

The psychologist's role should be that as a consultant to the surgeon. The relationship should be such that the psychologist can freely discuss his or her opinion as to the suitability of a patient to undergo and/or benefit from spine surgery. Preoperative counseling may help to prepare the patient. Not all patients are ready to undergo recommended procedures in the hoped-for postoperative changes. Indeed, some authors have proposed and validated several stages individuals go through in preparing to make change.[53] Patients in what is referred to as a "precontemplative" or "contemplative" stage are likely to be more dubious than those in the "action" phase. In addition, many psychologists will have training in experimental methods that could be beneficial in assisting to establish a presurgical evaluation protocol and a follow-up mechanism for outcomes assessment.

Real time communication among professionals helps the patient to develop a sense of security and comprehensiveness of care. Occasionally, elective spinal surgery should be postponed pending treatment of relevant psychological issues. Conducting hospital rounds jointly preoperatively and postoperatively provides an opportunity for immediate discussion and comparison of observations.

Guidelines as to when a psychological consultation may be indicated are listed in Table 4-3. It is helpful for the physician to prepare the patient for a psychological consult by indicating the information may be very beneficial at improving outcomes. The few minutes it may take to explain the rationale to the patient will pay enormous dividends in patient acceptance and productivity of the consultation.

Where possible, the surgeon should make specific requests as to areas of concern of the psychological consultant, such as presence of a mood disturbance that would interfere with the outcome. The possibility of an underlying personality disorder, history of drug or alcohol addiction/misuse, and role of psychological factors in pain, may also be relevant. Requesting a "psychological consult," especially from someone unfamiliar with the surgeon's own philosophy regarding the role of psychological issues, may yield disappointing results. Whether the consultation is done on an inpatient or outpatient setting, adequate time should be allowed. It may take more than one session. Ideally, the goal should be the development of an appropriate treatment algorithm rather than a go, no-go response. Providing feedback to the consultant as to the usefulness of the information will help to shape the evaluation process.

PSYCHOLOGICAL CONSULTATION AND REPORT

The psychological consultation will generally consist of a 1-hour interview combined with testing. Tests may include that of general personality, mood, pain, and to some degree functioning/disability. A comprehensive consultation report may seem somewhat lengthy and can approach three to six pages. However, it is important to identify and review sources of potential difficulties including the patient's personal history, medical background, history of injuries, treatment history and outcome, attribution/expectations, and the like. Indeed, if we listen long and hard enough, the patient may in fact provide the diagnosis.

● **TABLE 4-2** • Tests Grouped by Their Key Function

Key Function	Examples
Pain (qualitative characteristic)	McGill Pain Questionnaire; Numerical rating scales; Visual analog scales; Verbal rating scales; Pain drawings; North American Spine Society Questionnaire
Mood and personality overall psychological functioning	MMPI-2; Symptom Checklist 90-R; Beck Depression Inventory; Spielberg State-Trait Anxiety Inventory; Million Behavioral Health Inventory (MBHI); Illness Behavior Questionnaire (IBQ); Personality Assessment Inventory (PAI)
Pain beliefs and coping	Multidimensional Pain Inventory; Coping Strategies Questionnaire; Pain Self-Efficacy Questionnaire; Survey of Pain Attitudes; Sickness Impact Profile (SIP)
Level of functioning/perceive disability	Multidimensional Pain Inventory; Oswestry Disability Questionnaire; Sickness Impact Profile (SIP); Short-Form Health Survey (SF 36); Pain Disability Index; Roland-Morris Disability Scale
Cognitive functioning	Mini-Mental State; MicroCog; Neuropsychological Tests

TABLE 4-3 • Indications for Considering Psychological Consult

1. Outcome of diagnostic testing, suspected pathology, signs and symptoms do not fit
2. Greater than or equal to three Waddell signs
3. Markedly unusual reaction either positive or negative to medicine/treatments
4. Suspicion of emotional "instability"
5. "Personality" concerns
6. Suspicion of poor/inadequate/inappropriate coping, fears, beliefs, distress, expectations, and/or attributions

A well-thought-out consultation should provide insights as to the patient's history, expectations, attitude regarding proposed treatment, potential "risk factors," and the patient's goals/motivation as well as any treatment recommendations. Patients readily recite outcomes statistics, presumably given to them by practitioners, that cannot be confirmed in the literature. These outcomes statistics should be noted as they may represent unrealistic expectations that could lead to poor outcomes and patient dissatisfaction. Some individuals will benefit from a postoperative series of cognitive/behavioral interventions to minimize the development of a "chronic pain syndrome/pattern."

One of the most common contributing factors to poor functional outcomes is "kinesophobia," wherein patients develop a conditioned fear of activity anticipating increased pain, and therefore succumb to a very sedentary lifestyle resulting in deconditioning and other maladaptive physical and behavioral habits. Prearranging a rehabilitation/behavioral postoperative program for the more susceptible patients may prevent this.[54]

Patient "satisfaction" is often not associated with degree of pain relief or more common objective outcome measures. Instead, it appears to be related to two other factors: one, the correlation between patient expectations and actual outcome; second, the degree to which the patient perceives that the practitioner or team has attempted to help them. This may explain why so many patients, despite a less than desirable outcome, are very satisfied with the surgery and in fact under similar conditions would elect to have it again.

MECHANISM OF ACTION

The mechanism(s) by which psychological factors exert their influence can include behavioral/environmental, cognitive/affective, and neurochemical/physiologic. In the setting of depression, for example, the patient's inactivity, low motivation, and dysphoric attitude may be a consequence of inadequate positive reinforcement and stimulation from the environment. At the cognitive/affective level, depression is often associated with feelings of helplessness and catastrophic thinking, which can obviously impact on multiple outcomes of surgery. One would, hopefully, hesitate to proceed with an elective surgical procedure in a patient who anticipated the worse possible scenario. Finally, at the neurochemical/psychological level, abnormalities in neu-

ropeptides such as substance P and neurotransmitters including serotonin and norepinephrine contribute not only to disturbance in mood, but heightened levels of and reaction to nociceptive input.

The "placebo response" is often interpreted as indicative of the patient's psychological susceptibility. The process, however, is much more complicated. Benedetti and colleagues, for example, were able to evidence a "placebo response" in one part of the body but not in another.[55] Bandura and colleagues showed that administering naloxone, an opioid antagonist, reversed the increased pain tolerance created by administering a placebo with cognitive coping skill development.[56] Observing that this increased pain tolerance was naloxone reversible led to the conclusion that it must in part be related to endogenous opioid activation related to enhanced "self-efficacy." More recently, de la Fuente-Fernandez and colleagues demonstrated alteration in the release of dopamine from the disease-compromise nigrostriatal system in patients with Parkinson's disease following the administration of a placebo.[57] The degree to which this may be explained by cognitive factors such as "expectations" or conditioned effects remains unclear. However, the elusiveness of the explanation does not diminish the impressiveness of the findings. Placebos have also been noted to be beneficial in reducing postoperative swelling[58] and respiratory depression.[55]

The role of psychological factors, particularly in the experience of pain, is quite complex.[10] The impact of learning theory and conditioning is often underappreciated and frequently viewed in the limited context of behavior modification wherein some observable behavior is altered by providing a reward. Indeed, there is strong evidence of neurochemical and even synaptic alterations in the central nervous system in response to conditioning processes.[59] The concept of conditioned anxiety such as that experienced by a claustrophobic patient as a consequence of previous entrapment in a confined space, seems quite palatable. Similarly, the same conditioning process may account for observed activation of "craving centers" in the brain as assessed by brain imaging techniques when cocaine addicts are merely shown a videotape of drug paraphernalia.[60] In like manner, "conditioned nociception" or what on occasion has been referred to as the "corticalization of pain," may explain the persistence of complaints following the presumed offending spinal lesion.

The advancement in imaging including positron emission tomography, functional MRI, and quantitative audio radiologic imaging of regional cerebral blood flow has provided invaluable and heretofore unavailable information regarding processing mechanisms in the central nervous system particularly as it relates to pain.[61] One of the earlier and perhaps more legendary of these studies was that of Rainville and colleagues in which pain unpleasantness, associated with anterior cingular gyrus activity, was modulated through the use of hypnosis while little effect was noted on pain intensity, a somatosensory function.[62] The importance of this is self-evident. Careful observation reminds us how often two patients with near identical pathophysiology have such remarkable differences in their response pattern to pain. Indeed, it may be this affective component that results in the experience of nociception becoming disabling. This would help to explain the frequency with which depression is associated with poor surgical outcome even in the presence of a technically adequate spine surgery and improved radiologic findings.

Schofferman and colleagues emphasized the role of "risk factors" in outcomes following spine surgery.[33] Estimates range from 28% to 48% of patients in heterogenous chronic pain populations reporting a history of sexual and/or physical abuse. How events that have occurred perhaps decades before surgery may influence the experience of pain and outcomes of surgery remains unclear. However, at least three possibilities exist. One, that previous abuse may be associated with greater psychiatric morbidity, which in turn would negatively impact surgical outcome. Patients with histories of abuse, in fact, do demonstrate greater somatization and psychological distress upon testing.[43,63] The second possibility relates to observed changes in brain morphology. Reduced hippocampal volume has been identified in patients with histories of abuse.[64,65] The hippocampus is one of several limbic structures that serves the behavioral inhibition system and memory.[66] Increased activity in this system associated with negative emotionality may lead to heightened arousal and attention to nociception. Third, changes in neurohormonal activity including the hypothalamic–pituitary–adrenal axis has been observed.[67] This alteration was noted to be associated with history of sexual abuse and independent of the presence or absence of a psychiatric diagnosis.

CONCLUSIONS

Spine surgery continues to be a necessary and effective approach in treating patients with structural abnormalities including instability and compressive lesions. The majority of patients report substantial benefit. A relatively small but significant percent of patients are unimproved or worsened. Psychological factors may be influential in both the "responders" and "nonresponders." Psychological evaluations and interventions may further enhance the outcomes of those already reporting a favorable response. Such interventions may also minimize the number and degree of failures. The mechanism(s) by which a patient's history, current psychological status, and psychological intervention impact the individual's behavioral, emotional, and physiological functioning remains complex but is giving way to systematic study. The science of patient selection and management must advance as well as the more technological aspects of spine surgery for the patient to derive maximum benefit.

REFERENCES

1. Hall H. Surgery: indications and options. Neurol Clin 17:113–130, 1999.
2. CSAG Clinical Standards Advisory Group. Report of Back Pain. London, HMSO, 1994, pp 65–72.
3. Kastuik JP. Spine surgery in the future. Spine 17:S66–S70, 1992.
4. Davis RA. Long-term outcome analysis of 984 surgically treated herniated lumbar discs. J Neurosurg 80:415–521, 1994.
5. Junge A, Frolich M, Aherns S, et al. Predictors of bad and good outcome of lumbar surgery: A prospective clinical study with 2 years followup. Spine 21:1056–1065, 1996.
6. Carragee EJ, Kim DH. A prospective analysis of magnetic imaging findings in patients with sciatica and lumbar disc herniation: correlation of outcome with disc fragment and canal nephrology. Spine 22:1650–1660, 1997.
7. Deutsch AL, Howard M, Dawson EG, et al. Lumbar spine following surgical discectomy: magnetic resonance imaging features and implications. Spine 18:1054–1060, 1993.
8. Gibson JN, Grant IC, Waddell G. The Cochran review of surgery for lumbar disc prolapse and degenerative lumbar spondylosis. Spine 24:1820–1832, 1999.
9. Block AR, Gatchel RJ, Deardorff W, Guyer RD. The Psychology of Spine Surgery. Washington, DC, APA Books, 2003.
10. Price DD. Psychological Assessment of Pain and Analgesia. Seattle, International Association for the Study of Pain Press, 2000.
11. Crombie IK, Davies HT, Macrae WA. Cut and thrust: antecedent surgery and trauma among patients attending a chronic pain clinic. Pain 76:167–171, 1998.
12. Gentry WD, Newman MC, Goldner MI, et al. Relationship between graduated spinal block technique and MMPI for diagnosis and prognosis of chronic low back pain. Spine 2:210–213, 1977.
13. Watkins RG, O'Brien JP, Draugelis R, Jones D. Comparison of preoperative and postoperative MMPI data in chronic back patients. Spine 11:385–390, 1986.
14. Doleys DM, Doherty DC. Psychological and behavioral assessment. In Raj PR (ed). Practical Management of Pain (3rd ed). St Louis, Mosby, 2000, pp 408–438.
15. Moeller H, Hedlund R. Pain drawings in adult spondylolisthesis predicts the treatment outcome or fusion. Presented at North American Spine Society meeting, Chicago, 1999.
16. Moeller H, Hedlund R. Fusion or conservative treatment in adult spondylolisthesis: a perspective randomized study. Acta Orthop Scand 65:13–27, 1994.
17. Hueppe M, Uhlig T, Fogelsang H, Schumacker P. Personality traits, coping styles, and mood in patients awaiting lumbar disc surgery. J Clin Psychol 56:119–130, 2000.
18. Berger E. Late postoperative results of 1000 work related lumbar spine conditions. Surg Neurol 54:101–106, 2000.
19. Taylor ME. Return to work following back surgery, a review. Am J Industrial Med 16:79–88, 1989.
20. Hodges SD, Humphreys SC, Eck JC, Covington LA, Harrom H. Predicting factors of successful recovery from lumbar spine surgery among worker's compensation patients. J Am Osteopath Assoc 101:78–83, 2001.
21. Trief PM, Grant W, Fredrickson B. Perspective study of psychological predictors of lumbar surgery outcome. Spine 25:2616–2621, 2000.
22. Schade V, Semmer M, Main CJ, Hora J, Boos N. The impact of clinical, morphological, psychosocial and work related factors on the outcome of lumbar discectomy. Pain 80:239–249, 1999.
23. Junge A, Dvorak J, Aberns S. Predictors of good and bad outcome of lumbar disc surgery, a perspective clinical study with recommendations for screening to avoid bad outcomes. Spine 20:460–468, 1995.
24. Tandon T, Campbell F, Ross ER. Posterior lumbar interbody fusion: association between disability and psychological disturbance in non compensation patients. Spine 24:1833–1838, 1999.
25. Spengler BM, Quellette EA, Battie M, Zeh J. Elective discectomy for herniation of a lumbar disc. J Bone Joint Surg 72:230–237, 1990.
26. Greenough CG, Peterson MD, Hadlow S, et al. Instrumented posterior lateral fusion: results and comparison with anterior interbody fusion. Spine 23:479–486, 1998.
27. Kjellby-Wendt G, Styf JR, Carlsson SG. The predictive value of psychometric analysis in patients treated by extirpation of lumbar intervertebral disc herniation. J Spinal Disord 12:375–379, 1999.
28. Douglas TS, Mann NH, Hodge RL. Evaluation of preoperative patient education and computer assisted patient instruction. J Spine Disord 11:29–35, 1998.
29. Phelan EA, Deyo RA, Cherkin DC, et al. Helping patients decide about back surgery: a randomized trial of an instructive video program. Spine 26:206–211, 2001.
30. Iversen MD, Daltrey LH, Fossel AH, Katz JN. The prognostic importance of patient preoperative expectations of surgery for lumbar spinal stenosis. Patient Educ Counseling 34:169–178, 1998.
31. Cashion EL, Lynch WJ. Personality factors and results of lumbar disc surgery. Neurosurgery 4:141–145, 1979.
32. Pearce JM. Aspects of the failed back syndrome: role of litigation. Spinal Cord 38:63–70, 2000.
33. Schofferman J, Anderson D, Smith G, et al. Childhood psychological trauma and chronic refractory low back pain. Clin J Pain 9:260–265, 1993.
34. Carragee EJ, Chen Y, Tanner CM, et al. Provocative discography after limited lumbar discectomy: a controlled, randomized study of pain response in symptomatic and asymptomatic subjects. Spine 25:3065–3071, 2000.

35. Samwel H, Slappendel R, Crul BJ, Voerman VF. Psychological predictors of the effectiveness of radio frequency lesioning of the cervical spinal dorsal ganglion (RF-DRG). Eur J Pain 4:149–155, 2000.
36. Graver V, Haaland AU, Magnaes B, Loeb M. Seven-year clinical follow-up after lumbar disc surgery: results and predictors of outcome. Br J Neurosurg 13:178–184, 1999.
37. Doleys DM, Brown J. MMPI profile as an outcome "predictor" in the treatment of non-cancer pain patients utilizing intrathecal opioid therapy. Neuromodulation 4:93–97, 2001.
38. Frymoyer JW. Back pain and sciatica. N Engl J Med 318:291–296, 1988.
39. Coskun E, Suzer T, Topuz O, et al. Relationships between epidural fibrosis, pain, disability, and psychological factors after lumbar disc surgery. Eur Spine J 9:218–223, 2000.
40. Mannion RJ, Woolf CJ. Pain mechanisms and management: a central perspective. Clin J Pain 16:S144–S156, 2000.
41. Block AR. Presurgical Psychological Screening in Chronic Pain Syndromes: A Guide for the Behavioral Health Practitioner. Mahwah, NJ, Erlbaum Press, 1996.
42. Rush AJ, Polatin P, Gatchel RJ. Depression and low back pain: establishing priorities in treatment. Spine 25:2566–2571, 2000.
43. Polatin PB, Kinney RK, Gatchel RJ, et al. Psychiatric illness and chronic low back pain: the mind and the spine—which goes first? Spine 18:66–71, 1993.
44. Beck AT, Steer RA, Garbin MG. Psychometric properties of the Beck Depression Inventory and 25 years of evaluation. Clin Psychol Rev 8:77–95, 1998.
45. Zung WWK. A self-rating depression scale. Arch Gen Psychiatry 12:63–80, 1965.
46. Diagnostic and Statistical Manual of Mental Disorders (DSM-IV) (4th ed). Washington, DC, American Psychiatric Association, 1994.
47. Keller LS, Butcher JN. Assessment of Chronic Pain Patients with the MMPI-2. Minneapolis, University of Minnesota Press, 1991.
48. Fishbain D, Goldberg M, Meagher R, Steele R, Rossomoff H. Male and female chronic pain patients categorized by DSM-III psychiatric diagnostic criteria. Pain 26:181–197, 1986.
49. Jamison RW (ed.) Addiction and pain. Clin J Pain (Suppl) 18:S1–S115, 2002.
50. Barsky A. The patient with hypochondriasis. N Engl J Med 345:1395–1399, 2001.
51. Doleys DM, Coleton M, Tutak U. The use of intraspinal infusion therapy with non-cancer pain patients: followup and comparison of worker's compensation versus non-worker's compensation patients. Neuromodulation 1:149–159, 1998.
52. Willis KD, Doleys DM. The effects of long-term intraspinal infusion therapy with non-cancer pain patients: evaluation of patients, significant other, and clinical staff appraisals. Neuromodulation 2:241–253, 1999.
53. Kerns RD, Rosenberg R. Predicting responses to self management treatment of chronic pain: application of the pain stages of change model. Pain 85:49–55, 2000.
54. Ostelo RW, Koke AJ, Beurskens AJ, et al. Behaviorally/graded activity compared with usual care after first disc surgery: considerations in the design of a randomized clinical trial. J Manipulative Physiol Ther 23:312–319, 2000.
55. Benedetti F, Amanzio M, Baldi S, et al. The specific effects of prior opioid exposure on placebo analgesia and placebo respiratory depression. Pain 75:313–319, 1998.
56. Bandura A, O'Leary A, Taylor CB, Gauthier J, Cossard D. Perceived self-efficacy and pain control: opioid and non-opioid mechanisms. J Personality Social Psychol 53:563–571, 1987.
57. de la Fuente-Fernandez R, Ruth TJ, Sossal V, et al. Expectations and dopamine release: mechanism of the placebo effect in Parkinson's disease. Science 293:1164–1166, 2001.
58. Ho KH, Hashish I, Solmon P, Freeman R, Harvey W. Reduction of postoperative swelling by a placebo effect. J Psychosom Res 32:197–205, 1988.
59. Birmbauer N, Flor H. A leg to stand on, learning creates pain. Behav Brain Sci 20:441–442, 1997.
60. Childress AR, Mozley PD, McElgin W, et al. Limbic activation during cue-induced cocaine craving. Am J Psychiatry 156:11–18, 1999.
61. Casey KL, Bushnell MD (eds). *Pain Imaging*. Seattle, IASP Press, 2000.
62. Rainville P, Duncan GH, Price DD, Carrier B, Bushnell MC. Pain affect encoded in human anterior singular gyrus but not somatosensory cortex. Science 277:968–971, 1997.
63. Weiss ER, Longhurst JG, Mazure CM. Childhood sexual abuse as a risk factor for depression in women: psychological and neurological correlates. Am J Psychiatry 156:816–828, 1999.
64. Bremner JD, Randall P, Vermetten E, et al. Magnetic resonance imaging-based measurement of hippocampal volume in post traumatic stress disorder related to childhood physical and sexual abuse-a preliminary report. Biol Psychiatry 41:23–32, 1997.
65. Stein M, Koverola C, Hanna C, Torchia MG, McClarty B. Hippocampal volume in women victimized by childhood sexual abuse. Psychol Med 27:951–959, 1997.
66. Schacter DL, Wagner AD. Remembrance of things past. Science 285:1503–1504, 1999.
67. Heim C, Newport DJ, Heit S, et al. Pituitary–adrenal and autonomic responses to stress in women after sexual and physical abuse in childhood. JAMA 284:592–597, 2000.

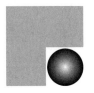

CHAPTER 5

Pharmacologic Therapies for Pain

J. DAVID HADDOX, DDS, MD, DABPM, MRO

The use of pharmacologic agents to induce analgesia is considered a routine part of surgical practice, yet many busy clinicians rely on outdated rote protocols learned in residency that may not serve the best interests of the patients who present for care. An understanding of the various types of analgesics available, including some nonpharmacologic agents, can improve care of patients undergoing perioperative or nonsurgical care by a neurologic surgeon.

Today, the physician has more classes and types of analgesic medications available than ever before. Learning how to use several from each class effectively is the foundation for improved pain care. This chapter, rather than attempting to be an exhaustive review, will focus on each type of analgesic, singling out a few representative drugs, with an attempt to provide salient information that will allow effective use of these various medications.

GENERAL PRINCIPLES

A premise to rational pharmacologic treatment of pain that is essential, and often confusing, is the distinction between efficacy and potency. *Efficacy*, in sum, is the ability of a drug, irrespective of dose, to achieve a certain effect. That is, will a specific drug cause a given effect, given enough of the drug? Opioids, of the pure μ-agonist variety, are all equally efficacious. Morphine, fentanyl, and oxycodone will all achieve the same degree of analgesia in a population (although there are some individual patients who may tend to do better with one or the other drug in a given situation). Nonsteroidal anti-inflammatory drugs (NSAIDs), however, do not have the same efficacy as opioids. With pain of mild-to-moderate intensity, they may work as well as a pure μ-agonist, but with higher intensities of pain, requiring upward titration of dose, NSAIDs will plateau in the degree of analgesia they can produce, whereas opioids will not. In other words, as pain increases, opioids can be titrated to the desired effect, assuming other, unwanted effects are managed so that the patient tolerates them. NSAIDs can be titrated to a recommended maximum dose, beyond which no more analgesia ensues, regardless of increases in dose. The mixed-opioid agonist-antagonists (such as penta-zocine), likewise, are less efficacious than pure μ-agonists. Because the antagonist effects predominate at higher doses, the mixed drugs in essence partially cancel their analgesia effects, demonstrating a "ceiling effect," that is, a limit to efficacy.

Potency, however, refers to the amount of a specific drug it takes to achieve a target effect. Thus, because it takes fewer molecules of fentanyl than morphine to achieve the same degree of analgesia, morphine is less potent than fentanyl. However, both fentanyl and morphine have equal *efficacy*. That is, titrated properly, in the population, they both will achieve the same degree of analgesia.

Another principle that is clinically relevant to the use of pharmaceutical agents to treat pain is that of the elimination half-life. A drug's half-life influences its recommended dosing frequency and determines how long after initiation until steady state is achieved. As a rule, it takes four to five half-lives to achieve steady state. Thus, if a drug has a half-life of approximately 4 hours, and it is given around the clock at an appropriate dosing interval, it will reach steady state in approximately 1 day (4 hours × 5 half lives = 20 hours). Thus, the total daily dose of the drug can be titrated on a daily basis, without fear of unsuspected accumulation producing unwanted effects a few days hence. If, however, a drug has a half-life of 2 days, it takes approximately 8 to 10 days to achieve steady state, making daily adjustments in dose riskier because the physician is increasing the dose before steady state has been achieved, risking overshoot when steady state finally ensues. In a clinical situation like this, the physician should use a short-acting, quickly eliminated drug to titrate frequently against the background of analgesia provided by the longer-acting drug, to allow the serum level of the longer half-life drug to get to steady state, so an intelligent assessment of its effect and the need for dosage adjustment can be made. Once steady state of the longer-acting drug is assured, assessment of the degree of pain control achieved by using both the longer and shorter-acting drugs can be made. If it is satisfactory, the amount of the shorter-acting drug required can be converted into an equianalgesic amount of the longer-acting drug and this can be added to the daily regimen, with careful follow-up over the next several days to ensure that the "equianalgesic" dose calculated from reference tables is appropriate for that individual patient.

NONSTEROIDAL ANTI-INFLAMMATORY DRUGS AND ACETAMINOPHEN

These types of nonopioid analgesics are often considered first-line analgesics. They enjoy the lack of significant abuse potential and do not induce the development of analgesic tolerance.[1] Numerous studies over decades, coupled with clinical experience, leave no doubt as to their analgesic efficacy. They are routinely used by physicians, and many are available over-the-counter—a source that must be taken into account when prescribing these as single-entity agents, or as a component of combination analgesics, because some of the toxicities of these drugs are dose-dependent.

Acetylsalicylic acid (ASA) and the other NSAIDs act by reducing prostaglandin synthesis through inhibition of the cyclo-oxygenase (COX) enzymes. Prostaglandins are nearly ubiquitous and serve a variety of functions, both beneficial and harmful. With tissue injury, arachidonic acid is released from disrupted cell membranes by the action of phospholipases. It is converted into prostaglandin H_2 (PGH_2) by COX. There have now been two similar, but distinct, isoforms of COX identified, COX-1 and COX-2. Both catalyze the conversion of arachidonic acid into PGH_2. Specific prostaglandin synthases then convert PGH_2 into different prostanoids in different tissues. In platelets, it is converted to thromboxane A_2 (TxA_2) by thromboxane synthase, whereas in the stomach, it is converted to PGE_2. TxA_2 is a potent stimulator of platelet aggregation, whereas PGE_2 is intimately involved in gastric protection by contributing to the protective mucous layer and stimulating bicarbonate secretion in the duodenum.[1] The prostanoids have roles in nociception, as well, sensitizing peripheral afferent terminals to the presence of histamine and bradykinin. In addition to their peripheral actions, they have central modulating effects on nociceptive transmission, such as being potential N-methyl-D-aspartate (NMDA) receptor inhibitors, inhibitors of central prostaglandin synthesis, and activators of serotonergic pathways.[2]

Thus, the therapeutic effects of the NSAIDs and, some suggest, acetaminophen, are mediated via this inhibition of prostaglandin activity. However, many of the side effects of the NSAIDs are also mediated in a similar fashion. Based on the knowledge that the different isoforms of COX exist and mediate different processes, several drugs are available now that selectively, or more accurately, preferentially inhibit COX-2, which is responsible for inflammatory processes and the pain that results from them. These drugs, called COX-2 inhibitors or coxibs, may offer some advantages in some clinical settings.

A limiting factor for the clinical utility of the drugs in this group is the presence of a ceiling effect on analgesia. That is, these drugs have a dose-dependent effect on pain up to a certain point, and then further increases in dose, even to the point of toxicity, will not induce more analgesia. Thus, these drugs have use in the treatment of mild-to-moderate pain but, by themselves, are not useful in patients with more severe pain.

While side effects will be discussed in relation to specific medicines below, an unexpected adverse event associated with NSAIDs of particular interest to neurologic surgeons is the development of aseptic meningitis. This has been reported with a number of medications in this class, including one of the coxibs, rofecoxib.[3]

Acetaminophen

Acetaminophen (US abbreviation: APAP; UK official generic name: paracetamol) is an antipyretic analgesic with no effect on platelet function or inflammatory processes. Its effects are thought to be due to central inhibition of prostaglandin function.[4] It is effective for mild-to-moderate pain. Taken within the intended dose range, acetaminophen is typically safe. Because of the lack of significant inhibition of peripheral COX, it does not promote bleeding, thus is safe to use in the perioperative period.

All sources of acetaminophen (single entity, over-the-counter, plus prescribed as part of a combination analgesic, such as hydrocodone/APAP) should not exceed 4000 mg daily. The recommended figure is lower in the setting of a patient who drinks alcoholic beverages regularly.[5] The main safety concern is dose-related hepatic toxicity. When seen, it is usually in the setting of overdose, alcoholism, fasting, or with concurrent administration of drugs that induce some components of the cytochrome P-450 (CYP 450) family of enzymes. APAP itself is not hepatotoxic. However, its metabolite, N-acetyl-p-benzoquinoneimine (NAPQI) causes hepatocellular necrosis. At normal doses, approximately 96% of APAP is metabolized by the liver, with most by either sulfation or glucuronidation. Only approximately 4% is metabolized by the CYP 450 system to the toxic intermediate NAPQI, which is rapidly converted to a nontoxic metabolite by glutathione conjugation. In an overdose, the routine metabolic pathways become saturated and metabolism is shunted to the CYP 450 system (2E1 and 1A2) and increased amounts of NAPQI are created. Glutathione stores become consumed and NAPQI accumulates.[4]

With chronic alcohol consumption, CYP 450 2E1 is increased and glutathione stores are reduced. At least one manufacturer indicates a three-drink per day threshold for seeking advice from the physician before consuming over-the-counter acetaminophen.[5] Isoniazid also increases 2E1. The levels of 1A2 are also increased by isoniazid, as well as barbiturates, caffeine, carbamazepine, phenytoin, and rifampin.[4]

Overdose symptoms are relatively nonspecific and include nausea, vomiting, diaphoresis, and general malaise. Symptoms may not manifest immediately, but can be delayed by 2 to 3 days after ingestion. Treatment of overdose includes the use of N-acetylcysteine.[5]

Aspirin

Aspirin, or ASA, is one of the first chemicals synthesized that had any significant medicinal value. It is the prototypical NSAID, being a nonselective COX inhibitor at usual analgesic doses, although it may somewhat selectively inhibit COX-1 at doses typically used to reduce platelet aggregation therapeutically.[6] Aspirin is an antipyretic, an anti-inflammatory, and an analgesic agent.

Aspirin is a very effective analgesic for mild-to-moderate pain. Like all the drugs in this section, it can have opioid-sparing effects because it works through a mechanism distinct from opioids, and it works largely in the periphery, reducing the amount of nociceptive signals generated, so that less opioid is needed centrally to cause the same reduction in perceived pain.

In addition to antithrombogenic effects and its gastrointestinal effects, it is associated with a specific allergic reaction that occurs rarely, but is not dose-related. This is the phenomenon of bronchospasm in the setting of an asthmatic with nasal polyps, the so-called "aspirin triad."[4] It is also contraindicated in the pediatric setting in the treatment of viral infections because it increases the risk for the development of Reye's syndrome.

Other Nonselective Cyclo-oxygenase Inhibitors

Ibuprofen is the prototype of this group, which also includes ketoprofen, naproxen, indomethacin, piroxicam, and diclofenac. These drugs all share certain characteristics similar to those of aspirin, without the peculiar cautions of Reye's syndrome. Patients with the aspirin triad should not take these medicines; other allergic reactions are possible with any of the class.

These drugs are also effective in the treatment of mild-to-moderate pain and are frequently used in the treatment of pain from the arthritides. The use of these drugs has been invaluable in the fight to control human suffering, but their side effects have also induced significant health consequences. It has been estimated that the use of nonselective COX-inhibitor NSAIDs cause over 100,000 hospitalizations and 16,500 deaths per year from gastrointestinal complications alone.[7,8] Not surprisingly, NSAID use increases with age, and it is estimated that 10% to 20% of patients older than 65 years of age have a current prescription for an NSAID.[4] This, coupled with the fact that the elderly, for a number of pharmacokinetic reasons, are more susceptible to NSAID-induced toxicities, demands caution when using this class of drug in the elderly patient, especially on a chronic basis, because many of the toxicities have an insidious development, announced by a catastrophic event.[1,2]

The adverse renal effects of nonselective COX inhibitors can come about in several ways. Chronic interstitial nephritis or papillary necrosis can occur with prolonged use. At particular risk for NSAID-induced renal failure are those patients with reduced circulating volume who have become dependent on prostaglandin-mediated renal vasodilatation to maintain renal blood flow.[2,6]

The NSAIDs can, however, be very useful in the treatment of pain, even when another type of analgesic, such as an opioid, is needed. Experience in the treatment of pain from cancer has shown that pain generated from a process with an inflammatory component, such as pathologic fracture, will respond with less opioid if an NSAID is concurrently administered.[2]

Selective Cyclo-oxygenase-2 Inhibitors

Celecoxib, rofecoxib, and valdecoxib are now marketed in the United States. They are all indicated for treatment of signs and symptoms of osteoarthritis, rheumatoid arthritis, and primary dysmenorrhea. In addition, rofecoxib and celecoxib are indicated for the management of acute pain. Celecoxib has been shown to reduce the prevalence of colon polyps in patients with familial adenomatous polyposis.[9]

All share the warning about the aspirin triad. Like the nonselective COX inhibitors, they have a ceiling effect with regard to the maximum analgesic effect. Subjects taking rofecoxib in one study had a significantly greater risk of experiencing a serious cardiovascular thrombotic event than those taking naproxen sodium.[10] Death rates from cardiovascular events were similar, however, so the clinical significance of this observation is still awaiting elucidation. Celecoxib is the only coxib that is contraindicated in patients with allergy to sulfonamides.

All have been shown to have a lower, but not zero, incidence of significant gastrointestinal adverse events compared to nonselective COX inhibitors. The coxibs have been shown to be associated with lower incidences of endoscopically confirmed gastric lesions than comparative nonselective NSAIDs, thus they are thought to be generally safer, especially for long-term use. This does not mean, however, that patients are not at risk for significant adverse gastrointestinal events or renal effects similar to those observed with the nonselective NSAIDs.

ANTIDEPRESSANT AGENTS

Medications marketed for their efficacy in treating depression are also very useful in the treatment of patients with pain. Antidepressant drugs can be helpful in treating pain (especially neuropathic pain) with or without concurrent depression, anxiety, insomnia, urinary incontinence, and, of course, depression.[11] The older medicines in this class, such as amitriptyline, have a broad spectrum of pharmacologic effects that can be useful or undesirable, depending on the patient, the problem, and the concomitant medications.

The side effects vary by subclass, with the tricyclic compounds generally having antimuscarinic profiles (xerostomia, constipation, impaired visual accommodation, worsening of narrow-angle glaucoma) and cardiac side effects (hypotension, prolonged Q-T interval), and the selective serotonin reuptake inhibitors (SSRIs) having appetite suppression and sexual dysfunction as some of their significant undesirable profiles. In an overdose, the lethality of the older drugs far surpasses the newer ones; thus, lower amounts should be prescribed when suicidal ideation is elicited or anticipated. One peculiar side effect that required revised labeling involves hepatic failure associated with nefazodone.[12]

In general, the use of an antidepressant as an adjuvant medication in the treatment of pain should follow two rules: (1) select a medicine that targets the specific symptom, or group of symptoms in the person, taking into account such factors as age, preexisting pathology, and concomitant medicines; and (2) start low and go slow. There is no correlation between serum level and pain efficacy for any of the drugs in this class.

For example, the use of a drug such as amitriptyline may not be the best choice for an elderly man presenting with new-onset pain in the trigeminal territory who has no other neurologic findings and a normal-appearing magnetic resonance image, due to the risk of inducing urinary obstruction. Even if a person such as this had no reported urinary problems, the odds are that he has some element of benign prostatic hypertrophy; thus, amitriptyline should be avoided.

Nortriptyline, which has a lesser antimuscarinic profile, would be a consideration, but is not free from risk of inducing urinary obstruction.

A typical starting dose of a tricyclic antidepressant is 10 mg at night, approximately 1 hour before bedtime. Because the older drugs all have half-lives of about a day, the dose may be increased in 10-mg increments every 4 to 5 days without risk of undetected accumulation. The older antidepressants are affected by coadministration of the newer medications, so that adding an SSRI can cause substantial elevation of the serum level of a tricyclic antidepressant drug.[13] It is common for patients to experience daytime sedation for a few days following initiation of dose, or significant dose increases. Tolerance to this develops fairly predictably. Another common side effect is rapid eye movement sleep rebound, characterized by vivid dreaming near awakening.

The SSRIs typically are given in the morning, but this can vary by drug and patient. The evidence for their analgesic effects is not nearly as convincing as that with the older tricyclic drugs, but they remain useful for their efficacy in treating depression, which commonly occurs in the setting of pain.

Trazodone, neither a tricyclic nor an SSRI, is not very effective in causing analgesia, but it is sedating and has fewer antimuscarinic side effects than amitriptyline, so it can be useful for its hypnotic properties. It is best administered after a meal or light snack because its absorption is enhanced by concomitant food administration and, thus, more predictable serum levels are obtained when administered consistently with food. The sleep latency can vary remarkably in clinical use, from 30 minutes to several hours. Thus, as with all antidepressants, the choice of drug, choice of dose, and choice of time of administration must be customized for each patient. Trazodone has been associated with priapism, and should not be given to patients recovering from myocardial infarction.

ANTICONVULSANT DRUGS

The anticonvulsant drugs have long been used in the treatment of pain by neurologic surgeons. Their use and side effect profiles are well described. Carbamazepine, a molecule with structural similarities to amitriptyline, is indicated for the treatment of trigeminal neuralgia and was the first anticonvulsant to carry an indication for a painful condition. Unlike the antidepressant drugs, the anticonvulsant drugs are not useful for the treatment of somatic or visceral pain. The anticonvulsant agents are now a varied class with quite distinct mechanisms of action and side effect profiles. A few representative compounds will be presented.

While phenytoin (previously known as diphenylhydantoin) was used to treat certain pains in the past, it was surpassed by carbamazepine, which has been shown to be effective in the treatment of trigeminal and glossopharyngeal neuralgias, and has been used in a wide array of other neuropathic conditions. The risk of hematologic side effects associated with the use of carbamazepine (aplastic anemia and agranulocytosis) caused it to be supplanted in many practices with the advent of gabapentin, currently the most popularly prescribed anticonvulsant for pain.

Gabapentin, designed to resemble gamma-aminobutyric acid (GABA), was studied and originally marketed as an adjunctive anticonvulsant. Experience rapidly proved, however, that it was a very effective analgesic for conditions in which neuropathic pain was a significant contributor to the overall clinical setting, such as postherpetic neuralgia, a condition for which it is indicated.[14–16] Gabapentin has several advantages over other drugs in this class. First, it is not metabolized, so there is no concern about accumulation of active metabolites. However, gabapentin is cleared renally, so dosage adjustment based on renal impairment is necessary. Second, it has almost no drug-drug interactions, so it is safe to use in many patients who are taking other medications related to their pain or other medical conditions. Third, it has a very low side effect profile, with fatigue, somnolence, dizziness, ataxia, nystagmus, and tremor being most commonly reported. The mechanism of action remains unclear. Gabapentin is not a GABA agonist, nor is it metabolized into GABA. It does not bind at the GABA receptor, nor does it affect the reuptake or metabolism of GABA.

Gabapentin is absorbed by a transport mechanism that can be saturated; thus, it has a dose-dependent oral bioavailability. A dose of 400 mg is approximately 25% less bioavailable than of a dose of 100 mg. The overall bioavailability, throughout the dose range, is approximately 60%, but decreases with increasing doses due to saturation of the transport mechanism. Above approximately 800 mg per dose, there is little additional absorption of gabapentin. Thus, because it is commonly dosed up to four times per day, the recommended maximum daily dose is approximately 3600 mg.

OPIOIDS

The oldest class of analgesic medicines is still the most effective for many situations. Yet, unlike the medicines mentioned thus far, their effective application is hampered by misunderstanding and myth. Also, there are unique laws, regulations, and policies that impose restrictions on the medical use of the opioids, and other controlled substances, that do not apply to the other drugs in this brief review.

Morphine, codeine, and thebaine are naturally occurring opioids and are isolated from the sap of the opium poppy. Fentanyl, meperidine, and methadone are synthetic opioids. Oxycodone, hydromorphone, and hydrocodone are semisynthetic opioids, so called because they are made by chemically modifying thebaine. While the opioids differ in potency, requiring different doses to achieve the same effect, the pure μ-agonists do not differ in efficacy. There are opioids, however, that are not pure μ-agonists, but rather are mixed agonists-antagonists (pentazocine, nalbuphine, butorphanol) or partial agonists (buprenorphine). The use of these drugs in a patient who has been exposed to pure μ-agonists on an ongoing basis can precipitate a withdrawal syndrome. The partial agonists and the mixed agonist-antagonists do not have the same efficacy as the pure μ-agonists. That is, they have a ceiling effect such that, beyond a certain dose, no more analgesia ensues.

Almost all types of pain, from nearly all causes, respond well to opioids, although higher doses may be needed for the treatment of neuropathic pain. They all have similar side effect profiles for the most part, although there are some idiosyncrasies that will be highlighted. Class side effects are respiratory depression (reduced response to $PaCO_2$), nausea, vomiting, itching, sedation, euphoria or dysphoria, miosis, and constipation.

The legal issues surrounding the use of these drugs involve federal law, which "sets the floor," and state laws, regulations, and medical board policies, which "set the ceiling." That is, state laws can be more restrictive, but not less restrictive, than federal laws. In other words, where there is a disparity between federal and state drug law or regulation, the more restrictive one prevails. Thus, a drug such as morphine, which is scheduled under federal law as a schedule II (or class II, abbreviated as C-II) controlled substance, must be at least a schedule II substance in every state, whereas a drug such as carisoprodol, which is not scheduled federally, is scheduled as a controlled substance in some states (in Georgia, for example, it is a class III medicine). There are also federal laws governing refills (class III, no more than five refills, with the last one dispensed before 6 months of the date of the original prescription; class II, no refills allowed) and telephonic prescriptions (class II, emergency only; class III to V, oral prescription in person or by telephone has the same force and effect as a written or facsimile copy). Medical licensing boards also have policies that affect the way these medicines are used. For a complete listing of every state's policy, the neurologic surgeon should consult the Database of State Laws, Regulations and Other Official Governmental Policies on the web site maintained by the University of Wisconsin's Pain and Policy Studies Group.[17]

The safe and effective use of opioids requires knowledge of the patient, the pain problem (intensity, pattern, type, expected course), concurrent diseases, concomitant medications, and an understanding of the patient's history, especially with regard to a family or personal history of substance abuse or addiction disorders.

Most physicians do not distinguish between physical dependence, an expected effect of certain types of medications used for a certain time (opioids, benzodiazepines, beta blockers, clonidine, caffeine, vasoconstrictive nasal decongestants, or ocular products), and the disease of addiction. Physical dependence is induced by repeated exposure to medicines that cause the body to adapt to their presence. As long as these medications are 1) continued as therapeutically indicated, 2) not reversed by the administration of an antagonist (for example, naloxone, or a mixed agonist-antagonist opioid), or 3) tapered slowly when no longer needed, the likelihood that the patient in whom physical dependence has developed will experience a withdrawal syndrome is minimal. Thus, the development of physical dependence as a consequence of medical therapy has almost no significance to the average patient. Only when withdrawal is induced, by careless action of a healthcare practitioner or the patient, does the presence of physical dependence have any health consequences.

Addiction, however, is a disease process. It has been defined by the American Academy of Pain Medicine, the American Pain Society, and the American Society of Addiction Medicine as "a primary, chronic, neurobiologic disease, with genetic, psychosocial, and environmental factors influencing its development and manifestations. It is characterized by behaviors that include one or more of the following: impaired control over drug use, compulsive use, continued use despite harm and craving."[18] The reason that most healthcare professionals confuse addiction with physical dependence is simply that most patients with addiction that present for treatment have also developed physical dependence to the substance(s) that they are abusing. Frequently, the withdrawal syndrome is the reason for presenting for care.

If one thinks about the number of drugs to which a person can develop physical dependence, and the use of these drugs by the population, it is easy to see that a substantial portion of the populace is physically dependent on something. Yet, the fraction of persons who are addicted to drugs other than alcohol is somewhat small, estimated at between 5% and 6%.[19] The development of addiction to opioid analgesics in properly treated patients with pain has been reported to be rare. However, data are not available to establish the true incidence of addiction in patients with chronic pain.

A condition that may appear to be addiction, at first glance or to the uneducated practitioner, has been called "opioid pseudoaddiction."[20] In the case of pseudoaddiction, a patient is experiencing pain that is inadequately treated. The patient may become increasingly demanding, become a "clock-watcher," or exhibit other behaviors that are typically attributed to "drug seeking." In fact, in the case of pseudoaddiction, the patient is not seeking drugs per se, but is seeking relief from pain that is being poorly managed by a healthcare professional. In the case of pseudoaddiction, when appropriate pain care is instituted, by whatever means, the behaviors cease. In the case of addiction, however, giving the person more drugs only temporizes the situation until they are consumed. Another important distinction between patients who are appropriately treated and those with untreated addiction disorders is how the drug affects the person, once they have access to it. The patient will control the use of the medicine, once it is has been effectively titrated, while the person with addiction will be consistently unable to control their use of the drug. In addition, the quality of life of the nonaddicted patient will be stabilized and improved while using the medicine, while the quality of life of the addicted person will inevitably decrease because of their interaction with the drug.

It is very important in clinical medicine, then, to have a clear differentiation in one's mind among patients who have pain and developed physical dependence to a medicine that is prescribed and taken as directed, patients whose pain is poorly managed and demonstrates the phenomenon of pseudoaddiction, addicts who are also physically dependent on the substance they are abusing, and addicts who are not physically dependent on the substance they are abusing (early cocaine addict, for example).

To use opioid analgesics in a clinically rational manner, there are certain principles that apply. The first of these is the concept of *minimum effective analgesic concentration*, or MEAC. This is the minimum blood level of a medicine that is necessary for clinically significant analgesia. There is also a level above which side effects will begin to occur. It is likely that the blood level for individual opioid side effects (nausea, sedation, pruritus) may be variable. The difference between the MEAC and the side effect level is known as the therapeutic range or therapeutic window (Fig. 5-1).

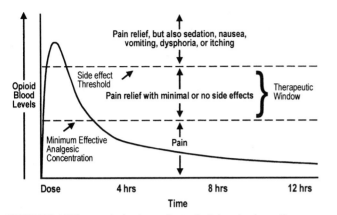

FIGURE 5-1 When a single dose of a typical drug is given, the concentration of the drug rises to a peak, and then gradually tapers off until it no longer produces a beneficial response. The level must exceed minimum effective analgesic concentration for analgesia to ensue, but side effects occur above a certain threshold that varies among patients. The goal for effective analgesia is to keep the blood level within the therapeutic window at all times. This is a stylized representation of an ideal situation. Individuals vary considerably, thus it is possible that for some patients the therapeutic window may be so narrow that the dose needed to reach analgesia will also be attended by unacceptable side effects.

It is critical to understand that the MEAC will vary with the following three factors: the patient, the perceived pain intensity, and the medication. That is, two patients with the same height and weight, with stable pain of 7 on a 10-point scale, may require different doses of morphine to achieve equivalent reductions in pain. Likewise, the dose of fentanyl for each to achieve equivalent reductions in pain will vary, although the morphine-to-fentanyl conversion ratio between the two patients, while variable, will tend to fall within the range of values in the equianalgesic tables commonly available. If either patient now has his or her pain under stable control, but then is subjected to an acute exacerbation of pain, such as a visit to the physical therapist, the MEAC increases and the patient will require more analgesic to remain comfortable and actively participate in the therapy. Thus, the goal of analgesic therapy, in theory, is to maintain a blood level that is above MEAC, but below that for significant side effects, or to keep the blood level of the opioid within the therapeutic window.

The second principle is that around-the-clock pain requires around-the-clock analgesia. Many pain problems, such as postoperative pain and chronic pain, are experienced by the patient nearly constantly. Other pains may fluctuate predictably, such as with activity (so-called incident pain), with time of day (early morning exacerbation of pain and stiffness with rheumatoid arthritis), or may have no predictable pattern of fluctuation. The traditional dosing of analgesics is inadequate to maintain blood levels above MEAC consistently. As an example, a common mistake in the setting of prolonged perioperative pain after a major spinal surgery is to provide the patient with a prescription for an immediate-release opioid in combination with APAP on either an as-needed basis or a fixed schedule of every 4 to 6 hours. These medicines, while effective for intermittent pain, short-term pain, or exacerbations of pain, are considered by pain specialists as being inappropriate for the treatment of nearly constant or longer-term pain problems, due to the "roller coaster"

Intermittent Dosing of IV, IM, or po (IR)

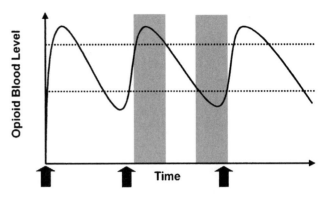

FIGURE 5-2 In the case of repeated administration (*dark arrows*) of an intravenous (IV), intramuscular (IM), or oral, immediate-release (IR) traditional opioid-acetaminophen combination analgesic, a "roller coaster" pattern of blood levels occurs. The blood level exceeds minimum effective analgesic concentration shortly after dosing, inducing analgesia, then exceeds side effect threshold (*first gray bar*), resulting in a pain-free, but nauseated, sedated, or itching patient, then it falls below side effect threshold, resulting in a comfortable patient (*area between gray bars*), then the level falls below minimum effective analgesic concentration, but the ordered or prescribed dosing interval is beyond the known duration of action of the medication, resulting in return of pain (*second gray bar*). This pattern repeats over time, such that the patient is uncomfortable (either pain or side effects) at various times during the daytime, and wakes up in pain several times at night.

effect of blood levels demonstrated in Figure 5-2. Other common clinical scenarios are depicted in Figures 5-3 through 5-5.

The third principle is that different patients with differing pain syndromes may respond differently to different medications. The first factor to consider is what type, or types, of pain is the patient experiencing? If a patient has nociceptive

IV Patient-Controlled Analgesia (PCA)

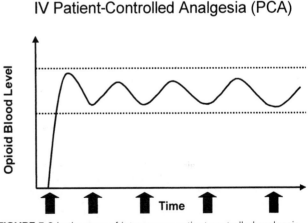

FIGURE 5-3 In the case of intravenous patient-controlled analgesia, the patient, who knows more about their pain intensity than anyone, is put in charge of medicating themselves within limits set by the physician. Following a loading dose (*first dark arrow*) to ensure the patient's blood level rises above minimum effective analgesic concentration, the patient-controlled analgesia pump is programmed with parameters that allow the patient to inject small doses of medication periodically to keep the blood level in the therapeutic window.

Depiction of blood profile of a long-acting opioid

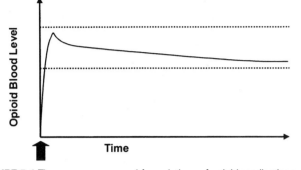

FIGURE 5-4 There are now several formulations of opioid medications available that provide longer durations of opioid blood levels than traditional immediate-release opioid medications. The theory behind these is to, in essence, emulate the smooth blood levels created by patient-controlled analgesia or a steady-state infusion of opioids.

pain, such as that from non-neural tissue trauma, postsurgical pain, non-neurologic oncologic pain, osteoarthritis, or chronic musculoskeletal pain, medicines such as an NSAID or an opioid may be appropriate, depending on the severity of the pain. In these cases, inflammatory processes are occurring in the periphery and are resulting in sensitized nerves; that is, nerves that generate action potentials in response to much less intense stimuli than they would in a normal state. These inflammatory processes may be occurring at an otherwise subclinical level, in that there may be no classic signs of inflammation. For example, an incision that appears clinically to be without signs of infection has created an "inflammatory

"Oral PCA"

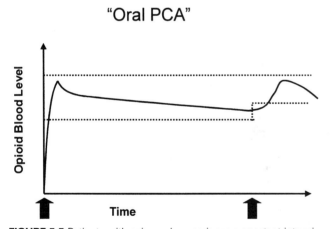

FIGURE 5-5 Patients with pain rarely experience a constant intensity. In this figure, a long-acting opioid is given at a dose that produces a blood level that is within the therapeutic window (*first arrow*). Later in the day, however, the patient goes to physical therapy, with the increased activity causing an exacerbation in pain and, therefore, raising the minimum effective analgesic concentration. To accommodate this, a dose of an immediate-release opioid is provided to raise the blood level above the new minimum effective analgesic concentration transiently (*second arrow*). When the transiently increased blood level from the immediate-release dose returns to the previous level, the transient increase in pain has subsided as well, so the residual blood levels from the long-acting opioid manage the baseline pain.

soup" at the cellular level, with release of mediators of inflammation, which sensitize nociceptive neurons. With an NSAID, the peripheral effects reduce sensitization in the periphery and, therefore, reduce the nociceptive traffic coming from the site of injury. However, they may not stop all the traffic. An opioid, which exerts its most significant analgesic action in the central nervous system (CNS), can address that traffic that gets to the dorsal horn. Thus, the use of an NSAID may have an opioid-sparing effect, resulting in lower opioid doses (with lower side effects) than if the opioid was used alone.

If the patient has a significant neuropathic pain, which is not due to inflammatory processes, but nervous system injury or disease, the antidepressant and antiepileptic medicines can be of great benefit. The antidepressant drugs, especially the older generation medicines, are of benefit when the pain is perceived as a constant pain, often described in terms of "burning," "stinging," or "prickly." If the pain is perceived as having a lancinating component, an anticonvulsant might work better than, or in addition to, and older generation antidepressant. Opioids rarely should be the first-line approach to neuropathic pain, but they can have significant use in carefully selected patients[21,22] and should be considered for patients who do not respond to, or cannot tolerate, antidepressant or anticonvulsant drugs.

The fourth principle is that all opioids cause side effects. The most serious acute side effect is respiratory depression. Respiratory depression from opioids is characterized by a respiratory pattern peculiar to opioids, typified by a marked slowing in respiratory rate, with deep, sighing breaths. This pattern can be altered, however, when other CNS depressants are contributing to respiratory depression. The risk factors for respiratory depression are an opioid-naïve state, minimal or no pain, old age, and concomitant administration of other drugs with CNS depressant properties. Fortunately, if opioids are judiciously titrated to analgesic effect, respiratory depression is rarely seen clinically. Also, especially in the setting of pain, tolerance to the respiratory depression effects of opioids occurs rapidly, often within a few days. Pain is also a powerful stimulus of respiratory drive.

Virtually every patient taking opioids for any time experiences constipation. Every patient for whom opioids are prescribed must also have a bowel regimen recommended. This regimen should include maintaining hydration, the use of stimulant laxatives, and good bowel hygiene. A common mistake in the setting of opioid-induced constipation is to recommend only stool softeners. While softeners can be useful as an adjunct therapy, they fail to provide any stimulation of bowel motility. Because opioids decrease bowel propulsive forces, stimulant laxatives are generally required. While high-fiber diets can be useful in maintaining bowel regularity in the general population, it is unwise to begin a high-fiber regimen in the setting of opioid-induced constipation, because this will increase the bulk of the stool, but will not increase propulsive action, because the opioids attenuate it. Unlike respiratory depression, tolerance to the constipating effect of opioids never develops reliably.

The fifth principle is that different classes of analgesics exert their effects through different mechanisms and, therefore, it may be advantageous to design a "balanced analgesic regimen" for an individual patient, not unlike the concept of balanced anesthesia in the operating environment where the anesthesiologist uses different medications to accomplish distinct, but complementary, pharmacologic effects in the patient. Thus, in the situation where the pain is thought to have primarily somatic genesis, the use of drugs such as NSAIDs that decrease peripheral sensitization (and therefore decrease the generation of nociceptive traffic) could be used, along with a local anesthetic, if clinically applicable (e.g., infiltration of skin before laminectomy incision) to diminish transmission of nociceptive traffic, along with an opioid to modulate the traffic that makes it into the dorsal horn. In the setting of a pain that is primarily neuropathic and has a constant burning quality, an older generation antidepressant may be a first-line therapy. Anticonvulsant drugs can often be helpful in the setting of neuropathic pain that has a lancinating quality. Both can be used to treat pains that have both features. As noted previously, opioids may be required to treat neuropathic pain effectively, often in addition to antidepressant or anticonvulsant drugs.

The sixth principle is to manage common comorbidities, such as insomnia. The National Sleep Foundation reports that one of the most common causes of insomnia is pain.[23] Virtually every person presenting with chronic pain also has insomnia. Sometimes, merely treating the pain effectively normalizes sleep. However, it is often advantageous to treat the insomnia primarily, instead of waiting for a secondary benefit of analgesic therapy. A person who is sleeping well will be more able to participate in rehabilitative and cognitive therapies than one who is sleep-deprived. The sedating, older antidepressants can be useful for this purpose. Trazodone, which is sedating but has no analgesic properties, has fewer antimuscarinic side effects than amitriptyline, but has the peculiar side effect of priapism. While this is rare, its presence should be actively sought. Most patients tolerate trazodone well, because of the relative lack of other side effects commonly seen with the older antidepressant drugs. The bioavailability of trazodone is positively affected by food, so to get the most consistent serum levels, it should be taken with some food. The dose of all antidepressant drugs should be gradually escalated, taking into account the elimination half-life, and allowing five half-lives between dose escalations to ensure that the new dose is being instituted after the patient has reached steady state on the previous dose. Timing of nocturnal doses of antidepressant drugs will also vary between patients, with most finding approximately 1 hour before intended bedtime to be optimal.

The seventh principle is compliance with prevailing laws, regulations, policies, and guidelines. Laws and regulations governing the prescribing of controlled substances are at two levels: federal and state. The federal laws and regulations (Comprehensive Drug Abuse Prevention and Control Act of 1970, 21 USC 801, et seq., and its enabling regulations, 21 CFR 1300-end) in essence set the "floor," while state laws set the "ceiling"; that is, the federal law and regulations dictate the minimum compliance level; state laws can be more restrictive (but not *less* restrictive) than federal law. Under federal law, controlled substances are classified into five classes or schedules. Schedule I drugs (C-I) have high abuse potential and no legitimate medical use. Drugs such as crack cocaine, heroin, and LSD are in schedule I. Medicines in schedule II (C-II) are drugs with significant abuse potential

that do have legitimate medical use, and include opioids such as fentanyl, hydromorphone, methadone, morphine, and oxycodone, and other medicines such as methylphenidate and phenmetrazine. Schedule III (C-III) drugs have less abuse potential than those in schedule II and include medicines such as hydrocodone-acetaminophen combinations, anabolic steroids, and dronabinol. Schedule IV (C-IV) drugs have even less abuse potential. Acetaminophen with codeine is the most common opioid in this class, which also contains the benzodiazepines. Schedule V (C-V) drugs have even less abuse potential, based primarily on the amount of opioid contained within the compounds. This class contains some of the antitussive and antidiarrheal drugs. Dispensing of the remainder of prescription, or so-called "legend," drugs is not as tightly controlled under federal law, requiring in most instances, only a valid prescription before dispensing to the consumer.

There are different federal regulations that apply to the different schedules of controlled substances. For example, the medicines in C-II cannot have refills designated and cannot be dispensed on the basis of oral prescription (except in certain emergency circumstances). C-III medicines can be refilled, but all refills must be dispensed within 6 months of the date of the original prescription. The medicines in C-III can also be dispensed by oral or telephone order from an authorized prescriber. Interestingly, there are no other time or quantity limits on the dispensing of controlled substances under federal law and regulation.

States, however, as mentioned, can be more restrictive in their laws and regulations than federal law and regulation. For example, emergency oral prescribing of C-II medicines is not allowed under any circumstances in Kentucky; prescriptions for C-II medicines expire after 72 hours in Oklahoma; and South Carolina has a quantity limit for C-II medicines. Some states have moved drugs into higher schedules than they are scheduled federally, for example, carisoprodol, an entity that is not scheduled federally, is a C-III in Georgia and a C-IV in Ohio.

In addition to state law and regulation, there can be guidance, policy, or regulation from the medical licensing board. It is imperative that the prescribing practitioner becomes familiar with the laws, regulations, and policies that prevail in the state in which they practice. A very useful resource for this material is the web site maintained by the Pain and Policy Studies Group at the University of Wisconsin.[17]

The final principle is simply this: rarely can patients be managed with a "cookie cutter" approach, because of the variables mentioned previously. Thus, it is important to individualize therapy in every case, taking into account the severity of pain, the type of pain, the predicted time-severity course of pain, the coexisting diseases, the other medications, the patient's history, and the prevailing laws.

SUMMARY

Most neurologic surgeons deal with pain on a regular basis, be it the reason for referral or as a postoperative phenomenon. Pain assessments are now considered standard of care. There are a number of different classes of medicines that provide analgesia. Some simple principles have been laid out in this chapter. The surgeon should become facile with a typical medicine in each class, and then expand their expertise to other members of the class. Familiarity with and practical application of the array of medications that have analgesic potential is essential to provide competent, effective, compassionate pain care.

REFERENCES

1. Bell GM, Schnitzer TJ. COX-2 inhibitors and other nonsteroidal anti-inflammatory drugs in the treatment of pain in the elderly. Clin Geriatr Med 17(3):489–502, 2001.
2. Jenkins CA, Bruera E. Nonsteroidal anti-inflammatory drugs as adjuvant analgesics in cancer patients. Palliative Med 13:183–196, 1999.
3. Bonnel RA, Villalba ML, Karowski CB, et al. Aseptic meningitis associated with rofecoxib. Arch Intern Med 162:713–715, 2002.
4. Barkin RL. Acetaminphen, aspirin, or ibuprofen in combination analgesic products. Am J Therapeutics 8:433–442, 2002.
5. McNeil Consumer Products. Regular Strength Tylenol® (acetaminophen) Tablets Package Insert in: Physician's Desk Reference. Montvale, NJ, Medical Economics, 2002.
6. Sharma S, Prasad A, Anand KS. Nonsteroidal anti-inflammatory drugs in the management of pain and inflammation: a basis for drug selection. Am J Ther 6:3–11, 1999.
7. Wolfe MM, Lichentenstein DR, Singh G. Gastrointestinal toxicity of nonsteroidal antiinflammatory drugs. N Engl J Med 340:1888–1899, 1999. [Erratum, N Engl J Med 341:548, 1999.]
8. Bombardier C, Laine L, Reicin A, et al. Comparison of upper gastrointestinal toxicity of rofecoxib and naproxen in patients with rheumatoid arthritis. N Engl J Med 343:1520–1528, 2000.
9. Stratton MS, Alberts DS. Current application of selective COX-2 inhibitors in cancer prevention and treatment. Oncology (Huntington) 16(5 Suppl 4):37–51, 2002.
10. Mukhergee D, Nissen SE, Topol EJ. Risk of cardiovascular events associated with selective COX-2 inhibitors. JAMA 286(8):954–959, 2001.
11. Fishbain DA. The association of chronic pain and suicide. Sem Clin Neuropsychiat 4(3):221–227, 1999.
12. Stewart DE. Hepatic adverse reactions associated with nefadozone. Can J Psychiat 47(4):375–377, 2002.
13. Virani A, Mailis A, Shapiro LE, et al. Drug interactions in human neuropathic pain pharmacology. Pain 73:3–13, 1997.
14. Rose MA, Kam PC. Gabapentin: pharmacology and its use in pain management. Anaesthesia 57(5):451–462, 2002.
15. Rice AS, Maton S. Postherpetic Neuralgia Study Group. Gabapentin in postherpetic neuralgia: a randomised, double blind, placebo controlled study. [Clinical Trial. Journal Article. Multicenter Study. Randomized Controlled Trial.] Pain 94(2):215–224, 2001.
16. Backonja M, Beydoun A, Edwards KR, et al. Gabapentin for the symptomatic treatment of painful neuropathy in patients with diabetes mellitus: a randomized controlled trial. JAMA 280(21):1831–1836, 1998.
17. University of Wisconsin Pain and Policy Studies Group. Database of State Laws, Regulations and Other Official Governmental Policies. Available at: www.medsch.wisc.edu/painpolicy/.
18. ASAM/AAPM/APS Consensus Document. Available at: www.pain-med.org/productpub/statements/pdfs/definition.pdf.
19. Portenoy RK. Opioid therapy for chronic nonmalignant pain: clinician's perspective. J Law Med Ethics 24:296–309, 1996.
20. Weissman DE, Haddox JD. Opioid pseudoaddiction: an iatrogenic syndrome. Pain 36(3):363–366, 1989.
21. Watson CP, Babul N. Efficacy of oxycodone in neuropathic pain: a randomized trial in postherpetic neuralgia. Neurology 50(6):1837–1841, 1998.
22. Gimbel JS, Richards R, Portenoy RK. Controlled-release oxycodone for pain in diabetic neuropathy: a randomized controlled trial. Neurology 60:927–934, 2003.
23. National Sleep Foundation. Common causes of insomnia. Available at: www.sleepfoundation.org/publications/sleepandpain.html#5.

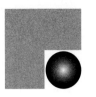

SECTION II

Pain Syndromes of Neurosurgical Importance

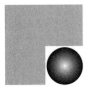

C H A P T E R 6

Myofascial Pain Syndromes

HUBERT L. ROSOMOFF, MD, D MED SCI, FAAPM,
AND RENEE STEELE-ROSOMOFF, BSN, MBA

The observation by Mixter and Barr in 1934 that proposed that the herniated disk would produce what we now call a *root syndrome* or *radiculopathy* was an attractive hypothesis whose validity appeared to be substantiated by surgical removal of the herniation with resultant resolution of the symptoms.[1] However, whether a herniated disk does, in fact, produce pain was questioned by Rosomoff in a signal publication in 1985.[2] This article was a reasoned set of observations combined with clinical and experimental evidence that supported the contention that herniated disks with nerve root compression do not always produce pain. Rather, soft tissue pathology can produce equivalent symptoms, and alternative nonsurgical methods provide successful treatment, even when manifest disk herniations or lumbar stenosis are present and are left uncorrected.

Some descriptions of patient histories with low back pain sound like the classic herniated disk, but could just as easily be representative of lumbar myofascial pain syndromes, in which pain distribution is identical and there is paucity of neurologic change.[3] The soft tissue examination demonstrates outstandingly painful, tender, or trigger points in the muscular system with limited motion in the back, hips, and legs, mimicking the herniated disk syndrome. Granted, the examination of the patient with a spinal disorder depends on a full assessment of neural function, but the examination cannot be concluded without a detailed examination of the soft tissues surrounding the spine, and in the lumbar area, the hips, and buttocks. Approximately 75% of the motion segment in the lower half of the body is through hip motion with the spine contributing 25%. As such, abnormality of muscular function in these areas must be clearly identified and treated, regardless of any necessity for operative intervention.

It is the premise of this chapter that disordered soft tissue structures are responsible for initiating biochemical alterations associated with hyperalgesia and chronic pain. These structures are extraspinal, both lumbar and cervical, in the surrounding paraspinal muscles, neck, shoulders, buttocks, hips, and legs. These peripheral sites and syndromes are treatable by alternative medical approaches, and treatment restores function and alleviates pain without the need for correcting the intraspinal pathologic entities that have been traditionally designated as the cause of pain and neurologic deficit. This biochemical process is called inflammation and may have both a central and peripheral component in which the related muscular groups become the target for dysfunction. Importantly, spinal pain must be distinguished from buttock and hip pain, which patients often describe to their physicians erroneously as being pain in the back (i.e., spinal pain). The history of pain with sitting and pain with weight bearing are the clues to direct the physician to examine the hips and buttocks with weight bearing such as standing and walking and, similarly, neck and shoulder pain must direct examination to the muscles in these areas, outside the spine.

Biochemically, cell membranes of the injured soft tissues break down to arachidonic acid, which is then biosynthesized into prostaglandins, thromboxane, monohydroxy fatty acids, and leukotrienes.[4–6] These individually and collectively are involved in the reactions to injury, producing hyperalgesia, vascular instability, and an inflammatory reaction, with loss of function.[7] The symptoms produced depend on the relative proportions of these substances at the site of injury. For example, prostaglandins produce vasodilatation, and the area feels warm. Thromboxane produces vasoconstriction, and the part feels cold. The leukotrienes produce inflammation leading to the development of focal tender or trigger points. These substances, when interacted with polypeptides, such as bradykinin and histamine, or in the presence of excessive mechanical stimulation, create a nociceptive impulse transmitted to the central nervous system.[8] These chemical reactions are inhibited by steroids, aspirin, and related products, effects that then provide a rationale for pharmacologic treatment.[9] Even more interesting, however, is the reversal of these same phenomena by focal physical forms of therapy, such as application of ice, which, parenthetically, has been well established as a method for limiting or averting tissue reaction to injury.[10] Vigorous activation of the musculoskeletal system also limits the reaction to injury because enkephalins are released at two to three times the baseline levels. This response serves as an endogenous pain control system.[11] It follows, then, that therapeutic application of these basic principles should lead the physician to prescribe the use of ice and vigorous exercise as alternatives to the traditional trials of bed rest, analgesic, and muscle relaxants.

There further ensues a number of secondary effects, such as sustained muscle contraction, referred pain, and autonomic reflex change. These phenomena, in fact, are major components of the chronic state. The muscle contraction is not reflex, as was once thought. It is, in fact, a chemical phenomenon, wherein the traumatized muscle releases calcium ions that combine with adenosinetriphosphatase to create an uncontrolled contraction, leading to pain, tenderness, vasoconstriction, and decreased blood supply, resulting in an energy-deficit contracture.[12] It is this inflammatory reaction and accompanying decreased muscle length that produce the restricted range of joint movement and tendon and fascial shortening. The result is functional disability and chronicity. Moreover, the autonomic counterpart can be so extreme as to be mistaken for reflex sympathetic dystrophy or complex regional pain disorders. Of further clinical interest is that immobilization, a traditional mode of treatment, and emotional tension are prime contributors to the production of disability; hence, the conclusion that acute treatment programs should avoid immobilization, and chronicity may be prevented by incorporating alternative relaxation and behavioral modification techniques to eliminate tension and stress when these elements are recognized.

Physicians frequently do not seek or do not report in detail abnormal movements of the back; soft tissue abnormalities; restricted ranges of motion in the neck, back, hips, or legs; or the presence of muscle tenderness and/or trigger points as might be seen with myofascial syndromes. To this end, it is mandatory that a soft tissue examination be done and all musculoskeletal abnormalities be identified. This is particularly important because myofascial syndromes may masquerade as disk syndromes. When done thoroughly, a comprehensive physical examination can reveal multiple areas of tenderness, trigger points, and restricted ranges of motion in the neck, back, hips, and legs. These can perpetuate mechanical dysfunction, continued strain, muscle fatigue, and pain. The difference, with respect to restricted ranges of motion and muscle tightness in the chronic state, is the ease of reversibility during the acute phase and the extreme difficulty of stretching contracted painful muscles in the chronic state. Even when this is recognized, many physical medicine facilities instruct their therapists to stop when stretching reaches the point of discomfort; when, in fact, stretching is only productive when the well-trained therapist pushes beyond the pain to achieve gradual and progressive release and lengthening of the pathologic structures.

COMMON MYOFASCIAL SYNDROMES: LOWER QUADRANTS

Quadratus Lumborum Syndrome

Pain usually begins with a quick, stooping movement when the torso is twisted, as in gardening and scrubbing the floor. Superficial pain is perceived at the iliac crest or greater trochanteric area, sometimes in the lower abdomen and groin. There also may be pain deep over the sacroiliac joint area and in the mid buttock. Symptoms are manifest with walking, twisting, stooping, turning in bed, and rising from a chair. Coughing or sneezing aggravates the pain, so that this phenomenon is not a necessary sign of free fragment disk herniation. Pain is felt in climbing steps, and there may be severe pain at night that awakens the patient. The examination finds guarded movements when walking, lying, or rising. There is a pelvic tilt when standing. There is limited flexion and extension in the spine with paraspinal tenderness. There sometimes is a leg length discrepancy, and the radiologic studies may show a small hemipelvis (Fig. 6-1).

Iliopsoas Syndrome

Iliopsoas syndrome is associated with the quadratus lumborum syndrome. This syndrome also may produce ipsilateral paraspinal pain or anterior thigh pain, or both. Gait is carried out with external rotation and flexion at the hip. Posture is stooped, with a flattened lordotic curve, and extension is limited due to contracture of the iliopsoas muscle. There may be tenderness deep in the femoral triangle, as well as deep in the pelvis (Fig. 6-2).

Gluteal Muscle Syndromes

Gluteal muscle syndromes produce leg extension pain in the sciatic distribution. The gluteus maximus produces pain in the buttock, coccyx, medial sacrum, and lateral iliac crest; the gluteus medius produces pain more deeply in the midbuttock and posterior thigh area; and the gluteus minimus produces pain in the lower buttock, posterior thigh, and calf or lateral thigh and leg radiating toward the ankle. It is easy to see how these syndromes can be confused with so-called classic descriptions of L5 or S1 radiculopathies (Fig. 6-3).

Piriformis Syndrome

Piriformis syndrome produces low back and sacroiliac-type pain with discomfort deep in the buttock, hip, posterior thigh, and, again, sciatic referred extension pain down the leg. There is tenderness over the sciatic notch and weak abduction and external rotation at the hip. The diagnosis is best made by feeling the tight piriformis muscle by way of a rectal examination, but this diagnosis can be often inferred from the clinical history, and treatment is similar to that of the gluteal syndromes (Fig. 6-4). It is the gluteal and piriformis syndromes that produce restrictive ranges of motion about the hips, which contribute to weight-bearing pain. These abnormalities are seen in nearly all of the chronic low back disorders. They are uncommonly sought and uncommonly diagnosed.

A simple way to demonstrate hip restriction is with a modified form of the Patrick's test. The patient lies on his back and the thigh is externally rotated at the hip. The knee is flexed and the ankle is placed just below the patella of the opposite knee. The distance from the lateral edge of the knee to the table is measured. The normal distance is 1 to 3 inches. If greater than 3 inches, there is a serious abnormality of hip rotation (Fig. 6-5). Many years of reviewing recorded examinations for low back disorders attests to physicians and therapists failure to record such an observation, which emphasizes the need for understanding this mechanism for low back pain and, beyond that, its treatment. Unless these mechanical impairments of posture, gait, movement, and weight displacement are addressed therapeutically, the patient will remain in pain. Moreover, this treatment should be combined with a functional restoration program to prevent recurrent pain and disability.

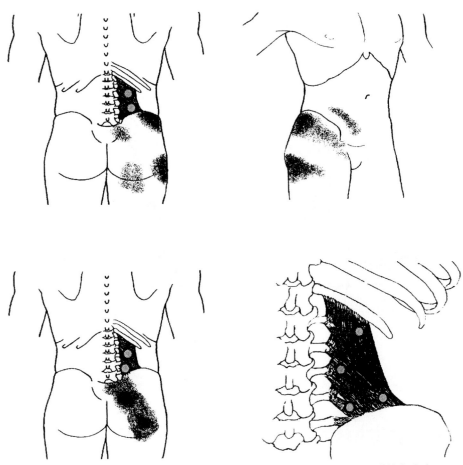

FIGURE 6-1 Quadratus lumborum muscle. (✱) represents tender/trigger point; *solid/stippled areas* represent pain pattern.

Rectus Abdominis Syndrome

Rectus abdominis syndrome is seen with a protuberant abdomen and soft musculature, giving rise to pain in the low and mid back areas. Examination of the abdomen will elicit pain posteriorly when the origin and insertion of the recti muscles are pressed with elevation of the extended lower extremities below and elevation of the shoulders above (Fig. 6-6).

COMMON MYOFASCIAL SYNDROMES: UPPER QUADRANTS

Levator Scapulae Syndromes

Levator scapulae syndromes present with a stiff neck and referred pain to the root of the neck, scapula, and shoulder. This is often caused by sustained shoulder elevation, cramped position, fatigue, and overuse as with tennis, swimming, or concentrated spectatorship. The symptoms are a stiff neck with pain and decreased range of motion, particularly in lateral flexion and there may be trigger points in the lateral trapezius muscle or at the angle of the scapula (Fig. 6-7).

Rhomboid Syndrome

Rhomboid syndrome produces pain between the shoulders with referred pain to the medial scapula and suprascapular areas. This is caused by poor posture, particularly now seen with prolonged use of computers. The symptoms are that of "tired shoulders" and back pain. There are tender points along the medial scapula up to the angle of the scapula (Fig. 6-8).

Supraspinatus Syndrome

In supraspinatus syndrome, pain is experienced at the shoulder and posterior arm, often confused with a pronator cuff tear. The pain is referred to the mid deltoid, lateral arm, forearm, and elbow. This is caused by carrying heavy objects with the arm hanging or with lifting overhead. Symptoms are pain on abduction of the shoulder, adduction of the arm behind the back, and difficulty reaching overhead. Women commonly have this syndrome when putting up their hair or fastening their brassiere. Trigger points are found in the supraspinatus muscles and suprascapular notch (Fig. 6-9).

Infraspinatus Syndrome

Pain is in the shoulder and lateral arm with reference to the shoulder joint, lateral arm and forearm, lateral hand, posterior

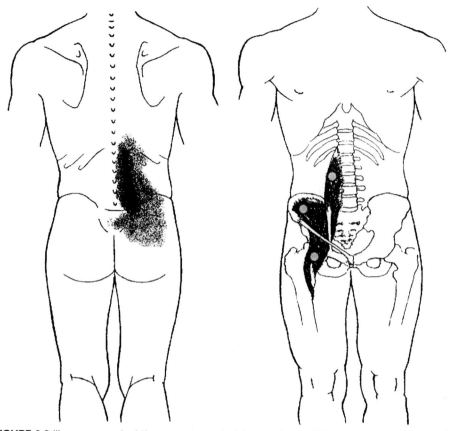

FIGURE 6-2 Iliopsoas muscle. (✳) represents tender/trigger point; *solid/stippled areas* represent pain pattern.

cervical areas, and medial scapula. This is caused by an overload in reaching up and posteriorly. Symptoms are an inability to reach the back pocket, fastening the bra, combing hair, and brushing teeth, and this is associated with the supraspinatus, teres minor, deltoid, biceps, and pectoral myofascial syndromes (Fig. 6-10).

Biceps Brachii, Brachialis Syndromes

Pain is perceived in the anterior shoulder over the bicipital tendon radiating toward the thumb with referred pain in these areas and in the suprascapular area. This is caused by heavy lifting with the arm flexed and supinated at the elbow. Symptoms are restricted motion of the shoulder with numbness and paresthesias in the first and second digits. Tender points are over the bicipital tendon and distal third of the muscles. This is commonly confused with a C6 radiculopathy (Fig. 6-11).

SECONDARY EFFECTS

Reduced physical functional capacities and performance may lead an individual to become depressed and anxious, particularly when he or she has a nonadaptive personality style. Fear may become a formidable barrier if the perception is that a permanent injury has occurred that, by activation, may produce

further loss of function. To this can be added the problems of dependencies, such as narcotics, barbiturates, and muscle relaxants, supplemented by alcohol. Patients also become dependent on back braces, regional injections, stimulators, and other such equipment, further reinforcing their perceptions that they are seriously disabled. Marital problems, role reversal, and disruption of the family unit may also occur. Low self-esteem, guilt, loss of motivation, and often, suicidal ideation are seen in these patients. Loss of identification is not limited to the shift in the patient's position in the family circle; it is compounded by a loss of vocational identification for those previously employed. Patients become more focused on their pain; they feel helpless, hopeless, and are said to be disability oriented. Social withdrawal takes place, and patients become isolated from family, friends, and previous activities. Prolonged immobilization compounds the pain-depression cycle. Physical, behavioral, and socioeconomic factors compound one another, and the family circle commonly reinforces the ensuing disability by subjugating their own needs while assuming the patient's responsibilities. They, too, become frightened, angry, and protective. The progression of events has now evolved into major behavioral reactions. Repeated unsuccessful attempts to relieve the patient of his or her pain and mental burdens through a series of unrewarding treatments, including bed rest, traction, ineffective physical therapy, interventional injections, drugs, radiography, myelography, and unsuccessful surgery, result in a fearful, untrusting, uncooperative patient. This iatrogenic failure frustrates the physician, who then advises the patient to

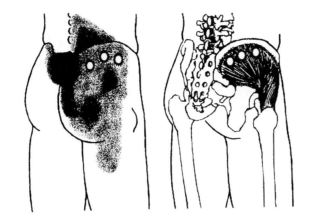

GLUTEUS MINIMUS

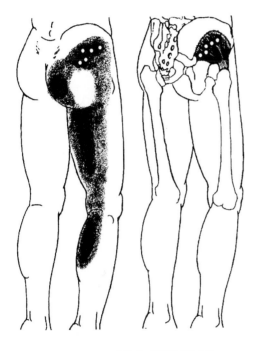

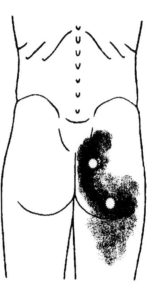

GLUTEUS MEDIUS   GLUTEUS MAXIMUS

FIGURE 6-3 Gluteal muscle. (✻) represents tender/trigger point; *solid/stippled areas* represent pain pattern.

seek psychiatric help because he or she has not responded to prolonged medical or surgical treatment, further implying that "it's all in the patient's head." If the patient is receiving workers' compensation, an employer may be compounding the issue by an uncaring attitude, unsympathetic pose, or threat to fire the worker and/or refusal to modify the job to accommodate the injury. Moreover, a well-intentioned lawyer may discourage the patient concerning rehabilitation efforts and a weary insurance adjuster, who has authorized many forms of treatment approaches in hopes of bringing the claim to closure, also begins to doubt the patient's claim of unsuccessful treatment. The overall result is a patient who now has chronic pain and is impaired physically; is weak and inactive; is drug- and alcohol-dependent, hostile, untrusting, and frightened; believes

he or she is helpless and hopeless; is unable to live independently; has marital and sexual problems; is anxious, depressed, and angry; has no job and no motivation; and is disabled and disability oriented. Where does one start to treat such a complex person?

TREATMENT OVERVIEW

The management of the back-injured individual is far from simple. An early referral to an experienced medical provider may prevent the simple lumbar sprain from becoming a

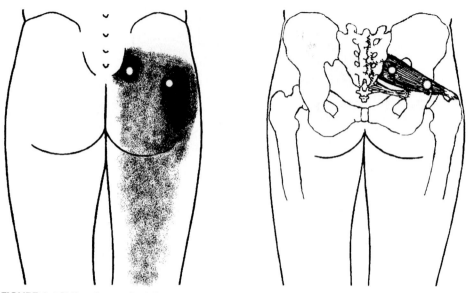

FIGURE 6-4 Piriformis muscle. (✱) represents tender/trigger point; *solid/stippled areas* represent pain pattern.

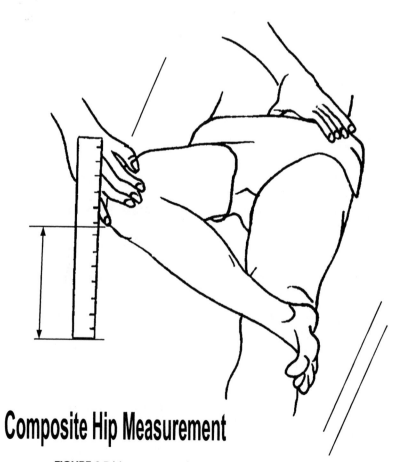

Composite Hip Measurement

FIGURE 6-5 Measurement of composite range of hip motion.

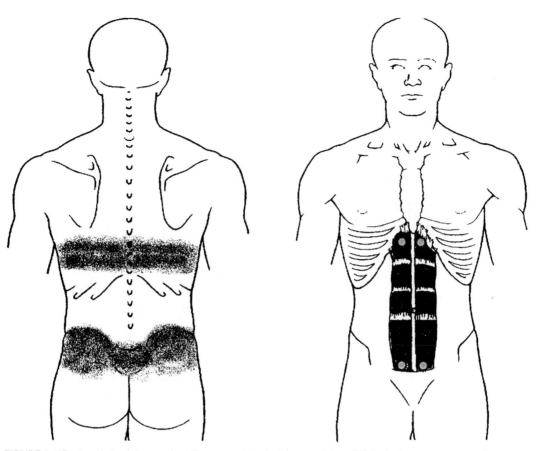

FIGURE 6-6 Rectus abdominis muscle. (✱) represent tender/trigger point; *solid/stippled areas* represent pain pattern.

catastrophe. Moreover, this early referral may avoid the behavioral consequences that are prone to develop, thus preventing chronicity.

The patient with failed back syndrome or low back loser is a victim of the system, and the cost for early multidisciplinary treatment is less than the cost that the victim exacts if the loser profile develops.[13] The treatment system, therefore, should be capable of identifying these problems early, and then deal with them in a comprehensive way. These problems can be categorized as sensory, perceptual, psychologic, psychosocial, and environmental.

The immediate natural reaction of humans to injury and pain is rest or immobilization. Persistent immobility increases pain; causes disuse, atrophy, and weakness; slows healing; and demineralizes bone, resulting in functional disability. Conversely, activity increases endorphin levels, which becomes an endogenous source of pain control, decreasing pain and facilitating healing. Furthermore, working through pain produces the phenomenon of stress-induced analgesia.[14]

Stress-induced analgesia is a keystone to successful treatment. If stress, that is, pain, is applied continuously without interruption, pain transmission will cease. In simplistic terms, it is like an overload to an electrical system, which blows the fuse or circuit breaker. The patient is pain-free for a period, which is a golden opportunity to apply usually pain-provoking therapy, like muscle stretching, before the circuit resets. Coupled with exercise-induced endorphin release, treatment can be advanced, but the patient and the treating

professional must overcome the natural fear of pain, which is frequently equated with injury.

Most therapists are taught to limit or halt treatment when the patient complains of pain, which, by this concept, is when treatment should begin. To progress functionally, it is necessary to activate muscles intensively 8 to 10 hours per day. Not only is there a decrease in pain, but there is also an effect on depression. A sense of well being is induced, mobility is increased, and analgesic intake is decreased. Importantly, drug withdrawal is eased, and detoxification can be achieved quickly with a minimum of side effects. With this conceptual background, let us discuss the role of the pain specialist and pain center.

The data of the usual clinical course show that 74% of the initial group of patients with nonspecific "spinal" pain have good pain control and can return to their previous productive lives (Fig. 6-12). Twenty-five percent, however, experience persistent symptoms beyond the first 4 weeks. These individuals should be reevaluated, specifically for myofascial syndromes. Plain radiographs may now be indicated to be certain that an occult lesion has not been overlooked and a sedimentation rate is appropriate to rule out inflammation or infection. Conservative measures, particularly physical therapy, should be pursued in a more intense fashion. Occupational therapy may be added to review those factors that may be influencing the outcome; that is, proper body mechanics and work-site factors that come under the aegis of ergonomics.

During the next 3 weeks, 9% of patients spontaneously recover, leaving 16% with pain and disability. If this process

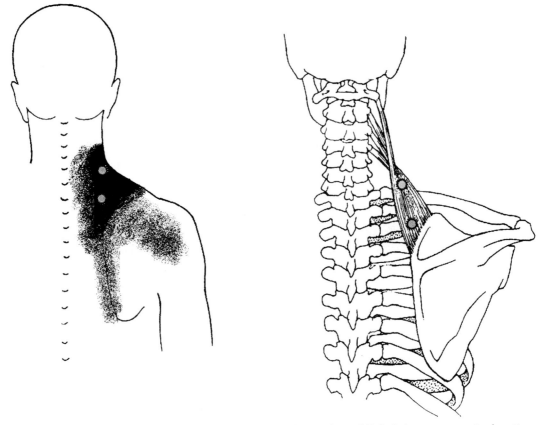

FIGURE 6-7 Levator scapulae muscle. (✳) represents tender/ trigger point; *solid/stippled areas* represent pain pattern.

does not resolve within the next 3 weeks, then consultation with a specialist is indicated. This should be with a musculoskeletal expert who could be a spine surgeon or pain medicine specialist to identify, specifically, myofascial syndromes that may have been overlooked or never treated, or other psychosocial barriers to recovery. It is important that the consultants understand the rehabilitation model, because the so-called minimally invasive techniques that are now commonly being applied are usually unproductive or not indicated.

In the period from 7 weeks to 3 months, another 4% of patients return to work, leaving 12% who remain symptomatic. Although originally proposed that a multidisciplinary team, which should include a neurosurgeon, reevaluate the patient at 3 months to include the psychological aspects of pain and ergonomic assessment, it is clear now that the 7-week mark is probably the better time to start this process, because it becomes more cost effective if done earlier. The process at 3 months results in another 5% of patients who return to work, leaving 7% of the original population with now chronic pain.[15] It should be pointed out that none of the task forces that has studied this problem have been willing to deal with the patient with chronic pain, but this is a most costly group of patients who cannot be ignored. It is time that they be evaluated by a multidisciplinary pain center that is comprehensive in its approach.

Treatment goals of multidisciplinary pain facilities have been stated as follows: reduction or elimination of pain; reduction or elimination of medication intake; correction of physical abnormalities, like posture, gait, and range of motion; reduction of psychiatric or psychological impairment, or both; education of chronic pain patients in the roles that emotions, behavior, and attitudes play in improvement of activities of daily living; improvement of level of function in social, familial, and household roles; improvement or restoration, or both, of strength and functional status; restoration of vocational and avocational role functions; and education on the ways of maintaining rehabilitation gains and avoidance of reinjury.[16] Initially, the efficacy of multidisciplinary pain facilities in treating chronic pain was questioned. Evidence from well-designed outcome studies, however, indicates that multidisciplinary pain facilities do return chronic pain patients to work.[17] The increased rates of return to work are due to treatment and the benefits of treatment are not temporary.[18]

Physicians should differentiate clearly between acute pain and chronic pain.[19] Chronic pain is a continuous noxious input, like that of acute pain, but modulated and compounded by the prolonged or recurrent nature of the chronic state and complicated by a multitude of economic and psychosocial factors.

Patients with chronic pain perceive their pain as a disability limiting their functional status.[20,21] Drug abuse, dependence, and addiction are reported in the range of 3.2% to 18.9%. Although these diagnoses are reported in a significant percentage of patients with chronic pain, little evidence proves that addictive behaviors are common.[22] At issue is whether patients with physician-perceived drug problems are best

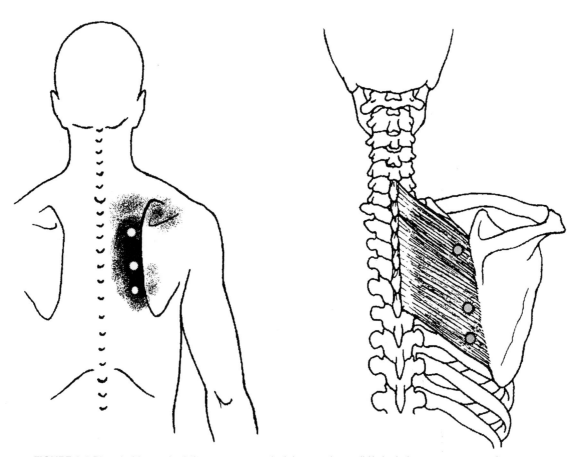

FIGURE 6-8 Rhomboid muscle. (✱) represents tender/trigger point; *solid/stippled areas* represent pain pattern.

treated at pain treatment facilities or drug and alcohol treatment facilities. Detoxification in pain treatment facilities where simultaneous pain treatment is available appears to be the better route. Physicians' perception of drug problems, therefore, is an indication for pain treatment facility referral.

Patients with chronic pain being treated at pain centers have been reported to experience a wide range of psychiatric conditions. These include depression, drug dependence abuse and/or addiction, anxiety, irritability and/or anger, suicidal or homicidal ideation, and memory and/or concentration problems. These data are supported by epidemiologic community studies, which indicate a strong relationship between chronic pain and depression.

The issue of depression is important, not only as a potential target symptom for treatment, but also because it is possible that coping strategies may differ in depressed chronic pain patients. Patients with chronic pain may over-rely on passive avoidance coping activities in response to life stresses, including pain. These coping activities may be a function of depressed mood.[13] It is likely that faulty coping activities are best addressed in a pain center setting, where patients can be taught to improve their coping abilities. Therefore, severe depression is an indication for pain treatment facility referral, but a facility with on-site psychiatric treatment should be chosen.

Failed back syndrome has been described as *persistent or recurrent back pain, sciatica, or other impairments that exist after back surgery or noninterventional treatment.*[23] Failed back syndrome can occur in as many as 40% of post-operative patients, and this syndrome represents the reason for a large number of pain center admissions. It is also claimed that these patients are characterized by drug misuse, reactive psychiatric problems, and unappreciated psychiatric and psychosocial problems that existed before surgery. Reoperations on this group of patients usually meet with limited success. The second operation may be only successful for 40% to 50% of patients, whereas the third and fourth operations are successful for 20% to 30% and 10% to 20% of patients, respectively.

It has been demonstrated that some of these patients have disturbed neck, shoulder, back, or hip muscles and loss of muscular support. These abnormalities may lead to increased biomechanical strain that results in disability. Improvement with pain facility treatment for patients who have had a number of surgical procedures can be as successful as for patients without surgeries.[13] Patients with one or more unsuccessful neck or back surgeries are candidates for pain treatment facility referral, especially if behavior abnormalities or drug problems, or both, are present.

Some patients who are thought to have surgically remediable conditions sometimes refuse or are denied surgery for medical reasons. These patients can be placed into a physically supervised exercise and conditioning problem. At 1-year follow-up, 84% of all such patients are improved.[24] Thus, a patient who refuses surgery or is a candidate for surgery, but has risky concomitant medical problems, should be considered alternatively for possible pain facility referral.

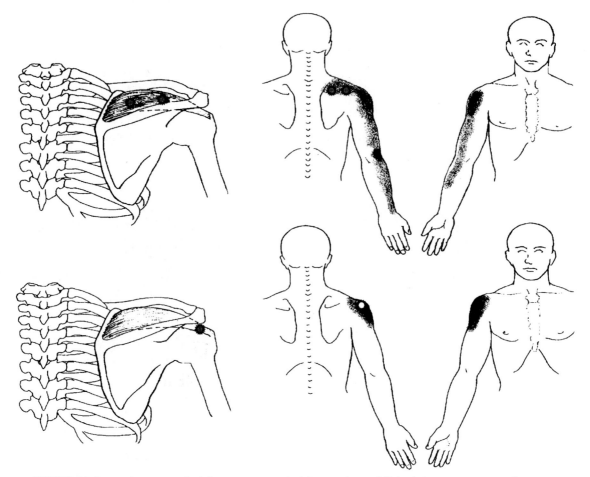

FIGURE 6-9 Supraspinatus muscle. (✱) represents tender/trigger point; *solid/stippled areas* represent pain pattern.

A particular body of literature alleges that many patients experiencing chronic low back pain cannot be assigned a diagnosis conforming to a specifically defined disease. The lack of "objective" physical findings in such patients has led to the designation of chronic intractable benign pain. This type of pain is thought to be a central phenomenon, which is made worse by sensory input. Poor adaptation makes pain the focus of the patient's life. Patients so classified are often evaluated for behavioral abnormalities and often become candidates for the diagnosis of psychogenic pain. Presumably, no physical findings indicative of an organic dysfunctional or pathologic process are present. Such a presumption is not supported by facts.

In a study that addressed this issue, 90 patients with back pain were isolated from a group of 283 patients with mixed chronic pain who conformed to the diagnosis of chronic intractable benign pain.[25] None had neurologic deficit; all radiologic studies were unremarkable. Almost all (97.6%) had tender or trigger points and multiple other non-neurologic abnormalities. Seven categories of abnormalities were identified: tender or trigger points, decreased range of motion, nondermatomal sensory abnormalities, contracted muscles, abnormal gait, miscellaneous physical signs, and decreased range of motion at the hips. Patients had an average of three of the seven categoric findings led by myofascial syndromes and other soft tissue changes. Almost one half (45.6) had non-

dermatomal sensory changes; this condition is physiologic dysfunction, not malingering or hysteria.

The investigators made the following conclusions:

1. Patients with chronic intractable benign pain without objective findings can be shown regularly to have musculoskeletal disorders.
2. Myofascial syndromes are the source of nociception in these patients.
3. Criteria for the specific diagnosis of myofascial pain syndrome are demonstrable in 97.6% of the patients.
4. Multiple physical findings (average = 3.1) are usual.
5. Myofascial abnormalities are objective findings.

THE MULTIDISCIPLINARY TEAM

The Rosomoff Comprehensive Pain and Rehabilitation Center has more than 80 full-time personnel in six divisions:

1. Neurologic surgery service primarily as consultants
2. Physical medicine and rehabilitation directing the application of all physical medicine modalities and treatments
3. Nurses trained in rehabilitation and behavior modification who monitor patient progress and serve as case managers

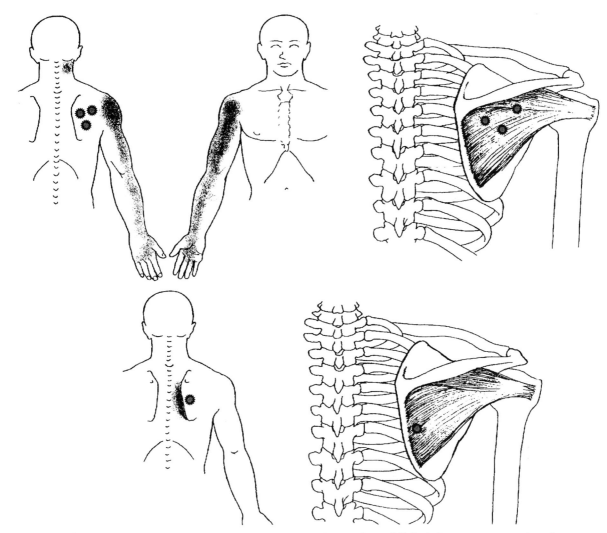

FIGURE 6-10 Infraspinatus muscle. (✱) represents tender/trigger point; *solid/stippled areas* represent pain pattern.

4. A behavioral division, which has psychiatrists and psychologists who are assigned as counselors to each patient and who administer biofeedback, behavioral modification, or other applicable techniques
5. Vocational rehabilitation specialists who evaluate and direct job placement
6. An ergonomic division that stimulates the job and adapts the patient or work site, or both, while computing daily achievement goals

The average program, including the evaluation, lasts 4 weeks on an inpatient or outpatient basis, or a combination thereof. Inpatient status is preferred for difficult, complicated cases, but it is not always possible, as dictated by reimbursement status. It should be understood clearly that, in a tertiary referral center, few "simple," early primary care–type patients are seen. We receive the most complex, "court of last resort," salvage cases.

Physical Medicine and Rehabilitation

Physical medicine has the goal of restoring body function to normal, or its closest equivalent. Because myofascial contracture is a common denominator in the low back disorders that we see, the first phase of management is muscle stretching and restoration of full range of motion in the joints of the hips, back, and lower extremities. This therapy includes gait retraining, because of acquired maladaptive patterns; postural adjustment; proper use of effective modalities; elimination of adjunct equipment, when possible; strength and endurance conditioning, with instruction of body mechanics; prevention of reinjury; vocational and avocational requirements; sexual counseling; and, lastly, a home maintenance program.

Modalities, when evaluated as unimodal therapy, may not show clear-cut evidence of effectiveness. They appear to be useful, however, in combination, which makes statistical evaluation more difficult. Nonetheless, scientific rationale exists for some. Ice application with lowering of temperature is known to decrease nerve conduction to the point of anesthesia, and the inflammatory reaction is contained with a reduction of chronic changes.[26–28] To be effective, the body part should be packed in ice for periods in excess of 30 minutes. Heat seems to soften muscle preparatory to stretching, but is not therapeutic. An adjunct vapo-coolant helps to block the stretch reflex and makes lengthening easier.

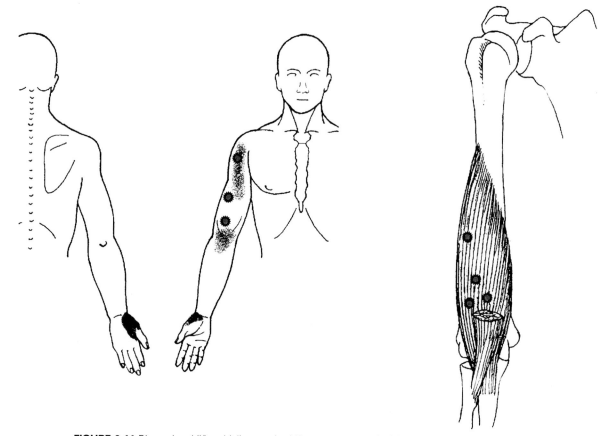

FIGURE 6-11 Biceps brachii/brachialis muscle. (✱) represents tender/trigger point; *solid/stippled areas* represent pain pattern.

Traction is useful for certain specific indications. Conceptually, we apply traction to stretch muscle groups, not to distract the spine or to release nerve entrapment. We do not believe that distraction can be effected with the weights that we use, and the principle of entrapment is not tenable. Therefore, traditional pelvic or leg traction is not used. Gravity traction is applied for iliopsoas contractures in the patient with a spinal flexion deformity or inability to extend the back, or both.

Autotraction is an important technique that allows three-dimensional placement of the spine by rotating, flexing, or extending the unit as the patient imposes his or her own body force by pushing and pulling.[29] The self-applied force of autotraction does not exceed that which could be potentially injurious, but it releases tight paraspinal muscles. Autotraction does not decompress the nerve root, as was the concept of its originators.[30,31]

Trigger point desensitization is indicated. Liberal use of ice is the preferred method of treatment, but like the other modalities (i.e., ultrasound, electrical stimulation, and neuroprobe), it is only an adjunct to stretching. Heat and neuromuscular massage also are used, but, again, as adjunct treatment to enhance muscle lengthening and supple movement.

Transcutaneous electrical neural stimulation (TENS) is used infrequently and only in patients who are TENS responders and who can be assisted with a difficult detoxification for which the TENS gives short-term relief as the drugs are withdrawn. TENS is not given to the patient beyond this period; it has no role in long-term therapy. Conceptually, we are aiming for resolution of the painful disorder by physical restoration, not by an attempt at distraction or at coping by learning to live with pain.

Passive, then active, range-of-motion exercises are essential, especially around the hips and, in particular, the hip rotators. Hamstring lengthening is another mandate, because hamstring tightness affects back movement. Full ranges of back motion are the ultimate goal, so flexion and extension exercises are instituted without prejudice for the proponents of either type. Both flexion and extension exercises are necessary.

A full compendium of exercises is used, as described in any standard physical therapy textbook, to establish full ranges of motion through the lower body with supple muscles and fluid movement. As this is being achieved, muscle strengthening and cardiovascular conditioning are added to the regimen with monitoring of those patients who have associated medical problems.

Movement therapy is an interesting adjunct because patients with pain often perform to music when, seemingly, they cannot move their bodies on command. When a specific muscle group is weak, functional electrical neuromuscular stimulation and muscle reeducation are implemented.[32] This technique can produce rapid and dramatic increases in muscle recruitment patterns and muscle strength, and foot-drop braces can be discarded.

Occupational therapy concentrates on body mechanics. Sitting, standing, walking, lifting, and driving tolerances are

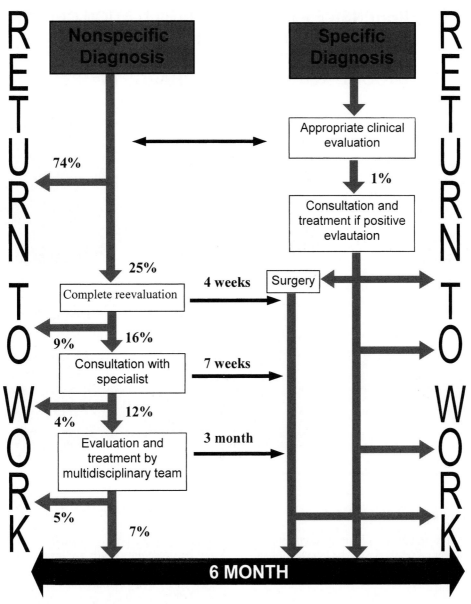

FIGURE 6-12 Critical path for the management of low back pain.

established and brought to normal levels of function. Pacing of activity is taught. Assistive equipment is used infrequently and only on specific indication. Energy-saving techniques are taught. Posture and gait are corrected because most patients are found to have poor posture and maladaptive gaits and fall due to contractures around the hips, knees, and ankles.

Activities of daily living are reviewed for home and work, looking for the proper use of body mechanics, with correction as needed. Driving evaluation is conducted and proper transfers are taught. Diversionary activities are reviewed and eye, hand, and leg coordination and tolerances are established. Education and vocational goals are set and job simulation is begun.

Job simulation and work conditioning are other concepts that we introduced to pain center management in the late 1970s. This is the ultimate goal of achievement for the working-aged group, but it does not exclude students or the elderly, who receive instruction for their individual needs. With respect to these problems, the occupational and physical therapists team with vocational counselors and ergonomists to develop the treatment plan.

Vocational Rehabilitation

Vocational rehabilitation counselors analyze factors of employment, such as age, education level, work history, supervisory and peer relationships, job requirements, job skills, transferable skills, date and circumstances of injury, return to work since injury and, most importantly, motivation, compliance, and job satisfaction. This type of program cannot be successful without the patient's full attention or effort. If the patient does not give both, the patient will be discharged from treatment. The vocational goal is full

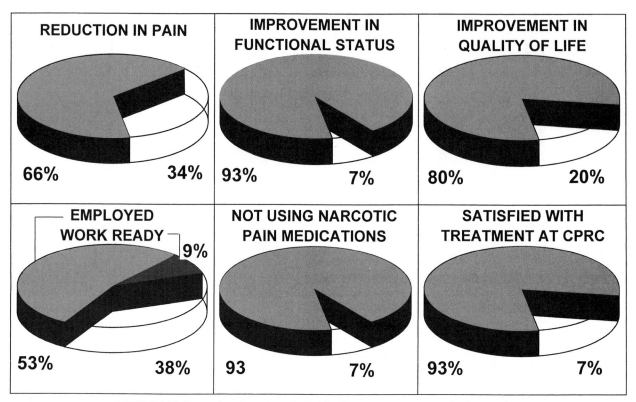

COMPREHENSIVE PAIN AND REHABILITATION CENTER
PROGRAM EVALUATION SYSTEM
November 1989 through March 1999
OUTCOME RESULTS AT DISCHARGE (N=1831)

REDUCTION IN PAIN
66%   34%

IMPROVEMENT IN FUNCTIONAL STATUS
93%   7%

IMPROVEMENT IN QUALITY OF LIFE
80%   20%

EMPLOYED WORK READY — 9%
53%   38%

NOT USING NARCOTIC PAIN MEDICATIONS
93   7%

SATISFIED WITH TREATMENT AT CPRC
93%   7%

FIGURE 6-13 Comprehensive pain and rehabilitation center program evaluation results.

functional activity and return to previous employment. Retraining is recommended rarely. Even the heaviest physical activity capacities have been achievable in most patients.

Behavioral Management

Behavioral management is a key issue. Nearly 20% of Americans experience one or more emotional disorders, so the patient with low back injury may be harboring such a problem. Our study of pain population patients found 62.5% to have anxiety disorders and 56.2% to have current depression.[33] The conditions were commingled with other less prevalent disorders. Only 5.3% of 283 patients were found to have no psychiatric diagnosis.

This study questions the criteria for the diagnosis of psychogenic pain. Pure psychogenic pain is probably rare when defined as a psychological factor directly leading to pain. However, all pain, as perceived by the patient, is real, regardless of cause. Most bodily pain is a combination of factors (e.g., physical stimuli and mental events). Mental and emotional states may be from a situation arising out of circumstances of the moment, from a background of personal experiences with pain from personality characteristics and/or the impact of prolonged intractable pain.

Behavioral analysis considers compliance, achievement level before injury activity level after injury, functional capacities, anxiety, depression, personality disorders, marital status, role reversal, and family history. Psychological services offer biofeedback and relaxation training. Group and family therapy deal with social interactions, return to environment, employment, and disability versus wellness with an emphasis on function, not pain.

Individual counseling is given when needed for anxiety, depression, fear of withdrawal, and poor coping skills, including sexual counseling. Every patient has an assigned counselor who monitors daily progress and reinforces the goal of physical restoration. Relaxation training includes coping approaches, muscle reeducation, meditation and distraction, guided imagery, autosuggestion, hypnosis, and tape supplements, which enhance live therapy. Stress management is incorporated into the behavioral sessions.

Weekly family groups explore the goals of the patient with the spouse or other family members. How to respond to pain without fear is discussed. Communication is an important subject. The roles of the various family members are defined, including distribution and responsibility. Experiences and frustrations are shared. These sessions facilitate the return to home, hopefully to an environment that now fosters wellness, not disability.

Biofeedback may be a pain control method, but we use it as a muscle tension and relaxation technique. Surface electromyographic biofeedback is used to regulate muscle tension, especially when an activity may, by experience, have been pain-provoking. Reduction of muscle tension correlates well with reduction of pain.[34]

The behavioral staff regulates tapering from drugs. As stated earlier, this process is carried out rapidly while pursuing intense activation. Endorphin release helps ameliorate withdrawal, and symptoms are generally minimal.

Ergonomics

In the early 1980s, industrial engineering and ergonomics were introduced into the pain center.[35] Ergonomics studies the worker in his or her environment, trying to match the physical capabilities to the industrial task. This process may require limited designing and redesigning of the workplace and the tools that are used. The goal is to condition the worker with regard to strength, posture, and flexibility, while eliminating fatigability.

The engineers see the human body as a machine, working with levers and acting as a mechanical crane. Proper lifting dictates carrying the weight close to the body; the more bulky the weight, the more difficult it is to carry, and the less efficient the handling of manual materials. The objectives are human comfort, optimum efficiency of the man-machine system, safety and prevention, health, and work satisfaction. Work satisfaction is an important issue. Human performance evaluations track overall strength, pace, reactions, hand steadiness, flexibility, level of cooperation, level of effort, ranges of motion gait, posture, and pain level. The bottom line is to make the achievement level match or exceed the task demand.

The ergonomists also analyze the patient's anthropometric measurements, from which stress points are identified. Patients are then taught the correct layouts for chairs, desks, home furniture, work-site equipment, and condition to prevent reinjury.

By the time of discharge, patients may have achieved the best physical condition in their lifetimes. Usually, by 1 week, patients are ambulatory and approaching independence in activities of daily living with decreasing levels of pain. They are approaching full ranges of motion with increasing strength in 2 to 3 weeks. Relief of pain is not the end point, but functional restoration is. At the end of 4 weeks, sometimes 6 weeks, the patients have achieved full functional levels of activity. If a neurologic deficit has been present, motor strength may recover in 2 to 3 weeks, sensation in 2 to 3 months, and reflexes in 3 months. Complete pain relief is attained in one third of patients; in the remainder, the pain may dissipate or become controllable for functional comfort. At discharge, the majority are able to resume full function and return to previous activities, despite residual pain.

PAIN CENTER EFFECTIVENESS

Are multidisciplinary pain centers effective? The answer is yes, by virtue of pain elimination, reduction, or tapering from opioid medication, increase in functional activity, return to work, decreased use of the healthcare system, closure of disability claims, and proved cost-effectiveness.[36] Treatment at multidisciplinary pain clinics, based on a meta-analysis of 3080 patients, found savings in medical expenditures equal to $9,548,000 and savings in indemnity expenditures equal to $175,225,000, with a total savings of $184,772,050.

Data from the University of Miami Comprehensive Pain and Rehabilitation Center are displayed in Figure 6-13, 92% improvement in functional status, a 66% reduction in pain, and a 62% return to employment or a work-ready state, together with a 93% patient satisfaction rate with treatment, are strong testimony to the effectiveness of multidisciplinary pain center treatment.

As favorable as these data are, questions still require resolution, and some patients have problems that cannot be eliminated with the available time limits. Room for improvement always exists. We submit, however, that the multidisciplinary, comprehensive approach to the management of low back disorders is the mode of treatment for these complex patients.

SUMMARY

We have emphasized prominence, misdiagnosis, and undertreatment of myofascial components of refractory low back pain syndromes; erroneous past tendency to focus on alleged observance of a lack of objective findings as support for a psychogenic formulation; importance of comprehensive evaluation and treatment defined as *including careful physical examination and treatment planning, as well as attending psychosocial vocational and ergonomic factors;* data supporting substantial functional restoration and decreased future medical usage deriving from intensive comprehensive rehabilitation approaches such as we have described. Not only is this an acceptable alternative to interventional treatments and surgery, its use will enhance surgical outcomes when used preoperatively, but also assure surgical success when implemented postoperatively. The myofascial syndromes are always present with spinal disorders. If not addressed, the best surgical technique will fail to relieve the pain because both the intraspinal and extraspinal causative factors must be eliminated, else assuredly, failed back syndromes will ensue at prohibitive costs to both human suffering and socioeconomic consequences.

REFERENCES

1. Mixter WJ, Barr JS. Rupture of the intervertebral disc with involvement of the spinal canal. N Engl J Med 211:210–215, 1934.
2. Rosomoff HL. Do herniated disks produce pain? Clin J Pain 1:91–93, 1985.
3. Travell JG, Simons DG. Myofascial Pain and Dysfunction: The Trigger Point Manual. Baltimore, Williams & Wilkins, 1983.
4. Granstrom E. Biochemistry of the prostaglandins, thromboxanes, and leukotrienes. *In* Bonica JJ, Lindblom U, Iggo A (eds). Advances in Pain Research and Therapy (vol 5). New York, Raven, 1983, pp 605–615.
5. Juan H. Prostaglandins as modulators of pain. Gen Pharmacol 9:403–409, 1978.
6. Moncada S, Ferreira SH, Vane JR. Pain and inflammatory mediators. *In* Vane JR, Ferreira SH (eds). Inflammation Handbook of Experimental Pharmacology. Berlin, Springer, 1978, pp 558–616.
7. Higgs GA, Moncada S. Interactions of arachidonate products with other pain mediators. *In* Bonica JJ, Lindblom U, Iggo A (eds). Advances in Pain Research and Therapy. New York, Raven, 1983, pp 617–626.

8. Ferreira SH. Prostaglandins: peripheral and central analgesia. *In* Bonica JJ, Lindblom U, Iggo A (eds). Advances in Pain Research and Therapy. New York, Raven, 1983, pp 597–603.

9. Higgs GA, Flower RJ, Vane JR. A new approach to anti-inflammatory drugs. Biochem Pharmacol 28:1959–1961, 1977.

10. Rosomoff HL, Clasen RA, Harstock R, et al. Brain reaction to experimental injury after hypothermia. Arch Neurol 13:337–345, 1965.

11. Carr DB, Bullen BA, Skrinar GS, et al. Physical conditioning facilities the exercise-induced secretion of beta-endorphin and beta-hypoprotein in women. N Engl J Med 305:560–563, 1981.

12. Cailliet R. Soft Tissue Pain and Disability. Philadelphia, FA Davis, 1980, pp 1–313.

13. Rosomoff HL. Nonoperative treatment of the failed back syndrome presenting with chronic pain. *In* Long DM, Decker BC (eds). Current Therapy in Neurological Surgery. Toronto, BC Decker, 1985, pp 200–202.

14. Lewis JW, Cannon JT, Liebeskind J. Opioid and non-opioid mechanisms of stress analgesia. Science 208:623–625, 1980.

15. Spitzer WO, LeBlanc FE, Dupuis M, et al. Scientific approach to the assessment and management of activity-related spinal disorders: a monograph for clinicians. Report of the Quebec Task Force on Spinal Disorders. Spine 12:51–59, 1987.

16. Fishbain DA, Rosomoff HL, Steele-Rosomoff R, Cutler BR. Types of pain treatment facilities and referral selection criteria. Arch Fam Med 4:58–66, 1995.

17. Fishbain DA, Rosomoff HL, Goldberg M, et al. The prediction of return to work after pain center treatment: a review. Clin J Pain 9:3–15, 1993.

18. Cutler BR, Fishbain DA, Rosomoff HL, et al. Does non-surgical pain center treatment of chronic pain return patients to work? A review and meta-analysis of the literature. Spine 19:643–652, 1994.

19. Fishbain DA, Rosomoff HL. What is chronic pain? Clin J Pain 6:164–166, 1990.

20. Turk DC, Matyas TA. Pain related behaviors: communication of pain. APS J 1:109–111, 1992.

21. Riley JF, Adhera DIT, Follick MJ. Chronic low back pain and functional improvement: Assessing beliefs about their relationship. Arch Phys Med Rehabil 69:579–584, 1988.

22. Fishbain DA, Steele-Rosomoff R, Rosomoff HL. Drug abuse, dependence, and addiction in chronic pain patients. Clin J Pain 8:77–85, 1992.

23. Long DM, Filtzer DL, Bendebba M, et al. Clinical features of the failed back. J Neurosurg 69:61–71, 1988.

24. McCoy CE, Selby D, Henderson R, et al. Patients avoiding surgery: Pathology and one-year lift status follow-up. Spine (Suppl):S198–S200, 1991.

25. Crue BL, Pinsky JJ. An approach to chronic pain of non-malignant origin. Postgrad Med J 60:858–864, 1984.

26. Rosomoff HL, Fishbain D, Goldberg M, et al. Physical findings in patients with chronic intractable benign pain of the back and/or neck. Pain 37:279–287, 1989.

27. Rosomoff HL. The effects of hypothermia on the physiology of the nervous system. Surgery 40:328–336, 1956.

28. Rosomoff HL, Clasen RA, Hartstock R, et al. Brain reaction to experimental injury after hypothermia. Arch Neurol 13:337–345, 1965.

29. Larsson U, Choler U, Lidstrom A, et al. Autotraction for treatment of lumbago-sciatica: a multicentre controlled investigation. Acta Orthop Scand 51:791–798, 1980.

30. Lind GAM. Auto-Traction: Treatment of Low Back Pain and Sciatica. Sweden: Sturetryckeriet, Diss. Link6ping, Link6ping University, 1974.

31. Natchev E. A manual on autotraction treatment for low back pain. Folksam Sci Council Publ B:171, 1984.

32. Abdel-Moty E, Khalil TM, Rosomoff RS, et al. Computerized electromyography in quantifying the effectiveness of functional electrical neuromuscular stimulation. *In* Asfour SS (ed). Ergonomics/Human Factors IV. New York, Elsevier, 1987, pp 1057–1065.

33. Fishbain DA, Goldberg M, Meagher R, et al. Male and female chronic pain patients categorized by DSM-III psychiatric diagnostic criteria. Pain 26:181–197, 1986.

34. Khalil T. Asfour SS, Waly SM, et al. Isometric exercise and biofeedback in strength training. *In* Asfour SS (ed). Trends in Ergonomics/Human Factors IV. New York, Elsevier, 1987, pp 1095–1101.

35. Khalil TM, Asfour SS, Moty EA, et al. New horizons for ergonomics research in low back pain. *In* Eberts RE, Eberts CG (eds). Trends in Ergonomics/Human Factors 11. New York, Elsevier, 1985, pp 591–598.

36. Turk DC. Efficacy of multidisciplinary pain centers in the treatment of chronic pain. *In* Cohen MJM, Campbell IN (eds). Pain Treatment Centers at a Crossroads: A Practical and Conceptual Reappraisal. Progress in Pain Research and Management (vol 7). Seattle, IASP Press, 1996, pp 257–273.

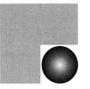

C H A P T E R 7

Failed Back Surgery Syndrome

KENNETH A. FOLLETT, MD, PhD

Failed back surgery syndrome (FBSS) is a condition that is all too familiar to most spine surgeons and physicians who manage patients with pain. The term *failed back surgery syndrome* is applied to those individuals who have persistent or recurrent back and/or extremity pain after spinal surgeries performed to relieve a complaint of pain or to correct neurologic or orthopedic abnormality. Use of the term *failed back surgery syndrome* or *postlaminectomy syndrome* as a diagnosis should be discouraged. These terms are nondescriptive because they encompass a large, heterogeneous group of disorders. When they are used as diagnoses for individual patients, they obscure the fact that specific, identifiable abnormalities are responsible for symptoms in many individuals. A specific diagnosis is preferable because it can guide further evaluation and treatment. Furthermore, the terms *failed back surgery syndrome* or *postlaminectomy syndrome* should not be considered "end-stage" diagnoses, with the implication that nothing further can be done for the patient.

Estimates of the incidence of FBSS range from 5% to 50%, depending on the criteria used to define success or failure. Overall, approximately 15% of patients who undergo spinal surgery will have persistent or recurrent symptoms.[1] Symptoms can arise from many sources, including organic (biologic or physiologic) and/or psychological (including subtle or overt psychological or psychiatric dysfunction and issues of secondary gain such as socioeconomic factors).[2] FBSS is best viewed as a spectrum of abnormalities ranging from purely organic to purely psychological, but in most cases consists of physiologic abnormality complicated by psychosocial factors. In this regard, FBSS is an excellent prototype of chronic pain as a biopsychosocial disorder.[3] The significance of psychological factors in chronic pain disorders cannot be overstated, and is described in detail in other chapters.

ETIOLOGY OF THE FAILED BACK SURGERY SYNDROME

To treat patients with FBSS appropriately, a specific explanation for failure must be determined. If a physician cannot determine why the previous procedure(s) failed, then subsequent treatments and procedures, including repeat spinal surgery, are likely to fail as well, and will quite likely fail for the same reasons that caused the initial failure. Many conditions can lead to or contribute to FBSS (Tables 7-1 to 7-4).[2] The large number of causes can make it difficult to determine the specific etiology in a given patient. To simplify the process of establishing a diagnosis and developing a treatment plan, symptoms can be categorized according to time of onset after previous surgery, location (primarily axial versus primarily appendicular), and pain characteristics (primarily nociceptive/somatic versus neuropathic). Identifying these general factors is a useful first step in determining the cause of symptoms because the major classes of abnormalities presenting early after previous surgery are different from those presenting late, and those abnormalities causing primarily back pain or nociceptive pain are different from those causing extremity pain or neuropathic pain.

The time of onset of symptoms relative to previous surgery is an important consideration because many causes of failure present stereotypically at specific intervals after surgery. The temporal presentation of symptoms can be grouped into the intervals of immediate failure (no relief of symptoms following surgery), early postoperative failure (several days to weeks), intermediate failure (several weeks to months), or late failure (months to years after surgery).[2] In general, the longer the interval between previous surgery and the onset of recurrent symptoms, the greater the likelihood that a structural, surgically correctable lesion can be identified as the source of recurrent symptoms.

A lack of even transient pain relief after lumbar spine surgery (i.e., immediate failure) has many potential causes (Table 7-1). Incorrect diagnosis, especially overt misdiagnosis, is an uncommon but important cause of immediate failure because of potentially serious consequences.[4,5] The evaluation of patients with symptoms referable to the back or spinal column should always include special attention directed toward detecting serious pathologic conditions such as tumor (including tumors of the spinal column or adjacent soft tissues, abdomen, pelvis, retroperitoneum) and infection (e.g., osteomyelitis, diskitis, epidural abscess). Immediate failure of surgery to relieve radicular symptoms should lead to consideration of noncompressive etiologies of radiculopathy

● **TABLE 7-1** • Temporal Onset of Symptoms in Failed Back Surgery Syndrome: Immediate Failure

Back Pain		Leg Pain	
Instability	Epidural fibrosis	Retained disk fragment	Arachnoiditis
Deconditioned back	Arachnoiditis	Far lateral disk	Arachnoid cyst
Meningeal irritation	Infection (diskitis, osteomyelitis, epidural abscess)	Far out syndrome	Synovial cyst
Arachnoid cyst	Pseudomeningocele	Wrong level decompressed	Neuritis (e.g., herpetic)
Diskogenic pain	Myofascial syndrome	Inadequate decompression	Conjoined root
Infection	Graft donor site pain	Lateral recess stenosis	Peripheral neuropathy
Facet arthropathy	Spondylosis	Retained foreign body	Piriformis syndrome
Muscle spasm	Spondylolysis	Pseudomeningocele	Delayed decompression
Loose hardware	Spondylolisthesis	Root sleeve meningocele	Battered root syndrome
Transaponeurotic fat herniation	Psychosocial	Diabetic mononeuropathy	Psychosocial
Wrong level fused	Patient expectation	Nerve root fibrosis	Patient expectation
Insufficient levels fused	Tumor (primary or metastatic, bone, soft tissue, retroperitoneal)	Nerve root injury	Facet fracture
Trauma (contusion, sprain, fracture)		Tumor (primary or metastatic, bone, neural, soft tissue)	
Fasciitis		Loose hardware with root impingement	
Graft donor site pain			

Modified from Follett KA, Dirks BA. Etiology and evaluation of the failed back surgery syndrome. Neurosurg Q 3:40–59, 1993.

and neuropathy as the cause of symptoms, such as metabolic (e.g., diabetic), viral, traumatic, vascular, and inflammatory processes.

Immediate failure may occur in patients who are not informed adequately about the expected outcomes of surgery, or whose goals for surgery are not met. For example, patients who are not advised that diskectomy may relieve radicular pain but not improve axial back pain may be disappointed if back pain persists after surgery. There are few, if any, pain-related conditions (including pain of spinal origin) for which a surgeon can tell a patient to expect complete pain relief after surgery. Despite this, when some patients with persistent pain are asked what they were told preoperatively to expect from surgery, they state they were told they would be "cured." This mismatch between expectations and outcomes leads to dissatisfaction with care and leads to an interpretation of failure of the treatment (D. Doleys, personal communication, 2000).

Improper patient selection can result in complete failure of the surgery to relieve symptoms and is one of the most common causes of failure.[4,6] Some patients with FBSS can be demonstrated, in retrospect, to have not met accepted criteria for surgical intervention.[4,7] Commonly, physical examination fails to demonstrate a cause for the persistent symptoms in these individuals,[4] and many are found to have psychological or psychiatric dysfunction that contributes to, or may be the sole cause of, their pain complaints.[4,8,9] Personality disorders, depression, somatization, conversion hysteria, and anxiety neuroses are common comorbidities in patients with chronic pain, may have a profound adverse impact on the success of surgical procedures, and must be recognized and addressed before operative intervention.[4]

Technical difficulty during surgery may cause failure in appropriately selected operative candidates. The wrong level or side might be operated on, especially in patients in whom intraoperative radiographic localization is difficult (for example, in obese individuals), in microsurgical cases, in patients with spinal segmentation defects, or in the setting of conjoined roots.[10] Surgery may be unsuccessful because of failure to recognize the full scope of the patient's pathology or failure to recognize the primary pathology if it is not obvious (e.g., disk fragments in the neural foramen, kinking of nerve root by the adjacent pedicle, root compression by articular process, spinal stenosis, and/or extraforaminal disk herniation).[11] Technical difficulties such as excessive bleeding that obscures the surgical field[2] or inadequate exposure will predispose to failure.[3]

Overt operative complications are unusual in first-time surgeries, with an incidence of approximately 5%, but may occur in as many as 17% of repeat surgeries.[12] Among operative complications, the "battered root syndrome," is one of the most common, reported to occur in as many as 12% of cases of diskectomy.[3,13] Battered root syndrome typically presents as incomplete postoperative resolution of radicular symptoms, sometimes with increased neurologic deficit (often attributed to root swelling).[14] It has been attributed to excessive retraction, bleeding, or use of cottonoid patties.[10] Frank nerve injury (e.g., avulsion of a conjoined root)[10] is rare (0.4% to 4% of cases). Other operative complications that may present within the immediate postoperative period include gross instability following extensive facetectomy or facet damage, postoperative hematoma, infection, or pseudomeningocele.

● T A B L E 7 - 2 • Temporal Onset of Symptoms in Failed Back Surgery Syndrome: Early Failure

Back Pain		Leg Pain	
Patient expectation	Pseudomeningocele	Patient expectation	Arachnoid cyst
Psychosocial	Infection (diskitis, osteomyelitis, epidural abscess)	Psychosocial	Pseudomeningocele
Deconditioned back	Loose hardware	Loose hardware	Root sleeve meningocele
Arachnoid cyst		Facet fracture	Recurrent disk
		Infection	

Modified from Follett KA, Dirks BA. Etiology and evaluation of the failed back surgery syndrome. Neurosurg Q 3:40–59, 1993.

Spinal fusions may fail for many of the same reasons that cause failure of decompressive surgeries, including improper diagnosis, improper patient selection, inadequate or incomplete surgery (e.g., too few levels fused), and technical errors. There are additional causes of persistent pain that are unique to fusion procedures. Patients may have persistent pain at the graft donor site, or nerve injury may occur at the donor site[15] (e.g., injury to cluneal nerves during harvest of iliac crest from a posterior approach). Facet fracture, pedicle screw malpositioning,[16] or slippage of a laminar hook may cause nerve root injury. Methylmethacrylate as a primary means of stabilization or as a salvage technique for stripped screws may damage neural elements through compression or heat.[17] Roots may be damaged also by graft extrusion after posterior lumbar interbody fusion (PLIF) or from retraction of the thecal sac during exposure of the disk space.[17,18]

Pain that recurs within the first few days or weeks following surgery ("early failure") (Table 7-2) shares some of the same causes as those which lead to immediate failure, including improper patient selection. Some patients will do well for a few days or weeks because of a "placebo" response[6]; others may overstate their early pain relief because they don't want to disappoint their physicians. Operative complications are a common cause of failure within this "early" time frame. Infections, which occur in as many as 5% of first-time spine surgeries and 17% of repeat surgeries,[12] pseudomeningoceles, and postoperative instability or recurrent disk herniation[19] may become symptomatic. Pain may occur if a bone graft becomes dislodged, hardware breaks or becomes dislodged, or if a neuroma forms at the site of an injured cutaneous nerve.[15] Pain may worsen as patients begin to normalize their

activity after surgery, especially in patients who became physically "deconditioned" before surgery.

As the interval between surgery and recurrent pain lengthens, the causes of recurrent pain begin to entail different problems from those that cause earlier failure (Table 7-3). Patients who have recurrent symptoms or new pain in the "intermediate failure" time frame, several weeks to several months after surgery, may have been improperly selected as operative candidates and will have had temporary relief as a placebo response. On the other hand, many individuals within this time frame will experience pain as a direct or indirect result of their operative procedures. Epidural fibrosis and arachnoiditis are particularly important causes of failure that present within this interval.[13,16,20,21–23] These conditions may result from excessive retraction, bleeding, or from inflammatory response to debris from cottonoid patties.[24] Epidural fibrosis is estimated to occur in as many as 6% to 8% of cases, and arachnoiditis in as many as 12% to 16% of lumbar spine surgeries.[3,4] These problems may be even more common after spinal fusion,[18,25] especially PLIF, which can require significant retraction of the thecal sac to gain access to the disk space. Patients with pain related to epidural fibrosis describe good initial relief of pain but over the following few weeks have recurrent pain, which may be similar or identical to their preoperative pain, especially if surgery was decompression (diskectomy or laminectomy) for radiculopathy due to compressive lesion. Pain may occur in new distributions if epidural fibrosis or arachnoiditis develop as a result of manipulation of the thecal sac (e.g., PLIF). Recurrent disk herniation at the same or at a new level occurs following as many as 13% of disk surgeries[3] and may present during the intermediate time frame.[13,22]

● T A B L E 7 - 3 • Temporal Onset of Symptoms in Failed Back Surgery Syndrome: Intermediate Failure

Back Pain		Leg Pain	
Loose hardware	Patient expectation	Loose hardware	Patient expectation
Deconditioned back	Epidural fibrosis	Facet fracture	Synovial cyst
Adjacent level disk degeneration	Arachnoiditis	Adjacent disk degeneration	Epidural fibrosis
Disk disruption under fusion	Spondylolysis	Graft donor site pain (scar)	Arachnoiditis
Pseudarthrosis	Spondylolisthesis		
	Fusion fracture		

Modified from Follett KA, Dirks BA. Etiology and evaluation of the failed back surgery syndrome. Neurosurg Q 3:40–59, 1993.

Pseudarthrosis may be a common cause of fusion failure,[21,26] with an incidence of 5% to 40%.[17] Pseudoarthrosis cannot be identified clearly until the fusion has had adequate time to mature, typically 6 months or longer, but may become symptomatic within the intermediate time frame. The role of pseudoarthrosis in causing new or recurrent pain after spinal surgery is unsettled. Many patients with pseudarthrosis are asymptomatic[9,27,28] and repair of pseudarthrosis does not usually relieve chronic pain.[18,29]

Patients with FBSS who present with late failure are those who do well for months or years following surgery, after which time pain recurs (Table 7-4). It is this group of patients in whom the likelihood of identifying structural pathology as the cause of recurrent symptoms is greatest. Some of these patients will be symptomatic from entirely new disease, others from progression of the underlying disease that led to the previous operation (e.g., osteoarthritis). In some instances, late failure may be related to the previous operative procedure. Instability may account for as many as 18% of failures after diskectomy, and may be even more common after laminectomy.[29,30] Fusion can result in "transitional" syndromes (accelerated degenerative changes at motion segments adjacent to the fusion) and may lead to recurrent back pain.[3,27] Disk space collapse, hypermobility, osteophyte formation, stenosis (sometimes caused by graft overgrowth), and frank segmental instability (seen in as many as 50% of old fusion patients)[31] may develop following fusion. Acquired spondylolysis[9] and abutment syndromes[17] following fusion may also lead to recurrent pain, as can pseudarthrosis[21,26] and fracture of fusion mass.[25]

EVALUATION OF THE PATIENT WITH FAILED BACK SURGERY SYNDROME

Successful treatment of patients with failed back surgery syndrome requires that the cause of recurrent symptoms be determined, that is, a *specific* diagnosis must be established. This can be difficult given the multifactorial etiology of FBSS. Diagnosis is further complicated by the difficulty of determining whether complaints of pain and neurologic abnormalities predate surgery or arose as a result of, or following surgery (i.e., which are old and which are new symptoms). It is helpful, and frequently essential, to review old records pertaining to the patient's pain complaint. Preoperative and postoperative data should be compared to determine which complaints

and findings (subjective, physical, and radiographic) are long-standing, which may have arisen as a result of the previous operative procedure(s), and which are new and unrelated to previous surgery.[2] The cause of failure of previous procedures must be determined to avoid failure of subsequent procedures for the same reasons.

The history and physical examinations provide the foundation for diagnosis. The patient's history is particularly important, because it will usually provide sufficient information to make a diagnosis. Attention should be directed toward eliciting symptoms of neurologic abnormality, systemic illness, or other serious underlying abnormality ("red flags" suggestive of cancer, infection, or other serious disorder), or orthopedic abnormalities. The interval from surgery to recurrent symptoms should be ascertained. The location of pain (e.g., axial, proximal extremity, nondermatomal, radicular) and character of pain, that is, primarily nociceptive ("aching," "throbbing") versus neuropathic ("burning," "shooting") provide important clues to help the examiner determine whether the organic problem is predominantly musculoskeletal/myofascial or neurogenic, or a combination of both. Symptoms of sensory change or weakness, and the specific location of such symptoms should be identified. With careful questioning, it should be possible to distinguish symptoms that predate previous surgical procedures from those arising as a result of, or subsequent to, previous operative procedures. Psychosocial factors, which can have a major impact on a chronic pain complaint and its successful treatment, must not be overlooked. These issues are described in detail in Chapters 1 and 4.

The physical examination should be directed toward confirming or refuting the preliminary diagnosis established by the history. Care should be taken to identify serious underlying abnormalities such as infection or tumor. Myofascial pain syndromes (described in detail in a preceding chapter) are very common in people with FBSS. This disorder can cause sciatic-like symptoms that mimic radiculopathy, and special emphasis must be directed toward identifying or excluding myofascial pain as the cause of radicular or pseudo-radicular complaints. Careful, systematic palpation may reveal tenderness, muscle spasm, or trigger points consistent with a myofascial syndrome. The presence of nonorganic signs (Waddell's incongruencies) such as abnormally dramatic behavior during the examination can alert the examiner to the presence of psychosocial problems that may contribute to the pain complaint.[32] Range of motion and strength should be assessed. Limitation of spinal motion is a nonspecific finding,

● **TABLE 7-4** • Temporal Onset of Symptoms in Failed Back Surgery Syndrome: Late Failure

Back Pain		Leg Pain	
Adjacent level instability	Fusion fracture	Stenosis (central, lateral, under fusion)	Adjacent disk degeneration
Spondylolysis	Pseudarthrosis		Loose hardware
Spondylolisthesis	Disk disruption under fusion	Recurrent disk herniation	Synovial cyst
Abutment syndrome	Loose hardware	Disk herniation under fusion	
Compression fracture above fusion	Facet syndrome	Instability	

Modified from Follett KA, Dirks BA. Etiology and evaluation of the failed back surgery syndrome. Neurosurg Q 3:40–59, 1993.

often associated with myofascial pain, but also associated with psychosocial problems.[17] Tension signs are useful indicators of physiologic dysfunction in FBSS patients because they typically resolve after successful treatment of a compressive root lesion. The significance of abnormalities identified on the physical examination can be difficult to determine because as many as 30% to 50% of patients with preoperative neurologic deficits will have persistent deficits even after an operation that successfully relieves their pain.[9,33] Review of previous medical records may be required to determine whether abnormalities are old or new, static or changing.

Most patients will have undergone previous diagnostic testing (e.g., radiographic studies, electrophysiologic studies). These studies should be reviewed to place new complaints into context against old abnormalities. New radiographic, electrophysiologic, and invasive tests should be performed selectively to support or refute the diagnosis established on the basis of the history and physical examinations. Radiographic studies are particularly important in determining the presence of a surgically correctable structural lesion.[2] Imaging studies that may be useful include plain spine radiographs, myelogra-phy, computed tomographic (CT) scans, magnetic resonance imaging (MRI), diskography, and nuclear medicine scans (Table 7-5).

Plain spine radiographs are readily available, relatively inexpensive, and well tolerated. They are especially useful for assessing bone abnormalities such as fracture or dislocation, instability (with flexion/extension views), pseudarthrosis, and failure of instrumentation (e.g., broken or dislodged pedicle screw or rod, jumped laminar hook). Radiographic changes associated with degenerative disease of the spine are very common findings on plain radiographs and should not be misinterpreted as the etiology of symptoms. Disk degeneration and spondylosis can be seen on plain radiographs in 75% of the general population by the seventh decade, are equally common in symptomatic and asymptomatic individuals, and their role in the pathogenesis of chronic pain is not easily determined.[9,26,31,34] In contrast, findings of spondylolisthesis and spondylolysis correlate more closely with persistent pain, particularly after spinal surgery. Postoperative spondylolis-thesis is twice as common in patients with poor outcome after laminectomy[30] and spondylolysis, seen in 2.5% of patients

● **T A B L E   7 - 5** • Radiographic Evaluation of Neck and Back Pain*

Parameter	Plain Radiographs	MRI	CT†	Myelography	Nuclear Medicine	Diskography
Alignment	+++	++	+	+	−	−
Cortical bone imaging	+++	−	+++	−	−	−
Cancellous bone imaging	+	+++	++	−	−	−
Soft tissue (ligament, muscle)	−	+++	++	−	−	−
Infection (diskitis, osteomyelitis)	+	+++	+	−	+	−
Intradural or extradural tumor	−	+++	++	+	−	−
Osseous tumor	+	+++	+++	−	+	−
Canal stenosis	−	+++	+++	++	−	−
Foraminal stenosis	−	++	+++	−	−	−
Facet hypertrophy	+	++	+++	+	−	−
Disk space narrowing	+++	+++	+	−	−	+
New disk herniation	−	+++	++	+	−	++
Recurrent disk	−	+++	++	+	−	+
Lateral disk	−	+++	++	−	−	−
Disk morphology	−	+++	+	−	−	+++
Pseudarthrosis	+	−	++	−	+	−
Instability (functional images)	++	−	−	+	−	−
Nerve roots	−	+++	+	+	−	−
Arachnoiditis, epidural fibrosis	−	+++	++	++	−	−
Provocative test	−	−	−	−	−	+++
Invasiveness	+++	+++	+++	+	+	−
Availability	+++	++	++	++	++	−
Cost	+++	−	+	−	+	+

From Follett KA, Dirks BA. Etiology and evaluation of the failed back surgery syndrome. Neurosurg Q 3:40–59, 1993, with permission.
* Least advantageous (−) to most advantageous (+++).
† With intravenous or intrathecal contrast material, when appropriate.
CT, Computed tomography; MRI, magnetic resonance imaging.

after lumbar fusion, is associated often with unsatisfactory outcomes.[26,35] Plain radiographs may reveal translational instability, which is generally more common in symptomatic than asymptomatic patients.[36]

MRI is the most useful imaging technique for assessing recurrent symptoms in patients with FBSS. It is well tolerated except for a small percentage of patients who require sedation before confinement in the scanner. Its greater expense, relative to other imaging studies, is offset by its greater sensitivity in detecting abnormalities. With gadolinium enhancement when appropriate, MRI can depict disk herniation, inflammation, infection (osteomyelitis, epidural abscess, etc.), epidural fibrosis, arachnoiditis, canal or foraminal stenosis, pseudomeningocele, and neoplasm.[2] MRI does not image cortical bone directly, and supplemental CT scanning may be necessary to completely delineate the nature of an abnormality. A combination of T2-weighted MRI, used as a "myelogram," and CT scanning to demonstrate bone detail, can be used in patients who require myelography but cannot undergo the procedure (e.g., dye allergy, coagulopathy). Gadolinium-enhanced MRI is particularly useful in differentiating recurrent disk herniation from postoperative epidural fibrosis, two common causes of FBSS, with a sensitivity and specificity of nearly 100%.[37,38] Epidural fibrosis generally enhances following gadolinium administration whereas disk herniation does not (although a rim of enhancement may be seen around herniated disk material).[2] MRI is exquisitely sensitive in showing degenerative change, which is common in asymptomatic individuals, so abnormal findings must be interpreted cautiously and in the context of the clinical problem.[2] Normal postoperative soft tissue changes complicate interpretation of early postoperative MRI scans, and MRI is most accurate when delayed at least 6 weeks from the surgical procedure.[38,39]

Myelography has become less important in the evaluation of patients with neck and back pain since the advent of MRI. Occasionally, myelography may present a clearer image of root sleeve cutoff or arachnoiditis. Myelography is most useful when combined with CT scanning. Postmyelogram CT scans provide substantial information about extradural compression of the thecal sac and roots. Myelogram/CT scanning is particularly useful when compression arises from bony abnormalities, which are not always apparent on MRI studies, but is of limited use for the evaluation of extradural soft tissue abnormalities such as differentiation of epidural fibrosis from recurrent disk herniation. In general, myelography will not reveal abnormalities not shown on a good quality MRI scan, and myelography is rarely indicated if a technically satisfactory MRI does not reveal significant abnormalities.

CT scanning can be a useful adjunct for the evaluation of patients with FBSS,[40] but has also become a secondary diagnostic tool since the advent of MRI. It is widely available, noninvasive, of moderate cost, and well tolerated by patients. Up to 60% of cases of FBSS have been attributed to bony abnormalities (usually incomplete decompression of lateral recess stenosis),[3] which are readily shown on CT studies. The use of CT in demonstrating soft tissue abnormalities is limited. While such abnormalities can be detected, it can be difficult to differentiate recurrent disk herniation from epidural fibrosis by CT alone. The sensitivity and specificity of CT scanning can be increased with the use of intravenous contrast agents[40–43] or instillation of intrathecal contrast material.

Diskography has become a popular technique for the evaluation of patients with pain of presumed spinal origin. However, the reliability and usefulness of diskography is unsettled for patients who have not had back surgery[44,45] and its role may be even more uncertain in the evaluation of patients with FBSS. Diskography can be used to study disk morphology, especially when used in conjunction with postdiskography CT scanning,[46] and also as a provocative test. As a provocative test, pain on injection of the disk should mimic the pain for which the patient is undergoing evaluation (i.e., pain should be "concordant"). When considering diskography for the evaluation of back pain, it is important to recognize that injection of disks in unoperated patients can produce pain.[47,48] False-positive results are common,[49] and there is a significant correlation between positive diskography results and the presence of psychiatric dysfunction.[50,51] In the setting of previous spine surgery, the reliability of diskography is even less certain. Because disk surgery necessarily alters the normal disk morphology, diskography for evaluation of disk morphology may not be valid for studying previously operated disks. As a provocative test, diskography is commonly positive in operated disks in asymptomatic individuals,[51] which brings into question the diagnostic significance of positive results in operated patients. As an invasive procedure, diskography has more risks than noninvasive imaging studies, including a 2% to 4% risk of diskitis, and concern has been expressed regarding radiation exposure during the procedure.[46,48]

In addition to the difficulty in establishing the use of diskography as a diagnostic test, there is a lack of consensus that diskography improves surgical outcomes. Some reports indicate that diskography offers no benefit in improving outcomes,[45,52] while others show a clear-cut benefit to diskography as an aid to management, for example, in the identification and treatment of "chemo-sensitive" disks.[45,53] The majority of patients with diskogram-positive back pain may improve with nonoperative care.[54] A "negative" diskogram may be more useful than a positive diskogram by eliminating a suspect disk as a source of pain.[2] Negative diskography also serves as a prognostic indicator of outcome following surgery: patients who undergo fusion after negative diskograms do poorly, compared to those who have positive diskograms.[55]

Radionuclide scans can be used for the evaluation of several specific abnormalities that lead to persistent back pain. These conditions include inflammation, occult fracture, pseudarthrosis, and instability (especially in the absence of frank instability on flexion/extension radiographs). Most fusions show increased tracer uptake for as long as 2 years. Isolated "hot spots" within the area of generalized increased uptake, or localized tracer accumulation greater than 2 years postoperatively suggest pseudarthrosis.[17] Single-photon emission CT scanning may provide additional localizing value.[56]

Electrophysiologic studies (electromyography, nerve conduction studies) can be useful in establishing the presence of mono- or poly-radiculopathy or peripheral neuropathy. Interpretation of results in postsurgical patients is confounded by the relatively common occurrence of residual abnormalities after previous surgery.[2] For instance, paraspinous muscle activity is typically abnormal for up to 3 to 4 years following posterior lumbar surgeries because of muscle denervation.[57] The results of electrical studies must be compared to previous studies, if available, and are most useful in the setting of new neuropathic symptoms.[2]

Other diagnostic tests, such as hematologic analysis (e.g., complete blood cell count, sedimentation rate, c-reactive protein) to look for evidence of infection or inflammatory disorders, may be useful when these abnormalities are suspected based upon the history and physical examinations. Diagnostic selective nerve and facet blocks may help differentiate potential causes of pain but their use in assessing operated levels is impaired because postoperative scarring alters infiltration of local anesthetics at the site.[17] Trigger point injections may aid in diagnosis of myofascial syndromes.[2]

Psychological evaluation is appropriate for many patients with FBSS, particularly those in whom no clear-cut organic cause for persistent or recurrent symptoms can be found, because many patients with FBSS harbor psychological or psychiatric disorders.[4,9] Psychological evaluation is particularly important (and often mandated by insurance carriers) for individuals being considered for pain-relieving surgery such as spinal cord stimulation or intrathecal analgesic administration. "Nonorganic" signs[32] correlate with general somatic and neurotic symptoms, disability behavior, and pain drawings[58] and are readily observed by most physicians.[2] The presence of nonorganic signs does not preclude the possibility that the patient has pain related to a surgically correctable lesion; however, these signs should alert the physician to possible psychological dysfunction and should trigger referral for psychological evaluation. Anxiety and depression are common accompaniments of chronic pain and by themselves do not necessarily indicate that the pain complaint has a significant psychogenic component. On the other hand, major untreated depression or anxiety have a significant adverse impact on responses to treatment of pain and, when present, must be addressed as part of the overall treatment program. The profound impact of psychological factors in chronic pain require that physicians be alert for evidence of dysfunction, and refer patients for formal psychological or psychiatric assessment when such dysfunction is suspected. Identification of psychological dysfunction is especially critical because many of these patients will argue persuasively for a surgical or interventional treatment for their pain, even when such treatments are not indicated on medical grounds.

TREATMENT OF FAILED BACK SURGERY SYNDROME

Options for treatment of symptoms associated with FBSS include reparative techniques (e.g., repeat surgery) and symptomatic therapies (interventional and noninterventional techniques). It is important, regardless of whether the ultimate treatment is surgical or nonsurgical, that goals of therapy be established before deciding on a course of treatment. The outcomes goals should be realistic, and they should be relevant to the patient and to the physician. Goals of treatment will vary among patients; the treatment plan should be developed with the intent of achieving the goals established for the individual patient.

Based upon the evaluation, as described previously, a diagnosis for the cause of symptoms should be established. Serious underlying pathology (e.g., infection, tumor) must be identified and addressed, if present. Attention should be directed next toward identifying the presence of a surgically correctable lesion. A surgically correctable lesion can be treated directly but in many cases it may be more appropriate to treat symptomatically using more conservative strategies (e.g., medications, spinal cord stimulation, intrathecal analgesic administration). If no surgically correctable lesion is identified, then treatment must proceed using therapies aimed at alleviating the symptoms. The treatment plan should be individualized and may vary substantially from one patient to the next, but in all cases must address each of the factors contributing to the pain, including both physical and emotional/socioeconomic issues. The following discussion will present an overview of strategies for treating pain associated with the failed back surgery syndrome. Details of specific therapies are available in other chapters.

Surgery is not indicated for patients with nonspecific chronic back or neck pain. Indiscriminate surgery does not provide good outcomes and is potentially harmful to patients. In a third-party assessment of outcomes of first-time lumbar fusion for pain, the majority of patients stated their back and/or leg pain was worse after surgery, and that quality of life was no better after surgery.[59] In general, the success rates of repeat surgery decrease with each successive operation, and the likelihood of surgical complication or worsening of pain increases with each successive operation.[60,61] In many cases, reoperation is no more successful in providing relief of pain than therapy directed specifically at pain management.[62] On the other hand, properly selected candidates for repeat surgery can have outcomes similar to those of carefully selected patients undergoing first-time surgeries. In fact, for carefully selected patients who have clearly concordant clinical and radiographic findings indicating the presence of a surgically correctable lesion, outcomes are better in those who undergo surgery than in those who are treated nonoperatively.[63] This is especially true for those individuals with a long interval between surgery and recurrent symptoms, who, as a group, will have the greatest likelihood of harboring surgically correctable disease. If a patient meets the indications for operative intervention, it should not be denied solely on the basis of the patient having had previous spinal surgery. If surgery is contemplated, the patient's pain complaint, abnormalities on physical examination, and supporting diagnostic studies (e.g., radiographs, electrophysiologic studies) should corroborate each other, and other factors contributing to the pain, including psychosocial problems, should be assessed and managed appropriately. Even patients with apparent surgically correctable pathology may have other conditions contributing to the pain complaint (e.g., myofascial pain). These associated conditions may not improve with surgery and, if not identified and treated, may lead to failure of repeat surgery to provide adequate relief of symptoms.

There is a tendency in many pain management circles to try to identify a physiologic "pain generator" in every patient. This approach, based on the "medical model" of chronic pain, minimizes the significance of psychological, social, and economic factors in chronic pain. Physicians inadvertently promote "medicalization" of chronic pain by ordering multiple tests and recommending repeated evaluations. Over time, patients who are subject to multiple tests and evaluations may begin to suspect that something must be wrong, and if they finally see the right physician, or have the right test, the cause of the pain will be identified. This leads to further "doctor shopping," repetitive care, and inappropriate treatment, all of which are expensive, potentially harmful, and delay proper treatment. If careful evaluation reveals no surgically correctable abnormalities, it is important that a frank discussion be held with the patient to inform him or her of this fact and to advise the patient that attention will be directed toward treatment of the pain rather than further searching for a surgical problem. Patients with maladaptive personality disorders and/or psychiatric dysfunction, in particular, may tend to ignore advice to pursue nonsurgical, conservative measures. These individuals can push physicians into performing surgery when it is not appropriate, and special efforts must be taken to educate them regarding the nature and treatment of chronic pain. Many patients, in particular those with little or no evidence of organic etiology of pain, will benefit from enrollment in a multidisciplinary and/or cognitive-behavioral–based pain management program (discussed in detail in a subsequent chapter). Unfortunately, such programs are not widely available, especially in smaller communities. Outcomes of treatment in behavior-based, multidisciplinary programs can equal those achieved with other approaches (i.e., interventional therapies) and should be remembered as an option for patients who are not appropriate candidates for other treatment programs.[64,65]

Treatment of persistent or recurrent symptoms frequently requires a combination of medications, passive and active physical medicine modalities, and behavioral and interventional therapies. Fundamental to the treatment of FBSS is the need to recognize that chronic pain should not be treated the same as acute pain. Acute pain signals acute tissue injury. Treatment of acute pain involves strategies aimed at promoting rest and tissue healing. In contrast, chronic pain typically leads to decreased activity and progressive deconditioning and needs to be approached through a program of reconditioning and mobilization. Therapies relevant to treatment of acute pain can be detrimental to the treatment of chronic pain.[66]

Patient education about the nature of chronic pain is an important part of treatment. Some patients interpret the presence of pain as a sign that their bodies are being injured or damaged, or that they are in imminent danger of harming themselves if they are physically active, and they avoid physical activity. This leads to further deconditioning and greater pain. Other patients may be willing to increase daily activities or participate in reconditioning programs but experience increased pain (which may worsen, especially early in the course of reconditioning) and refrain from further activity. Once serious or progressive pathology has been eliminated as a cause for pain, patients need to be instructed and reassured that chronic pain is not, in itself, dangerous or harmful ("hurt does not equal harm"), and they should be encouraged to increase their physical activities.

Physical therapy for reconditioning to improve range of motion and strength of painful areas is important in the treatment of chronic back and neck pain. Aggressive strengthening exercises may provide significant pain relief, even to the degree that surgery may not be necessary for patients who are deemed surgical candidates.[67] Most patients can be given instructions for home exercise programs (for stretching, range of motion, and strengthening) by their physicians (e.g., with the aid of "low back pain" brochures widely available).

Specific care by a physical therapist is not always necessary, but evaluation and short-term management by a physical therapist may be useful in helping a patient establish an ongoing home exercise program, or for the patient who needs directed guidance to remain compliant with a home exercise program. Long-term treatment under the auspices of a physical therapist is rarely indicated in chronic pain management. More aggressive reconditioning may be necessary using functional training such as "back schools" or work hardening programs, in which efforts are made to mimic a patient's work environment. Home traction devices may provide symptomatic benefit for some patients with chronic pain by helping stretch and relax muscles.

Recognition of an underlying myofascial syndrome, which is very common in patients with chronic back or neck pain, is important because therapy directed toward the myofascial pain syndrome can provide dramatic relief of symptoms.[68] The key to treatment of many myofascial pain syndromes is passive stretch and mobilization. A commonly used treatment is "spray and stretch," in which vapocoolant spray (e.g., fluorimethane) is applied to the skin surface, providing analgesia, which facilitates stretching of muscles to full length. Spray-and-stretch therapy can often be performed by the patient in the home after the technique has been demonstrated. Trigger points, if identified, may be dry needled or injected with saline, local anesthetics, and/or steroids.[68,69] Spray and stretch generally inactivates trigger points more quickly and with less patient discomfort than injection but may be especially effective if done immediately after trigger point injection.[69] In addition to establishing a good home exercise program for the patient, transcutaneous electrical nerve stimulation (TENS) is often helpful for the treatment of myofascial pain. Various medical approaches including nonsteroidal anti-inflammatory drugs (NSAIDs), tricyclic antidepressants, or judicious use of muscle relaxants may be necessary.

Medication therapy is the mainstay of treatment for many individuals with FBSS. The treating physician should determine whether the pain problem is nociceptive/somatic, neuropathic, or a mixed nociceptive/neuropathic disorder. Pharmacologic therapy should be tailored to address the type of pain. Detailed discussion of pharmacologic treatment is provided in an earlier chapter. In general, nociceptive/somatic pain (i.e., "tissue pain") is treated with anti-inflammatory agents and analgesics such as opiates, with or without adjuvant medications such as antidepressant drugs. In contrast, neuropathic pain is often treated more effectively with anticonvulsant and antidepressant medications. In particular, lancinating, paroxysmal pain (described by patients as "electrical shocks" or "shooting" pain) may respond to anticonvulsant therapy. Constant dysesthetic pain (typically described by patients as "burning") may respond to treatment with antidepressant medications such as amitriptyline. Many pain problems will require treatment with combinations of classes of medications.

NSAIDs provide pain relief to many patients, and they warrant use on a trial basis. Several weeks of use may be required before pain relief begins to develop.[70] Some patients obtain better pain relief with one NSAID than another, and trials with several different classes may be necessary to find the most effective one for a given patient.[70] Many physicians prescribe antidepressant drugs (e.g., amitriptyline) to patients with chronic pain. Doses that seem effective in relieving pain are lower than those required for antidepressant activity (e.g., 10 to 100 mg of amitriptyline per day), suggesting that pain relief may occur via neurochemical changes not directly related to depression.[71]

Opioid (narcotic) analgesics may be appropriate on an "as-needed" basis for patients who have occasional exacerbations of pain. Some patients may benefit from long-term, scheduled opioid use.[72–74] The risk of addiction from chronic opioid use is low, but patients should be carefully selected for this form of therapy, and long-term opioids should be part of a multimodal approach to therapy. When given on a chronic basis, opioids should be given on a scheduled basis rather than "as needed," and a sustained release formulation (pill or transdermal patch) is preferred. The indications for chronic opioid administration and the treatment protocol (e.g., dose schedule, who may prescribe refills, frequency of refills) should be carefully documented in the patient's medical record when using chronic opioid agents, and consideration should be given to using a "contract" with the patient if questions arise regarding his or her potential compliance with the opioid program.[72,74]

The usefulness of epidural steroid injections in management of chronic pain is controversial. Epidural steroid injections may be beneficial in reducing pain related to inflammation of tissues, including radicular pain that may arise from root inflammation.[75,76] Epidural steroids relieve radicular pain better than axial pain.[75] There is no clear indication for epidural steroids for the treatment of nonspecific neck or back pain.

A variety of nonpharmacologic therapies are useful adjuvants in many patients. These include orthoses, TENS, relaxation/biofeedback, hypnosis, and acupuncture. Orthoses (e.g., back braces, cervical collars) restrict mobility and may lead to further stiffness and increased pain, but in some instances they may be beneficial if used during activities that patients routinely find uncomfortable. As with other adjuvant therapies, the use of orthoses should be individualized according to the needs of the patient.

Neurosurgical procedures intended to provide symptomatic relief of chronic pain may be appropriate for some patients. Spinal cord stimulation (discussed in detail in a subsequent chapter) can help patients with persistent neuropathic pain (e.g., radicular pain from epidural fibrosis) but does not seem useful for nociceptive pain. The historical success rate of spinal cord stimulation in relieving chronic pain is approximately 50% to 70%.[62,77–79] A major limitation of spinal cord stimulation in treating chronic pain has been difficulty in providing relief of axial (truncal) pain. Consequently, a patient with back pain and radiating leg pain may obtain relief of leg pain but not back pain, and overall pain relief and functional status may not improve significantly. Other shortcomings of spinal cord stimulation systems such as mechanical failure[79] have been diminishing in frequency as electronics and hardware have improved. With the introduction of dual channel stimulation systems, better relief of axial pain may be obtained.[80] Technologic improvements, in conjunction with careful patient selection, may lead to higher success rates than are reported traditionally.

Intraspinal analgesic infusion therapy via implanted infusion pump (discussed in detail in a subsequent chapter), traditionally used for cancer-related pain, has been used to manage chronic pain of nonmalignant origin.[81–83] In fact, the most common application of intrathecal analgesic therapy is for treatment of pain related to FBSS. In general, outcomes studies indicate that approximately 60% to 80% of patients have good pain relief with intrathecal analgesic administration, with associated improvements in activities of daily living and mood.[81,82] Although the standard measure of "success" is 50% or greater reduction of pain, patients with less than 50% improvement in pain may be satisfied with the result of intrathecal analgesic therapy.[83] The degree of pain relief afforded to an individual patient varies according to the nature of the pain complaint and the patient. Long-term outcomes studies indicate that pain relief is similar regardless of the nature of pain (i.e., nociceptive, neuropathic, visceral)[81,82]; however, anecdotal experience suggests that patients with nociceptive pain tend to respond favorably to continuous spinal analgesic administration whereas those with neuropathic pain respond less well to the commercially available agent (morphine sulfate), more often require adjuvant intrathecal agents (i.e., medications such as bupivacaine or clonidine, which are not approved by the US Food and Drug Administration for intrathecal use), and require more intense management. As with other forms of surgical therapy, patients must be selected carefully for infusion therapy, and they should undergo a temporary trial of intrathecal analgesic to confirm relief of symptoms before implantation of the permanent system.

Destructive procedures for chronic nonspecific pain are not indicated in general. Facet denervation (discussed in a subsequent chapter) may be appropriate for individuals with axial pain who respond to well-placed selective facet blocks; however, long-term relief is not always accomplished following such procedures. Peripheral ablative procedures (e.g., ganglionectomy, rhizotomy) are not indicated for the relief of nonmalignant pain because the effectiveness is short-lived. Central ablative procedures such as cordotomy are not usually offered for the treatment of nonmalignant pain, especially if there is a significant component of neuropathic pain, due to lack of proven long-term efficacy and the risk of inducing postlesion dysesthetic pain.

In summary, the failed back surgery syndrome describes a heterogeneous population of patients with recurrent or persistent pain after spinal surgery. Successful treatment requires careful, thorough evaluation of the cause of symptoms, determination of a specific diagnosis, and formulation of a treatment regimen based on the diagnosis and goals of therapy. The approaches to treatment are as varied as the patients and must be individualized to meet the needs and goals of each patient. For individuals with identifiable surgically correctable abnormalities who meet accepted criteria for surgical intervention, repeat surgery can be offered with a reasonable likelihood of success. On the other hand, for some of these individuals, symptomatic treatment (e.g., medication therapy, spinal cord stimulation, intrathecal analgesic administration) may be more appropriate than repeat surgery. Surgery should not be offered to patients in the absence of clear-cut indications. Patients not meeting indications for repeat surgery should be engaged in programs designed to address the major factors underlying their persistent pain complaints, which may include both physiologic and psychosocial abnormalities. Many patients will require multimodal or multidisciplinary treatment. Physicians who have completed specialized training in comprehensive management of chronic pain (e.g., diplomats of the American Board of Pain Medicine) may facilitate the care of these individuals. Physicians managing the treatment of these individuals should remember that the goals of treatment of chronic pain can be moving targets; as one problem is corrected, another may arise. As is true of many patients with chronic pain, individuals with pain associated with the failed back surgery syndrome benefit from on-going reassessment and adjustment of their treatment programs to optimize recovery.

REFERENCES

1. La Rocca H. Failed lumbar surgery syndromes: causes and correctives. *In* Bridwell KH, DeWald RL (eds). The Textbook of Spinal Surgery. Philadelphia, JB Lippincott, 1991, pp 719–738.
2. Follett KA, Dirks BA. Etiology and evaluation of the failed back surgery syndrome. Neurosurg Q 3:40–59, 1993.
3. Burton CV, Kirkaldy-Willis WH, Yong-Hing K, et al. Causes of failure of surgery on the lumbar spine. Clin Orthop 157:191–199, 1981.
4. Long DM, Filtzer DL, BenDebba M, et al. Clinical features of the failed–back syndrome. J Neurosurg 69:61–71, 1988.
5. Wiesel SW, Feffer HL, Borenstein DG. Evaluation and outcome of low-back pain of unknown etiology. Spine 13:679–680, 1988.
6. Spengler DM, Freeman C, Westbrook R, et al. Low-back pain following multiple lumbar spine procedures. Failure of initial selection? Spine 5:356–360, 1980.
7. Fager CA, Freidberg SR. Analysis of failures and poor results of lumbar spine surgery. Spine 5:87–94, 1980.
8. Bouras N, Bartlett JR, Neil-Dwyer G, Bridges PK: Psychological aspects of patients having multiple operations for low back pain. Br J Med Psychol 57:147–151, 1984.
9. Frymoyer JW, Hanley EN Jr, Howe J, et al. A comparison of radiographic findings in fusion and nonfusion patients ten or more years following lumbar disc surgery. Spine 4:435–440, 1979.
10. Gill K, Frymoyer JW. The management of treatment failures after decompressive surgery. *In* Frymoyer JW (ed). The Adult Spine: Principles and Practice. New York, Raven Press, 1991, pp 1849–1872.
11. MacNab I. Negative disc explorations: an analysis of the causes of nerve-root involvement in sixty-eight cases. Clin Orthop 53:891–903, 1971.
12. Stolke D, Sollmann W-P, Seifert V. Intra- and postoperative complications in lumbar disc surgery. Spine 14:56–59, 1989.
13. Frymoyer JW. The role of spine fusion. Question 3. Spine 6:284–290, 1981.
14. Finnegan WJ, Fenlin JM, Marvel JP, et al. Results of surgical intervention in the symptomatic multiply-operated back patient. J Bone Joint Surg 61A:1077–1082, 1979.
15. Frymoyer JW, Howe J, Kuhlmann D. The long-term effects of spinal fusion on the sacroiliac joints and ilium. Clin Orthop 134:196–201, 1978.
16. Weinstein JN, Spratt KF, Spengler D, et al. Spinal pedicle fixation: reliability and validity of roentgenogram-based assessment and surgical factors on successful screw placement. Spine 13:1012–1018, 1988.
17. Kostuik JP, Frymoyer JW. Failures after spinal fusion. Causes and surgical treatment results. *In* Frymoyer JW (ed). The Adult Spine: Principles and Practice. New York, Raven, 1991, pp 2027–2068.
18. Wetzel FT, La Rocca H. The failed posterior lumbar interbody fusion. Spine 16:839–845, 1991.
19. Armstrong JR. The causes of unsatisfactory results from the operative treatment of lumbar disc lesions. J Bone Joint Surg 33B:31–35, 1951.
20. Cauchoix J, Ficat C, Girard B. Repeat surgery after disc excision. Spine 3:256–259, 1978.
21. Frymoyer JW, Hanley E, Howe J, et al. Disc excision and spine fusion in the management of lumbar disc disease: a minimum ten-year followup. Spine 3:1–6, 1978.
22. Greenwood J, McGuire TH, Kimball F. A study of causes of failure in the herniated intervertebral disc operation: an analysis of sixty-seven reoperated cases. J Neurosurg 9:15–20, 1952.
23. Weir KA, Jacobs GA. Reoperation rate following lumbar discectomy. An analysis of 662 lumbar discectomies. Spine 5:366–370, 1980.
24. Hoyland JA, Freemont AJ, Denton J, et al. Retained surgical swab debris in post-laminectomy arachnoiditis and peridural fibrosis. J Bone Joint Surg 70B:659–662, 1988.
25. Laasonen EM, Soini J. Low-back pain after lumbar fusion. Surgical and computed tomographic analysis. Spine 14:210–213, 1989.
26. Frymoyer JW, Matteri RE, Hanley EN, et al. Failed lumbar disc surgery requiring second operation: a long-term follow-up study. Spine 3:7–11, 1978.
27. Goldner JL. The role of spine fusion. Question 6. Spine 6:293–303, 1981.
28. Lehmann TR, La Rocca HS. Repeat lumbar surgery. A review of patients with failure from previous lumbar surgery treated by spinal canal exploration and lumbar spinal fusion. Spine 6:615–619, 1981.
29. Lehmann TR, Spratt KF, Tozzi JE, et al. Long-term follow-up of lower lumbar fusion patients. Spine 12:97–104, 1987.
30. Johnsson K-E, Redlund-Johnell I, Uden A, et al. Preoperative and postoperative instability in lumbar spinal stenosis. Spine 14:591–593, 1989.
31. Markwalder T-M, Reulen H-J. Diagnostic approach in instability and irritative state of a "lumbar motion segment" following disc surgery–failed back surgery syndrome. Acta Neurochir (Wien) 99:51–57, 1989.
32. Waddell G, McCulloch JA, Kummel E, et al. Nonorganic physical signs in low-back pain. Spine 5:117–125, 1980.
33. Weber H. Lumbar disc herniation. A controlled, prospective study with ten years of observation. Spine 8:131–140, 1983.
34. Torgerson WR, Dotter WE. Comparative roentgenographic study of the asymptomatic and symptomatic lumbar spine. J Bone Joint Surg 58A:850–853, 1976.
35. Nachemson AL. The lumbar spine. An orthopaedic challenge. Spine 1:59–71, 1976.
36. Friberg O. Functional radiography of the lumbar spine. Ann Med 21:341–346, 1989.
37. Hueftle MG, Modic MT, Ross JS, et al. Lumbar spine: postoperative MR imaging with Gd-DTPA. Radiology 167:817–824, 1988.
38. Ross JS, Mararyck TJ, Scrader M, et al. MR imaging of the postoperative spine: assessment with gadopentetate dimeglumine. AJR 155:867–872, 1990.
39. Ross JS, Masaryk TJ, Modic MT, et al. Lumbar spine: postoperative assessment with surface-coil MR imaging. Radiology 164:851–860, 1987.
40. Heithoff KB, Burton CV. CT evaluation of the failed back surgery syndrome. Orthop Clin North Am 16:417–444, 1985.
41. Braun KF, Hoffman JC Jr, Davis PC, et al. Contrast enhancement in CT differentiation between recurrent disk herniation and postoperative scar: prospective study. AJNR 6:607–612, 1985.
42. Firooznia H, Kricheff II, Rafii M, et al. Lumbar spine after surgery: examination with intravenous contrast-enhanced CT. Radiology 163:221–226, 1987.
43. Schubiger O, Valavanis A. CT differentiation between recurrent disc herniation and postoperative scar formation: the value of contrast enhancement. Neuroradiology 22:251–254, 1982.
44. Nachemson A, Zdeblick TA, O'Brien JP. Controversy—Lumbar disc disease with discogenic pain. What surgical treatment is most effective? Spine 21:1835–1838, 1996.
45. Resnick DK, Malone DG, Ryken TC. Guidelines for the use of discography for the diagnosis of painful degenerative lumbar disc disease. Neurosurg Focus 13:1–9, 2002.
46. Ford LT. Discography and intradiscal therapy. *In* Bridwell KH, DeWald RL (eds). The Textbook of Spinal Surgery. Philadelphia, JB Lippincott, 1991, pp 695–710.
47. Holt EP Jr. The question of lumbar discography. J Bone Joint Surg 50A:720–726, 1968.
48. Nachemson A. Editorial comment. Lumbar discography – where are we today? Spine 14:555–557, 1989.
49. Carragee EJ, Tanner CM, Yang B, et al. False-positive findings on lumbar discography. Reliability of subjective concordance assessment during provocative disc injection. Spine 24:2542–2547, 1999.
50. Carragee EJ, Paragioudakis SJ, Khurana S. 2002 Volvo Award winner in clinical studies: Lumbar high-intensity zone and discography in subjects without low back problems. Spine 25:2987–2992, 2000.
51. Carragee EJ, Chen Y, Tanner CM, et al. Provocative discography in patients after limited lumbar discectomy: a controlled, randomized study of pain response in symptomatic and asymptomatic subjects. Spine 25:3065–3071, 2000.
52. Madan S, Gundanna M, Harley JM, et al. Does provocative discography screening of discogenic back pain improve surgical outcome? J Spinal Disord 15:245–251, 2002.
53. Derby R, Howard MW, Grant JM, et al. The ability of pressure-controlled discography to predict surgical and non-surgical outcomes. Spine 24:364–372, 1999.

54. Rhyne AL, Smith SE, Wood KE, et al. Outcome of unoperated discogram-positive low back pain. Spine 20:1997–2001, 1995.
55. Colhoun E, McCall I, Williams L, et al. Provocation discography as a guide to planning operations on the spine. J Bone Joint Surg 70B:267–271, 1988.
56. Lusins JO, Danielski EF, Goldsmith SJ. Bone SPECT in patients with persistent back pain after lumbar spine surgery. J Nucl Med 30:490–496, 1989.
57. See DH, Kraft GH. Electromyography in paraspinal muscles following surgery for root compression. Arch Phys Med Rehabil 56:80–83, 1975.
58. Wynn Parry CB, Girgis F. The assessment and management of the failed back, Part II. Int Disabil Stud 10:25–28, 1988.
59. Franklin GM, Haug J, Heyer NJ, et al. Outcome of lumbar fusion in Washington State workers' compensation. Spine 19:1897–1904, 1994.
60. Waddell G, Kummel EG, Lotto WN, et al. Failed lumbar disc surgery and repeat surgery following industrial injuries. J Bone Joint Surg 61A:201–207, 1979.
61. Lehman TR, La Rocca HS. Repeat lumbar spine surgery. A review of patients with failure from previous lumbar surgery treated by spinal canal exploration and lumbar spinal fusion. Spine 6:615–619, 1981.
62. North RB, Kidd DH, Lee MS, et al. A prospective, randomized study of spinal cord stimulation versus reoperation for failed back surgery syndrome: initial results. Stereotact Funct Neurosurg 62:267–272, 1994.
63. Ackerman SJ, Steinberg EP, Bryan RN, et al. Persistent low back pain in patients suspected of having herniated nucleus propulsus: radiographic predictors of functional outcomes – implications for treatment selection. Radiology 203:815–822, 1997.
64. Becker N, Sjogren P, Bech P, et al. Treatment outcome of chronic non-malignant pain patients managed in a Danish multidisciplinary pain center compared to general practice: a randomized controlled trial. Pain 84:203–211, 2000.
65. Guzman J, Esmail R, Karjalainen K, et al. Multidisciplinary bio-psycho-social rehabilitation for chronic low back pain. Coch Database System Rev 1:CD000963, 2002.
66. Loeser JD, Bigos SJ, Fordyce WE, et al. Low back pain. *In* Bonica J, Loeser JD, Chapman CR, Fordyce WE (eds). The Management of Pain, ed 2. Philadelphia, Lea & Febiger, 1990, pp 1448–1483.
67. Nelson BW, Carpenter DM, Dreisinger TE, et al. Can spinal surgery be prevented by aggressive strengthening exercises? A prospective study of cervical and lumbar patients. Arch Phys Med Rehabil 80:20–25, 1999.
68. Travell JG, Simons DG. Myofascial Pain and Dysfunction. The Trigger Point Manual. Baltimore, Williams & Wilkins, 1983, pp 5–44.
69. Travell JG, Simons DG. Myofascial Pain and Dysfunction. The Trigger Point Manual. Baltimore, Williams & Wilkins, 1983, pp 45–102.
70. Benedetti C, Butler SH. Systemic analgesics. *In* Bonica J, Loeser JD, Chapman CR, Fordyce WE (eds). The Management of Pain, ed 2. Philadelphia, Lea & Febiger, 1990, pp 1640–1675.
71. Monks R. Psychotropic drugs. *In* Bonica J, Loeser JD, Chapman CR, Fordyce WE (eds). The Management of Pain, ed 2. Philadelphia, Lea & Febiger, 1990, pp 1676–1689.
72. Burchman SL, Pagel PS. Implementation of a formal treatment agreement for outpatient management of chronic nonmalignant pain with opioid analgesics. J Pain Symptom Manage 10:556–563, 1995.
73. Portenoy RK. Opioid therapy for chronic nonmalignant pain: a review of the critical issues. J Pain Symptom Manage 11:203–217, 1996.
74. Turk DC. Clinicians' attitudes about prolonged use of opioids and the issue of patient heterogeneity. J Pain Symptom Manage 11:218–230, 1996.
75. Ferrante FM, Wilson SP, Iacobo C, et al. Clinical classification as a predictor of outcome after cervical epidural steroid injection. Spine 18:730–736, 1993.
76. Weinstein SM, Herring SA, Derby R. Contemporary concepts in spine care: epidural steroid injections. Spine 20:1842–1846, 1995.
77. Barolat G. Current status of epidural spinal cord stimulation. Neurosurg Q 5:98–124, 1995.
78. Gybels JM, Sweet WH. Neurosurgical Treatment of Persistent Pain. Basel, Switzerland, Karger, 1989, pp 293–302.
79. Turner JA, Loeser JD, Bell KG. Spinal cord stimulation for chronic low back pain: a systematic literature synthesis. Neurosurgery 37:1088–1095, 1995.
80. Van Buyten J-P, Van Zundert J, Milbouw G. Treatment of failed back surgery syndrome patients with low back and leg pain: a pilot study of a new dual lead spinal cord stimulation system. Neuromodulation 2:258–265, 1999.
81. Winkelmüller M, Winkelmüller W. Long-term effects of continuous intrathecal opioid treatment in chronic pain of nonmalignant etiology. J Neurosurg 85:458–467, 1996.
82. Paice JA, Penn RD, Shott S. Intraspinal morphine for chronic pain: a retrospective, multicenter study. J Pain Symptom Manage 11:71–80, 1996.
83. Anderson VC, Burchiel KJ. A prospective study of long-term intrathecal morphine in the management of chronic nonmalignant pain. Neurosurgery 44:289–300, 1999.

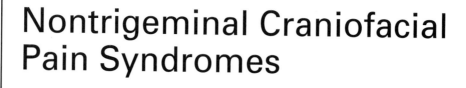

C H A P T E R 8

Nontrigeminal Craniofacial Pain Syndromes

RICHARD K. OSENBACH, MD

Pain in the head and face is a common problem that can be extremely distressing to the patient and is often frustrating for the physician treating the patient. Trigeminal neuralgia (TN) is probably the most common and well-recognized craniofacial pain syndrome. In addition, many patients suffer injury to one or more branches of the peripheral trigeminal system that results in a neuropathic facial pain syndrome that is most accurately termed *trigeminal neuropathic pain* (TNP). However, there are numerous other pathological conditions that produce craniofacial pain (Table 8-1).[1] These "nontrigeminal" pain syndromes, although individually less common, collectively represent an important group of conditions that are not uncommonly seen in the average medical practice. Unfortunately, many nontrigeminal pain syndromes lack the classical features of trigeminal neuralgia, making accurate diagnosis difficult for even the most skilled practitioner of pain medicine.

The purpose of this chapter is to review the diagnosis and treatment of some of the more common nontrigeminal craniofacial pain syndromes. TN and TNP will not be discussed except in the context of differentiating these conditions from other craniofacial pain syndromes.[1,2]

APPROACH TO THE PATIENT WITH CRANIOFACIAL PAIN

The single most important aspect in the evaluation of the patient with craniofacial pain is to establish the correct diagnosis. While this may seem simple enough, in practice, securing the correct diagnosis can be time-consuming, difficult, and frustrating. Nonetheless, successful treatment hinges on accurate diagnosis. Although surgical procedures such as microvascular decompression and retrogasserian radiofrequency rhizotomy may be highly effective for trigeminal neuralgia, they are ineffective and ill-advised for *most* nontrigeminal pain conditions. Accurate diagnosis of craniofacial pain begins with a careful detailed history covering all aspects of the pain including circumstances of onset, location, duration, temporal course, severity, quality, precipitating and aggravating factors, associated neurologic symptoms, and response to medications.

One of the most useful factors in differentiating the various syndromes is the temporal characteristics of the pain; that is, is the pain paroxysmal or constant? In fact, differentiation based solely upon temporal characteristics of the pain can be extremely useful in excluding certain pain syndromes. For example, TN is *classically* described as intermittent or paroxysmal while atypical facial pain (AFP) is nearly always described as constant. However, regardless of the syndrome, one observation would appear to be a major determinant of surgical efficacy; that is, the more paroxysmal pain dominates the clinical picture, the more likely it is that surgery may be beneficial.

GLOSSOPHARYNGEAL NEURALGIA

Clinical Features

Glossopharyngeal neuralgia (GPN) is a disabling syndrome characterized by pain that is perceived *primarily* in the sensory territory of the glossopharyngeal nerve. It has a peak incidence during the fifth to seventh decades. GPN shares some clinical features characteristic of TN.[3–6] The pain is typically unilateral, sharp, and lancinating, begins suddenly, and lasts for a few seconds to minutes before subsiding as quickly as it began. The pain may occur spontaneously or can be precipitated by activities such as swallowing. Episodes of pain not uncommonly occur in clusters separated by several minutes and are generally so severe that patients cease all activity. The clusters characteristically occur in an irregular fashion spaced over days, weeks, or months. Early on, pain-free intervals may be relatively long, but as GPN evolves and becomes more chronic, the clusters become more frequent.

There are also important distinctions between TN and GPN. TN is approximately 70 to 100 times more common than GPN. TN is slightly more common in females (3:2) while GPN occurs without a gender predilection. Interestingly, GPN occurs more often on the left side (3:2), while right-sided pain in more common with TN (5:3). Bilateral involvement, uncommon in both conditions, is only half as common in

● TABLE 8-1 • Common Causes of Craniofacial Pain

Neuropathic pain

Idiopathic trigeminal neuralgia
Secondary trigeminal neuralgia
Trigeminal neuropathic pain
Postherpetic neuralgia
Geniculate neuralgia
Vagal-glossopharyngeal neuralgia
Occipital neuralgia

Headache syndromes

Classic migraine (migraine with aura)
Common migraine (migraine without aura)
Migraine variants
Muscle tension headache
Post-traumatic headache
Cluster headache
Chronic paroxysmal hemicrania
Headache caused by other disorders

Pain due to tumors of the head and neck
Myofascial pain disorders

Temporomandibular joint disorders

Dental and periodontal pain

Pulpitis and periodontal abscess
Bruxism
"Burning tongue syndrome" (glossodynia)

Ocular and periocular pain

Tolosa-Hunt syndrome
Orbital apex syndrome
Cavernous sinus syndrome
Parasellar syndrome
Corneal problems (foreign body, keratitis)
Angle closure glaucoma
Optic neuritis
Orbital cellulitis

Pain due to aural diseases

Ramsay-Hunt syndrome
Otitis externa and interna
Bullous myringitis
Tumors
Mastoiditis

Disorders of the midface

Paranasal sinusitis
Trauma
Tumors

GPN (2%) as in TN (4%), and usually occurs in sequence rather than simultaneously. Finally, the clinical presentation of GPN tends to be much more variable and atypical than that of classical TN. Indeed, some authors have indicated that GPN is more often atypical than not.[7] For example, the pain of GPN is not uncommonly constant and may be variously described as aching, a pressure sensation, or even burning. Moreover, the pain can sometimes persist without relief for periods of several days to a few weeks. Approximately 10% of patients with GPN also suffer from concomitant TN.

Etiology and Pathogenesis

Although the pain of GPN *most often* occurs within the territory of the glossopharyngeal nerve, the location of the pain can be variable. The variability of the pain associated with GPN can only be appreciated through a familiarity with the anatomy of the glossopharyngeal nerve. The glossopharyngeal nerve carries general somatic sensory input from the external and middle ear, the posterior third of the tongue, and the pharynx. Consequently, the pain in GPN may be perceived in any of these areas. Two types of GPN have been described. Classic GPN is characterized by pain in the posterior portion of the tongue and/or tonsillar region. There is also an otalgic variety in which the pain is primarily located in the ear, and some patients may actually experience pain in both locations. The clinical presentation may be further clouded by the fact that around 10% of patients with GPN also have concomitant TN. The diagnosis of GPN can be secured by anesthetizing the posterior pharynx with a 10% solution of cocaine, which should relieve the pain of GPN for several hours, even if precipitated by swallowing or tactile stimulation of a trigger zone.

Although the majority of cases of GPN are considered idiopathic, structural lesions of the posterior fossa (excluding cases believed to be caused by vascular compression) can also produce the syndrome. In approximately 5% to 8% of patients with TN, a structural lesion in the cerebellopontine angle is believed to be the cause of the pain (so-called secondary TN). Similarly, a small percentage of patients may suffer from secondary GPN due to a structural lesion that affects the glossopharyngeal nerve, usually in the region of the jugular foramen. However, the structural lesions associated with GPN are remarkably different than those associated with TN. The structural lesions responsible for secondary TN are most often benign intradural tumors or occasionally vascular lesions, whereas secondary GPN is more often caused by a malignant neoplasm that affects the nerve extracranially. Infections or other inflammatory processes may also underlie GPN but are rare in patients with TN. Glossopharyngeal neuralgia can rarely be caused by compression of the nerve by an elongated styloid process.[8] Finally, although multiple sclerosis is found in 2% to 3% of patients with TN, it is almost never encountered in patients with GPN.

Treatment

As with other pain syndromes, nonoperative treatment should be attempted before considering surgery. Pharmacologic therapy of GPN is similar to that for TN. Antiepileptic drugs (AEDs) such as carbamazepine (Tegretol), oxcarbazepine (Trileptal), gabapentin (Neurontin), and so on may be effective at the outset, but their efficacy tends to fade so that surgical treatment must be considered.

Surgical treatment of GPN includes (1) microvascular decompression (MVD), (2) intracranial rhizotomy, and (3) percutaneous glossopharyngeal rhizotomy.[3,4,6,9–13] As with TN, it has been suggested that the majority of cases of idiopathic GPN are caused by vascular compression of the glossopharyngeal and vagal rootlets as they enter the medulla at the root entry zone, most often by the posterior inferior cerebellar artery (PICA) although other vessels may not infrequently be involved. Jannetta initially demonstrated vascular compression in 15 of 17 patients with GPN who underwent posterior fossa exploration, and then about a decade later reported on 28 patients with GPN in whom vascular compression was noted in 100% of cases.[10] Based on the observations by Jannetta as well as others, MVD has been adopted as the primary surgical therapy for GPN by many surgeons who have reported similar findings and results.[9–12]

Unfortunately, there are some patients in whom vascular compression is conspicuously absent in spite of a careful and diligent search. In the absence of obvious vascular compression, intracranial rhizotomy to include the glossopharyngeal *and* upper vagal rootlets should be considered.[4] Intracranial rhizotomy has its origin in the 1920s when Adson performed the first open intracranial preganglionic rhizotomy.[7] Unfortunately, the procedure was complicated by serious intraoperative hemorrhage that led to the death of the patient several hours following surgery. Dandy performed the first successful glossopharyngeal rhizotomies for GPN and reported excellent pain relief.[5] Dandy believed that the open intracranial procedure was superior to extracranial division of the glossopharyngeal nerve in the neck because interrupting the nerve proximal to the ganglion seemed to prevent recurrence of the pain. Furthermore, the procedure was highly selective, thus avoiding injury to other nerves. Although the original operation was limited to division of the glossopharyngeal rootlets, it later became apparent that inclusion of the upper vagal rootlets was necessary for more complete and long-term pain relief. Rushton and colleagues reported on a series of 217 patients with GPN treated over a 50-year period at the Mayo Clinic.[3] Seventy-one initially underwent intracranial glossopharyngeal rhizotomy. These authors also came to appreciate that inclusion of the upper vagal rootlets was necessary for success. Ultimately, 110 (85%) of 129 patients who underwent surgery were judged to have achieved "good" pain relief.

Sectioning of the glossopharyngeal nerve and upper one third of the vagus produces surprisingly little neurologic dysfunction. The most common postoperative problem is not surprisingly swallowing dysfunction, which may occur in up to 20%.[3] Obviously, in the rare patient with bilateral GPN, bilateral rhizotomies are contraindicated because this could lead to severe swallowing dysfunction. One of the major side effects that must be anticipated is the intraoperative hemodynamic changes that may often occur with manipulation and division of the ninth and tenth cranial nerves. Hypotension and tachycardia may occur and the surgeon should always inform the anesthesiologist when the vagal-glossopharyngeal complex is being manipulated. Of equal significance is the occurrence of hypertension at the point when the glossopharyngeal nerve is cut. This response is the result of interruption of the afferent vasodepressor impulses that originate from the carotid sinus and travel to the brainstem in the ninth nerve. This response may be so robust as to require the administration of antihypertensive agents to prevent the complications of acute hypertension.

Percutaneous glossopharyngeal rhizotomy can be considered as an alternative to open intracranial rhizotomy. Several techniques have been developed to destroy the fibers of the glossopharyngeal nerve within the pars nervosa of the jugular foramen including injection of alcohol or the use of radiofrequency current. The major risk of percutaneous glossopharyngeal rhizotomy is intracranial hemorrhage due to inadvertent placement of the needle into the intracranial space. The use of

computed tomography can facilitate introduction of the electrode into the proper location.[13] Gybels and Sweet used percutaneous rhizotomy as their initial procedure for the treatment of GPN.[14] They contend that by using the anterior approach, it is virtually impossible to enter the intracranial cavity, making the risk of hemorrhage from needle puncture nearly nonexistent. These authors also point out that the inferior ganglion of the ninth cranial nerve and the nodose ganglion of the vagus nerve lie below the jugular foramen, and consequently, a lesion in this area is central or proximal to the majority of the cells of origin in both nerves. The authors summarized the outcomes of 21 patients from eight series between 1977 and 1988 treated in this manner, noting that the patients generally "did well."[14] Complications included intraoperative bradycardia, hypotension, postoperative dysphagia, and vocal cord paralysis.

GENICULATE NEURALGIA (INTERMEDIUS NEURALGIA)

Anatomy and Pathophysiology

Geniculate or intermedius neuralgia is a relatively rare paroxysmal pain syndrome characterized by intermittent, sharp pain in the distribution of the sensory component of the facial nerve. More than six decades ago, J. Ramsey Hunt conducted extensive studies of the functional anatomy of the facial nerve and the various pain syndromes presumably related to its dysfunction, and concluded that there are four distinct pathways that comprise the facial nerve sensory system.[15] The first is comprised of afferent fibers from the geniculate ganglion that provide sensation to the tympanic membrane, a small cutaneous area of the external ear, and the inner ear. The second pathway includes sensory fibers that supply the orbit, posterior nasal region, and palate. These fibers travel in the greater superficial petrosal nerve and pass through the sphenopalatine ganglion to be distributed to their respective areas of sensory innervation. The third sensory component concerned with general somatic sensation includes fibers concerned with sensibility of the face originating in the geniculate ganglion and traveling with the facial nerve to the muscles of facial expression. The fourth pathway is largely concerned with the special sensation of taste and involves the chorda tympani but also contains some fibers that provide general sensory input from the anterior two thirds of the tongue.

Geniculate neuralgia can be classified according to etiology into primary, secondary, and reflex forms or according to the distribution the pain into otalgic and prosopalgic forms based upon the sensory distribution of the facial nerve described previously.[16] The pathophysiology of geniculate neuralgia is *presumed* to be analogous to that of TN and GPN, and indeed, compression of the nervus intermedius by vascular loops has been identified in a number of patients who have undergone posterior fossa exploration for this condition.[17]

Clinical Features and Diagnosis

Many features of the pain are reminiscent of those associated with TN. Most patients with idiopathic or primary geniculate neuralgia experience brief episodes of severe lancinating pain deep in the ear and posterior auricular region, so-called otalgic geniculate neuralgia.[18] The pain is nearly always unilateral. Attacks of pain may occur spontaneously or can be triggered by non-noxious stimuli such as tactile stimulation within the ear canal, swallowing, or talking. The pain may last from a few seconds to several minutes, then resolve, leaving the patient pain-free between attacks. Some patients may experience associated symptoms such as salivation, tearing, a bitter taste, tinnitus, and vertigo during the attack. The occurrence of these associated symptoms is believed to result from some type of central connections of the nervus intermedius or perhaps irritation of other components of the facial and vestibulocochlear nerves. However, objective neurologic findings are conspicuously absent.

The correct diagnosis of true idiopathic otalgic geniculate neuralgia is difficult because many conditions can produce pain in and around the ear and in the face. Likewise, prosopalgic geniculate neuralgia is difficult to substantiate as facial pain is a symptom common not only of TN but numerous other conditions such as sphenopalatine neuralgia, cluster headache, atypical facial pain, and carotidynia, to name just a few. Although each of these syndromes are said to possess certain features that set it apart from others, in practice, the symptoms overlap significantly and the supposedly distinguishing features are often spurious.

Otalgic geniculate neuralgia can also occur as a secondary effect of herpetic inflammation of the geniculate ganglion, so-called Ramsay-Hunt syndrome. In such cases, the characteristic vesicular eruption that involves the pinna, eardrum, and external ear canal discloses the diagnosis. The pain of geniculate herpes differs from that of primary geniculate neuralgia in that it is more often a constant burning pain as contrasted with the typical sharp neuralgic pain most often associated with primary intermedius neuralgia.

Surgical Treatments

Assuming primary aural pathology has been excluded and pharmacologic therapy has been attempted and failed, surgery may be considered. Although vascular compression has been presumed to be the etiology of pain in nonherpetic cases of geniculate neuralgia, the relative importance of vascular compression has yet to be determined. Indeed, there exist far fewer cases of geniculate neuralgia that come to surgery than TN or for that matter even GPN. Moreover, there are relatively few cases in which the precise vascular relationships to the nervus intermedius been examined in detail.[19]

Taylor, in 1909, was one of the first individuals to operate on a patient with otalgia that he believed represented "tic douloureux of the sensory filaments of the facial nerve."[20] After exposing the facial-vestibulocochlear complex, Taylor divided the nervus intermedius, facial nerve, and upper fascicle of the acoustic nerve and reported that the pain was relieved. In 1969, White and Sweet summarized the cases operated upon by Taylor along with eight additional cases of geniculate neuralgia.[21] Based primarily on observations that cutting the nervus intermedius relieved the pain *or* that stimulation of the nerve actually could invoke the pain, they concluded that the nervus intermedius was somehow involved in the mechanism of aural pain.

Rupa and colleagues reported 18 patients with otalgia who underwent a total of 31 surgical procedures.[17] Seventeen patients were treated with sequential rhizotomy while a single patient underwent MVD as the only procedure. These authors sectioned a number of nerves either singly or in combination including the nervus intermedius (n = 14), geniculate ganglion (n = 10), glossopharyngeal nerve (n = 14), vagus nerve (n = 11), tympanic nerve (n = 4), and chorda tympani (n = 1). Vascular loops were identified in nine patients and these individuals also underwent MVD. This inclusive approach resulted in pain relief in 72% of patients who were observed for an average of just over 3 years.

Given the difficulty with the diagnosis and the lack of data regarding surgery for geniculate neuralgia, it is not possible to advocate one specific surgical procedure for this condition. A reasonable approach might be to explore the posterior fossa with the intent of identifying a site of vascular compression. If there is undeniable evidence of vascular compression, then it would seem reasonable to perform MVD without sectioning the nervus intermedius. However, if no evidence of vascular compression is found, then nervus intermedius rhizotomy should be considered. For patients who initially enjoy pain relief following MVD but in whom pain recurs, re-exploration with division of the nervus intermedius can be considered.

OCCIPITAL NEURALGIA

Occipital neuralgia is a condition characterized by pain in the distribution of the greater and/or lesser occipital nerves. Classic occipital neuralgia presents with fairly clear-cut stereotypical features. Unfortunately, many other conditions including tension headache, migraine, and cervical strain may also produce or be associated with chronic occipital and suboccipital pain and are incorrectly diagnosed as occipital neuralgia. The latter conditions should be easily differentiated from occipital neuralgia by the absence of the electric shock-like pain that characterizes occipital neuralgia.

Anatomy and Pathophysiology

Knowledge of the anatomy of the upper cervical nerves and their central connections is essential to understand the clinical picture of occipital neuralgia and to differentiate this condition from other suboccipital pain syndromes.[22] The greater occipital nerve (GON) originates from the large dorsal medial branch of the C2 spinal nerve. The GON initially runs transversely covered by the suboccipital musculature and then turns and courses cephalad. At the nuchal line, the nerve pierces the aponeurotic attachments of the trapezius and sternocleidomastoid muscles and divides into terminal branches that provide sensory innervation to the scalp from the occipital region and the area above the mastoid to the vertex and occasionally as far forward as the coronal suture. The lesser occipital nerve arises primarily from the cervical plexus contribution of the ventral ramus of C2. It emerges from the investing fascia of the posterior triangle of the neck and travels along the posterior border of the sternocleidomastoid before dividing into terminal sensory branches that supply the area over the mastoid eminence and posterior aspect of the pinna. A portion of the latter area may also be supplied by the C3 dermatome.

The primary nociceptive afferent fibers that enter the spinal cord through the C2 root synapse with second-order neurons in the substantia gelatinosa of the upper cervical dorsal horn. Remember that the descending spinal trigeminal tract containing nociceptive input from the head and face merges with the substantia gelatinosa in the upper cervical cord. It has therefore been suggested that nociceptive information from the face and upper cervical dermatomes may actually converge at this level and may explain why some patients with occipital neuralgia have pain referred to the temple or retroorbital region in the distribution of the trigeminal nerve.

Diagnosis and Management

Occipital neuralgia may be caused by a myriad of underlying problems such as inflammation, metabolic disorders, and physical trauma including traction, compression, and entrapment (Table 8-2).[23,24] True occipital neuralgia must be distinguished from other occipital pain syndromes. Occipital neuralgia can be categorized as either "neuralgic" or "nonneuralgic" based on clinical presentation. The pain of classical "neuralgic" occipital neuralgia is almost always unilateral, and is most often described as a sharp, shooting, electric-like sensation that occurs in the distribution of the GON and radiates toward the vertex. The attacks of pain are fairly stereotypical and can sometimes be triggered by cervical motion and/or palpation along the course of the GON. The attacks of pain may occur in bursts that last for several seconds. Between painful attacks, the patient may be free of symptoms or may experience a continuos dull headache in the suboccipital region. In some patients, the neuralgic pain may be accompanied by other symptoms particularly following acute cervical strain. However, the paroxysmal lancinating component of the pain remains the key to correct diagnosis.

Patients with true occipital neuralgia may demonstrate signs of neurologic dysfunction in the C2 nerve root distribution although the presence of neurological findings is not required for the diagnosis.[25] There may be objective sensory loss in the distribution of the GON of which the patient is often unaware. Some patients may demonstrate hyperpathia without frank sensory loss and in some cases Tinel's sign can be elicited by percussion over the GON.

In contrast, there exists a large group of patients that describe their pain as dull, aching, throbbing, pounding, or as a pressure sensation. These patients with "non-neuralgic" occipital pain generally complain of a more constant pain that does not vary significantly in intensity. These patients more often complain of more diffuse pain that may be bilateral and involve adjacent areas such as the neck, shoulders, temple, forehead, and so on. These patients not uncommonly also relate constitutional or visual symptoms.

Diagnostic evaluation of the patient with suspected occipital neuralgia should include imaging studies of the craniovertebral junction (CVJ). Plain radiographs with dynamic views or computed tomography may sometimes identify a bony anomaly or atlantoaxial instability as the underlying cause for the pain.[26,27] Magnetic resonance imaging of the CVJ and upper cervical spine will exclude more ominous problems such as an intraspinal tumor, vascular lesion, or Chiari type I

● TABLE 8-2 • Underlying Causes of Occipital Neuralgia

Congenital
Chiari I malformation
Traumatic
C1–2 instability
Fractures of C1
Osseous abnormalities
Osteoarthritis
C1–2 arthrosis syndrome
Hypertrophic facet joint
Inflammatory
Rheumatoid arthritis with cranial settling
Gout
Myofascial pain
Tumors
Cervical spinal cord tumors
Metastatic neoplasms
Posterior fossa tumors
Vascular lesions
Arterial or venous compression
Postoperative
Ventriculoperitoneal shunts
Retromastoid craniectomy
Mastoidectomy
Metabolic
Diabetic neuropathy
Miscellaneous
Spasmodic torticollis
Entrapment syndrome
Idiopathic

malformation. Laboratory studies are helpful in excluding inflammatory and metabolic problems. If an underlying cause is identified, then treatment should be directed toward correcting that particular problem. Assuming no underlying cause can be identified, then treatment is focused on the pain.

The initial treatment of idiopathic occipital neuralgia should be conservative and may include modalities such as immobilization with a cervical collar, nonsteroidal anti-inflammatory drugs (NSAIDs), muscle relaxants, transcutaneous electrical nerve stimulation, nerve blocks, and acupuncture.[24] A trial of therapy with one or more AEDs may be effective although the efficacy of these agents has not been as well studied for occipital neuralgia as TN. Tricyclic antidepressants (TCAs) may be useful although in the author's experience the TCAs seem to be somewhat more beneficial in patients who experience a more constant burning type of pain while AEDs are often more effective for intermittent, sharp, neuralgic type of pain. However, not uncommonly, combining one of the TCAs with an anticonvulsant will produce a degree of analgesia that exceeds that which can be achieved with either agent alone.

The true sensitivity and specificity of diagnostic blocks is unknown, especially in the absence of placebo controls.

Notwithstanding these limitations, local anesthetic blocks are easy to perform, are minimally invasive, and can be both diagnostic as well as therapeutic. For maximum accuracy and specificity, occipital nerve block should be performed with a minimal volume of local anesthetic (0.5 to 1.0 cc). When performed as a therapeutic maneuver, a steroid preparation such as depomedrol or Celestone may be added to the solution injected. Occasionally, some patients will report pain relief far in excess of the duration of the block and a few patients will obtain long-term benefit although in my experience, this is exceptional.

Patients with intractable occipital neuralgia who fail nonoperative therapy may be candidates for surgery of the C2 pathways and numerous surgical options have been described for treatment of this condition.[24,28–32] Decompression and neurolysis of the GON, which is presumed to be entrapped, can be performed although there are few reports of any long-term success with this approach.[29] Indeed, there has been significantly more experience with destructive procedures such as occipital neurectomy, dorsal root ganglionectomy, and intradural rhizotomy. More recently, peripheral nerve stimulation techniques have been used for the treatment of this condition.

Peripheral neurectomy of the GON or its branches is a safe and relatively simple procedure that produces variable results. In patients who have undergone successful, well-done, repetitive diagnostic occipital nerve blocks, occipital neurectomy appears to result in good initial pain relief but recurrence is common.[30] Perhaps the major reason why pain recurrence is so high is related to regeneration of the nerve with formation of a painful neuroma. Additionally, peripheral neurectomy does not address any potential dysfunction of more proximal neural elements that may be involved in the generation and maintenance of pain. Intradural dorsal rhizotomy is designed to eliminate the afferent input to the spinal cord and has been reported successful in up to 50% of patients.[24] However, intradural rhizotomy is a more formidable procedure than occipital neurectomy and is associated with a higher morbidity. Moreover, there is anatomic evidence in animals that as many as 30% of nociceptive afferent fibers may enter the spinal cord through the ventral root. If this is in fact true in humans, this may explain the failure of dorsal rhizotomy because selective section of the dorsal roots would fail to eliminate these ventral nociceptive afferent fibers. The shortcomings of occipital neurectomy and intradural rhizotomy can be circumvented by dorsal root ganglionectomy. Ganglionectomy eliminates the cell bodies of the primary nociceptive afferent fibers and at least theoretically prevents regeneration of these fibers. Dorsal root ganglionectomy is performed under general anesthesia with the patient prone. The C2 ganglion lies between C1 and C2 immersed in a venous plexus that must be coagulated to expose the ganglion. Once exposed, the ganglion is excised by dividing the neural elements proximal and distal to the ganglion. Observations by Lozano and colleagues indicate that C2 ganglionectomy is effective in 90% of patients who experience neuralgic type of pain but is ineffective in patients without the paroxysmal lancinating pain component.[33] More recently, peripheral nerve stimulation has been advocated as a treatment for occipital neuralgia.[34] Under local anesthesia, a wire-type of electrode is inserted subcutaneously and oriented transversely around the level of C1. Test stimulation is performed to ensure coverage of the pain topography with stimulation-induced paresthesias. Patients who experience adequate pain reduction during an appropriate length screening trial then undergo implantation of a permanent system. Occipital nerve stimulation has the advantage of being reversible, testable (at least to certain degree), and does not involve destruction of neural structures with the production of sensory loss. Although this procedure appears attractive, long-range follow-up will be necessary to determine if the benefit is durable. A final option is to perform high cervical spinal cord stimulation using paddle electrode placed retrograde beneath the posterior arch of C1 and the lamina of C2. Using electrodes in this location it is possible to achieve stimulation into the occipital and suboccipital regions and even into the lower jaw in some cases.

MISCELLANEOUS NON-NEOPLASTIC CRANIOFACIAL PAIN SYNDROMES

There are many other conditions for which craniofacial pain is a prominent feature. A comprehensive review of all of these conditions is outside the scope of this chapter. Following is a brief description of some of more well-recognized, albeit uncommon, syndromes.

Sphenopalatine Neuralgia

The sphenopalatine or pterygopalatine ganglion contains synapses of parasympathetic fibers that originate from the facial nerve and are then transmitted to the ganglion through the greater superficial petrosal nerve and to some extent the nerve of the pterygoid canal. Sphenopalatine neuralgia (a.k.a. Sluder's syndrome, lower-half headache) is a rare pain syndrome characterized by pain in the middle portion of the face.[1] Various causes have been suggested including spread of adjacent paranasal sinus infection with concomitant vasoconstriction, nasal pathology with resultant stimulation of the pterygopalatine ganglion, and a vasodilator syndrome. Patients experience spontaneous unilateral pain in the middle third of the face that often originates near the root of the nose. The pain can spread to the eye, upper teeth, palate, or pharynx. Customarily, no trigger zone can be identified. Autonomic symptoms such as lacrimation, rhinorrhea, and salivation may accompany the pain.

Treatment of sphenopalatine neuralgia consists of blockade of the pterygopalatine ganglion by local anesthetics. This can be accomplished using several techniques including topical transnasal application or blockade through a lateral approach.[35] In selected patients with persistent pain, the ganglion may be destroyed using percutaneous radiofrequency thermocoagulation or by alcohol neurolysis.

Vidian Neuralgia

Vidian neuralgia, also known as Vail's syndrome, is similar to sphenopalatine neuralgia.[1] The nerve of the pterygoid canal or vidian nerve contains postganglionic sympathetic fibers that originate in the superior cervical plexus, become part of the internal carotid plexus and pass through the pterygopalatine ganglion as the vidian nerve. Vidian neuralgia is more common in females and consists of attacks of unilateral pain, frequently nocturnal, involving the nose, eye, ear, head, or neck. The condition is believed to be caused by irritation or inflammation of the vidian nerve. Frank sinus infection should be excluded. Blockade of the pterygopalatine ganglion described previously may be diagnostic as well as therapeutic.

Carotidynia

Carotidynia is a unilateral syndrome that consists of intense throbbing episodes of pain in the region of the carotid artery. The most intense pain is located over the lateral neck, near the angle of the jaw, and the ear. The usual onset is during the fourth decade, with women affected more often than men. The pain is usually intermittent but may occur over a long period and then spontaneously remit. The carotid artery is usually tender and palpation may trigger the pain. The patient usually has difficulty turning the head contralateral to the pain and there is often associated muscle stiffness and referred pain to the head. Similar to cluster headache, an attack of carotidynia can be aborted by inhalation of 100% oxygen. It is important to exclude other pathological conditions such as aneurysm, carcinoma, and inflammatory disorders of the neck, mandible, lateral pharynx, and salivary glands. The treatment of carotidynia mirrors that of migraine and includes ergotamine derivatives, beta blockers, and the like. In some patients, stress reduction techniques, such as biofeedback and hypnosis, may prove beneficial.

Superior Laryngeal Neuralgia

Superior laryngeal neuralgia shares some of the characteristic features of trigeminal and glossopharyngeal neuralgia. Patients experience intermittent attacks of unilateral, severe, lancinating pain that originates near the lateral aspect of the thyroid cartilage or the piriform sinus and radiates outward toward the angle of the jaw and occasionally to the ear. A trigger zone is thought to be present in the larynx and the pain may be triggered by swallowing, yawning, sneezing, or tactile stimulation of the skin covering the hyoid bone. The condition must be differentiated from glossopharyngeal or hyoid neuralgia. Additionally, a careful otolaryngologic examination should be conducted to exclude primary laryngeal pathology. The diagnosis may be confirmed by local anesthetic blockade of the superior laryngeal nerve. Initial treatment involves the use of anticonvulsants such as carbamazepine. Patients who fail medical therapy and in whom intractable symptoms develop can be considered for microvascular decompression of the upper vagal rootlets. If no clear compression is identified, the upper vagal fibers along with the glossopharyngeal nerve may be divided.

FACIAL PAIN AND MALIGNANCY

Malignant involvement of structures of the head and neck can be a particularly challenging problem both for the patient and physician. Given that the face is the most expressive part of the human body, it is not surprising that malignant tumors that involve head and facial structures provoke tremendous fear and anxiety.

Mechanisms of Cancer Pain of the Head and Neck

Pain can be associated with any type of malignant tumor that involves structures of the head and neck. Effective pain management requires a general understanding of the growth characteristics and patterns of spread of various types of tumors. Head and neck tumors produce pain through several mechanisms including stimulation of nerve endings in mucous membranes, compression and/or invasion of sensory nerves, ulceration and infection, bony invasion and destruction, and as a complication of oncologic therapy.[36]

Stimulation of free nerve endings in the mucosa and submucosa is often one of the initial signs of tumor growth. Stimulation of these nociceptors generally produces a superficial pain, often causing a local constant burning sensation. Malignant tumors that arise from the mucous membranes are primarily squamous cell carcinomas. These tumors tend to ulcerate although the ulceration per se does not necessarily produce the pain. Rather, local irritants activate nociceptors to produce the pain. Additionally, ulcerated tissue often becomes secondarily infected, leading to inflammation and edema that further potentiates the pain. Pain related to ulceration and inflammation is aggravated by movement of the affected area and varies from site to site. Invasion or compression of the trigeminal nerve or any of its peripheral branches is another cause of pain. The pain will generally be felt in the area innervated by the particular portion of the nerve that is involved. Bone invasion by tumor does not initially produce pain. However, as the tumor grows it causes the periosteum to expand, which stimulates the nociceptive afferents that innervate this structure. The pain is usually localized to the site of involvement but can be referred to a more distant area. Another way in which bony involvement causes pain is secondary bacterial invasion with development of osteomyelitis. Finally, pain may occur as a complication or sequela of treatment of the underlying tumor. Radical surgical resection of head and neck cancer often requires that nerves be transected to achieve a total resection. This can lead to the formation of painful neuromas. Mucositis is a common complication of chemotherapy either administered alone or in combination with radiation therapy. Some patients will also develop an outbreak of herpes zoster in the area involved by the tumor and go on to develop postherpetic neuralgia.

Primary Oncologic Therapy

The initial management of pain related to head and neck cancer is to consider primary treatment strategies directed at the tumor.[37,38] This may involve a combination of primary resective surgery, radiation therapy, and chemotherapy. This approach is based not only on an attempt to "cure" the tumor but also on the assumption that reduction in the size of the tumor will lead to a reduction in pain.

Radical surgical resection is the primary therapy for a large number of malignant head and neck tumors including those involving the larynx, hypopharynx, mouth, mandible, and paranasal sinuses.[37,38] Indeed, early surgery with or without radiation may be curative in some cases. Surgery may also be indicated for patients that have received radiation and present with a recurrence. Bone invasion especially in combination with radionecrosis of bone is a frequent cause of pain. In such cases, resection of the involved bone is the most direct and rapid method of eliminating the pain. Surgery can be particularly effective for the following:

1. Recurrent cancer involving the oral cavity (tonsil, base of tongue, retromolar space, or anterior pillar) associated with radionecrosis
2. Osteoradionecrosis of the mandible with or without tumor recurrence
3. Recurrent tumor or the nasal cavity and paranasal sinuses
4. Recurrence of lymph node metastases in the neck after both initial surgery and radiation[38]

Radiation therapy alone or combined with surgery is often the initial treatment for some malignant tumors of the head and neck.[39] Radiation is an important adjunct in the treatment of cancer pain. Even in advanced tumors that are not amenable to radical resection, radiation therapy is often beneficial in controlling pain, especially in radiosensitive tumors including undifferentiated carcinomas of the tonsil, nasopharynx, and paranasal sinuses, as well as ulcerating tumors of the tongue and mouth. Not uncommonly, pain is the result of recurrent cancer that has previously been treated with surgery and radiation. In such cases, further radiation may be ineffective and even counterproductive because an excessive dose can lead to radionecrosis and ultimately increase pain. In such cases, the question of whether to give additional radiation must be carefully weighed and performed only if poor results would be anticipated from alternative treatments or when the possibility of a cure may still exist.[38]

The rationale for chemotherapy is again based on the assumption that there is a correlation between reduction in tumor burden and alleviation of pain. Indeed, palliative chemotherapy has been utilized for many years in cancer of the head and neck although the results have been inconsistent and in many cases suboptimal.[40]

Neurosurgical Management

Although the majority of patients with craniofacial pain related to malignancy can be effectively managed with medical therapy alone, some continue to have intractable disabling pain that requires a more aggressive approach. One of the major obstacles to the effective treatment of pain experienced by patients with advanced cancer is therapeutic nihilism. Unfortunately, once it has been determined that the patient has an incurable disease and that further therapeutic maneuvers will be ineffective, an erroneous assumption is all too often made that death from certain types of cancer is inevitably painful. Such could be farther from reality. All patients with cancer should receive aggressive and effective pain relief throughout their entire disease process regardless of the stage of disease or their functional status. Indeed, the philosophical as well as practical approaches to pain management should be identical regardless of whether the disease is potentially curable or whether the patient is suffering from a terminal illness. Even in the terminal patient, effective reduction of pain is possible and often enables the patient to be more functional and improves the quality of life that remains. Consequently, surgical intervention for pain control when medical therapy has failed should not be viewed

as an overly aggressive approach, but as a viable option for effective pain management.

Many surgical procedures have been developed for the treatment of pain in general and facial pain in particular. Many of the surgical procedures that are effective in the treatment of facial pain target various portions of the trigeminal system. Although peripheral destructive procedures are highly effective for trigeminal neuralgia, these procedures for the most part are only temporarily effective in patients with invasive head and neck cancer and have a propensity to produce deafferentation pain. Consequently, many of the surgical procedures that have been shown to be effective in treating cancer pain in the head and neck have targeted more central structures of the trigeminal system within the brainstem and upper cervical spinal cord.

Intraventricular Opiates

Following the discovery of opiate receptors in the brain and spinal cord in the 1970s, it was found that intrathecal administration of opiates resulted in a rapid and profound analgesia that was reversible with naloxone. Similar observations were subsequently made in humans and since the early 1980s spinal opiates have been a cornerstone in the armamentarium of pain management for patients with cancer. Intrathecal opiates are most commonly administered into the spinal fluid on a continuous basis using an implanted infusion pump. Unfortunately, spinal delivery may not be particularly effective in the treatment of pain in the head and neck region. Therefore, for patients with pain related to invasive cancer of the head and neck, intraventricular opiate therapy may offer a viable alternative for achieving pain control. The therapeutic basis underlying the local administration into the intraventricular cerebrospinal fluid (CSF) is based on studies that have demonstrated a high concentration of opiate receptors in the walls of the third ventricle and the periaqueductal gray matter. Administration of morphine directly into the cerebral ventricles produces widespread analgesia that is dose-dependent, stereospecific, and reversible by naloxone.

The use of intraventricular opiates (IVOs) should be based on strict criteria. This therapy should be restricted to patients with terminal head and neck cancer in whom oral narcotic therapy has failed. In general, patients with bilateral midline or diffuse pain that is not amenable to either percutaneous or open destructive procedures are the best candidates for IVO therapy. Patients with pain in the lower half of the body may also be considered for IVOs only after failure of or contraindications to the use of spinal opiates.[41]

Intraventricular opiates are generally administered as a daily bolus injection through an implanted ventricular catheter connected to a subcutaneous reservoir. A ventricular catheter is placed into the lateral ventricle in a standard fashion and positioned as close as possible to the foramen of Monro or if possible threaded into the third ventricle. The catheter is connected to a subcutaneous access port. The port is accessed percutaneously with a 25-gauge needle and several milliliters of CSF are gently aspirated; the CSF is kept to flush the catheter after instillation of the drug. It is critical that meticulous sterile technique be used each time the reservoir is accessed to avoid contamination. Preservative-free morphine is injected into the reservoir and gently flushed using the CSF that was withdrawn. Although the patient is likely not opiate naïve, one should begin with a relatively small dose of approximately 0.1 mg. The dose is incrementally escalated until pain control is achieved, usually approximately 1.0 mg, although some patients may ultimately require considerably more drug to achieve adequate analgesia. Typically, the onset of analgesia occurs between 15 and 30 minutes following administration with peak analgesic effect being reached by 60 minutes. The mean duration of analgesia is approximately 28 hours (range, 12 to 70 hours).[41] During the titration period, patients must be closely observed for signs of respiratory depression, which should be reversed if necessary using naloxone administered intravenously. During the titration period, nausea and vomiting are relatively common, occurring in approximately 30% of patients. This is usually fairly self-limited, can be managed with antiemetic preparations, and does not necessarily preclude continuation of therapy.

Lazorthes and colleagues reported their experience with IVO therapy in 82 patients with cancer pain.[41] The average follow-up was 9 weeks (range, 12 to 443 days). The initial daily dose of morphine was 0.3 mg (range, 0.1 to 2 mg). All patients reported complete analgesia within 1 hour of injection of the drug (average, 20 minutes) and an average duration of pain relief of 28 hours. The end point of the study was death due to the underlying cancer. Final assessment of the patients in this series over an average of 2.5 months indicated excellent or good analgesia in 66 patients (80%), moderate pain control in 14 patients (17%), and failure of treatment in 2 patients. As is the case with spinal opiates, dose escalation was common. For patients that survived for more than 60 days, there was a tenfold increase in the average final dose of morphine compared to the initial dose. The side effects of therapy were for the most part minor and included nausea, vomiting, headache, pruritus, urinary retention, dizziness, and disorientation. Major central side effects including respiratory depression occurred in only 3 of the 82 patients (4%) and were immediately reversed by naloxone with only minimal effects on the induced analgesia.

Lesions of the Spinal Trigeminal Tract and Nucleus

Open trigeminal tractotomy. Trigeminal tractotomy is designed to interrupt the primary nociceptive afferent fibers that descend in the brainstem to synapse with second-order neurons in the spinal trigeminal nucleus. Destruction of this pathway produces ipsilateral analgesia in all three divisions of the trigeminal nerve.[42] Trigeminal tractotomy as originally described by Sjöqvist is performed through a suboccipital craniotomy.[43] The cerebellar tonsil is elevated to expose the dorsolateral surface of the medulla, and the olive and obex, which serve as important anatomic landmarks, are identified. The descending trigeminal tract is sectioned by choosing an area approximately 8 to 10 mm above the obex and just posterior to the last vagal rootlet and making an incision 3.5 to 4 mm deep perpendicular to the direction of the fibers of the tract. A lesion created in this fashion reliably produces ipsilateral analgesia in all three divisions of the trigeminal nerve. Unfortunately, the procedure is technically demanding and associated with significant morbidity. The most common complications include ataxia (due to injury of the spinocerebellar tract) and dysphagia (related to injury of the nucleus ambiguous). Sjöqvist's

original procedure was modified to make the lesion more caudally at a point where the spinocerebellar tract is not as superficial and where the trigeminal tract is covered only by a few external arcuate fibers. Although a more caudal incision spares the spinocerebellar tract and results in significantly less ataxia, it is also more likely to result in incomplete and only temporary analgesia, particularly in the third division of the trigeminal nerve as well as the sensory territories of the facial, glossopharyngeal, and vagal nerves. To produce consistent analgesia in these areas, the lesion must be more rostral and closer to the obex.

The results of trigeminal tractotomy have been variable. Some authors have reported significant pain reduction in 90% to 100%; others have reported success in as few as 17% of patients despite complete facial analgesia.[42] Because of the high occurrence of complications, variable pain relief, the relatively frequent recurrence of pain, and the existence of other more successful and less morbid procedures, open trigeminal tractotomy currently has limited if any application and for the most part has been discarded by neurosurgeons.

Percutaneous trigeminal tractotomy and nucleotomy. Percutaneous trigeminal nucleotomy was first performed in 1967 by Crue and colleagues in a patient with facial pain related to carcinoma of the ethmoid sinuses.[44] In 1971, Fox described a percutaneous freehand approach to trigeminal tractotomy.[45] Both procedures are performed awake, the former aided by a stereotactic frame and the latter without. The target is selected by identifying anatomical landmarks after injection of contrast material into the cisterna magna. Both procedures utilize a radiofrequency (RF) lesion, which is always preceded by physiologic localization. Electrical stimulation at the target generally produces a dysesthetic sensation referred to the area supplied by the primary afferent projections. Ipsilateral arm paresthesias indicate the electrode is placed too medially in the nucleus cuneatus while contralateral upper extremity sensations imply the electrode is too anterior in the spinothalamic tract. Placement too far posteriorly in the corticospinal tract will elicit motor responses. During the past decade, Kanpolat and colleagues advocated the use of computed tomography for percutaneous freehand trigeminal tractotomy using special electrodes designed to eliminate artifact.[46]

The major difference between open trigeminal tractotomy and percutaneous nucleotractotomy is that the latter not only targets the descending primary afferent fibers but also the cell bodies of the second-order neurons that reside in the spinal trigeminal nucleus. Both stereotactic and freehand trigeminal tractotomy are effective in patients with cancer pain, providing immediate pain relief in 85% to 100% of patients. The procedure may also be effective in selected patients with neuropathic pain syndromes. Although treatment of noncancer pain syndromes with these procedures is sometimes beneficial in the short term, long-term results are disappointing. The major complications are related to inaccurate electrode placement and include ataxia that is frequent, albeit usually transient, and inadvertent contralateral sensory loss.

Caudalis DREZ lesions. Nashold and associates are largely responsible for introducing the concept of creating multiple small RF lesions in the lower portion of the spinal trigeminal nucleus or nucleus caudalis.[47] The nucleus caudalis is situated in a triangular area between the dorsolateral sulcus and the exit zone of the eleventh cranial nerve. Around the level of the C2 root, the nucleus merges with the dorsal horn of the upper cervical cord and is covered by a thin layer of the descending spinal trigeminal tract. As one moves rostrally near the obex, the spinocerebellar tract and external arcuate fibers overlie the nucleus.

The procedure is carried out with the patient prone under general anesthesia. The operation can be performed through either a bilateral or unilateral exposure. A small suboccipital craniectomy and C1 hemilaminectomy are performed and the dura opened. The usual precautions should be taken as with any intradural posterior fossa procedure. Using the operating microscope, the first step is to identify the major landmarks that will be used to guide the procedure. The rootlets of C2 lie just below the posterior arch of C1; one is able to identify the dentate ligament and fibers of the eleventh cranial nerve laterally. The obex can be visualized by gently retracting the medial dura. Special right-angled caudalis dorsal root entry zone (DREZ) electrodes have been designed for this procedure. A smaller electrode is initially used at the more caudal levels where the nucleus lies closer to the surface. Beginning immediately above the sensory rootlets of C2, lesions are made in a straight line at approximately 1-mm intervals for 15 seconds at 75 °C. At the level of C1, the nucleus is larger and thus a larger electrode is used. This electrode is also insulated except at the tip in order to prevent inadvertent injury to the more superficial spinocerebellar tract. The row of lesions is continued rostrally and curved slightly ventrally running 1 to 2 mm posterior to the line of the rootlets of the 11th nerve. The lesions are continued to the tuber cinereum or about 5 mm above the level of the obex. Although the number of lesions is not specifically set, roughly 10 lesions are made with the smaller electrode and 6 to 10 lesions with the larger electrode.[47] The most significant complication is ataxia, related to injury of the spinocerebellar pathway. The incidence of ataxia was previously around 50%; however, with use of the newer right-angled electrodes, the incidence of ataxia is substantially reduced. The recent use of trigeminal evoked potentials as an adjunct has also allowed identification of the somatotopic organization and selective destruction of portions of the nucleus caudalis based on the location of pain.

The major application of the caudalis DREZ procedure would appear to be for neuropathic pain syndromes such as anesthesia dolorosa, postherpetic neuralgia, pain related to brainstem infarction, and the like. It has not been used as frequently for cancer pain, which often has a large nociceptive component. Pain reduction has been reported between 25% and 100% in patients with cancer.[42] However, many patients with head and neck cancer pain have a significant component of deafferentation pain related to prior resective procedures and it would seem that caudalis DREZ might be useful in carefully selected patients.

Midbrain tractotomy. Mesencephalotomy or midbrain tractotomy is a very effective operation for the treatment of pain in the head, neck, and shoulder. Midbrain tractotomy is designed to destroy the second-order fibers that carry pain and temperature sensation in the spinothalamic and quintothalamic (trigeminothalamic) pathways. Although most commonly used for cancer pain, selected patients with pain of benign origin also achieve long-term pain relief with this procedure. Midbrain tractotomy is especially useful when caudalis DREZ has failed.

The procedure is performed stereotactically. The classical target is located 5 mm behind and inferior to the posterior commissure and 5 to 10 mm lateral to the midline.[48] The target is roughly in line with the inferior border of the superior colliculus. As with other stereotactic destructive procedures, it is critical to perform physiologic localization before making the lesion. Electrical stimulation in the area of the target at 100 Hz and very low thresholds most commonly produces a sensation of burning although a variety of sensations have been reported. If the target is too far ventral and rostral, it places the extraocular movements at risk while a target placed too inferiorly can risk auditory function. After performing a test lesion, a permanent lesion is made for 30 seconds at 80 °C. A second lesion is then made after withdrawing the electrode about 3 mm; a third lesion can sometimes be made more medially to affect the reticulothalamic tract and periaqueductal gray.

CLUSTER HEADACHE

Incidence and Pathophysiology

Cluster headache (CH) is a syndrome that occasionally comes to the attention of the neurosurgeon when the symptoms become refractory to all forms of medical therapy. Cluster headache is less common than migraine. It is significantly more common in males and there is some evidence to support a genetic predisposition to this condition.

Current theories about the etiology of CH have been nicely summarized by Menizabal and colleagues.[49] However, no single mechanism has been identified that adequately explains all of the clinic features of CH. The cyclical nature of CH has led some investigators to implicate the hypothalamus, particularly the suprachiasmatic region. Abnormal levels of melatonin as well as all of the customary pituitary hormones have been identified in patients with CH, although it is not clear whether these hormonal alterations represent a primary event or simply an epiphenomenon. Another theory has suggested the existence of a "generator" in the intracavernous portion of the carotid artery that in turn activates fibers within the carotid plexus. There is some evidence for a sterile inflammatory process within the cavernous sinus as the initial trigger for the headache. Changes in cerebral blood flow have been shown to occur in conjunction with CH although again it is not certain that these changes represent primary events. It does appear that prophylactic drugs block these vascular changes. Additional factors that may contribute to the mechanism of CH include hypoxemia, hypocapnia, and the immune system, the latter based on the identification of circulating immune complexes and interleukins in patients with CH.

Clinical Features

Cluster headache has a rather typical clinical presentation.[49,50] Patients affected by this condition experience sudden attacks of severe pain located in the temple, eye, or periocular region(s). In fact, the pain of CH is one of the most severe pains that a person can experience. The pain is usually described as excruciating, but unlike that of migraine it is usually nonthrobbing. An additional feature that differentiates CH from migraine is the absence of an aura affording the patient little warning before the headache begins. Although the pain is usually located in the trigeminal distribution, approximately 18% of patients experience symptoms in the head and neck that lie outside of this territory. In approximately 50% of patients, the headache tends to be nocturnal, although it is not uncommon to observe a circadian rhythm in some patients, with attacks occurring at a particular time of the day or night.[25]

The typical CH attack may be as short-lived as 5 minutes or may persist for several hours before subsiding spontaneously. During the attack, the patient may be extremely restless, may clutch their head, and even bang their head against a hard surface. The frequency of the attacks varies from a single episode every other day to several attacks that occur on a daily basis. One of the distinguishing features of CH is the association of autonomic findings during the attack. These usually are manifest as excessive parasympathetic activity relative to a partial sympathetic paresis. Frequent findings include excessive lacrimation, conjunctival hyperemia, rhinorrhea, nasal congestion, diaphoresis of the face and/or forehead, eyelid edema, and a partial or complete Horner's syndrome. As many as 70% of patients may also have tenderness in the region of the carotid artery in the neck similar to that found in patients with carotidynia.[49,50]

Cluster headache is classified according to its duration as either episodic or chronic based on the duration of the headache cycle.[25] Episodic CH occurs in cycles that last anywhere from 1 week to a year (typically 2 weeks to 3 months), with the cycles separated by pain-free intervals of 2 weeks or more. Chronic CH by definition persists for more than 1 year without remission or with remission lasting less than 14 days. Chronic CH may occur as such from the start or may evolve from episodic CH.

Alcohol and tobacco have been described as classic triggers for CH. Indeed, males that suffer from CH tend to have a high incidence of increased consumption of alcohol and tobacco products. Approximately 17% of patients with new onset of CH will produce a history of recent head trauma. Other "triggers" have also been described to include stress, extremes of temperature, sexual activity, and less commonly ingestion of certain types of foods.[49,50]

The differential diagnosis of CH includes other "cluster-like" syndromes including chronic paroxysmal hemicrania (CPH), cluster-tic syndrome, and SUNCT syndrome (short-lived unilateral neuralgiform headache with conjunctival tearing, sweating, and rhinorrhea).[49–53] CPH, which is more common in women, is characterized by short (5 to 10 minutes) attacks of stabbing pain in the periorbital region that occur between 5 and 20 times daily. By definition, CPH responds to indomethacin. Autonomic dysfunction may occur, but the main distinguishing feature is the high daily frequency of attacks (as many as 100 in some patients). Cluster-tic syndrome is a rare condition characterized by three different pain components. Two resemble trigeminal neuralgia and CH while the third type of pain is of a mixed nature, beginning as a neuralgic type of pain that is immediately followed by an ipsi-lateral headache accompanied by autonomic signs. *SUNCT syndrome* is a term that is limited to very short cluster-like attacks lasting on the average 10 to 60 seconds and occurring predominantly in men. The attacks may sometimes be triggered by chewing, eating certain types of foods, or by tactile stimulation of the nose, eyelid, or supraorbital area.[53]

Rarely, structural pathology of the central nervous system can produce a syndrome in which the pain closely resembles that of CH. Some of the conditions that have been associated with so-called symptomatic CH include meningiomas of the cavernous sinus, arteriovenous malformations, pituitary tumors, nasopharyngeal carcinoma, vertebral artery aneurysms, and metastatic lung cancer.[49] Symptomatic CH should be suspected when the clinical picture does not fit with that of classic CH. Often, the pain lacks the typical periodicity and there may be background pain between the attacks. The patient with symptomatic CH tends to respond less completely to the drugs that are typically effective. Finally, any neurologic signs other than miosis or ptosis should raise the suspicion of structural pathology.

Surgical Treatment

Primary management of CH is pharmacologic. However, in a small number of patients, the symptoms become intractable and disabling and surgical therapy can be considered. Surgery should only be considered for patients who are psychologically stable with unilateral pain who have undergone exhaustive medical therapy with all possible pharmacologic agents and whose pain is resistant to medical treatment. A number of surgical procedures have been tried for CH, most of which have been directed at trigeminal pathways.[54–59] The most common procedures are those that have proven useful for trigeminal neuralgia including glycerol rhizolysis, percutaneous RF rhizotomy, and MVD.

Retrogasserian RF rhizotomy has been one of the more effective surgical procedures for the treatment of intractable CH. This procedure in performed in a manner identical to that for TN. The patient is given a short-acting sedative for introduction of the needle into the foramen ovale. Using C-arm fluoroscopy, a needle is advanced into the foramen ovale. The stylet is withdrawn and replaced with the lesioning electrode. The patient is allowed to awaken and physiological testing is performed to localize the tip of the electrode to the proper trigeminal distribution. Once the proper position has been established, a lesion is created. Unlike TN, treating CH usually requires production of a rather complete analgesia to ensure adequate pain relief. Fortunately, even with complete facial anesthesia, anesthesia dolorosa is infrequent, occurring in only about 2% of patients.[54] In patients with pain confined to the orbital and periorbital regions, a lesion encompassing cranial nerves V1 and V2 will usually suffice. However, if the pain also occurs in the temples or the ear, the lesion should also include cranial nerve V3, because the auricular branch of the mandibular nerve supplies these areas.

The cluster attacks stop in the majority of patients following RF rhizotomy and are substantially improved in a smaller percentage of patients. However, the results are not completely satisfactory because there is an initial 15% failure rate that has been attributed to technical reasons. In the patients that initially enjoy pain relief, recurrence occurs in approximately 20%. In these patients, the procedure can be repeated. Mathew has pointed out that pain recurrence often occurs on the contralateral side and that a history of intermittent contralateral headache may be at higher risk to develop recurrence.[54] Consequently, it has been recommended to select only patients with strictly unilateral pain.

Another procedure that can be used is retrogasserian glycerol injection.[56] The technique is similar to RF rhizotomy except that instead of creating a thermal lesion, glycerol is instilled into the trigeminal cistern. Although glycerol rhizolysis has been shown to be effective, there are several disadvantages. First, the analgesia produced with glycerol injection is not as complete as that produced by RF lesioning, and hence, pain relief may be less satisfactory. Second, glycerol lesions are difficult to control whereas RF lesioning can be performed with a high degree of selectivity. Finally, glycerol may leak outside of Meckel's cave and produce chemical meningitis.

In addition to the procedure just described, other destructive operations have been used for treatment of CH including open trigeminal rhizotomy, peripheral trigeminal neurectomies, section of the greater superficial petrosal nerve or nervus intermedius, and lesion of the sphenopalatine ganglion.[54,57–59]

Based in part on the excellent results in patients with trigeminal neuralgia, MVD has been proposed as an effective surgical procedure in patients with chronic intractable CH.[60]

POSTTHERPETIC NEURALGIA

Postherpetic neuralgia (PHN) is a chronic pain disorder that follows an acute outbreak of herpes zoster or shingles. The eruption is caused by reactivation of the varicella-zoster virus or human herpesvirus-3, which had been dormant within sensory ganglia of the nervous system (trigeminal, geniculate, and dorsal root ganglia). Even after the acute rash subsides, pain may persist in the affected areas and the condition is known as PHN. Some studies have estimated the prevalence of PHN to range from 3% to 5% while other studies have indicated prevalence rates as high as 9% to 14%.[61] The prevalence of PHN has been estimated from 9% to 14%. The risk of developing PHN increases significantly with advancing age. The incidence is approximately 60% in patients age 60 and jumps to 75% in patients older than 70 years of age. In the head and face, shingles usually affects the ophthalmic territory of the trigeminal nerve, and consequently, PHN generally produces first division pain. In fact, patients with herpes zoster involving the trigeminal territory are at highest risk of developing PHN, although other areas may also be affected. Once the acute skin eruption resolves, the affected skin often exhibits a reddish or purple discoloration. Patients with PHN complain of severe constant pain that may have multiple components including constant burning, deep aching, stabbing, and gnawing. Some patients have severe dysesthesias and in extreme cases some patients have been known to scratch their skin to the point that it is eroded down to the bone. Although sensation may be normal, many patients have varying degrees of sensory loss from mild hypalgesia to complete anesthesia of the affected area.

Of all the chronic pain syndromes, PHN ranks among the most refractory to treatment. The usual medications customarily used for treatment of neuropathic pain should be tried, but pharmacologic therapy is not uncommonly unsuccessful.

Although traditional thinking has maintained that opioids are ineffective for neuropathic pain, that is not always the case. Indeed, some patients with neuropathic pain in general and PHN in particular may respond favorably to opioids, albeit at somewhat higher doses than are generally required for treatment of nociceptive pain.

Unfortunately, surgical treatment of PHN has been unrewarding.[61–63] Although numerous surgical approaches have been attempted, none have proven to be of consistent benefit. Indeed, it is true that nearly all of the surgical procedures that have been tried work in some patients; however, no procedure is effective in a large number of patients. In general, neuromodulation procedures are more desirable than destructive operations for the treatment of PHN, as is true for most deafferentation pain syndromes. Many patients with PHN already have evidence of deafferentation with varying degrees of sensory loss on the face. Consequently, destructive procedures on the peripheral trigeminal system (peripheral neurectomy, percutaneous RF rhizotomy, glycerol rhizolysis, stereotactic radiation surgery, etc.) that produce further sensory loss are almost never effective, not uncommonly make the situation worse, and are therefore contraindicated for this condition.

The cornerstone of surgical treatment for PHN involves neuromodulation using various types of electrical stimulation. For patients with relatively well-preserved sensation, it is possible to try peripheral nerve stimulation. A percutaneous electrode can be inserted beneath the skin just above the orbital rim to stimulate the supraorbital and supratrochlear nerves. Although the success rate for this may be relatively low, it is quite easy and associated with essentially no morbidity. Direct stimulation of the trigeminal ganglion has been attempted with varying degrees of success.[64] An electrode is inserted percutaneously through the foramen ovale using an approach identical to that for RF rhizotomy. Test stimulation is performed for a few days up to several weeks to determine effectiveness. If adequate pain relief is achieved, the electrode can be connected to an internal pulse generator (IPG) generally implanted beneath the clavicle. One of the major problems with this technique has been electrode stability. The electrodes tend to move or become dislodged, and it can be difficult to keep them in place for long periods.

Deep brain stimulation (DBS) was popular in the 1970s and subsequently was virtually abandoned for the treatment of chronic pain. However, with the recent resurgence of the technique for the treatment of movement disorders, the interest in DBS for the treatment of pain has also been rekindled. There are several anatomic pain targets used for DBS including the periaqueductal gray (PAG), periventricular gray (PVG), ventrocaudal nucleus of the sensory thalamus, medial lemniscus, and the sensory projection of the thalamus in the internal capsule. It is believed that stimulation of the PAG or PVG produces analgesia by activation of endogenous opioid systems and therefore stimulation of the PAG/PVG is best suited for primarily nociceptive pain that is opioid-responsive. In contrast, stimulation of the sensory thalamus is a paresthesia-producing stimulation similar to spinal cord stimulation and is more effective for neuropathic pain.[65] It is usually necessary for the patient, at least theoretically, to have some preservation of sensation to perceive the paresthesias from thalamic stimulation. In practice, it is relatively easy to insert an electrode into both targets and test both to determine which provides the best analgesia. Either one or both electrodes can then be connected to an IPG assuming that the screening trial has been successful.

More recently, motor cortex stimulation (MCX) has been advocated as a potential therapy for a variety of central deafferentation pain syndromes. The technique was introduced in the 1990s as a treatment for post-stroke and thalamic pain and has recently been utilized for a variety of other central and peripheral deafferentation pain syndromes including anesthesia dolorosa, trigeminal neuropathic pain, PHN, phantom pain, and pain following peripheral nerve injury.[66,67] The technique would appear to be especially applicable for individuals with significant sensory loss who may not be able to readily perceive the sensation produced by various forms of paresthesia-producing stimulation. Indeed, ability to perceive paresthesias is not required for successful MCX although it has been suggested that MCX may be less successful in patients who are completely anesthetic in their painful areas.

It has been suggested that pharmacologic characterization of the pain may be a useful predictor as to who will respond favorably to MCX.[68] This is done through intravenous (IV) infusion of barbiturates, ketamine, and morphine. Patients likely to benefit from MCX demonstrate reduction in pain with intravenous administration of barbiturates and/or ketamine. Patients who respond to IV morphine but not barbiturates or ketamine are less likely to get good pain relief with MCX. Although not currently used, the use of preoperative transcranial magnetic stimulation may ultimately provide a useful tool for selection of patients for MCX.

Although destructive procedures are generally contraindicated for the treatment of PHN, there are some data to suggest that some patients with PHN may benefit from caudalis DREZ ablation.[69] However, overall caudalis DREZ ablation is a procedure that can be associated with significant neurologic morbidity and therefore this operation should be reserved as a last resort for highly selected patients who have exhausted all other reasonable options including MCX and/or DBS.

ATYPICAL FACIAL PAIN

There exists a group of patients with a diverse group of facial pain problems that share common symptoms, but for whom an underlying cause for the pain cannot be identified and whose pain does not fit the clinical picture of any specific condition. These patients with so-called atypical facial pain represent a relatively large group of patients who are quite difficult to manage especially because there are no proven therapies. Some authors have included patients with pain following traumatic injury to a peripheral branch of the trigeminal nerve among those labeled as having atypical facial pain.[1] However, this type of pain is more properly classified as trigeminal neuropathic pain for which there is in most cases an underlying cause as well as a number of logical treatment options.[2]

Atypical facial pain occurs most often in young females and differs from classic trigeminal neuralgia in almost every aspect. The pain can be unilateral but is often reported as bilateral. It is generally reported as continuous and is usually described by adjectives such as burning and/or aching. Pain-free intervals are rarely reported. Although some patients may experience intermittent sharp pain that is superimposed on the constant background pain, the stereotypical paroxysmal neuralgic type of pain associated with typical TN is conspicuously absent. Although the distribution of the pain often is within the trigeminal territory, the pain not uncommonly extends beyond the trigeminal innervation to involve the ear, the upper neck, and the back of the scalp. Atypical facial pain is usually not triggered by stimuli outside of the painful area although stimuli within the area of pain are uncommonly reported to intensify the pain. The neurologic examination is usually normal although sensory testing may often reveal varying degrees of sensory loss.

Atypical facial pain is a condition with no obvious underlying cause. Hence, the diagnosis of atypical facial pain is usually one of exclusion. All patients should have a careful neurologic examination. A thorough oral and otolaryngologic examination should also be conducted to exclude any pathology in these areas. Finally, some type of imaging study of the head, preferably magnetic resonance imaging, is appropriate for patients with chronic atypical facial pain to completely exclude any structural pathology that might not be apparent on physical examination.

Treatment of the patient with atypical facial pain can be a tremendous challenge. Frequently, these patients have already seen numerous healthcare providers and often become extremely frustrated due to the fact that an underlying cause for their pain cannot be identified. Many of these patients have significant emotional stressors and other concomitant psychological factors that undoubtedly contribute to their chronic pain. Psychological counseling can be useful although many patients will interpret referral to a psychologist or psychiatrist as a suggestion that the pain is "in their head" and will continue to insist that a cause be identified when in fact none exists. Pharmacologic therapy can be attempted but is not terribly rewarding. It is critical to understand that the surgical procedures that are typically used for trigeminal neuralgia are almost uniformly unsuccessful in these patients. There have certainly been a few reports of successful treatment of atypical facial pain with microvascular decompression of the trigeminal nerve but this would seem to be the exception rather than the rule. Patients with atypical facial pain should not be offered destructive surgical procedures. Not only are these nearly uniformly unsuccessful, but they may produce deafferentation pain or anesthesia dolorosa.

REFERENCES

1. Bonica JJ. General considerations of pain in the head. *In* Bonica JJ (ed). The Management of Pain, ed 2. Philadelphia, Lea & Febiger, 1990, pp 651–675.
2. Burchiel KJ. Trigeminal neuropathic pain. Acta Neurochir (Suppl) 58:145–149, 1993.
3. Rushton JG, Stevens JC, Miller RH. Glossopharyngeal (vagoglossopharyngeal) neuralgia: a study of 217 cases. Arch Neurol 38:201–205, 1981.
4. Wilkins RH. Glossopharyngeal (vagoglossopharyngeal) neuralgia. *In* Barrow D (ed). Surgery of the Cranial Nerves of the Posterior Fossa. American Association of Neurological Surgeons Publications Committee, 1993, pp 245–252.
5. Dandy WE. Glossopharyngeal neuralgia (tic douloureux): its diagnosis and treatment. Arch Surg 15:198–214, 1927.
6. Onofrio BM. Glossopharyngeal rhizotomy. *In* Rengachary SS, Wilkins RH (eds). Neurosurgical Operative Atlas, vol 12. Baltimore, Williams & Wilkins, 1991, pp 323–326.

7. White JC, Sweet WH. Pain and the Neurosurgeon: a Forty-Year Experience. Springfield, Ill, Charles C Thomas, 1969, pp 265–302.

8. Grossmann E, Paiano GA. Eagle's syndrome: a case report. J Craniomandib Pract 16:126–130, 1998.

9. Jannetta PJ. Neurovascular compression in cranial nerve and systemic disease. Ann Surg 192:518–524, 1980.

10. Jannetta PJ. Cranial rhizopathies. *In* Youmans JR (ed). Neurological Surgery, ed 3. Philadelphia, WB Saunders, 1990, pp 4169–4182.

11. Kondo A. Follow-up results of using microvascular decompression for treatment of glossopharyngeal neuralgia. J Neurosurg 88:221–225, 1998.

12. Resnick DK, Jannetta PJ, Bissonnette D, Jho HD, Lanzino G. Microvascular decompression for glossopharyngeal neuralgia. Neurosurgery 36:64–69, 1995.

13. Arbit E, Krol G. Percutaneous radiofrequency neurolysis guided by computed tomography for the treatment of glossopharyngeal neuralgia. Neurosurgery 29:580–582, 1991.

14. Gybels JM, Sweet WH. Neurosurgical Treatment of Persistent Pain: Physiological and Pathological Mechanisms of Human Pain. Basel, Switzerland, Karger, 1989, pp 91–103.

15. Hunt JR. Geniculate neuralgia (neuralgia of the nervus facialis): a further contribution to the sensory system of the facial nerve and its neuralgic conditions. Arch Neurol Psychiatry 37:253–285, 1937.

16. Bruyn GW. Nervus intermedius neuralgia (Hunt). Cephalalgia 4:71–78, 1984.

17. Rupa V, Saunders RL, Weider DJ. Geniculate neuralgia: the surgical management of primary otalgia. J Neurosurg 75:505–511, 1991.

18. Loeser J. Cranial neuralgias. In Bonica JJ (ed). The Management of Pain, ed 2. Philadelphia, Lea & Febiger, 1990, pp 676–686.

19. Ouaknine GE, Robert F, Molina-Negro P, et al. Geniculate neuralgia and audiovestibular disturbances due to compression of the intermediate and eighth nerves by the postero-inferior cerebellar artery. Surg Neurol 13:147–150, 1980.

20. Clark LP, Taylor AS. True tic douloureux of the sensory filaments of the facial nerve. JAMA 53:2144–2146, 1909.

21. White JC, Sweet WH. Pain and the Neurosurgeon: A Forty-Year Experience. Springfield, Ill, Charles C Thomas, 1969, pp 257–265, 345–372, 622–627.

22. Bogduk N. The clinical anatomy of the cervical dorsal rami. Spine 7:319–330, 1982.

23. Hammond SR, Danta G. Occipital neuralgia. Clin Exp Neurol 15:258–270, 1978.

24. Lozano A. Treatment of occipital neuralgia. *In* Gildenburg PL, Tasker RR (eds). Textbook of Stereotactic and Functional Neurosurgery. New York, McGraw-Hill, 1998, pp 1729–1733.

25. International Headache Society, Headache Classification Committee. Classification and diagnostic criteria for headache disorders, cranial neuralgias, and facial pain. Cephalgia 8(Suppl)7:1–96, 1988.

26. Star MJ, Curd JG, Thorne RP. Atlantoaxial lateral mass osteoarthritis: a frequently overlooked cause of severe occipitocervical pain. Spine 17:S71–S76, 1992.

27. Ehni G, Benner B. Occipital neuralgia and the C1–2 arthrosis syndrome. J Neurosurg 61:961–965, 1984.

28. Stechison MT, Mullin BB. Surgical treatment of greater occipital neuralgia: an appraisal of strategies. Acta Neurochir (Wein) 131:236–240, 1994.

29. Poletti CE. Proposed operation for occipital neuralgia: C-2 and C-3 root decompression. Case report. Neurosurgery 12:221–224, 1983.

30. Oh S, Tok S, Allemann J, et al. Exeresis in occipital neuralgia. Neurochirurgie 26:47–50, 1983.

31. Dubuisson D. Treatment of occipital neuralgia by partial posterior rhizotomy at C1–3. J Neurosurg 82:581–586, 1995.

32. Horowitz MD, Yonas H. Occipital neuralgia treated by intradural dorsal nerve root sectioning. Cephalalgia 13:354–360, 1993.

33. Lozano A, Vanderlinden G, Rothbart P. Microsurgical C2 ganglionectomy for chronic intractable occipital pain (abstract). J Neurosurg 80:407A–408A, 1994.

34. Weiner RL, Reed KL. Peripheral neurostimulation for control of intractable occipital neuralgia. Neuromodulation 2:217–220, 1999.

35. Racz GB, Morton AB, Diede JH. Sphenopalatine ganglion block. *In* Waldman SD, Winnie AP (eds). Interventional Pain Management. Philadelphia, WB Saunders, 1996, pp 223–225.

36. Bonica JJ. Pain caused by cancer of the head and neck and other specific syndromes. *In* Bonica JJ (ed). The Management of Pain, ed 2. Philadelphia, Lea & Febiger, 1990, pp 793–811.

37. Million RR, Cassisi NJ, Wittes RE. Cancer in the head and neck. *In* DeVita VT Jr, Hellman S, Rosenberg SA (eds). Cancer: Principles and Practice of Oncology. Philadelphia, Lippincott, 1982, pp 301–395.

38. Molinari R. Oncologic therapy of pain in cancer of the head and neck. *In* Bonica JJ, Ventafridda V (eds). Advances in Pain Research and Therapy, vol. 2. New York, Raven, 1979, pp 523–531.

39. Kinzie J. Radiation therapy. *In* Moossa AR, Robson MC, Schimpff SC (eds). Comprehensive Textbook of Oncology. Baltimore, Williams & Wilkins, 1986, pp 677–682.

40. Williams SD. Head and neck cancer: role of chemotherapy. *In* Moossa AR, Robson MC, Schimpff SC (eds). Comprehensive Textbook of Oncology. Baltimore, Williams & Wilkins, 1986, pp 683–686.

41. Lazorthes Y, Sallerin B, Verdi JC. Intracerebroventricular administration of morphine for control of irreducible cancer pain. *In* Gildenburg PL, Tasker RR (eds). Textbook of Stereotactic and Functional Neurosurgery. New York, McGraw-Hill, 1998, pp 1477–1482.

42. Teixeira MJ. *In* Gildenburg PL and Tasker RR (eds). Textbook of Stereotactic and Functional Neurosurgery. New York, McGraw-Hill, 1998, pp 1389–1402.

43. Sjöqvist O. Studies on pain conduction in the trigeminal nerve: contribution to surgical treatment of facial pain. Acta Psychiatr Scand 17(Suppl):1–139, 1938.

44. Crue BL, Todd EM, Carregal EJA, Kilham O. Percutaneous trigeminal tractotomy. Bull LA Neurol Soc 32:86–92, 1967.

45. Fox JL. Intractable facial pain relieved by percutaneous trigeminal tractotomy. JAMA 218:1940–1941, 1971.

46. Kanpolat Y, Deda H, Akyar, et al. CT-guided trigeminal tractotomy. Acta Neurochirug (Wien) 100:112–114, 1989.

47. Nashold BS Jr, El-Naggar AO, Gorecki JP. The microsurgical trigeminal caudalis nucleus DREZ procedure. *In* Nashold BS, Pearlstein RD (eds). The DREZ Operation. American Association of Neurological Surgeon Publications Committee, 1996, pp 159–188.

48. Gorecki J. Stereotactic midbrain tractotomy. *In* Gildenburg PL, Tasker RR (eds). Textbook of Stereotactic and Functional Neurosurgery. New York, McGraw-Hill, 1998, pp 1651–1659.

49. Mendizabal JE, Umana E, Zweifler R. Cluster headache: Horton's cephalagia revisited. Southern Med J 91:606–617, 1998.

50. Sjaastad O. Cluster headache. Handbook Clin Neurol 48:217–246, 1986.

51. Benoliel R, Sharav Y. Paroxysmal hemicrania: case studies and review of the literature. Oral Surg Oral Med Oral Pathol 85:285–292, 1998.

52. Sjaastad O. Chronic paroxysmal hemicrania (CPH). Handbook Clin Neurol 48:257–266, 1986.

53. Benoliel R, Sharaz Y. SUNCT syndrome: case report and literature review. Oral Surg Oral Med Oral Pathol 85:158–161, 1998.

54. Mathew N. Treatment of headache. *In* Gildenburg PL, Tasker RR (eds). Textbook of Stereotactic and Functional Neurosurgery. New York, McGraw-Hill, 1998, pp 1735–1749.

55. Morgenlander JC, Wilkins RH. Surgical treatment of cluster headache. J Neurosurg 72:866–871, 1990.

56. Hassenbusch SJ, Kunkel RS, Kosmorsky GS, et al. Trigeminal cisternal injection of glycerol for treatment of chronic intractable cluster headaches. Neurosurgery 29:504–508, 1991.

57. Gardner WJ, Stowell A, Dutlinger R. Resection of the greater superficial petrosal nerve in the treatment of unilateral headache. J Neurosurg 4:105–114, 1947.

58. Meyer JS, Binns PM, Ericsson AD, et al. Sphenopalatine ganglionectomy for cluster headache. Arch Otolaryngol 92:475–484, 1970.

59. Ray BS. The surgical treatment of headache and atypical neuralgia. J Neurosurg 11:596–606, 1954.

60. Wilkins RH, Morgenlander JC. Results of surgical treatment of cluster headache: initial relief followed by recurrence. Neurosurgery 24:948–951, 1989.

61. Watson CP. Postherpetic neuralgia. *In* Burchiel KJ (ed). Surigcal Management of Pain. New York, Thieme, 2002, pp 393–400.

62. Friedman AH, Nashold BS Jr. Postherpetic neuralgia. *In* Wilkins RH, Rengechary SS (eds). Neurosurgery. New York, McGraw-Hill, 1985, pp 2367–2368.

63. Loeser JD. Herpes zoster and postherpetic neuralgia. Pain 25:149–164, 1986.

64. Broggi G, Franzini A, Ferroli P. Trigeminal stimulation. *In* Burchiel KJ (ed). Surgical Management of Pain. New York, Thieme, 2002, pp 903–907.

65. Rezai AR, Lozano AM. Deep brain stimulation for chronic pain. *In* Burchiel KJ (ed). Surgical Management of Pain. New York, Thieme, 2002, pp 565–576.

66. Tsubokawa T, Katayama Y, Yamamoto T, Hirayama T, et al. Treatment of thalamic pain by chronic motor cortex stimulation. Pacing Clin Electrophysiol 14:131–134, 1991.

67. Nguyen JP, Lefaucher JP, Le Guerinel C, et al. Motor cortex stimulation in the treatment of central and neuropathic pain. Arch Med Res 31:263–265, 2000.

68. Yamamoto T, Katayama Y, Hirayama T, Tsubokawa T. Pharmacological classification of central post-stroke pain: comparison with the results of chronic motor cortex stimulation therapy. Pain 72:5–12, 1997.

69. Bernard EJ Jr, Nashold BS Jr, Caputi F, Moossy JJ. Nucleus caudalis DREZ lesions for facial pain. Br J Neurosurg 1:81–91, 1987.

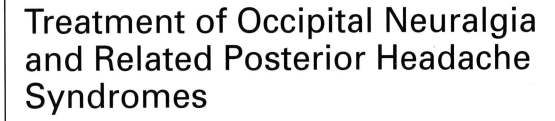

Treatment of Occipital Neuralgia and Related Posterior Headache Syndromes

RICHARD L. WEINER, MD, FACS

Occipital neuralgia (International Association for Study of Pain [IASP] class II-10)[1] in its purest form is a relatively rare headache disorder characterized by unilateral or bilateral paroxysmal, lancinating, deep, aching pain in the distribution of the second cervical dorsal root originating in the suboccipital area. It frequently follows the greater and/or lesser occipital nerves, which form from the posterior primary division of C2 radiating toward the scalp vertex. Pain may also extend to the fronto-orbital and retro-orbital areas of the head and face and associated symptoms may include hyperesthesia of the scalp, vertigo, tinnitus, and tearing. There is frequently focal nerve tenderness to palpation in the affected suboccipital site. Although the etiology remains unknown, there is a frequent correlation with head and neck trauma. Most patients will respond positively to a diagnostic nerve block. This syndrome is frequently mischaracterized and confused in the literature and in clinical practice with several far more prevalent and similar conditions all of which can be quite refractory to medical and surgical treatment.

Posterior region headaches more commonly present under the diagnosis of cervicogenic pain (IASP class VII-2)[1], occipital headaches, C2–3 mediated pain, and transformed migraine headaches. These are characterized as attacks of moderate to severe unilateral pain without change of side, ordinarily involving the whole hemicranium while starting in the posterior cervical or occipital region. The pain is generally constant, deep, dull, and steady but not excruciating. The pain begins in the neck or suboccipital area and extends to the forehead and temporal areas. There tends to be persistence and intensification of pain over time with attacks varying in duration from 1 to several days. Later phases include chronic daily headaches with more continuous pain greater than 15 days per month. There is general agreement that the targeted occipital headache is C2/C3 mediated and includes some combination of greater and/or lesser occipital nerve involvement.

ETIOLOGY

Occipital headaches can result from a variety of causes. Closed head injury and/or direct trauma to the occipital regions can produce unilateral or bilateral occipital nerve–mediated pain, which responds temporarily to local nerve blocks. Cervical strain, localized muscle tension/spasm, and focal lesions such as subcutaneous cysts are also frequently implicated. Much less commonly there can be involvement of the C2/C3 nerve root from ligamentous compression or foraminal spondylosis/stenosis. Idiopathic occipital headaches occur with significant frequency as well.

MEDICAL TREATMENT

Patients with posterior headache pain are usually referred to either the headache neurologist or anesthesia pain management specialist for diagnosis and treatment. The mainstay of therapy has been medication oriented and includes a combination of narcotic, non-narcotic, anti-inflammatory, neuroleptic, and antidepressant medications. Frequently, detoxification from excessive narcotic intake is required and helpful in reducing the intensity and frequency of pain. Steroid/local anesthetic nerve blocks can be both diagnostic and therapeutic, directed at either the occipital peripheral nerves or the C2/C3 extraforaminal root. Other treatments include cervical immobilization (collar), manipulative physical therapy, transcutaneous electrical nerve stimulation, ultrasound/heat, cryoprobe freezing, and alcohol neurolyis. Unfortunately, a significant number of patients become refractory to these relatively noninvasive treatment options.

SURGICAL TREATMENT

Occipital nerve neurolysis and/or neurectomy have been part of the neurosurgical armamentarium in treating intractable occipital headaches for many years. Although occasionally very effective, the not infrequent development of delayed deafferentation pain in the distribution of the affected occipital nerve limits the long-term usefulness of the procedure. C2 ganglionectomy[2] in post-traumatic C2 pain syndromes has resulted in an 80% good to excellent outcome with a 3-year follow-up. Nontraumatic C2 pain patients did not fare nearly as well and subtle but significant morbidity including post-operative dizziness or gait disturbances may be a persistent problem. C2 decompression can achieve up to a 79% success rate with 33% pain free and 46% adequate pain relief over 2 years.[3] C1/C2 fusion can correct focal instability and may be indicated on occasion. C1/C3 posterior rhizotomy via ventro-lateral DREZ lesioning at C1–3 can be an effective but highly invasive surgical technique.[4] Neurolysis of the greater occipi-tal nerve can be effective in the short run, but most patients tend to experience significant recurrences within 1 to 2 years.[5]

Experience with peripheral nerve electrical stimulation for painful mononeuropathies and complex regional pain syndromes involving one major peripheral nerve led to the sentinel observation that the subcutaneous tissues can conduct and propagate electrical impulses in a dermatomal and/or myotomal distribution of one or more occipital nerves. This has led to the development and refinement of a percutaneous neurostimulation procedure in which a stimulation electrode is implanted transversely into the subcutaneous space at the level of C1 as a minimally invasive treatment alternative for intractable occipital headache syndromes.[6]

Patient Selection

Beginning in late 1992, I began implanting percutaneous wire electrodes in a series of patients with refractory occipital headaches thought to be unresponsive to medication but with excellent if temporary response to occipital nerve steroid/anes-thetic block. All patients underwent successful percutaneous trial stimulation for up to 7 days before permanent implant and had acceptable behavioral and psychological profiling.

Implant Technique

Using local anesthesia at the incision site only, a vertical 2-cm incision is made at the level of the C1 lamina either medial and inferior to the mastoid process or in the midline posteriorly under fluoroscopic control extending to, but not into, the cervicodorsal fascia. The patient may be posi-tioned laterally or prone depending on the incision entry point. The subcutaneous tissues immediately lateral to the incision are undermined sharply to accept a loop of elec-trode created after placement and tunneling to prevent elec-trode migration. A Tuohy needle is gently curved to conform to the transverse posterior cervical curvature (bevel concave) and without further dissection is passed trans-versely in the subcutaneous space across the base of the affected greater and/or lesser occipital nerves, which at the level of C1, are located within the cervical musculature and overlying fascia. Single or dual quadripolar or octapolar electrodes may be passed from a midline incision to either affected side or alternatively placed to traverse the entire cervical curvature bilaterally from a single side or via two opposing incisions.

Rapid needle insertion usually obviates even a short-acting general anesthetic once the surgeon becomes facile with the technique. Following placement of the electrode into the Tuohy needle, the needle is withdrawn and the electrode con-nected to an extender cable for intraoperative testing.

Intraoperative Stimulation Testing

After lead placement, stimulation is applied using a temporary radio frequency (RF) transmitter to various select electrode combinations enabling the patient to report the stimulation location, intensity, and overall sensation while on the operat-ing table. Most patients have reported an immediate stimula-tion in the selected occipital nerve distribution with voltage settings from 1 to 4 volts with midrange pulse widths and fre-quencies. A report of burning pain or muscle pulling should alert the surgeon that the electrode is probably placed either too close to the fascia or too far above or below the C1 level and should be repositioned. Repeated needle passage for electrode placement can lead to subcutaneous edema and/or hematoma formation with loss of electrode conductivity, thereby blocking evaluation for permanent lead positioning.

Electrode Fixation and Tunneling

Probably the most important aspect of the procedure involves techniques to prevent electrode migration (pullback) from its transverse subcutaneous position in the highly mobile upper cervical region. Following successful stimulation, the elec-trode is sutured to the underlying fascia with the supplied sili-cone fastener and 2–0 silk sutures. A small dab of medical grade silicone glue is placed between the fastener and elec-trode using a small angiocatheter to ensure fixation. A loop of electrode is also sutured loosely in the previously prepared subcutaneous pocket to reduce migration risk. A short-acting general anesthetic is used to tunnel the electrode(s) or exten-der wire to the distal site for connection and implantation of the receiver or generator.

Power Plant Implantation

There are two options available for the system power source: an external RF transmitter/receiver system, or an implantable pulse generator. The RF system allows for more continuous higher voltage outputs at the expense of rechargeable 9-volt batteries and is US Food and Drug Administration approved for peripheral use. Most patients, however, opt for the implantable pulse generator system, which is an off-labeled application for peripheral use. With the voltage settings usually required for occipital stimulation, the lithium ion battery can last 5 to 7 years before replacement.

RESULTS

Implant experience from 1993 through 2000 has consistently shown an approximately 80% good and excellent long-term pain relief with a 10% fair and 10% poor response in over 60 implanted patients. The total headache years in this population was approximately 423 years with mean headache duration of 8 years in 77% females and 23% males. Almost half of the patient population exhibited some degree of bilateral pain with one side typically dominant. Preoperative visual analog score (VAS) scores ranged from 5 to 10 with a mean of 9. Postoperative VAS scores ranged from 0 to 10 with a mean of 3.

Stimulation Usage

Patterns of therapy usage varied among this patient population with some setting their device for continuous stimulation while others used the device only when symptomatic or to abort an impending headache. Common usage scenarios included:

- Stimulation to abort intermittent paroxysmal pain
- Attenuation of a migraine trigger
- Blockade of chronic and intermittent daily pain
- Blockade of exacerbations of continuous chronic pain

Complications

Most complications revolved around lead migration (7%) skewed more toward the early years of implant technique development. Lead breakage or disconnection (9%) is probably a function of the lead implant location in a highly mobile area. Infection was rare (3%) and a new implant in a previously infected site was successfully implanted and continues to function well.

Mechanism of Action

The mechanisms of action for the paresthesia patterns and pain relief obtained from this therapy are incompletely understood but would appear to involve the following elements:

- Subcutaneous electrical conduction
- Dermatomal stimulation
- Myotomal stimulation
- Sympathetic stimulation
- Local blood flow alteration
- Peripheral nerve stimulation
- Peripheral and central neurochemical mechanisms

Recent work with direct electrical stimulation of the greater occipital nerve has shown an increase in metabolic activity in the trigeminal nucleus caudalis and cervical dorsal horn cells in the cat by 220% ipsilateral to the stimulation and by a lesser amount contralaterally.[7] The dorsal horn activity was at the level of C1/C2 and interaction with the trigeminally innervated structures suggests that the frontally radiating occipital headaches occur as a consequence of overlap of nociceptive information processing at the level of the second-order neurons. Recent positron emission tomography scan studies in cluster headache patients demonstrate activation of the ipsilateral hypothalamic gray matter region during nitroglycerin spray–induced headaches.[8] These observations suggest the presence of a central trigger mechanism for a variety of headache pain conditions. Peripheral, subcutaneous electrical stimulation may influence blood flow within these activated regions via stimulation of the trigeminovascular system at the level of the upper cervical spine.

R E F E R E N C E S

1. Sanin LC, Matthew NT, Bellmeyer LR, AIi S. International Headache Society (IHS) Headache classification as applied to a headache clinic population. Cepalgia 14(6):443–446,1994.
2. Lozano AM, Vanderlinden G, Bachoo R, Rothbart P. Microsurgical C-L ganglionectomy for chronic intractable occipital pain. J Neurosurg 89(3):359–365, 1998.
3. Pikus HJ, Phillips JM. Outcome of surgical decompression of the second cervical root for cervicogenic headache. Neurosurgery 39(1):63–70, 1996.
4. Dubuisson D. Treatment of occipital neuralgia by partial posterior rhizotomy at C 1-3. J Neurosurg 82(4):581–586, 1995.
5. Bovim G, Fredriksen TA, Stolt-Nielsen A, Sjaastap O. Neurolysis of the greater occipital nerve in cervicogenic headache: a followup study. Headache 32(4):175–179, 1992.
6. Weiner RL, Reed KL. Peripheral neurostimulation for control of intractable occipital neuralgia. Neuromodulation 2:217–221, 1999.
7. Goadsby PJ, Knight YE, Hoskin KL. Stimulation of the greater occipital nerve increases metabolic activity in the trigeminal nucleus caudalis and cervical dorsal horn of the cat. Pain 73(1):23–28, 1997.
8. Goadsby PJ, Bahra A, May A. Mechanisms of cluster headache. Cephalgia 19(Suppl 23):19–21, 1999.

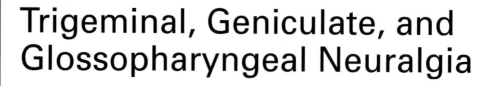

C H A P T E R   1 0

Trigeminal, Geniculate, and Glossopharyngeal Neuralgia

ANDREW S. YOUKILIS, MD, AND OREN SAGHER, MD

PATHOPHYSIOLOGY OF CRANIAL NEURALGIAS

The diagnosis and medical management of cranial neuralgias can be both one of the most frustrating and rewarding challenges in neurosurgical practice. Facial pain is an extremely vexing problem, with a wide variety of possible causes. It is important, therefore, for neurosurgeons to have a broad understanding of the etiologic underpinnings of the majority of facial pain syndromes. Good outcome depends on proper diagnosis and patient selection for any treatment regimen being considered. Fortunately, with an improved understanding of entities such as trigeminal neuralgia, our ability to diagnose and treat facial pain syndromes has improved remarkably over the past half century.

Many theories have been postulated to explain the cause of cranial neuralgias. One of the most common is based on the observation that demyelination of large-diameter A fibers is frequently found at the trigeminal root entry zone in patents with trigeminal neuralgia.[1] This theory holds that there is ephaptic transmission from these fibers to poorly myelinated Aδ and unmyelinated C fibers, which results in paroxysmal facial pain. It has been widely speculated that this demyelination comes from compression of the trigeminal nerve by an artery or vein at the root entry zone. Interestingly, autopsy series have shown that vascular compression is absent in a significant percentage of patients with trigeminal neuralgia. Conversely, these studies also note that vascular compression of the trigeminal nerve is often present in patients who have never suffered from trigeminal neuralgia.

Regardless of the etiology, patients with trigeminal neuralgia tend to present in a stereotypic fashion. The classic symptoms of trigeminal neuralgia include

1. Paroxysmal, "electric" pain in trigeminal distribution on one side of the face
2. Trigger areas, which when stimulated bring on this classic type of pain
3. Periods of remission and exacerbation

4. Pain that is typically more severe in the morning and absent during sleep
5. Periodic pain relief when treated with an adequate trial of carbamazepine

Controversy exists over the epidemiology of trigeminal neuralgia. Multiple studies show a trend toward a female predominance with as high as a 2:1 female-to-male ratio. In addition, the overwhelming majority of patients with the disease present at age 50 or older. The paroxysmal attacks appear to occur with a slightly increased tendency on the right side of the face; however, this as well is controversial. Multiple case studies corroborate that the location of the pain is more frequent in the V2, V3 distributions. Despite these trends, trigeminal neuralgia can appear in either gender, at any age, on either side of the face and in any distribution of the trigeminal nerve. For these reasons it is important to consider the diagnosis in any patient with paroxysmal facial pain. The neurologic examination and imaging studies are generally without demonstrable abnormalities. It is important to remember, however, that patients with multiple sclerosis or tumors of the cerebellopontine angle can present with classic features of trigeminal neuralgia. For this reason, imaging studies including magnetic resonance of the brain and posterior fossa should be performed as part of the initial evaluation.

The causes of facial pain are myriad, but can be roughly classified into several categories (Table 10-1). Although many types of facial pain fall outside the expertise or practice of neurosurgery, it is nevertheless important for the neurosurgeon to consider the differential diagnosis before embarking on medical or surgical therapy.

The diversity of possible causes in facial pain represents the first (and sometimes most difficult) hurdle to treatment. When an anatomic cause can be found, such as is the case in cancer of the head and neck, efforts can then focus on treatment of the lesion or on palliative treatment. However, when no such lesion is apparent, the neurosurgeon must rely on other, indirect, diagnostic clues. Such factors as distribution of pain, pain triggers, and quality of pain provide important information on the origin of the pain as well as the most appropriate treatment. Table 10-2 summarizes some of the salient features of commonly encountered facial pain syndromes.

● **TABLE 10-1** • Facial Pain Etiologies

Culprit	Examples
Nerve	Trigeminal neuralgia Postherpetic neuralgia Trigeminal neuropathic pain Glossopharyngeal neuralgia Sphenopalatine neuralgia Geniculate neuralgia (Ramsay Hunt)

Teeth and Jaw	Dentinal, pulpal, or periodontal
	   pain temporomandibular
	   disorders

Sinuses and aerodigestive tract	Sinusitis Head and neck cancer
Eyes	Tolosa-Hunt Syndrome Optic neuritis Iritis Glaucoma
Vessels	Giant cell arteritis Migraine Cluster headache (?)
Psyche	Psychogenic facial pain ?Atypical facial pain

TRIGEMINAL NEURALGIA VERSUS ATYPICAL FACIAL PAIN

Diagnostic uncertainty may arise when a patient presents with what appears to be trigeminal neuralgia with atypical features. Certain authors differentiate between *typical trigeminal neuralgia* (TTN) and *atypical trigeminal neuralgia* (ATN). Fromm notes that a certain percentage of patients initially present with a prodromal continuous, dull, aching pain in the jaw or teeth that is not brought on by typical trigger zones.[2] These patients generally go on to develop more classic, paroxysmal pain in the same division of the trigeminal nerve, months or years later. It is also possible that people with TTN develop atypical features and neuropathic characteristics to their pain over time. It is important to note, however, that while patients with ATN may present with atypical features, their response to initial medical management does not differ from patients with TTN.[2]

The term *atypical facial pain* (AFP) has historically been used to define facial pain of psychogenic origin. While this may be true in the majority of these patients, the ambiguity of this term itself demonstrates our lack of understanding of facial pain syndromes in general. For this reason, many patients become labeled with this diagnosis for lack of a better understanding of the true etiology of their problem. The presentation of patients with AFP can therefore be extremely variable. Their pain can range from a dull ache to a sharp, tearing sensation. Their suffering is usually constant with intermittent exacerbations, and the pain generally does not obey dermatomal or anatomic boundaries. The trigger for its onset is usually emotional or stress-related. Unlike patients with trigeminal neuralgia, these patients are often seen rubbing or massaging the area of their pain for symptomatic relief. In general their symptoms respond more readily to antidepressants than they do to anticonvulsant-type medications.[1]

Patients with AFP oftentimes exhibit a characteristic personality type. They generally develop mistrust for their care providers because nothing that has been done for them has relieved their pain significantly. There is often a discrepancy between the florid description of their suffering and the relative lack of outward manifestation of their pain. Unlike the intermittent, paroxysmal nature of trigeminal neuralgia, this pain permeates every aspect of the patients' lives.

The variable presentation of patients with AFP has compelled investigators to search for etiologies other than facial

● **TABLE 10-2** • Diagnostic Clues in Facial Pain

Diagnosis	Pain Character	Pain Distribution	Pain Triggers	Other Clues
Trigeminal neuralgia	Paroxysmal, lancinating	Trigeminal *only* V2 most frequent	Touch, chewing, talking, etc.	
Glossopharyngeal neuralgia	Paroxysmal, lancinating	Ear, throat	Swallowing	

Trigeminal neuropathic pain	Constant, burning,
	  dull throbbing
		Trigeminal *only*	None	History of trigeminal
				  nerve injury

Postherpetic neuralgia	Constant, crawling
	May have paroxysmal
	  component
		Trigeminal *only*
		V1 most frequent
			Touch	History of herpes zoster
				  ophthalmicus

Anesthesia dolorosa	Constant, burning, itching
	  in an insensate region
		Trigeminal *only*	None	History of trigeminal
				  nerve lesion

Malignancy	Constant, but may have
	  paroxysmal component
		In area of neoplasm
		  or referable to nerve
		  compression
			Possible if
			  trigeminal nerve
			  involved
				Head/neck neoplasm

Atypical facial pain	Constant	Nonanatomic, often
		  bilateral
			None	Prominent psychiatric
				  component

pain of psychogenic origin. It is interesting to note that a percentage of patients who undergo section of the portio major of the trigeminal nerve continue to perceive light touch in a trigeminal distribution. Certain authors have identified alternate pain pathways such as afferent anastomoses between the portio major and portio minor, nervus intermedius, and eighth cranial nerve, which could be responsible for this preserved sensation. These anatomic variations raise some concern regarding Bell's thesis of the "three divisions of the trigeminus." Keller and Van Loveren postulate that "perhaps some of the neuralgias currently categorized as atypical may be reassigned to the domain of the facial nerve rather than to the more stereotypic classification, pain of psychogenic origin."[3]

EVALUATION OF CRANIAL NEURALGIAS

When a patient presents with facial pain symptoms that do not follow the classic features of trigeminal neuralgia described above, the clinician must begin to explore other possible etiologic clues. This is especially true for pain that is constant, pain that is not confined to the dermatomal distribution of the trigeminal nerve, and pain that does not respond initially to carbamazepine. Patients with trigeminal neuropathic pain often present with a constant, burning pain and history of an injury to one or more peripheral divisions of the trigeminal nerve. Postherpetic neuralgia is generally preceded by a vesicular rash and is most often confined to the ophthalmic branch of the trigeminal nerve only. Other possibilities such as temporal arteritis, cluster headache, temporomandibular joint dysfunction and atypical odontalgia can be initially misconstrued as trigeminal neuralgia if the physician does not specifically rule out their identifying features.

Geniculate neuralgia was first described by Hunt in 1937.[4] Patients with this disorder generally present with symptoms referable to the nervus intermedius, subserving the autonomic and sensory functions of the facial nerve. Pain is primarily retroorbital and otalgic in nature. The pain may be associated with ipsilateral signs of autonomic dysfunction such as increased tearing, rhinorrhea, and nasal congestion. For this reason geniculate neuralgia is thought to be linked to cluster headache. Surgical intervention for this syndrome, including sectioning of the nervus intermedius, has shown mixed results at best.[5]

In a similar fashion, patients with glossopharyngeal neuralgia present with pain in the sensory distribution of the ninth cranial nerve, primarily otalgic and pharyngeal in distribution. Like trigeminal neuralgia, the pain is usually paroxysmal in nature, with pain-free periods as well. Similarly, this pain can be structural (related to a tumor, cyst, arteriovenous malformation) or idiopathic in nature. Variability of symptoms is much more common and acceptable, however, in glossopharyngeal neuralgia than it is in typical trigeminal neuralgia.[6] Initial treatment, like that of trigeminal neuralgia, is medical and patients usually respond to carbamazepine. In cases of clear-cut vascular compression, patients usually respond well to microvascular decompression. Sectioning of the glossopharyngeal nerve, both intracranially and percutaneously has also been performed with good results.[7]

MEDICAL MANAGEMENT

The initial treatment of most facial pain syndromes is usually medical. Treatment, however, must be diagnosis-driven. Therefore, pain due to a head or neck neoplasm may be best treated by treatment of the lesion. Similarly, psychogenic pain is best addressed by treatment of the underlying psychiatric condition. In this next section, we will discuss the most common medications utilized in the treatment of cranial neuralgias.

Anticonvulsants

Following Trousseau's observation that trigeminal neuralgia resembled the epilepsies in its paroxysmal presentation, a number of anticonvulsants have been used in its treatment. Potassium bromide was first used successfully in the treatment of trigeminal neuralgia.[1] In 1942, Bergouignan described the use of phenytoin for the treatment of trigeminal neuralgia.[8] However, it was the development of a new Ciba-Geigy anticonvulsant in 1961 that revolutionized the treatment of facial pain.[9] Later known as carbamazepine, this medication still constitutes the linchpin of medical therapy in many facial pain syndromes. Other anticonvulsants have been subsequently developed and tested in the treatment of facial pain. Among these, only baclofen has remained a first-line therapy in trigeminal neuralgia. Table 10-3 outlines the typical anticonvulsant medications used in the treatment of facial pain.

The mode of action of anticonvulsants in the treatment of facial pain is not entirely clear. However, animal studies have indicated that both carbamazepine and baclofen act to enhance inhibitory neuronal activity in the trigeminal nucleus oralis.[10] Because it appears that this sensory nucleus plays an important role in trigeminal neuralgia, it is likely that the action of anticonvulsants at the level of the brainstem sensory nuclei is at least partially responsible for their beneficial effects.

In addition to their important therapeutic role in trigeminal neuralgia, anticonvulsants are used to treat other paroxysmal facial pain syndromes. Paroxysmal components in trigeminal neuropathic pain, malignant facial pain, and postherpetic neuralgia are typically treated with anticonvulsants.

Experimental studies evaluating the mechanism of action of drugs effective in trigeminal neuralgia have helped to elucidate a theory for the pathophysiology of the disorder. However, the definitive cause of trigeminal neuralgia remains to be determined. Theories of the pathogenesis of trigeminal neuralgia will be addressed more comprehensively elsewhere; however, drug actions will be briefly reviewed here.

Most experimental studies have focused on neurons in the nucleus oralis of the trigeminal nuclear complex.[2] This region receives heavy input from the perioral region, a frequent trigger zone for the paroxysms of pain in trigeminal neuralgia. Carbamazepine and phenytoin have been shown to facilitate inhibition of input to the nucleus oralis after electrical stimulation of the maxillary nerve in experimental animals. Testing of baclofen in the animal model has also shown this effect.[10] This led to the clinical testing and success of baclofen in the therapy of trigeminal neuralgia. Taken together, these lines of evidence support the hypothesis that there is a deficiency in segmental inhibition at the trigeminal

● **TABLE 10-3** • Trigeminal Neuralgia: Medical Therapy

Drug	Dosing	Common Adverse Reaction	Severe Adverse Reaction	Contra-Indication
Carbamazepine (Tegretol)	Starting dose: 100–300 mg/day Therapeutic range: 800–1200 mg/day	Dizziness, somnolence, nausea, vomiting, diplopia, rash	Hematopoietic (aplastic anemia), dermatologic (Stevens-Johnson), congestive heart failure	Previous myelosuppression, adverse reaction to tricyclic medications
Phenytoin (Dilantin)	Starting dose: 200 mg/day Therapeutic range: 5–7 mg/kg/day	Nystagmus, ataxia, dizziness, lethargy, incoordination, dysarthria, rash, gingival hyperplasia	Hepatitis, Stevens-Johnson	Hydantoin hypersensitivity
Baclofen (Lioresal)	Starting dose: 30 mg/day Therapeutic range: 50–80 mg/day	Lethargy, ataxia, gastrointestinal distress, nausea	Withdrawal seizures, hallucinations	
Clonazepam (Klonopin)	1.5–6 mg/day (divide dose to minimize sedation)	Central nervous system depression	Lethargy, rash, fatigue, thrombocytopenia	Benzodiazepine sensitivity, liver disease, narrow angle glaucoma
Oxcarbazepine (Trileptal)	Starting dose: 300 mg/day Therapeutic range: 800–1200 mg/day	Dizziness, somnolence, nausea, vomiting	Unknown	Unknown
Sodium valproate (Depakote)	Starting dose: 600 mg/day Therapeutic range: 600–1200 mg/day	Tremor, nausea, vomiting, weight gain, alopecia, irritability	Hepatotoxicity	Liver disease

nucleus contributing to the pathogenesis of trigeminal neuralgia. Nevertheless, there is also evidence that peripheral nerve irritation or injury also contributes to or results in loss of the central inhibitory mechanisms.[11,12]

Carbamazepine

Carbamazepine is a tricyclic drug related structurally to the antidepressant imipramine. It was first synthesized in 1961[13] and subsequently found to be effective in seizure disorders, affective disorders, and trigeminal neuralgia. After oral ingestion, the drug is absorbed from the gastrointestinal tract with peak blood levels generally achieved 2 to 8 hours after the dose. Drug is distributed into all tissues and is approximately 70% to 80% protein bound in blood. Initially, there is a linear relationship between dose and plasma concentration. During chronic therapy, carbamazepine typically causes autoinduction of hepatic metabolism. Therefore, while initial elimination half-life is 20 to 40 hours, later in treatment it can become as short as 11 hours. This effect on metabolism is thought to be responsible for significant fluctuation in serum concentration of drug during maintenance therapy. Side effects and drug efficacy are known to correlate with serum concentration of drug. In the past a divided dosing strategy has been used to limit peak serum concentration of drug. More recently, a new formulation of controlled-release carbamazepine has been marketed. This allows less frequent dosing and more stable blood levels of drug. A study using the

controlled-release formulation has shown a significant reduction in serum concentration fluctuations.[14]

The first reports of the use of carbamazepine for treatment of trigeminal neuralgia were published in 1962.[9,15] Following this there were many open trials initially in Europe and later in the United States. The early trials were frequently uncontrolled and difficult to interpret. Furthermore, follow-up periods were short and often patients with atypical facial pain were included in the treatment groups. Better-controlled studies later confirmed the efficacy of carbamazepine in the treatment of trigeminal neuralgia.[16–20]

Initial response of trigeminal neuralgia to carbamazepine is virtually universal. Lack of response should lead the clinician to carefully reassess the diagnosis. However, despite the initially good response, a small percentage of patients are unable to tolerate the side effects of the medication. In addition, long-term studies have demonstrated a gradual decline in efficacy with time. The initial response rate is usually in the 80% range,[20] but by 10 years from the start of therapy, only about 50% of patients respond to carbamazepine therapy.[21]

Currently, carbamazepine is the initial drug of choice for the management of trigeminal neuralgia. The initial dose in an average-size adult is 200 mg per day, increasing by 200 to 300 mg per day until pain relief is achieved. Early dose-related side effects may be minimized by a gradual escalation to therapeutic dose range. A typical dose range that results in pain control is between 800 and 1200 mg per day. The dose may need to be increased after several weeks of therapy because of hepatic enzyme induction. At this point, it may also prove beneficial to take a greater proportion of a divided dose in the evening to ensure adequate serum concentration of drug for pain control the following morning.

Before initiating therapy with carbamazepine, a baseline complete blood cell count and liver and renal function tests should be obtained. These studies should be repeated every 2 weeks for the first 2 months of therapy and then four times per year thereafter. Drug should be discontinued if the peripheral white blood cell count drops below 3000 cells per microliter (see subsequent section).

Between 20% and 40% of patients treated with carbamazepine experience some form of drug-related side effect. Early dose-related side effects commonly include somnolence, dizziness, nausea, and nystagmus. These occur more commonly in the elderly and when dose escalates rapidly. Dermatologic reactions occur in approximately 5% to 10% of patients and include rash, erythema multiforme, and rarely Stevens-Johnson syndrome. The most common idiosyncratic side effects are hematologic and occur 2% to 6% of the time. The most serious of these is aplastic anemia, which, while rarely encountered, necessitates the regular monitoring of a hematologic profile as described previously. Other infrequent side effects include hepatotoxicity, hyponatremia, and congestive heart failure.

Because carbamazepine induces hepatic drug metabolism, it has interactions and effects on many commonly used drugs. Serum concentrations of clonazepam, valproate, primidone, and other antiepileptic drugs are often decreased due to enzyme induction. Carbamazepine has no significant interaction with baclofen. Phenytoin and carbamazepine compete for a common catabolic pathway. Therefore, phenytoin levels typically rise in combination therapy with carbamazepine, although the autoinduction of hepatic catabolic pathways makes the effect somewhat unpredictable, requiring careful monitoring of blood levels. Lamotrigine and valproate have been shown to inhibit metabolism of the bioactive carbamazepine epoxide, thus potentiating toxicity without necessarily changing serum concentration of drug. A comprehensive review of interactions is beyond the scope of this chapter, and the reader is encouraged to refer to one of the numerous sources available.[1,2,22]

Phenytoin

Phenytoin (diphenylhydantoin) was first synthesized in 1908 and tested for use as a hypnotic. It is a white crystalline powder, insoluble in water. After oral absorption, peak serum concentration is generally reached in 4 to 8 hours. The time taken to reach serum peak concentration is independent of dose. Phenytoin is absorbed in the small intestine and bound 90% to serum proteins, primarily albumin. Drug is metabolized in the liver. When the catabolic pathway becomes saturated, phenytoin levels rise with zero-order kinetics. Therefore, small increments in dose can result in large changes in serum concentration.

The efficacy of phenytoin in trigeminal neuralgia was initially reported in 1942.[8] Patients who respond to therapy generally experience pain relief within 2 days of onset of therapy. The dose to achieve pain control is usually in the 5 to 7 mg/kg

per day range. There have been no controlled trials to date comparing phenytoin with carbamazepine for trigeminal neuralgia.[23,24] Reports of efficacy with phenytoin describe a response rate of anywhere from 25% to 60% of patients.[25] These are certainly less than the response rates reported in the literature for carbamazepine. Thus, phenytoin has not typically been the initial drug of choice for the treatment of trigeminal neuralgia.

The most frequently encountered dose-dependent side effects of phenytoin are ataxia, drowsiness, nystagmus, and diplopia. Other common side effects include gingival hyperplasia, acne, and hirsutism. Morbilliform rash can occur commonly. Manifestations of systemic hypersensitivity include Stevens-Johnson syndrome, hepatitis, a lupus-like syndrome, and folate-responsive megaloblastic anemia.

Drug interactions with phenytoin are quite frequent. The drug is loosely bound to hepatic cytochrome P-450 and thus is susceptible to competitive displacement. Because phenytoin is a potent hepatic enzyme inducer, metabolism of numerous drugs is altered. Serum levels of phenytoin should be carefully monitored when medications with known interactions are added or withdrawn.[1]

Baclofen

Baclofen became available in 1972. Structurally, it is an analogue of the inhibitory neurotransmitter gamma aminobutyric acid (GABA). After oral ingestion, baclofen is rapidly absorbed via the gastrointestinal tract and serum peak concentration is achieved in 2 to 3 hours. It has a variable half-life in general ranging from 3 to 4 hours. Drug is excreted unchanged by the kidneys.[2]

In laboratory studies, baclofen has similar features to carbamazepine and phenytoin. In a cat model, baclofen was found to promote segmental inhibition at the nucleus oralis of the trigeminal brainstem complex.[26] After this encouraging experimental data, baclofen was used in a series of clinical trials and found to have efficacy in trigeminal neuralgia. To date, there have been several trials, including a blinded crossover trial with carbamazepine, which have shown the efficacy of baclofen.[26-29] In long-term follow-up, resistance to therapy with baclofen develops in 30% of patients.[26] There appears to be a synergism between baclofen and either carbamazepine or phenytoin, and therefore combination therapy in specific cases is a reasonable option.[30] Because baclofen is formulated as a racemic mixture, the issue of which isomer is most effective has been examined. In these experimental series, the L-baclofen isomer has been found to be significantly more effective and better tolerated than the racemic form.[31,32]

The initial dose of baclofen is 10 mg three times per day. The dose should be incrementally increased until pain relief is achieved or toxicity is encountered. Typical daily maintenance dose required in trigeminal neuralgia is 50 to 60 mg per day.

Common side effects of baclofen include somnolence, dizziness, and gastrointestinal distress. These are usually dose-dependent. Baclofen does not have the potentially life-threatening adverse effects of carbamazepine or phenytoin, and is typically very well tolerated. Because of the low toxicity profile, some clinicians use it as first-line therapy in trigeminal neuralgia despite its lower efficacy. Withdrawal of medication should be gradual to prevent seizures or hallucination. Baclofen does not have known interactions with other medications.[2]

Oxcarbazepine

Oxcarbazepine is a derivative of carbamazepine and has been marketed outside the United States since 1991. The drug is metabolized rapidly to a pharmacologically active compound whose half-life is 14 to 26 hours. Clinical studies, primarily in epilepsy, have shown less significant toxicity when compared to carbamazepine.[33–35] The degradation pathway for oxcarbazepine differs from that for carbamazepine and does not induce hepatic enzyme systems.

Most studies evaluating the efficacy of oxcarbazepine to date are directed at patients with epilepsy. There has been a small trial of oxcarbazepine in patients with trigeminal neuralgia refractory to carbamazepine therapy. All patients had a good response.[36] A second crossover trial from carbamazepine to oxcarbazepine also showed promising results.[37] Dosing with oxcarbazepine is similar to that for carbamazepine. Higher doses of oxcarbazepine are often tolerated due to an improved side effect profile.

Although beyond the scope of this chapter, it is important to mention that other medications such as clonazepam, sodium valproate, capsaicin, salicylates, and ophthalmic and local anesthetics are frequently used in cases of refractory cranial neuralgias. Other medications such as antidepressants, neuroleptics, and opioids can be used in conjunction with standard therapies for more atypical presentations.

OVERVIEW OF SURGICAL TREATMENT OPTIONS

While medical management of facial pain syndromes remains the mainstay of initial treatment, there are a variety of safe and effective surgical options for patients who fail medical management. While other chapters in this text will provide a more in-depth assessment of the various surgical approaches for cranial neuralgias, we will present here a brief overview of the surgical treatment options.

Surgical management can be generally divided into *denervating* and *nerve-sparing* procedures. Although currently not commonly used, peripheral denervating procedures (supraorbital, infraorbital, and submental) and more proximal trigeminal rhizotomy (subtemporal and posterior fossa) were once quite commonplace. These denervating procedures have been largely supplanted by percutaneous procedures including radiofrequency (RF) and glycerol or balloon compression rhizolysis. The success of these procedures is to a certain degree dependent on the production of an area of numbness in the distribution of the patient's pain. The majority of percutaneous procedures can be performed on an outpatient basis without general anesthesia. Under mild sedation, a trocar is inserted through the cheek and fluoroscopically guided through the foramen ovale into the region of the gasserian ganglion. For RF rhizolysis, a lesion is made after stimulation confirms the tip of the needle to be in the proper distribution. Glycerol rhizolysis involves instillation of anhydrous glycerol

through the trocar after cisternogram is performed in the sitting position with contrast material. Balloon compression uses a Fogarty catheter that is inflated at the entry of the trigeminal nerve into the cistern. The latter two procedures are more frequently recommended in cases of cranial nerve V1 trigeminal pain as the incidence of corneal anesthesia is thought to be less than that of RF rhizolysis in this particular distribution.[38–40]

Since its popularization by Janetta in the 1970s,[41] microvascular decompression (MVD) has become a mainstay of surgical management in trigeminal neuralgia. Unlike the *denervating* percutaneous techniques mentioned above, MVD has the advantage of being a *nerve-sparing* procedure, focused at the hypothesized source of the problem, and is not dependent on the production of facial numbness. While the risks of this procedure are obviously elevated in comparison (see below), several series have shown MVD to have a lower long-term rate of recurrence in comparison with the percutaneous procedures.[42,43]

In the past 5 years, stereotactic radiation surgery has evolved as a new treatment option for trigeminal neuralgia.[44,45] Controversy exists as the nature of this technique precludes physiologic confirmation of lesion location before placement. Nonetheless, preliminary reports have suggested a high rate of initial pain control, a low incidence of facial numbness, and a low rate of short-term recurrence.[46] Long-term follow-up of radiation surgery is not yet available to fully evaluate the long-term results and risks of this procedure.

TREATMENT OUTCOMES

As mentioned previously, approximately 80% of patients with trigeminal neuralgia can be treated successfully with medical management. Due to side effects and tachyphylaxis, successful medical management 10 years after initiation decreases to less than 50%.[20,21] Table 10-4 provides an overview analysis of surgical outcome and morbidity for comparison.

TREATMENT ALGORITHM

For patients who have been carefully evaluated and diagnosed with trigeminal neuralgia, appropriate initial therapy is carbamazepine. It would be reasonable to consider baclofen initially, especially in elderly or frail patients, with the understanding that efficacy, along with toxicity, is less. Either drug should be titrated until pain relief is achieved or side effects ensue. If pain remains refractory, a combination therapy with baclofen and carbamazepine or phenytoin should be tried, given the synergism of these medications. If combination therapy proves ineffective, consideration should be given to either a second-line medication or surgical therapy. Once pain relief is achieved for a period of several months, attempts can be made to wean from medical therapy. If pain recurs, therapy must be reinstituted. Medication trials are also appropriate for those patients in whom recurrent pain develops after surgical procedures. As previously mentioned, the

● **TABLE 10-4** • Outcome Analysis

	Glycerol Rhizolysis	Radiofrequency Rhizolysis	Balloon Compression	Radiosurgery[44]	Microvascular Decompression[48,49]
Initial pain relief	91%	98%	93%	94%	98%
Recurrence at 2 years	54%	20–23%	21%	54% pain free 88% with 50–100% relief	15%
Complications					
Masseter weakness	1.7%	7–24%	66%	–	0%
Dysesthesias	16%	11–24%	19%	6%	0.5%
Corneal anesthesia	3.7%	3–7%	1.5%	–	0.05%
Keratitis	1.8%	0.6–1%	0%	–	0%
Anesthesia dolorosa	1.8%	0.2–1.5%	0.1%	–	0%
Cranial nerve deficit	0%	0%	0%	–	3%
Ipsilateral hearing loss	–	–	–	–	0.8–1.98%
CSF leak	–	–	–	–	1.85–2.44%
Mortality	0%	0%	0%	0%	0.2–0.6%

(Adapted from Taha[47])

diagnosis of trigeminal neuralgia should also be reconsidered in cases that do not show the typical initial response to medical therapy.

When patients fail medical management, either due to intolerable side effects or loss of effect, surgical options should be considered. For younger patients with few operative risk factors, MVD is usually recommended based on its high initial rate of success, low rate of recurrence, and lower risk of deafferentation-related complaints. For older patients with higher operative risk factors, the percutaneous route is generally recommended as first-line surgical therapy. It is unclear at this point whether radiation surgery offers any advantages over the more established surgical therapies.

While the medical and surgical results for the treatment of trigeminal neuralgia have improved dramatically over the past half-century, our ability to diagnose atypical facial pain syndromes is still quite poor. It is important for the neurosurgeon to recognize that patients who present with atypical symptoms generally respond poorly to the routine medical and surgical management aimed at patients with more classic signs of trigeminal neuralgia. Moreover, these patients may respond more favorably to antidepressants and psychiatric consultation.

CONCLUSION

Trigeminal neuralgia is a disease with relapses and remissions whose symptoms are not relieved by traditional medical approaches to pain management. While there is no cure for the disorder, effective medical and surgical interventions are available. Thus, it is a disease that requires rational medical decision making and a close alliance between those practitioners specializing in medical and surgical therapies.

Neurosurgeons are frequently called on to diagnose and treat facial pain. Although surgical options for specific facial pain syndromes are quite attractive, it is crucial that neurosurgeons be familiar with the myriad facial pain syndromes that do not respond to surgery. Moreover, it is important to arrive at a rational treatment regimen that addresses not only the cause of pain, but the character of the pain as well. A better appreciation of the neuroanatomic and chemical changes that occur in chronic pain has allowed us to rationalize our medical treatment of different pain syndromes. As our understanding of the neuroanatomy and pathophysiology of facial pain improves, so will our ability to offer more effective treatment, both medical and surgical.

REFERENCES

1. Zakrzewska JM. Trigeminal neuralgia. *In* Warlow CP, van Gijn J (eds). Major Problems in Neurology, vol. 28. London, WB Saunders, 1995.
2. Fromm GH, Sessle BJ. Trigeminal Neuralgia: Current Concepts Regarding Pathogenesis and Treatment. Boston, Butterworth-Heinemann, 1991.
3. Keller JT, Van Loveren H. Pathophysiology of the pain of trigeminal neuralgia and atypical facial pain: a neuroanatomical perspective. Clin Neurosurg 322:75–93, 1985.
4. Hunt JR. Geniculate neuralgia (neuralgia of the nervus facialis): a further contribution to the sensory system of the facial nerve and its neuralgic conditions. Arch Neurol Psychiatry 37:253–285, 1937.
5. Morgenlander JC, Wilkins RH. Surgical treatment of cluster headache. J Neurosurg 72(6):866–871, 1990.
6. Rushton JG, Stevens JC, Miller RH. Glossopharyngeal (vagoglossopharyngeal) neuralgia: a study of 217 cases. Arch Neurol 38(4):201–205, 1981.
7. Wilkins RH. Glossopharyngeal (vasoglossopharyngeal) neuralgia. *In* Barrow DL (ed). Trigeminal Neuralgia and Other Trigeminal Dysfunction Syndromes. AANS, 1993, pp 245–251.
8. Bergouignan M. Cures hereuses de neuralgie faciales essentielles par le diphenylhydantoinate de soude. Rev Laryngol Otol Rhinol 63:34–41, 1942.
9. Blom S. Tic douloureux treated with a new anticonvulsant. Arch Neurol 9:285–290, 1962.
10. Terrence CF, Sax M, Fromm GH, Chang CH, Yoo CS. Effect of baclofen enantiomorphs on the spinal trigeminal nucleus and steric similarities of carbamazepine. Pharmacology 27(2):85–94, 1983.
11. Burchiel KJ. Ectopic impulse generation in focally demyelinated trigeminal nerve. Exp Neurol 69:423–429, 1980.

12. Burchiel KJ. Abnormal impulse generation in focally demyelinated trigeminal roots. J Neurosurg 53:674–683, 1980.
13. Shindler W. 5H-Dibenz [b,f] azepines. Chem Abstr 55:1671, 1961.
14. Mckee PJW Blacklaw J, Butler E. Monotherapy with conventional and controlled release carbamazepine. Br J Clin Pharmacol 32:99–104, 1991.
15. Blom S. Trigeminal neuralgia: its treatment with a new anticonvulsant drug (G-32883). Lancet 1:839–840, 1962.
16. Campbell FG, Graham JG, Zilkha KJ. Clinical trial of carbamazepine in trigeminal neuralgia. J Neurol Neurosurg Psychiatry 29:265–267, 1966.
17. Killian JM, Fromm GH. Carbamazepine in the treatment of trigeminal neuralgia: use and side effects. Arch Neurol 129–136, 1968.
18. Rockliff BW, Davis EH. Controlled sequential trials of carbamazepine in trigeminal neuralgia. Arch. Neurol 15:129–136, 1966.
19. Sturman RH, O'Brien FH. Non-surgical treatment of douloureux with carbamazepine. Headache 9:88–91, 1969.
20. Rasmussen P, Rushede J. Facial pain treated with carbamazepine. Acta Neurol Scand 46:385–408, 1970.
21. Taylor JC, Brauer S, Espir LE. Long- term treatment of trigeminal neuralgia with carbamazepine. Postgrad Med J 57:16–18, 1981.
22. Masdeu JC. Medical treatment and clinical pharmacology. In Rovit RL, Murali R, Jannetta PJ (eds). Trigeminal Neuralgia. Baltimore, Williams and Wilkins, 1990.
23. Swedlow M, Cundill JD. Anticonvulsant drugs used in the treatment of lacerating pain. Anesthesia 36:1129–1132, 1981.
24. Chintz A, Sellinger DF, Greenhouse AH. Anticonvulsant therapy in trigeminal neuralgia. Am J Med Sci 252:62–67, 1966.
25. Braham J, Saia A. Phenytoin in the treatment of trigeminal and other neuralgias. Lancet 2:892–893, 1960.
26. Fromm GH, Terrence CF, Chattha AS. Baclofen in trigeminal neuralgia. Arch Neurol 37:768–771, 1980.
27. Fromm GH, Terrence CF, Chattha AS. Baclofen in the treatment of trigeminal neuralgia: double blind study and long-term follow-up. Ann Neurol 15:240–244, 1984.
28. Parmar BS, Shick KH, Gardlin IC. Baclofen in trigeminal neuralgia—a clinical trial. IJDR 1:109–113, 1989.
29. Steardo L, Leo A, Marrano E. Efficacy of baclofen in trigeminal neuralgia and some other painful conditions. Eur Neurol 23:51–55, 1984.
30. Baker KA, Taylor JW, Lilly GE. Treatment of trigeminal neuralgia: Use of baclofen in combination with carbamazepine. Clin Pharmacol 4:93–96, 1985.
31. Fromm GH, Terrence CF. Comparison of L-baclofen and racemic baclofen in trigeminal neuralgia. Neurology 37:1725–1728, 1987.
32. Sawynok J, Dickson C. D-baclofen is an antagonist at baclofen receptors mediating antinociception in the spinal cord. Pharmacology 31:248–259, 1985.
33. Houtkooper MA, Lammertsma A, Meyer JWA, et al. Oxcarbazepine: a possible alternative to carbamazepine. Epilepsia 28:693–698, 1987.
34. Reinikainen KJ, Keranen T, Halonen T, et al. Comparison of oxcarbazepine and carbamazepine: a double-blind study. Epilepsy Res 1:284–289, 1987.
35. Dam M, Ekberg R, Loyning Y, et al. A double-blind study comparing oxcarbazepine and carbamazepine in patients with newly diagnosed, previously untreated epilepsy. Epilepsy Res 3:70–76, 1989.
36. Zakrzewska JM, Patsalos PN. Oxcarbazepine: a new drug in the management of trigeminal neuralgia. J Neurol Neurosurg Psychiatry 52:472–476, 1989.
37. Remmilard G. Oxcarbazepine and intractable trigeminal neuralgia. Epilepsia 35:528–529, 1994.
38. Belber CJ, Rak RA. Balloon compression rhizolysis in the surgical management of trigeminal neuralgia. Neurosurgery 20(6):908–913, 1987.
39. Brown JA, Preul MC. Percutaneous trigeminal ganglion compression for trigeminal neuralgia. Experience in 22 patients and review of the literature. J Neurosurg 70(6):900–904, 1989.
40. Burchiel KJ. Percutaneous retrogasserian glycerol rhizolysis in the management of trigeminal neuralgia. J Neurosurg 69(3):361–366, 1988.
41. Jannetta PJ, Tew JM Jr. Treatment of trigeminal neuralgia. Neurosurgery 4(1):93–94, 1979.
42. Apfelbaum RI. A comparision of percutaneous radiofrequency trigeminal neurolysis and microvascular decompression of the trigeminal nerve for the treatment of tic douloureux. Neurosurgery 1(1):16–21, 1977.
43. Burchiel KJ, Steege TD, Howe JF, Loeser JD. Comparison of percutaneous radiofrequency gangliolysis and microvascular decompression for the surgical management of tic douloureux. Neurosurgery 9(2):111–119, 1981.
44. Kondziolka D, Lunsford LD, Flickinger JC, et al. Stereotactic radiosurgery for trigeminal neuralgia: a multi-institutional study using the gamma unit. J Neurosurg 84(6):940–945, 1996.
45. Young RF, Vermulen S, Posewitz A. Gamma knife radiosurgery for the treatment of trigeminal neuralgia. Stereotactic Functional Neurosurg 119:2–9, 1998.
46. Niranjan A, Lunsford LD. Radiosurgery: where we were, are, and may be in the third millennium [editorial]. Neurosurgery 46(3):531–543, 2000.
47. Taha JM, Tew JM Jr. Comparison of surgical treatments for trigeminal neuralgia: reevaluation of radiofrequency rhizotomy [see comments]. Neurosurgery 38(5):865–871, 1996.
48. McLaughlin MR, Jannetta PJ, Clyde BL, Subach BR, Comey CH, Resnick DK. Microvascular decompression of cranial nerves: lessons learned after 4400 operations [see comments]. J Neurosurg 90(1):1–8, 1999.
49. Barker FG 2nd, Jannetta PJ, Bissonette DJ, Larkins MV, Jho HD. The long-term outcome of microvascular decompression for trigeminal neuralgia [see comments]. N Engl J Med 334(17):1077–1083, 1996.

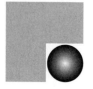

C H A P T E R 1 1

Central and Deafferentation Pain Syndromes

RICHARD K. SIMPSON JR, MD, PhD, FACS

The mechanisms responsible for pain and the variety of therapies available for pain management are discussed in numerous chapters within this text. This chapter focuses on the origin of central pain syndromes, the physiologic basis for their occurrence, and contemporary medical and surgical paradigms directed toward their management. Of note is the rather artificial distinction between the terms *central pain* and *deafferentation pain*. It is generally accepted that central pain refers to pain arising as a result of a lesion in the central nervous system, whereas deafferentation pain is attributed to injury of a peripheral nerve or nerve root.[1] Both mechanisms of pain likely reflect deafferentation of some sort whether it is based on peripheral afferent nerve fibers or to more centrally conducting sensory pathways in the spinal cord or brain.[2]

Several attempts have been made to redefine central pain based on both clinical and laboratory data. These include spontaneous, peripherally induced, and continuous or ongoing pain.[3] An additional classification system includes intermittent, steady, and evoked pain.[4] Another aspect often not included in these classification systems is the important behavioral component to central pain.[5] Most of the evidence regarding behavior has been collected from animals and includes autotomy or other forms of compulsive self-directed behavior.[6] Scratching, rubbing, biting, and licking of the affected area are forms of these pain-related behaviors that can be observed in humans.[7] Protection, guarding, and avoidance behaviors involving the affected area are also common in central pain syndromes that can manifest as persistent postural flexions.[8]

Historically, central pain has been referred to as deafferentation pain, dysesthetic pain, causalgia, anesthesia dolorosa, and even phantom limb pain when peripheral neural structures have been injured.[9] Central pain has also been referred to as post-stroke pain, thalamic pain, or spinal cord injury pain when central structures have been injured.[10] Because of the location of the neural damage, different treatment options exist. Therefore, it is appropriate to discuss central pain in terms of these distinctions until additional research can demonstrate genuine differences in their various mechanisms of production. This chapter presents several of the commonly recognized descriptive types of central pain syndromes. Included are spinal cord injury pain, post-stroke pain, and phantom limb pain.

Several options exist for patients suffering from central pain syndromes. These include both medical and surgical options. In the surgical group, these options include both ablative or destructive surgery and augmentative surgery. Indications for treatment for conditions of spinal cord injury pain, post-stroke pain, and phantom limb pain are relatively simple. If these patients have pain that is not tolerable without some sort of therapy, then therapy can be instituted. Medical management would be explored and medical regimens would be exhausted before surgical intervention would be entertained. If the patient had pain and desired intervention but did not respond to medical measures or could not tolerate the medicines, then that patient would be considered to be a potential surgical candidate.

As with the application of any form of surgical or medical treatment, careful patient selection is paramount for a reasonable likelihood of an effective outcome. The importance of this issue cannot be overstressed. Candidates must not have serious coexisting medical problems that could adversely influence the course of surgery or endanger the patient beyond acceptable operative risk. These patients should exhibit the necessary cognitive ability to fully understand the issue of informed consent, and should have adequate access to support for general care and transportation for follow-up clinic or hospital visits. Likewise, these patients should not be suffering from serious mental health issues, particularly poorly treated or untreated depression.

PATHOPHYSIOLOGY

Spinal Cord Injury Pain

It was in the early part of the past century that pain following spinal cord injury was clearly recognized. After WWI, Riddoch,[11] Holmes,[12] and Lhermitte[13] described this type of pain as not only unpleasant, but as a "dreadful sensation." As with all central pain phenomena, the pathophysiology of spinal cord injury pain is poorly understood. Several causes have been identified, including the most common, trauma, but also inflammatory, neoplastic, ischemic, and developmental such as a syrinx formation.[14] Central pain can be experienced by patients subjected to ablative spinal cord procedures such as cordotomy.[15] Patients typically describe the pain as diffuse and burning and a deep ache, with bouts of intermittent sharper pain particularly of a tingling quality. The pain is sensed generally at and below the level of spinal cord injury.

Cellular mechanisms for pain production of spinal cord injury pain are only now being explored. Mechanisms common to all forms of central pain phenomena are generally accepted as potentially the mechanism of pain after spinal injury. Injury to the spinothalamic tract has been implicated as a cause of such pain whether or not the dorsal columns have been described to be involved.[16] Both the cells of origin of this pathway and the terminal projections of the tract, particularly the thalamus, are possibly responsible.[17] It is more likely, since damage to the spinal cord results in interruption of multiple different pathways, that pain is produced from a number of different projection systems to a variety of targets in the brain.[18]

Cells in the dorsal horn of the spinal cord contributing to the ascending projections systems including the spinothalamic tract are somatically organized.[19] Cells in the superficial lamina (I and II) are high-threshold or nociceptive-specific cells.[20,21] Permeated through the lamina of the dorsal horn (I to VI) are cells of wide dynamic range or multireceptive cells.[22,23] These cell types have distinct roles in pain perception, the former more selective in nature for the detection of tissue damage; the latter of a nonspecific nature acting to condition or warn of impending damage.[24] In addition, cells in dorsal column nuclei that respond to painful stimuli have been recorded and obviously play a role in pain perception.[25] Interruption of the normal afferent inputs to dorsal horn or dorsal column nuclear cells from peripheral structures likely results in aberrant signal processing or an abnormal relay of information to higher structures that ultimately conclude as a central pain phenomenon.[26]

Many spinal cord pathways project centrally to structures involved in pain perception.[25] These pathways include the spinoreticular tract, which projects from the dorsal horn to numerous areas of the brainstem from the medulla to the mesencephalon.[27] Another pathway projecting in this fashion is cells forming the spinomesencephalic tract.[28] Other pathways include the spinoparabrachial system projecting primarily onto the midbrain and periaqueductal gray matter.[29] These projections are primarily contralateral and terminate particularly in the area of the superior colliculus and the pretectal nuclei as well as the periaqueductal gray matter and the parabrachial nuclei.[30]

Another complex fiber group is the spinopontoamygdaloid pathway, which also incorporates a spinohypothalamic component.[31] The cells of origin have large receptive fields and exhibit wind-up phenomenon.[32] This pathway likely contributes to the emotional and affective response to pain.[33] In addition, the autonomic responses to noxious stimulation may be mediated by this pathway.[34] Projections from this pathway also include the basal ganglia, particularly the globus pallidus ventralis, and the preoptic and septal nuclei.[35] Certainly, damage or destruction of one or more of these spinal cord pathways will contribute to abnormal perceptions that, in part, are

conceived as a deafferentation type of pain, a central pain, following spinal cord injury.[36]

Post-Stroke Pain

Central pain following a stroke has been recognized for nearly 100 years largely as a result of observations by Dejerine and Roussy.[37] The concept of central pain developed from these early observations and autopsy studies of three patients. Post-stroke lesions can be either ischemic or hemorrhagic.[38] Iatrogenic lesions can also produce this form of central pain, which is generally the result of tumor removal or stereotactic placement of a lesion.[39] Post-stroke lesions causing pain are not necessarily located in the thalamus. Lesions in the brainstem, pons, and even the cortex can produce central pain.[14]

A role exists for the dorsal column medial lemniscal system in the transmission of pain. Cells in the dorsal column nuclei receive unmyelinated C-type fibers carried within the dorsal columns and respond to nociceptive stimulation.[25] There is evidence that visceral pain is carried in fibers ascending in the medial aspect of the dorsal column system.[40] Activity from these cells then, in turn, activate dorsal column nuclear cells sensitive to noxious input and relay the activity to the ventrobasal complex.[41] In the ventrobasal complex, the receptive fields of these cells tends to be small and these cells appear to be intermingled with those receiving dorsal column medial lemniscal inputs.[42]

The receptive fields of cells in the posterior nuclear group tend to be large, have bilateral representation of the body, and frequently respond to non-noxious stimulation.[41] Sensitization of these cells and those in the ventrobasal group has been observed after prolonged noxious stimulation similar to that observed in the dorsal horn.[42] The close association of the cells in the ventrobasal and posterior nuclear groups responding to noxious stimulation to those chiefly responding to lemniscal inputs suggests that these areas contribute to the sensory discriminative features of pain behavior.

Cells in the central lateral nucleus and the nucleus submedius, in general, receive inputs from wide receptive fields and exhibit features of bilateral somatotopic representation.[43] The concept of spinothalamic tract projections traveling directly to the parafascicular and intralaminar nuclei is controversial.[44] Although historically taught as a primitive relay system from spinothalamic tract activity to diffuse projections to the cerebral cortex, it is more likely that these nuclei are involved in some aspects of the motor response to pain due to their dense projections to the basal ganglia.[45] The nucleus submedius, in contrast, does indeed receive direct projections from the spinothalamic tract.[43] This nucleus exhibits similar electrophysiologic features as the parafascicular and intralaminar nuclei. The ventral medial nucleus contains neurons that are sensitive to thermonociception and tends to project to the insula.[46]

Another small fiber tract with features similar to the dorsal column medial lemniscal system is the spinocervical tract.[47] This pathway commonly associated with non-primates is found in humans. Cells from the dorsal horn relay ascending fibers to the lateral cervical nucleus located at spinal levels C1 and C2. Cells from the lateral nucleus respond primarily to non-noxious cutaneous stimuli but also respond to noxious stimulation. Fibers from this nucleus project to the ventrobasal group and then relay to the somatosensory cortex.

Clearly, damage or destruction to the nuclei of the thalamus and other cortical and subcortical structures can result in abnormal firing patterns of surviving neurons. Such abnormal patterns of neuronal activity unmediated by surrounding damaged structures could give rise to painful sensations. Such pain is not only an abnormal sensation, it is easily provoked, often explosive in nature, unbearable, poorly localized, persistent, and can produce violent emotional reactions. It is as if the default mode to a disturbance in the ascending afferent system is to provide the most primitive form of sensation normally used for protection and preservation, that being pain.

Phantom Limb Pain

Phantom limb pain is the perfect example of a nervous system responding to damage in a manner that defies logic. Initial descriptions of such pain can be found in Weir Mitchell's discussions of post-battlefield injuries during the American Civil War.[48] After amputation, either surgical or traumatic, the vast majority of patients (up to 97%) experience phantom limb pain.[49] Phantom limb pain must be distinguished from an older term, *stump pain*.[50] Stump pain incorporates a number of potential causes that are not neuropathic or central in origin. Such causes can be related to the skin itself, the vasculature, bone, neuromas, and infections.[51]

Mechanisms of phantom limb pain are likely to incorporate those described earlier for spinal cord and post-stroke pain as well as those discussed in other chapters regarding neuropathic pain. However, there are likely to be some unique contributions to phantom limb pain from the peripheral nerves themselves. Neuromas can form from the damaged nerve endings that can spontaneously produce painful sensation and be hypersensitive.[52] Attempts by the body to reestablish connections through the injury can produce what has been described as chaotic reinnervation.[53] This can lead to the formation of ectopic excitation sites and ephaptic synapse formation.[54] Formation of the abnormal neural elements can induce a hypersensitivity to stimulation and likely an abnormal perception to nonpainful stimulation. Thus, phantom limb pain has many mechanisms in common with pain following peripheral nerve injury.

Phantom limb pain can be experienced by patients with root avulsions or as result of spinal cord injury.[55] Therefore, spinal mechanisms for pain production are likely to be involved. Disinhibition of dorsal ganglion cells or dorsal horn cells along with the abnormal firing patterns likely to be generated by the afferent loss may be reflected as a phantom pain.[56] In addition, because of the complex nature of this perception, higher cortical centers are likely to be involved as well.[57] Not only can cells of wide dynamic range, known to exist in the thalamus, be involved such as that mentioned with spinal cord injury pain, but neuronal plasticity of the cerebral cortex may play a role. Cortical reorganization of the cerebral cortex may occur after amputation.[58]

MEDICAL STRATEGIES

Spinal Cord Injury Pain

Spinal cord injury pain is exceedingly difficult to successfully treat by either medical or surgical means. However, before considering surgical options, several medical therapies should be tried. Diphenhydramine (Benadryl®) has been administered with some success.[59] In general, antidepressant medications, particularly amitriptyline, can be administered with some benefit to the patient. Others in this class include imipramine, fluphenazine, chlorpromazine, and benperidol.[14] Anticonvulsant therapy is a virtual mainstay in the medical management of spinal cord injury pain.[60] Older established drugs include diphenylhydantoin (Dilantin®), and carbamazepine (Tegretol®), as well as valproate (Depakote®). Newer anticonvulsants such as gabapentin (Neurontin®) have also been shown to be successful as treatment for spinal cord injury pain.[60]

Other drugs include mexiletine, which has properties similar to those of lidocaine, and potassium channel blockers such as 4-amino pyridine.[61] Baclofen, a GABA agonist; ketamine, an NMDA antagonist; clonidine; naloxone; L-dopa preparations; and many others have been used with some success.[62–64] Opiates have demonstrated rather limited use for spinal cord injury–induced pain.[65] These drugs are most effective when used in conjunction with nonsteroidal anti-inflammatory drugs.[66] These drugs and others are generally begun at a relatively low dose, then titrated to the maximally tolerated dose, if necessary, or until reasonable benefit is seen. Side effects and toxicity should be avoided, which can be difficult when complex drug regimens incorporating several drugs are used.

Post-Stroke Pain

Post-stroke pain, like all other manifestations of central pain phenomena, remains highly refractory to a number of medications. In general, the same medications for spinal cord injury–induced central pain can be used for patients suffering from post-stroke pain. For this particular pain syndrome, however, mexiletine has been found to be reasonably successful.[67] Clonazepam, trazodone, doxepin, and many other antidepressant drugs have yielded some success as well.[68] Other medications include serotonin agonists and tryptophan, which may provide some relief in these patients with very difficult conditions.[69] Anticonvulsant drugs including phenytoin, carbamazepine, valproate, phenobarbital, and a relatively new drug, gabapentin, have all been used with some success to treat this most difficult condition.[2] As with the treatment of spinal cord injury–induced pain, several other classes of drugs have been used with modest success. These include adrenergic, cholinergic, GABAergic, and glutaminergic agents, and a variety of opiates and their antagonists.[2]

Intervention for all forms of central pain often includes physical therapy, ultrasound, heat, massage, and orthotic devices.[70,71] The role of these therapies cannot be ignored. Likewise, common to all forms of central pain is the coexistence of depression and the need for psychiatric management of such patients. Apart from the benefits of antidepressant drugs mentioned above is psychiatric support.[72] Anxiety, loneliness, the feeling of abandonment and helplessness, and other psychosocial and economic issues can compound an already desperate situation. Certainly, maximizing the support elements, especially in the family, is necessary for improved function. Behavioral modification such as distraction, relaxation, or the use of biofeedback can be worthwhile. Acupuncture and hypnosis have been shown to be of value to some patients with post-stroke pain.[73] Many other forms of alternative medicine are often explored by these patients. Their efficacy has yet to be determined with clarity.

Phantom Limb Pain

Medical management of phantom limb pain can incorporate the therapeutic options outlined above for spinal cord injury and post-stroke pain syndromes. Transcutaneous electrical nerve stimulation (TENS) can be reasonably effective in the management of some of these patients.[74] Physical stimulation of the stump via thermal, mechanical, or electrical means can provide reasonable pain relief for many patients.[75] Other forms of therapy unique to this condition are direct intervention on the stump area, including stump revision.[76] Injections of fentanyl delivered intrathecally or to the stellate ganglion have been helpful.[77,78] Intravenous calcitonin has been shown to reduce the curious phenomenon of spinal anesthesia–induced phantom limb pain.[79] Opioids can also be of value.[80] Other authors have had success with intravenous sodium pentothal, oral carbamazepine, or topical capsaicin.[81–83] Clonazepam and ketamine have also been tried.[84,85] Actions directed toward the stump itself including correction of skin disorders; infection; and the prosthesis shape, design, and use are all important issues to be addressed in patients with phantom limb pain.

SURGICAL STRATEGIES

Spinal Cord Injury Pain

Spinal cord injury pain can be localized to the level of injury (transitional zone pain), areas at and/or below the level of injury, and injuries incorporating the cauda equina, such as the double lesion syndrome.[60] Other pains associated with spinal cord injury, such as musculoskeletal pain and spinal instability, can contribute to the overall pain complaint but are not discussed here as part of the features of central pain. Surgery for spinal cord injury pain or any other central pain should be a last resort, after all other reasonable options have been tried and failed. Failure can be due to a lack of satisfactory benefit despite maximizing the approach, or that the side effects are intolerable thus preventing the advancement of such a treatment option.

The primary ablative neurosurgical operation for spinal cord injury pain has been cordotomy. This procedure, developed in 1912 by Spiller and Martin for patients with spinal cord lesions, can be performed via open laminectomy or a percutaneous approach.[86] The open procedure is usually performed at the T1 to T2 level and is done bilaterally.[87] There are significant limitations to the open technique versus the percutaneous approach. These open procedures necessarily are done under general anesthesia. Accessing the appropriate target, generally the spinothalamic tract, is difficult to verify because no response to stimulation can be elicited. However, in cases of unusual anatomy or accompanying lesions, the open cordotomy is preferable. Although the spinothalamic tract is the primary target, the most effective cordotomy likely involves the spinotectal, spinoreticular, and dorsal and ventral spinocerebellar pathways.[88]

Percutaneous cordotomy remains an accepted form of central pain relief after exhausting all other measures. Popularized in the early 1960s by Mullan, this operation is done under sedation using x-ray and precision cordotomy electrodes.[89] Usually at the C1 to C2 level, a dorsal or lateral approach can be achieved. A low anterior approach at C5 to C6 can be done to prevent the complication of respiratory embarrassment that can result from procedures at C1 to C2. However, the dermatomal level of anesthesia is necessarily compromised by this lower approach. Patients with intermittent or shooting pain tend to respond better to cordotomy than those whose pain is predominately steady in nature. An unpleasant postoperative dysesthesia syndrome may develop in patients who undergo cordotomy.

Other types of destructive or ablative neurosurgical procedures for spinal cord injury pain include cordectomy and midline commissurotomy.[90,91] As with cordotomy, these lesions must take into consideration that the generators of the pain occur below the level of the therapeutic lesion, including, if possible, all of the collateral fibers. There is little reported experience with these two procedures. The dorsal root entry zone (DREZ) lesion, however, has been used successfully to treat these patients. This procedure is done in an open manner, with a heat generator (radiofrequency lesion needle electrodes or laser) or a sharp cut.[92,93]

These operations have been popularized by Nashold and Sindou, respectively, since the 1970s.[92,93] The techniques are similar in their approach to the generator of pain. Nashold's method calls for a small insulated needle to be inserted 2 mm into the spinal cord just medial to the dorsal rootlets at a 25% to 45% angle and aimed laterally. These lesions are made every millimeter along the affected segments of cord. Sindou's method uses a surgical cut at a 45% angle 2 mm into the cord at the line of entry of the dorsal rootlets over each affected dermatomal segment. These operations can be performed in a bilateral manner along numerous dermatomal segments.

Other surgical interventions that are augmentative rather than ablative include the use of epidural spinal cord stimulation and the use of an intrathecal drug delivery device. Epidural spinal cord stimulation involves either open or percutaneous placement of an electrode over the dorsal columns just above the affected site and tunneling of the stimulation electrode lead to a pulse generator placed in a subcutaneous pocket, generally in the trunk region.[94] Relying largely on the gate theory for effectiveness, the electrical output is adjusted to block aberrant transmissions from the pain generators to consciousness. The implanted drug delivery device involves placing an intrathecal catheter and attaching it to a subcutaneous pump that can be programmed to deliver the selected drug in a specified amount and pattern.[63] The result is targeted delivery of the drug via the cerebrospinal fluid (CSF), bypassing breakdown and side effect issues associated with oral or parenteral administration.

Post-Stroke Pain

There are few CNS areas to consider for either ablative or augmentative surgical approaches to patients suffering from post-stroke pain due to the far rostral location of the likely generators. Historically, however, lesions in the caudal nervous system such as cordotomy have been used to treat post-stroke pain referred to as thalamic pain.[38] The results have been reported to be short lived or disappointing. Depending on the location of the stroke, lesions can be produced in the bulbar trigeminal pathways, the bulbar and pontine spinothalamic tracts, and in tracts within the mesencephalon.[14] Contemporary use of these lesions as treatment for post-stroke pain is rare.

Thalamotomy, involving the medial or nonspecific nuclei and the ventrocaudal nuclei have all been targets for central pain management.[95] In particular, pulvinotomy has been used to treat thalamic pain with some success.[96] Other ablative procedures that have been attempted include resection of the sensory cortex ("topectomy").[97] Frontal leucotomy and cingulotomy have also been tried.[98] Lesions in the hypothalamus have been done as well.[99] These lesions are reserved for the most extreme cases of central pain management such as the post-stroke type. Side effects can be devastating and the degree of pain resolution can be poor. These lesions are generally created using a variety of stereotactic techniques and types of equipment. In general, a coordinate frame is placed on the patient's head, and a previously defined target is identified by imaging and or electrophysiologic recording. The patient is minimally sedated, and functional testing of the target is used and verified based on the patient's response. The target is then destroyed by heat or by cold. Recently, the gamma knife has been used to perform ablative procedures for central pain management.[100] Although less invasive, data regarding the long-term pain relief are forthcoming.

Augmentative procedures for post-stroke pain are limited as well. Intrathecal delivery of medication has not been sufficiently addressed with regard to post-stroke pain.[101] As additional drugs are added to the armamentarium, such a technique may become more useful. Thalamic placement of an electrode for deep brain stimulation has been used for post-stroke pain.[102] Additional sites for stimulation include the internal capsule and the periventricular and periaqueductal gray regions. Other intracranial sites have been stimulated for pain management but are rarely used. Recently, motor cortex stimulation has been shown to be useful in the most refractory central pain syndromes including thalamic syndrome or post-stroke pain.[103] By this method, an electrode is placed epidurally over the motor strip over the corresponding somatotopic region. The device is then managed similarly to a deep brain stimulator.

Phantom Limb Pain

Phantom limb pain has been managed much the same way as spinal cord injury pain. Again, the stump itself has to be evaluated, if it exists. Infection, flap problems, bone spurs, neuromas, prosthesis problems, and others may need to be surgically addressed.[76] Ablative procedures including cordotomy and DREZ are commonly used for phantom limb pain refractory to all other measures.[92,93] In addition, epidural spinal cord stimulation and the use of intrathecal drug delivery devices have been

used for these patients.[94,101] Intracranial lesions and placement of deep brain stimulators have also been utilized as treatment for phantom limb pain with some success.[102] The same techniques and principles outlined above for spinal cord injury pain apply to their use for phantom limb pain.

TREATMENT OUTCOMES

Spinal Cord Injury Pain

Accurate numbers that reflect the successful medical management of spinal cord injury pain are lacking. The incidence of spinal cord injury pain is high, nearly two thirds of all patients.[104] Over time, this rate drops to 25% at 5 years after injury.[105] Many patients perceive initial benefits from a number of the drugs outlined previously, and a large number have sustained medical relief of pain or their pain slowly resolves. Over time, some of these patients have significant breakthrough central pain that is long term in nature and intolerable in quality. These patients are considered surgical candidates.

Cordotomy has been an effective surgical treatment for spinal cord injury pain.[106] Tasker and North reported that of the 39 patients treated in this manner, 75% to 86% of patients obtained relief of the shooting type of pain, whereas only 27% experienced relief from the burning or tingling component to the pain.[87] Porter reported that 87% of 34 patients experienced significant early pain relief and 62% had long-term resolution of their pain.[106] In smaller series, White and Sweet, and Botterell had 50% and 57% of their patient series achieve long-term pain relief through a cordotomy.[38,107] Cordectomy provided pain relief to 70% to 100% of patients in a series of 19 spinal cord injuries by Jefferson.[108] These results held true if the cordectomy was done at T11 or below but not above that level. Virozub and colleagues reported that 13 of 24 spinal cord–injured patients with central pain responded to midline commissurotomy.[109]

Dorsal root entry zone lesions have been used to treat spinal cord injury pain. Friedman and Bullitt reported that 25 of 31 patients (80%) reported satisfactory transitional zone pain relief, whereas 8 of 25 patients (32%) reported relief of the more diffuse component of this central pain.[110] Wiegand and Winkelmuller reported that of their series of 20 patients, 50% obtained long-term pain relief.[111] These results were analogous to other reports of similar-size series by Nashold and Young.[111,112]

In contrast, stereotactic thalamotomy has not been shown to be particularly helpful for spinal cord injury–induced central pain. However, a renewed interest in thalamotomy for such pain has been kindled by Young and others by the use of radiation surgery, primarily the use of the gamma knife unit.[100] Thalamic stimulation, on the other hand, has provided relief to some of these patients. Of the 178 cases reported by Young and Rinaldi, 12 had spinal cord injury pain.[102] Approximately four-fifths of all patients had initial significant relief, with nearly two-thirds of these patients experiencing significant long-term relief. Hosobuchi reported similar results in a series of 122 patients with only a few suffering from spinal cord injury pain.[113]

Post-Stroke Pain

Results for the medical management of post-stroke pain are rather sketchy. Few large studies have been reported. Edmondson and colleagues, in 1993, reported successful management of four cases of post-stroke pain with intravenous lidocaine.[67] These patients were then maintained on oral mexiletine. Success rates for other medicines as treatment for post-stroke pain have not been clearly defined. Despite some success with medical therapy, surgical management is an option for these patients using either ablative or augmentative techniques.

The largest series of thalamotomy for post-stroke pain was reported by Amano and colleagues.[114] Forty-seven patients underwent thalamotomy for chronic pain. Of these, 10 were post-stroke or thalamic pain patients and were treated with a medial thalamotomy, incorporating the centromedian and parafasicular nuclei. Initially, 9 of the 10 patients had significant pain relief. Long-term pain relief was recognized in 7 of the original 10 patients. Ohye reported the results of 9 post-stroke patients treated with a more posterior or basal thalamotomy.[115] Four patients achieved satisfactory relief, but only for the deep rather than superficial component of their pain. A combination of both approaches as outlined by Gildenberg resulted in only 30% to 35% of patients with central pain obtaining significant relief.[116] Lesions in the posterior hypothalamus for post-stroke pain have been reported by Sano and colleagues.[117] His single case failed to respond to this form of ablative neurosurgery.

There exists only a limited experience with deep brain stimulation for post-stroke pain. Of the 178 patients treated by Young, only 14 had post-stroke or brain injury–induced pain.[102] Overall, of the patients with chronic pain treated in this series, 80.3% experienced pain relief during the testing phase and 62.2% experienced long-term pain relief. Worldwide, 964 chronic pain patients have been treated with deep brain stimulation as of 1997.[102] Approximately 50% of the patients with neuropathic or central pain syndromes have achieved long-term pain relief. Motor cortex stimulation, as reported by Tsubokawa and colleagues, was also successful as treatment for post-stroke or thalamic pain.[118] Of his 11 patients, 8 (73%) responded very successfully and 5 of these 8 continued to have long-term benefits.

Phantom Limb Pain

The success of medical management of phantom pain has not been sufficiently examined. In part, the difficulty in gauging the success of any therapy for phantom pain is due to the tendency for the severity of the condition to subside and the confounding painful influences of the stump itself. Nevertheless, Jaeger and Maier reported a high degree of success with calcitonin delivered intravenously.[119] Stannard and Nikolajsen reported that ketamine produced a significant degree of pain relief in most patients in their series.[85,120] However, relief from pain was relatively short. Intrathecal fentanyl dramatically reduced pain in all of eight patients in a series reported by Jacobsen and colleagues.[121]

Reports on the results from surgical experiences regarding phantom limb pain are limited. Denervation of the stump by peripheral neurectomy has yielded poor results and has largely been abandoned as a form of therapy. Cordotomy has been used for years to treat phantom limb pain with some success. Of 52 patients reviewed by Siegfried and Centinalp, 38% had good-to-excellent pain relief, and 44% had some-to-good pain relief.[122] Of 22 patients treated with the DREZ lesion for phantom pain, as reported by Saris and colleagues, 36% had satisfactory pain reduction.[123]

Although ablative surgery for phantom limb pain seems to lack general efficacy, augmentative procedures may provide improved outcomes. Epidural spinal cord stimulation was shown by Krainick and colleagues to provide good-to-excellent pain relief in 45% of 64 patients.[124] Another 11% of these patients had partial but good pain reduction. Long-term good-to-excellent benefits were seen in only 23% of patients. Siegfried and Centinalp reviewed the results of 148 patients with epidural spinal cord stimulation and found that 51% had good-to-excellent pain reduction and 18% had partial-to-good pain reduction.[122] Mundinger and Neumuller studied the results of thalamic deep brain stimulation on 14 patients with phantom limb pain.[125] Of these patients, nearly all (13) experienced satisfactory pain relief. Thalamotomy for phantom limb pain has not proven to be particularly successful. The sole case as reported by White and Sweet resulted in suicide.[38] As with the treatment of other manifestations of central pain, the role of intrathecal drug delivery devices for phantom limb pain has not been adequately addressed. Based on the results from the use of intrathecal fentanyl, as mentioned previously, additional trials for this condition need to be entertained. Phantom limb pain may be treated most successfully by preemptive analgesia methods.[75]

CONCLUSIONS

It is quite clear that central pain remains one of the most difficult conditions to treat, despite modern medicine. Currently available medical therapies fall far short of a reasonable goal of satisfactory pain relief in most patients. Certainly, as newer and more targeted drugs are developed, these numbers will improve. Agents directed against specific membrane receptors, cellular metabolism, and even against the intranuclear elements are currently being explored by my laboratory and those of others. Physicians treating patients who have central pain and the patients themselves have reason to be optimistic about the outcome of these efforts.

Regarding the surgical management of central pain, it is also quite clear that ablative neurosurgical treatment has not met its implied goals. In general, fewer than half, and in fact, probably much less than half of patients treated in this manner for central pain achieve long-term and satisfactory pain relief. The future of successful management of conditions such as pain after spinal cord injury, pain after stroke, and pain after amputation may lie with augmentative therapies. Central nervous system stimulation may prove vastly superior to ablation, particularly if the precise targets that produce relief can be discovered. In addition, target drug delivery of current and newly developed drugs may provide yet another and better dimension of central pain management.

REFERENCES

1. Meglio M. Evaluation and management of central and peripheral deafferentation pain. *In* Gildenburg PL, Tasker RR (eds). Textbook of Stereotactic and Functional Neurosurgery. New York, McGraw-Hill, 1998, pp 1631–1635.
2. Boivie J. Central pain. *In* Wall PD, Melzack R (eds). Textbook of Pain. Edinburgh, Churchill-Livingstone, 1999, pp 879–914.
3. Tasker RR. Deafferentation pain syndromes: introduction. Adv Pain Res Ther 19:241–257, 1991.
4. Tasker RR. Pain resulting from nervous system pathology (central pain). *In* Bonica JJ (ed). The Management of Pain. Philadelphia, Lea and Febiger, 1990, pp 264–280.
5. Ovelmen-Levitt J, Levitt M, Gorecki JP. Pathophysiology of central/neuropathic pain. *In* Gildenburg PL, Tasker RR (eds). Textbook of Stereotactic and Functional Neurosurgery. New York, McGraw-Hill, 1998, pp 1627–1630.
6. Levitt M, Levitt J. The deafferentation syndrome in monkeys: dysesthesias of spinal origin. Pain 10:120–147, 1981.
7. Vierck CJ. Can mechanisms of central pain syndromes be investigated in animal models: *In* Casey KL (ed). Pain and Central Nervous System Disease: The Central Pain Syndrome. New York, Raven, 1991, pp 129–141.
8. Bennett GJ. Neuropathic pain. *In* Wall PD, Melzack R (eds). Textbook of Pain. Edinburgh, Churchill-Livingstone, 1994, pp 201–224.
9. Mersky H, Bogduck N. Classification of chronic pain. Seattle, IASP, 1994, pp 1–222.
10. Bonica JJ. Introduction: semantic, epidemiologic, and educational issues. *In* Casey KL (ed). Pain and Central Nervous System Disease: The Central Pain Syndrome. New York, Raven, 1991, pp 13–29.
11. Riddoch G. The clinical features of central pain. Lancet 234:1093–1098, 1150–1156, 1205–1209, 1938.
12. Holmes 1919 from Pagni CA. Central pain due to spinal cord and brain stem damage. *In* Wall PD, Melzack R (eds). Textbook of Pain. Edinburgh, Churchill-Livingstone, 1989, pp 634–655.
13. Lhermitte J, Levy G, Nicolas M. Les sensations de decharges electriques, symptome precoce de la sclerose en plaque, Clinique et pathogenie. Presse Med 39:610–613, 1927.
14. Pagni CA. Central pain due to spinal cord and brain stem injury. *In* Wall PD, Melzack R (eds). Textbook of Pain. Edinburgh, Churchill-Livingstone, 1989, pp 634–655.
15. Nathan PW, Smith MC. Clinico-anatomical correlation in anterolateral cordotomy. *In* Bonica JJ, Liebskind JC, Albe-Fessard D (eds). Advances in Neurology. New York, Raven, 1979, pp 921–926.
16. Willis WD. The origin and destination of pathways involved in pain transmission. *In* Wall PD, Melzack R (eds). Textbook of Pain. Edinburgh, Churchill Livingstone, 1989, pp 112–127.
17. Poggio GF, Mountcastle VB. Functional organization of the thalamus and cortex. *In* Mountcastle VB (ed). Medical Physiology. St. Louis, CV Mosby, 1980, pp 271–298.
18. Willis WD. Neuronal mechanisms of pain discrimination. *In* Lund JS (ed). Sensory Processing in the Mammalian Brain. New York, Oxford University, 1991, pp 130–143.
19. Mountcastle VB. Neural mechanisms in somesthesis. *In* Mountcastle VB (ed). Medical Physiology. St. Louis, CV Mosby, 1980, pp 348–390.
20. Apkarian AV, Hodge CJ. Primate spinothalamic pathways: I. A quantitative study of the cells of origin of the spinothalamic tract. J Comp Neurol 288:447–473, 1989.
21. Apkarian AV, Hodge CJ. Primate spinthalamic pathways: II. The cells of origin of the dorsolateral and ventral spinothalamic pathways. J Comp Neurol 288:474–492, 1989.
22. Willis WD, Coggeshall RE. Sensory Mechanism of the Spinal Cord. New York, Raven, 1991.
23. Simone DA, Sorkin LS, Oh U, et al. Neurogenic hyperalgesia: Central neural correlates in responses of spinothalamic tract neurons. J Neurophysiol 66:228–246, 1991.
24. Koltzenburg M, Lundberg LER, Torebjork HE. Dynamic and static components of mechanical hyperalgesia in human hairy skin. Pain 51:207–219, 1992.
25. Mountcastle VB. Pain and temperature sensibilities. *In* Mountcastle VB (ed). Medical Physiology. St. Louis: CV Mosby, 1980, pp 391–427.
26. Simpson RK Jr. Peripheral Nerve Fiber Group and Spinal Cord Pathway Contributions to the Somatosensory Evoked Potential. Charleston, Medical University of South Carolina Press, 1980.
27. Haber LH, Moore BD, Willis WD. Electrophysiological response properties of spino reticular neurons in the monkey. J Comp Neurol 207:75–84, 1982.
28. Lima D, Coimbra A. Morphological types of spinomesencephalic neurons in the marginal zone (lamina I) of the rat spinal cord, as shown after retrograde labeling with cholera toxin subunit B. J Comp Neurol 279:327–339, 1989.
29. Slugg RM, Light AR. Spinal cord and trigeminal projections to the pontine parabrachial region in the rat as demonstrated with *Phaseolus vulgaris* leucoagglutinin. J Comp Neurol 339:49–61, 1994.
30. Hylden JLK, Hayashi H, Bennett GJ, Dubner R. Spinal lamina I neurons projecting to the parabrachial area of the cat midbrain. Brain Res 336:195–198, 1985.
31. Bernard JF, Besson JM. The spino(trigemino)-pontoamygdaloid pathway: electrophysiological evidence for an involvement in pain processes. J Neurophysiol 63:473–490, 1990.
32. Bernard JF, Besson JM. Convergence d'informations nociceptives sur des neurones parabrachio-amygdaliens chez le rat. Comptes Rendus Acad Sci 307:841–847, 1988.
33. Menetrey D, De Pommery J. Origins of spinal ascending pathways that reach central area involved in visceroception and visceronociception in the rat. Eur J Neurosci 3:249–259, 1991.
34. Burstein R, Cliffer KD, Giesler GJ. Direct somatosensory projections from the spinal cord to the hypothalamus and telencephalon. J Neurosci 7:4159–4164, 1987.
35. Burstein R, Dado RJ, Cliffer KD, Giesler GJ. Physiological characterization of spinohypothalamic tract neurons in the lumbar enlargement of rats. J Neurophysiol 66:261–284, 1991.
36. Cliffer KD, Burstein R, Giesler GGJ. Distributions of spinothalamic, spinohypothalamic, and spinotelencephalic fibers revealed by anterograde transport of PHA-L in rats. J Neurosci 11:852–868, 1991.
37. Dejerine J, Roussy G. La syndrome thalamique. Rev Neurol 12:521–532, 1906.
38. White JC, Sweet WH. Pain and the neurosurgeon. A forty year experience. Springfield, Ill, Charles C Thomas, 1969.
39. Tasker RR. Cardosa de Carvalho GT. Central pain of spinal cord origin. *In* North RB, Levy RM (eds). Neurosurgical Management of Pain. New York, Springer-Verlag, 1997, pp 111–119.
40. Gildenberg PL, Hirshberg RM. Limited myelotomy for the treatment of intractable cancer pain. J Neurol Neurosurg Psychiatry 47:94–96, 1994.
41. Al-Chaer ED, Lawand NB, Westlund KN, Willis WD. Visceral nociceptive input into the ventral posterolateral nucleus of the thalamus: a new function for the dorsal column pathway. J Neurophysiol 71:92–105, 1996.
42. Al-Chaer ED, Lawand NB, Westlund KN, Willis WD. Pelvic visceral input into the nucleus gracilis is largely mediated by the postsynaptic dorsal column pathway. J Neurophysiol 71:106–123, 1996.
43. Blommqvis A, Ericson AC, Broman J, Craig AD. Electron microscopic identification of lamina I axon terminations in the nucleus submedius of the thalamus. Brain Res 585:425–430, 1992.
44. Bowsher D. Some afferent and efferent connections of the parafascicular centre median complex. *In* Purpura DP, Yahr MD (eds). The Thalamus. New York, Columbia University Press, 1966, pp 99–108.
45. Dong WK, Ryu H, Wagman IH. Nociceptive responses of neurons in medial thalamus and their relationship to spinothalamic pathways. J Neurophysiol 41:1592–1613, 1978.
46. Craig AD, Bushnell MC, Shang ET, Blomqvist A. A thalamic nucleus specific for pain and temperature sensation. Nature 372:770–773, 1994.
47. Truex RC, Taylor MJ Smythe MQ, Gildenberg PL. The lateral cervical nucleus of the cat, dog, and man. J Comp Neurol 139:93–104, 1965.
48. Nathanson M. Phantom limbs as reported by S. Weir Mitchell. Neurology 38:504–505, 1988.
49. Tasker RR. Chronic pain syndromes of the nervous system. Phantom and stump pain. *In* North RB, Levy RM (eds). Neurosurgical Management of Pain. New York, Springer, 1997, pp 100–105.
50. Jensen TS, Krebs B, Nielsen J, Rasmussen P. Immediate and long-term phantom limb pian in amputees: incidence, clinical characteristics and relationship to preamputation limb pain. Pain 21:267–278, 1985.
51. Jensen TS, Nikolajsen L. Phantom pain and other phenomena after amputation. *In* Wall PD, Melzak R (eds). Textbook of Pain. Edinburgh, Churchill-Livingstone, 1999, pp 799–814.
52. Nystrom B, Hagbarth KE. Microelectrode recordings from transected nerves in amputees with phantom limb pain. Neurosci Lett 27:211–216.
53. Sunderland S. Nerves and Nerve Injuries. Baltimore, Williams & Wilkins, 1978.

54. Devor M, Rappaport ZH. Pain and the pathophysiology of damaged nerve. *In* Fields HL (ed). Pain Syndromes in Neurology. London, Butterworths, 1990, pp 47–83.

55. Melzac R, Loeser JD. Phantom body pain in paraplegics: evidence for a central pattern generating mechanism for pain. Pain 4:195–210, 1978.

56. Nordenbos W. Pain. Amsterdam, Elsevier, 1959.

57. Davis KD, Kiss ZH, Luo L. Phantom sensations generated by thalamic microstimulation. Nature 391:385–387, 1998.

58. Flor H, Elbert T, Muhlnickel W. Cortical reorganization and phantom phenomena in congenital and traumatic upper-extremity amputees. Exp Brain Res 119:205–212, 1998.

59. Yashon D. Spinal Injury. Norwalk, Conn, Appleton-Century-Crofts, 1986, pp 381–406.

60. Beric A. Spinal cord damage: injury. *In* Wall PD, Melzack R (eds). Textbook of Pain. Edinburgh, Churchill-Livingstone, 1999, pp 915–927.

61. Hansebout RR, Blight AR, Fawcett S, Reddy K. 4-Aminopyridine in chronic spinal cord injury: a controlled, double-blind, crossover study in eight patients. J Neurotrauma 10(1):1–18, 1993.

62. Middleton JW, Siddall PJ, Walker S, Molloy AR, Rutkowski SB. Intrathecal clonidine and baclofen in the management of spasticity and neuropathic pain following spinal cord injury: a case study. Arch Phys Med Rehabilitation 77(8):824–826, 1996.

63. Loubser PG, Akman NM. Effects of intrathecal baclofen on chronic spinal cord injury pain. J Pain Symptom Management 12(4):241–247, 1996.

64. Nagaro T, Shimizu C, Inoue H, et al. The efficacy of intravenous lidocaine on various types of neuropathic pain. Jpn J Anesthesiol 44(6):862–867, 1995.

65. Siddall PJ, Gray M, Rutkowski S, Cousins MJ. Intrathecal morphine and clonidine in the management of spinal cord injury pain: a case report. Pain 59(1):147–148, 1994.

66. Hendler N. Pharmacotherapy of chronic pain. *In* North RB, Levy RM (eds). Neurosurgical Management of Pain. New York, Springer-Verlag, 1997, pp 117–129.

67. Edmondson EA, Simpson RK, Stubler DK, Beric A. Systemic lidocaine therapy for poststroke pain. South Med J 86:1093–1096, 1993.

68. Leijon G, Boivie J. Central post-stroke pain–the effect of high and low frequency TENS. Pain 38:187–191, 1989.

69. Leijon G, Boivie J. Central post-stroke pain–a controlled trial of amitriptyline and carbamazepine. Pain 36:27–36, 1989.

70. Rosomoff HL, Seres J. Rehabilitation and treatment outcomes. *In* North RB, Levy RM (eds). Neurosurgical Management of Pain. New York, Springer-Verlag, 1997, pp 117–129.

71. Lehmann JF, deLateur BJ. Ultrasound, shortwave, microwave, laser, superficial heat and cold in the treatment of pain. *In* Wall PD, Melzack R (eds). Textbook of Pain. Edinburgh, Churchill-Livingstone, 1999, pp 1383–1397.

72. Hendler N. Psychological and psychiatric aspects of pain. *In* North RB, Levy RM (eds). Neurosurgical Management of Pain. New York, Springer-Verlag, 1997, pp 22–36.

73. Macdonald AJR. Acupuncture analgesia and therapy. *In* Wall PD, Melzack R (eds). Textbook of Pain. Edinburgh, Churchill-Livingstone, 1989, pp 634–655.

74. Katz J, Melzack R. Auricular transcutaneous electrical nerve stimulation (TENS) reduces phantom limb pain. J Pain Symp Management 2:73–83, 1991.

75. Weinstein SM. Phantom limb pain and related disorders. *In* Backonja MM (ed). Neuropathic Pain Syndromes. Neurologic Clinics. Philadelphia, WB Saunders, 1998, pp 919–935.

76. Baumgartner R, Riniker C. Surgical stump revision as a treatment of stump and phantom pains. Results of 100 cases. *In* Siegfried S, Zimmermann M (eds). Phantom and Stump Pain. Berlin, Springer-Verlag, 1981, pp 118–122.

77. Jacobsen L, Chabal C, Brody MC. Relief of persistent postamputation stump and phantom limb pain with intrathecal fentanyl. Pain 37:317–322, 1989.

78. Wassef MR. Phantom pain with probable reflex sympathetic dystrophy. Efficacy of fentanyl infiltration of the stellate ganglion. Reg Anesth 22:287–290, 1997.

79. Fiddler DS, Hindman BJ. Intravenous calcitonin alleviates spinal anesthesia–induced phantom limb pain. Anesthesiology 74:187–189, 1991.

80. Portenoy RK. Pharmacologic Management of Neuropathic Pain. Neurology Alert Special. New York, American Health Consultants, 1992, pp 1–17.

81. Kayama K, Watanabe S, Tsuneto S, Takahashi H, Naito H. Thiopental for phantom limb pain during spinal anesthesia. Anesthesiology 69:598–600, 1988.

82. Patterson JF. Carbamazepine in the treatment of phantom limb pain. South Med J 81:1100–1102, 1988.

83. Rayner HC, Atkins RC, Westerman RA. Relief of local stump pain by capsaicin cream. Lancet 1:1276–1277, 1989.

84. Bartusch SL, Sanders BJ, D'Alessio JG. Clonazepam for the treatment of lancinating phantom limb pain. Clin J Pain 12:59–62, 1996.

85. Nikolajsen L, Hansen CL, Nielsen J, Keller J, Arendt-Nielsen L, Jensen TS. The effect of ketamine on phantom pain: a central neuropathic disorder maintained by peripheral input. Pain 67:69–77, 1996.

86. Spiller WG, Martin E. The treatment of persistent pain of organic origin in the lower part of the body by division of the antero-lateral column of the spinal cord. JAMA 58:1489–1490, 1912.

87. Tasker RR, North R. Cordotomy and myelotomy. *In* North RB, Levy RM (eds). Neurosurgical Management of Pain. New York, Springer-Verlag, 1997, pp 191–220.

88. White JC. Anterolateral chordotomy–its effectiveness in relieving pain of non-malignant disease. Neurochirurgia 6:83–102, 1963.

89. Mullan S, Harper PV, Hekmatpanah J, Torres H, Dobbin G. Percutaneous interruption of spinal pain tracts by means of a strontium-90 needle. J Neurosurg 20:931–939, 1963.

90. Wertheimer P, Lecuire J. La myelotomie commissurale posterieure. A propos de 107 observations. Acta Chir Belgica 52:568–574, 1953.

91. Dunward QJ, Rice JP, Ball MJ, Gilbert JJ, Kaufmann JC. Selective spinal cordectomy: clinicopathological correlation. J Neurosurg 56:359–367, 1982.

92. Nashold BS Jr. Neurosurgical technique of the dorsal root entry zone operation. Appl Neurophysiol 51:136–145, 1988.

93. Sindou M, Jeanmonod D. Microsurgical DREZotomy for the treatment of spasticity and pain in the lower limbs. Neurosurgery 24:655–670, 1989.

94. Barolat G. Experience with 509 plate electrodes implanted epidurally from C1 to L1. Stereotactic Functional Neurosurg 61(2):60–79, 1993.

95. Gorecki JP. Destructive lesions for persistent pain. *In* Gildenburg PL, Tasker RR (eds). Textbook of Stereotactic and Functional Neurosurgery. New York, McGraw-Hill, 1998, pp 1417–1424.

96. Siegfried J. Stereotactic pulvinarotomy in the treatment of intractable pain. Prog Neurol Surg 8:104–113, 1977.

97. Lende RA, Kirsh WM, Druckman R. Relief of facial pain after combined removal of precentral and postcentral cortex. J Neurosurg 34:537–543, 1971.

98. Ballantine HT, Cosgraove R, Giriunas I. Surgical treatment of intractable psychiatric illness anc chronic pain by stereotactic cingulotomy. *In* Schmidek H, Sweet W (eds). Operative Neurosurgical Techniques: Indications, Methods and Results. Philadelphia, WB Saunders, 1995, pp 1423–1430.

99. Sano K. Intralaminar thalamotomy (thalamolaminotomy) and posterior hypothalamotomy in the treatment of intractable pain. *In* Krayenbuhl H, Maspes PE, Sweet WH (eds). Progress in Neurological Surgery. Basel, Karger, 1977, pp 50–103.

100. Young RF, Jacques DB, Rand RW. Medial thalamotomy with the Leksell gamma knife for treatment of chronic pain. Acta Neurochir (Suppl) 62:105–110, 1994.

101. Penn RD, Paice JA. Chronic intrathecal morphine for intractable pain. J Neurosurg 67:182–186, 1987.

102. Young RF, Rinaldi PC. Brain stimulation. *In* North RB, Levy RL (eds). Neurosurgical Management of Pain. New York Springer, 1997, pp 283–301.

103. Tsubokawa T, Katayama Y, Yamamoto T. Chronic motor cortex stimulation for the treatment of central pain. Acta Neurochir 52(Suppl):137–139, 1991.

104. Stormer S, Gerner HJ, Gruninger W, et al. Chronic pain/dysaesthesiae in spinal cord injury patients: results of a multicentre study. Spinal Cord 35(7):446–455, 1997.

105. Johnson RL, Gerhart KA, McCray J, Menconi JC, Whiteneck GG. Secondary conditions following spinal cord injury in a population based sample. Spinal Cord 36(1):45–50, 1998.

106. Porter RW, Hohmann GW, Bors E, French JD. Cordotomy for pain following cauda equina injury. Arch Surg 92:765–770, 1966.

107. Botterell EH, Callaghan JC, Jousse AT. Pain in paraplegia: clinical management and surgical treatment. Proc R Soc Med 47:17–24, 1953.

108. Jefferson A. Cordectomy for intractable pain. *In* Lipton S, Miles J (eds). Persistent Pain. New York, Grune and Stratton, 1983, pp 115–132.

109. Virozub ID, Bublik LA, Chernovskii VI. Treatment of pain in vertebral-spinal cord injury by functional operations on the spinal cord. Zhurnal Voprosy Neirokhirurgii Imeni N – N – Burdenko (1):11–13, 1990.

110. Friedman AH, Bullitt E. Dorsal root entry zone lesions in the treatment of pain following brachial plexus avulsion, spinal cord injury and herpes zoster. Appl Neurophysiol 51:164–169, 1988.

111. Wiegand H, Winkelmuller W. Behandlung des deafferentierungsschmerzes durch hochfrequenzlasion der hinterwurzeleintrittszone. Deutsche Med Wochenschr 110: 216–220, 1985.

112. Young RF. Clinical experience with radiofrequency and laser DREZ lesions. J Neurosurg 72:715–720, 1990.

113. Hosobuchi Y. Subcortical electrical stimulation for control of intractable pain in humans. J Neurosurg 64:543–553, 1986.

114. Amano K, Kitamura K, Sano K. Relief of intractable pain from neurosurgical point of view with reference to present limits and clinical indications: A review of 100 consecutive cases. Neurol Med Chir 16:141–153, 1976.

115. Ohye C. Vim thalamotomy for the retreatment of central pain. *In* Proceedings of the 4th annual meeting of the Japanese Congress of Neurological Surgeons, Tokyo, 1985, pp 39–45.

116. Gildenberg PL. Functional neurosurgery. *In* Schmidek HH, Sweet WH (eds). Operative Neurosurgical Techniques. Indications, Method, and Results. New York, Grune and Stratton, 1983, pp 1001–1016.

117. Sano K, Sekino H, Amano K. Posteromedial hypothalamotomy in the treatment of intractable pain. Confin Neurol 37:285–290, 1973.

118. Tsubokawa T, Katayama Y, Yamamoto T. Chronic motor cortex stimulation in patients with thalamic pain. J Neurosurg 78:393–401, 1993.

119. Jaeger H, Maier C. Calcitonin in phantom limb pain: a double-blind study. Pain 48:21–27, 1992.

120. Stannard CF, Porter GE. Ketamine hydrochloride in the treatment of phantom limb pain. Pain 54:227–230, 1993.

121. Jacobsen L, Chabal C, Brody MC. A comparison of the effects of intrathecal fentanyl and lidocaine on established postamputation stump pain. Pain 40:137–141, 1990.

122. Siegfried J, Centinalp E. Neurosurgical treatment of phantom limb pain: a survey of methods. *In* Siegfried J, Zimmermann M (eds). Phantom and Stump Pain. Berlin, Springer-Verlag, 1981, pp 148–155.

123. Saris SC, Iacono RP, Nashold BS. Dorsal root entry zone lesions for post-amputation pain. J Neurosurg 62:72–76, 1985.

124. Krainick JU, Thoden U, Riechert T. Pain reduction in amputees by long-term spinal cord stimulation. J Neurosurg 52:346–350, 1980.

125. Mundinger F, Neumuller H. Programmed transcutaneous (TNS) and central (DBS) stimulation for control of phantom limb pain and causalgia: a new method for treatment. *In* Siegfried J, Zimmermann M (eds). Phantom and Stump Pain. Berlin, Springer-Verlag, 1981, pp 167–178.

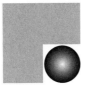

CHAPTER 12

Complex Regional Pain Syndrome

RICHARD W. ROSENQUIST, MD, AND NAEEM HAIDER, MD, MBBS

The diagnosis and treatment of complex regional pain syndromes (CRPS) types I and II (formerly known as reflex sympathetic dystrophy [RSD] and causalgia) have vexed medical practitioners. Reports of the condition were initially made by Paget in 1862, and the term *causalgia* appeared in descriptions by Mitchell and colleagues in 1864.[1] Over a century later, the pathophysiology of CRPS remains elusive. Numerous theories have developed concerning the mechanism for maintenance and spread of this disorder. These theories, along with descriptions of clinical symptoms or treatment response, have been used in an attempt to categorize the disorder into specific symptom patterns. Unfortunately, large numbers of patients are difficult to categorize into the various syndrome patterns described. As a result, systematic treatment approaches are lacking due to the complexity in assigning patients to one category or another. Not surprisingly, treatment outcome is highly variable.

TAXONOMY

CRPS types I and II have been described in many ways. The previous taxonomy of these pain syndromes (reflex sympathetic dystrophy and causalgia) was confusing as a clinical designation because they had been used so indiscriminately that it was no longer clear what was being diagnosed. RSD implied an autonomic disorder through the use of the term *sympathetic,* leading to indiscriminate use of sympathetic nerve block, both percutaneous and surgical. Some of the varied terms used to describe these syndromes are listed in Table 12-1.

Any link between nociceptive neurons and postganglionic sympathetic activity is inconsistent. Sympathetic blocks alter the syndrome temporarily on occasion and to little or no extent on others.[2–6] Despite evidence that adrenergic mechanisms may be involved, measures of sympathetic responses have shown normal results.[7,8] The term *RSD* has been used, without precision, to refer to soft tissue changes possibly related to the sympathetic nervous system, that may or may not be the result of a reflex and may occur later in the disorder.

In an attempt to reduce the current level of confusion and to revise terminology and criteria related to RSD, a special consensus workshop was held in Orlando in 1993. This workshop examined the terms *RSD, causalgia, sympathetically maintained pain (SMP),* and *sympathetically independent pain (SIP),* and considered the need for revision of the IASP taxonomy. The goal was to define various associated symptoms and findings of the disorders, to determine the value and role of various tests in the diagnosis of these disorders, and to develop an algorithm for diagnosis.[9]

CRPS was chosen to represent the many diverse descriptive terms in use. The word *complex* represents the varied clinical phenomena seen in each group. The "regional" distribution of symptoms and findings is a hallmark of the disorder. "Pain" is a cardinal symptom. Complex regional pain syndromes were divided into two types by this conference,[9] as shown in Table 12-2.

A third category was proposed to allow for patients who did not meet all criteria for CRPS I or II, and to allow collection of data that might otherwise go unrecorded in this syndrome[9]; this type is called CRPS NOS (not otherwise specified) and encompasses patients in whom symptoms and signs do not fulfill the criteria for CRPS I or CRPS II. Clinicians should apply NOS codes from the ICD-10 classification for those cases not meeting the diagnostic criteria of CRPS I and II.

Due to the frequency with which the term *reflex sympathetic dystrophy* and *causalgia* are used, albeit imprecisely, it was thought that immediate transition to the terms *CRPS type I and type II* was unrealistic. To facilitate a gradual conversion, the terms *RSD* and *causalgia* were retained parenthetically.[9] The appropriate use of this new system may allow greater clinical uniformity in the diagnosis of patients and differentiation of the type I and II subgroups.

EPIDEMIOLOGY

There is still no well-designed, prospective study in current literature that addresses the epidemiology of CRPS. The median age for patients in one prospective study was 41 years (range, 4 to 84 years old), with a mean duration of 405 days.[10] A retrospective study in US pain centers reported a mean age of 41.8 years (range, 18 to 71 years) and a mean duration of

● **TABLE 12-1** • Taxonomy of Complex Regional Pain Syndrome

Acute atrophy of the bone	Reflex neurovascular dystrophy
Algoneurodystrophy	Reflex sympathetic dystrophy
Causalgia	Shoulder-hand syndrome
Chronic traumatic edema	Sudeck's atrophy
Postinfarctional sclerodactyly	Sympathalgia
Posttraumatic dystrophy	Traumatic angiospasm
Posttraumatic osteoporosis	Traumatic vasospasm
Posttraumatic spreading neuralgia	

CRPS symptoms for 2.5 years before referral. Thirty-three percent of referrals were from surgeons and only 7% from the primary care physician.[11] These studies have identified a female-to-male ratio of 3:1 and 2.3:1, respectively.[10,11]

The majority of patients present with CRPS involving one extremity. There has been no predominant representation of either upper or lower limbs. Bilateral limb involvement has been reported in 11% to 16% of patients.[11,12] The female-to-male ratio increased from 3:1 to 4:1 with multiple RSD sites and the median age decreased from 41 to 35 years.[12]

The predominant inciting event in CRPS is trauma,[10] usually fractures, followed by surgery and inflammatory processes. In a US pain clinic study, 77% of the patients had a known inciting event. Unknown precipitating causes occurred in 10% to 23% of patients.[10,11]

CLINICAL FEATURES

CRPS presents with spontaneous pain with or without hyperalgesia that is typically associated with a triad of autonomic (sympathetic), motor, and sensory disturbances. The cardinal symptom is spontaneous pain. Patients frequently report worsening pain at night and it is unknown whether this represents a circadian change or is due to lack of sensory input. Pain is worsened by dependency and movement of the joints (pseudoarthritis). It is most commonly seen in the distal portion of an affected extremity following a noxious event. Sensory disturbances are not limited to pain. Dysesthesia is common, in which the skin may be either hyperesthetic or hypoesthetic, more pronounced on the dorsal than ventral surface. Mechanical allodynia, in which non-noxious mechanical stimuli elicit pain, is frequently absent during the onset of CRPS and usually occurs later in the disease.

Symptoms are not limited to a single extremity and may bear little relation to the severity of the initiating injury, occurring after minor injuries such as sprains, bruises, needle sticks, fractures, or an immune reaction. In addition, symptoms are frequently found in distal tissues not affected by the initiating lesion. It is the unfamiliarity with these syndromes, the lack of spatial connection with the lesion site, and the diffuse non-anatomic nature that makes the diagnosis easily missed.

Autonomic Disturbance

Distal portions of the extremity frequently exhibit edema, most prominently on the dorsum. Skin color is altered and may be red, mottled, slightly blue, or frankly cyanotic. Skin temperature difference is observed between affected and non-affected extremities in many patients. Limb temperature may not correspond with environmental temperature. Sudomotor activity is altered in approximately one-half of all patients with CRPS.[10] The alteration may result in increased or decreased sweating. Sudomotor changes do not concern most patients.[10]

● **TABLE 12-2** • Differentiation of Complex Regional Pain Syndromes

CRPS Type I (RSD)	CRPS Type II (Causalgia)
Type I is a syndrome that develops after an initiating noxious event	Type II is a syndrome that develops after nerve injury.
Spontaneous pain or allodynia/hyperalgesia occurs, is not limited to the territory of a single peripheral nerve, and is disproportionate to the inciting event.	Spontaneous pain or allodynia/hyperalgesia occurs and is not necessarily limited to the territory of the injured nerve.
There is or has been evidence of edema, skin blood flow abnormality, or abnormal sudomotor activity in the region of the pain since the inciting event.	There is or has been evidence of edema, skin blood flow abnormality, or abnormal sudomotor activity in the region of the pain since the inciting event.
This diagnosis is excluded by the existence of conditions that would otherwise account for the degree of pain dysfunction.	This diagnosis is excluded by the existence of conditions that would otherwise account for the degree of pain and dysfunction.

CRPS, Complex regional pain syndrome.

Motor Disturbance

Patients whose symptoms are consistent with CRPS may frequently display dystonia of the distal extremity. Movement of the affected extremity may be accompanied by a coarse nonphysiologic tremor, and motor strength may be reduced or lost altogether.[13]

Trophic Disturbance

Trophic changes seen with complex regional pain syndrome, such as grooving of the nails, hair growth, hair loss, skin texture changes, loss of subcutaneous tissue, and osteoporosis, are not usually present at the onset. The changes typically appear late in the disease course and are of little use in making an early diagnosis.[10,14]

PATHOPHYSIOLOGY

Several hypotheses have been devised regarding mechanisms involved in the generation and maintenance of this syndrome. The conceptual understanding of complex regional pain syndrome has been dynamic, varied, and contentious. The first real hypothesis was the "vicious circle" proposed by Leriche in 1939.[15] This was later expanded by Livingston in 1943 with the incorporation of the concept of abnormal firing in self-sustaining loops in the dorsal horn provoked by an irritative focus in small nerve endings or major nerve trunks.[16] This abnormal firing would then activate central projection fibers, giving rise to pain.

Many of the proposed hypotheses implicate sympathetic activity as part of the abnormal function manifested at the periphery.[17] There are several lines of evidence for the ability of the sympathetic nervous system to play a role in the generation of pain and other associated changes in some of the patients with complex regional pain syndromes based on clinical observations:

1. In 1948, Walker and Nulsen demonstrated that pain could be the result of the efferent actions of the sympathetic nervous system.[18] Patients undergoing preganglionic sympathectomy for the treatment of vascular disease or "causalgia" had electrodes left in place along the sympathetic chain. This allowed activation of the sympathetic ganglia now detached from the central nervous system in the postoperative period. Stimulation evoked pain in previously painful areas in patients with causalgia, but did not produce pain in patients with vascular disease. This demonstrated that sympathetic fibers could acquire the capacity to evoke pain. This was confirmed by White and Sweet in 1969.[19]
2. Pain may by relieved by the performance of local anesthetic sympathetic blocks or other sympatholytic procedures such as regional application of guanethidine or intravenous phentolamine.[20–24]
3. Pain may reinitiate or exacerbate by applying an alpha-adrenoceptor agonist either iontophoretically or via injection in a limb with superficial burning pain and hyperalgesia.[25–28]

4. Guanethidine elicits pain when injected intravenously in the affected extremity. This is thought to represent a response to norepinephrine released from postganglionic terminals.[29]

This evidence should not be misconstrued to imply that the sympathetic nervous system is causally involved in the generation of the pain and other associated phenomena in all patients with CRPS. In addition, because these descriptions are procedurally related, the potential role of a placebo effect cannot and should not be discounted.[30,31]

Any theory that attempts to explain the sympathetic nervous system's role in CRPS must explain the following:

1. How does the sympathetic nervous system become coupled in the periphery to primary afferent neurons producing the different components of pain observed in these patients?
2. Where are the sites of interaction between sympathetic efferent and sensory afferent fibers involved in pain sensation?
3. Which afferent fibers carry pain sensation in sympathetically maintained pain?
4. What occurs on the cellular level to explain the proposed sympathetic-afferent interactions?
5. How does the change of activity in sympathetic neurons relate to the production of blood flow changes, sweating, somatomotor changes, and trophic changes?

Research is being performed using animal models, which reproduce components of symptoms seen in complex regional pain syndrome but do not reproduce CRPS itself. The testable hypotheses evaluated on these models and the therapeutic strategies based on understanding obtained from this research require that clinical diagnoses match the components of the model evaluated. Figure 12-1 represents a general hypothesis about the neural mechanisms involved in the generation of CRPS I and II.[32]

DIAGNOSIS AND EVALUATION

The clinical signs and symptoms of CRPS are extremely variable. As a result, it is important to differentiate CRPS from other medical diagnoses. It is equally important that CRPS, which may develop as a consequence of, or alongside, other medical conditions, not be misdiagnosed or remain untreated. Examples of conditions that have similar features are presented in Table 12-3.

Diagnostic Criteria for Reflex Sympathetic Dystrophy

To develop a systematic and reproducible approach to the diagnosis of CRPS, systems have been developed, which incorporate clinical symptoms and signs with laboratory testing. One such system is demonstrated in Table 12-4.

Other scales have been developed to bring a more objective set of measurements to the diagnosis. Tables 12-5 and 12-6 present the published system based on the Mayo Autonomic Laboratory experience.

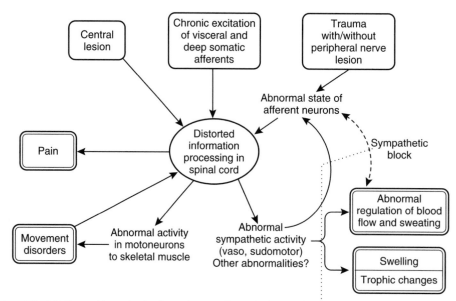

FIGURE 12-1 General hypothesis about the neural mechanisms of generation of CRPS I and II following peripheral trauma with and without nerve lesions, chronic stimulation of visceral afferent fibers (e.g., myocardial infarction) and deep somatic afferents, and, rarely, central trauma. The clinical observations are double-framed. Note the vicious circle (*arrows in bold black*). An important component of this circle is the excitatory influence of postganglionic sympathetic axons on primary afferent fibers in the periphery. (From Jänig W, Stanton-Hicks M (eds.). Reflex Sympathetic Dystrophy: A Reappraisal. San Diego, IASP Press, p.10.)

The current clinical approach to the diagnosis of RSD/SMP recommended by the Mayo group is to use a combined clinical and laboratory system with particular emphasis on:

1. Severity of pain
2. Distribution of pain (diffuse)
3. Allodynia on the RSD/SMPPSS combined with RSD/SMPLAB focuses on quantitative sudomotor axon reflex test asymmetry (QSART; measuring the sweat response evoked by transcutaneous iontophoresis of acetylcholine), resting sweat output (RSO), and skin vasomotor alterations.

This approach results in the following scale:

1. Definite RSD/SMP: allodynia to touch, pressure, and movement plus unilateral asymmetry of QSART (grade 3) or RSO (grade 3 asymmetry)
2. Probably RSD/SMP: RSD/SMPPSS (probable) plus any of the following on RSD/SMPLAB:
   a. QSART3 or RSO3
   b. QSART2 + RSO2 or VM2

3. Possible RSD/SMP: chronic limb pain plus QSART1 or RSO1 or VM1.[34]

The IASP published standardized, consensus-based diagnostic criteria for CRPS in 1994.[35] These criteria were intended to improve clinical recognition of the disorder and facilitate selection of more generalized samples for treatment outcome and basic science research. Subsequent work to validate them empirically has been limited, but has suggested several problems. A study by Bruehl and colleagues has explored the external validity of IASP diagnostic criteria for CRPS and compared them to proposed research diagnostic criteria.[36] A standardized evaluation of signs and symptoms of CRPS was conducted in 117 patients meeting IASP criteria for CRPS and 43 patients experiencing neuropathic pain with established non-CRPS etiology. Multiple discriminant function analyses were used to test the IASP diagnostic criteria and decision rules, as well as propose modifications of these criteria to discriminate between patients with CRPS and those experiencing non-CRPS neuropathic pain. Current IASP criteria and decision rules discriminate significantly between groups (Appendices A and B).

● **TABLE 12-3** • Conditions with Features Similar to Complex Regional Pain Syndrome	
1. Post-traumatic vasoconstriction from thrombophlebitis	8. Autoimmune disorders
2. Infection	9. Radiculopathy
3. Arthritis	10. Neuritis
4. Fracture radiculopathy	11. Herpetic neuralgia
5. Avulsion of nerve roots	12. Thoracic outlet syndrome
6. Soft tissue damage pain dysfunction syndromes	13. Myofascial pain syndromes
7. Tenosynovitis	14. Fasciitis

● TABLE 12-4 • Criteria for Diagnosis of Complex Regional Pain Syndrome

Clinical Symptoms and Signs	Laboratory Results	Interpretation
Burning pain	Thermometry/thermography	>6 Probable RSD
Hyperpathia/allodynia	Bone radiography	
Temperature/color changes	Three-phase bone scan	3–5 Possible RSD
Edema	Quantitative sweat test	
Hair/nail growth changes	Response to sympathetic blockade	<3 Unlikely RSD[33]

However, although sensitivity was high (0.93), specificity was poor (0.36) and a positive diagnosis of CRPS was likely to be correct in as few as 40% of cases. The addition of empirically based modifications to the criteria enabled discrimination between CRPS and non-CRPS groups ($P < .001$). The use of a decision rule, requiring at least two sign categories and four symptom categories to be positive, optimized diagnostic efficiency (Appendix C). In this setting, a diagnosis of CRPS was likely to be accurate in up to 84% of cases and non-CRPS neuropathic pain in up to 88% of cases. These results suggest that the current criteria may lead to overdiagnosis. Inclusion of modifications can improve their external validity.

Sensitivity and specificity of diagnostic criteria/decision rules to discriminate CRPS from non-CRPS neuropathic conditions. Numbers listed in the decision rules (Table 12-7) refer to number and sign and symptom categories (out of four possible categories) required to be present for the syndrome to be considered CRPS.

PSYCHOLOGY

There is no controversy regarding the emotional suffering and behavioral changes engendered by severe chronic pain. However, the role of psychological factors in CRPS is unclear at best and frequently contradictory with regard to clinical observations and psychometric testing. In a review of psychological issues in reflex sympathetic dystrophy, Covington draws the following conclusions[37]:

1. There is no good evidence that true RSD is a psychogenic condition.
2. It is highly likely that anxiety, stress, and chemical dependence increase nociception in RSD. Appropriate treatment with relaxation and antidepressants should help.
3. The severe pain of causalgia is the cause of psychiatric suffering and not the converse.
4. Pathologic signs and symptoms in RSD may be worsened by volitional or inadvertent behaviors, such as immobilization and disuse. These behaviors may be motivated by fear, misinformation, or regressive urges. Thus, although maladaptive, they may not indicate psychopathology.
5. Patients with conversion disorder and factitious illness may be erroneously diagnosed with RSD and thus receive inappropriate treatment. Their failure to respond may mislead professionals into the belief that RSD is a psychiatric condition.
6. Conversion/factitious mechanisms may be more likely to mimic RSD than other pain syndromes. If true, such cases should be relatively rare in the primary care setting and increasingly common in tertiary care and beyond.

● TABLE 12-5 • Reflex Sympathetic Dystrophy Probability Scoring System (Prospective Study)[a]

Parameter	Definite	Probable	Possible	Not RSD/SMP
Allodynia Touch (a) Pressure (b) Movement (c)	3/3	2/3	1/3	0/3
Vasomotor History (a) Examination (b)	4/4	≥2/4	≤1/4	0/4
Swelling History (a) Examination (b)				

[a]Grading is dependent on a combination of a and b.
The clinical diagnosis of RSD/SMP is based on a score of 0–7 as follows:

Score	Diagnosis
7	Definite RSD/SMP
4–6	Probable RSD/SMP
2–3	Possible RSD/SMP
0–1	Not RSD/SMP

● **TABLE 12-6** • Autonomic Laboratory Grading of RSD/SMP (RSD/SMPLAB; Prospective Study)

Autonomic Scoring Scale		
QSART	RSO	Vasomotor
Reduction-1 or Increase-1	Reduction-1 or Increase-1	Reduction-1 or Increase-1
Reduction-2 or Increase-2	Reduction-2 or Increase-2	Reduction-2 or Increase-2
Reduction-3 or Increase-3	Reduction-3 or Increase-3	Reduction-3 or Increase-3

An additional point is provided if the variation in temperature over the toe or finger pads between two sets of thermographic recordings is ≥2 °C.
The laboratory diagnosis RSD/SMP is based on the following:

Score	Diagnosis
>6	Definite RSD/SMP
4–6	Probable RSD/SMP
2–3	Possible RSD/SMP
0–1	Not RSD/SMP

We lack definitive information as to whether aberrant behavior following a trivial injury can produce RSD that otherwise would not occur. We also do not know whether high levels of state or trait anxiety can do so.

TREATMENT REGIMENS

Once the diagnosis of complex regional pain syndrome has been established, the far more difficult process of treating the patient must begin. This requires a multidisciplinary approach if there is to be any hope of success. Performance of blocks, implantation of devices, and time spent in an office are typically the smallest part of a successful treatment regimen. Treatment protocols generally revolve around pain relief from medications or sympatholysis, where appropriate; physical therapy; and psychological support. However, even the most carefully planned treatment protocol will not produce satisfactory results in all patients.

Pain relief has been achieved using sympatholysis and medications including:

1. Sympathetic ganglion blocks[38]
2. Sympathetic neurolytic blocks[39]
3. Percutaneous radiofrequency sympathectomy[40]
4. Epidural and intrathecal administration of local anesthetics, alpha-2 agonists, and opioids[41]
5. Intravenous regional administration of guanethidine, bretylium, and local anesthetics[24,27,42]
6. Systemic administration of alpha blockers such as phentolamine[43]
7. Surgical resection of the sympathetic chain[44,45]
8. Oral alpha blocking agents such as prazosin, terazosin, doxazosin, and phenoxybenzamine[46,47]
9. Topical clonidine[48]
10. Antiseizure medications such as Dilantin®, Tegretol®, and gabapentin[49]
11. Tricyclic antidepressants[50,51]
12. Nonsteroidal anti-inflammatory drugs[50,51]
13. Opioids[50,51]
14. Calcitonin[52]
15. Spinal cord stimulation techniques[53–55]

Sympatholysis and pain relief, although important, are but one piece of the treatment regimen. It is critical that these patients are rapidly evaluated and placed in an appropriate physical or occupational therapy program so that long-term joint and limb dysfunction can be minimized or avoided altogether. It also

● **TABLE 12-7** • Sensitivity and Specificity of Chronic Regional Pain Syndrome Differentiation

Criteria/Decision Rule[a]	Sensitivity	Specificity
IASP: ≥1 sign or symptom for both criterion 2 and 3	0.98	0.36
IASP: ≥1 sign for both criterion 2 and 3	0.82	0.60
Research criteria: ≥2 sign categories and ≥2 symptom categories	0.94	0.36
Research criteria: ≥2 sign categories and ≥3 symptom categories	0.85	0.69
Research criteria: ≥2 sign categories and ≥4 symptom categories	0.70	0.94
Research criteria: ≥3 sign categories and ≥2 symptom categories	0.76	0.81
Research criteria: ≥3 sign categories and ≥3 symptom categories	0.70	0.83
Research criteria: ≥3 sign categories and ≥4 symptom categories	0.86	0.75

[a]$P < .001$.

provides an objective functional measurement that may be used to follow response to the treatment regimen. These programs should include both passive and active range of motion, desensitization, coordination activities, aerobic and strength activities, treatment of myofascial pain disorders that may be secondary to the initial disorder, and finally work hardening as needed to maximize functional gain and return to work.

Surgical sympatholysis has been used for patients with CRPS with mixed results.[56] The predominant associative factor with failure in a retrospective review was time from onset of disease until blockade.[56] Critics have argued against permanent sympatholysis, citing that a strong placebo response can confound results.[57,58] Somatic afferent blockade may accompany sympathetic blockade in some cases, leading to confusion in regard to the true source of pain relief.[59] The possibility of somatic nerve blockade and placebo response as a means for pain relief with sympathectomy becomes more of a concern when surgical or permanent neurolysis is considered.[58] At this time, there is little evidence that permanent sympatholysis offers benefit to patients with CRPS that responds to temporary blockade.[58]

Spinal cord stimulation, available for longer than 30 years, has been used for a variety of conditions including complex regional pain syndrome.[53–55] In cases that fail conservative treatment using multidisciplinary pain protocols, implantable techniques as a part of an advanced multidisciplinary treatment plan may be considered.[60] Due to the nondermatomal presentation of symptoms involving one or two extremities, use of neuraxial electrodes allows for complete coverage of the affected region. This allows control of allodynia and hyperalgesia by means of paresthesias that can be targeted to affected regions. Using varying electrode combinations, with changes in amplitude and pulse width, effective pain relief can be obtained in many patients. Limited studies are available to demonstrate efficacy.[54,55] Randomized trials are even harder to come by. Most involve small numbers of patients observed for a limited period. However, in carefully selected patients, a reduction in pain and an improvement in quality of life can be obtained.[61] Most case series of patients implanted with spinal cord stimulators demonstrate a 60% success rate with regard to improvement in pain control over time.[62] Sympathectomy obtained with the use of spinal cord stimulation has not correlated with the relief of pain in this condition,[63] further confounding the role of the autonomic nervous system in the pathogenesis of the disease.

CONCLUSIONS

The diagnosis and treatment of complex regional pain syndromes remains extremely challenging. The development of the new taxonomy along with more clearly defined diagnostic criteria should help provide a basis on which to choose the most effective treatment regimens. In addition, the uniformity it provides may facilitate the application of mechanistic understanding and treatment modalities evaluated in laboratory models to patients who are truly suffering. It is crucial that proper diagnosis is pursued in all patients in whom the label of CRPS is entertained. In those patients diagnosed with CRPS, a multidisciplinary approach must be used to maximize treatment success.

REFERENCES

1. Mitchell SE, Morehouse CR, Keen WW. Gunshot Wounds and Other Injuries of the Nerves. Philadelphia, JB Lippincott, 1864.
2. Devor M, Basbaum AI, Bennet GJ, et al. Mechanisms of neuropathic pain following peripheral injury. In Basbaum AI, Besson JM (eds). Towards a New Pharmacotherapy of Pain. Dahlem Workshop Reports. Chichester, England, John Wiley, 1991, pp 417–440.
3. Janig W. Causalgia and reflex sympathetic dystrophy: in which way is the sympathetic nervous system involved? Trends Neurosci 8:471–477, 1985.
4. Janig W. The sympathetic nervous system in pain: physiology and pathophysiology. In: Stanton-Hicks M, Janig W, Boas RA (eds). Reflex Sympathetic Dystrophy. Boston, Kluwer, 1990, pp 41–54.
5. Janig W. Pain and the sympathetic nervous system: pathophysiological mechanisms. In Bannister R, Mathias CJ (eds). Autonomic Failure (3rd ed). Oxford, Oxford University Press, 1992, pp 231–251.
6. Blumberg H. Clinical and pathophysiological aspects of reflex sympathetic dystrophy and sympathetically maintained pain. In Janig W, Schmidt RF (eds). Reflex Sympathetic Dystrophy. Pathophysiological Mechanisms and Clinical Implications. Weinheim, Germany, VCH Verlagsgesellschaft, 1992, pp 29–49.
7. Campbell JN, Meyer RA, Raja SN. Is nociceptor activation by alpha-1 adrenoreceptors the culprit in sympathetically maintained pain? Am Pain Soc J 1:3–11, 1992.
8. Roberts WJ. A hypothesis on the physiological basis for causalgia and related pains. Pain 24:197–311, 1986.
9. Stanton-Hicks M, Janig W, Hassenbusch S, Haddox JD, Wilson P. Reflex sympathetic dystrophy: Changing concepts and taxonomy. Pain 63:127–133, 1995.
10. Veldman PH, Reynen HM, Artnz IE, et al. Signs and symptoms of reflex sympathetic dystrophy: prospective study of 829 patients. Lancet 342:1012–1016, 1993.
11. Allen G, Galer BS, Schwartz L. Epidemiogicical review of 134 patients with complex regional pain syndrome assessed in a chronic pain clinic. Pain 80:539–544, 1999.
12. Veldman PJM, Goris RJA. Multiple reflex sympathetic dystrophy. Which patients are at risk for developing a recurrence of reflex sympathetic dystrophy in the same or another limb. Pain 64:463–466, 1996.
13. Schwartzman RJ, Kerrigan J. The movement disorder of reflex sympathetic dystrophy. Neurology 40:57–61, 1990.
14. Campbell JN, Raja SN, Meyer RA. Painful sequelae of nerve injury. In Dubner R, Gebhart GF, Bond RF (eds). Proceedings of the Vth World Congress on Pain, Pain Research and Clinical Management, vol. 3. Amsterdam, Elsevier, 1988, pp 135–143.
15. Leriche R. La Chiurgie del la Douleur. Paris, Masson and Cie, 1939.
16. Livingstone WK. Pain Mechanisms, A Physiological Interpretation of Causalgia and Its Related States. London, Macmillan, 1943.
17. Evan JA. Reflex sympathetic dystrophy. Surg Clin North Am 26:780–790, 1946.
18. Walker AE, Nulsen F. Electrical stimulation of the upper thoracic portion of the sympathetic chain in man. Arch Neurol Psychiatry 59:559–560, 1948.
19. White JC, Sweet WH. Pain and the Neurosurgeon. Springfield, Ill, Charles C Thomas, 1969.
20. Bonica, JJ. Causalgia and other reflex sympathetic dystrophies. In Bonica JJ, Liebeskind JC, Albe-Fessard DG (eds). Advances in Pain Research and Therapy, vol. 3. New York, Raven, 1979, pp 141–166.
21. Hannington-Kiff JG. Pain Relief. Philadelphia, Lippincott, 1974.
22. Arner S. Intravenous phentolamine test: diagnostic and prognostic use in reflex sympathetic dystrophy. Pain 46:17–22, 1991.
23. Raja SN, Treede RD, Davis KD, Campbell JN. Systemic alpha-adrenergic blockage with phentolamine: a diagnostic test for sympathetically maintained pain. Anesthesiology 74:691–698, 1991.
24. Hord AH, Rooks MD, Stephens BO, Rogers HG, Fleming LL. Intravenous regional bretylium and lidocaine for treatment of reflex sympathetic dystrophy: a randomized, double-blind study. Anesth Analg 74:818–821, 1992.
25. Wallin G, Torebjork HE, Hallin RG. Preliminary observations on the pathophysiology of hyperalgesia in the causalgic pain syndrome. In Sottermann Y (ed). Sensory Functions of the Skin in Primates. Oxford, Pergamon, 1976, pp 498–499.
26. Torebjork E. Clinical and neurophysiological observations relating to psychophysiological mechanisms in reflex sympathetic dystrophy. In Stanton-Hicks M, Janig W, Boas RA (eds). Reflex Sympathetic Dystrophy. Boston, Kluwer Academic, 1990, pp 71–80.
27. Torebjork E, Wahren LK, Wallin G, Hallin R, Koltzenburg M. Noradrenalin-evoked pain in neuralgia. Pain 63:11–20, 1995.

28. Wahren LK, Gordh T, Torebjork E. Effects of regional intravenous guanethidine in patients with chronic neuralgia of the hand: a follow-up study over a decade. Pain 62:379–385, 1995.
29. Blumberg H, Janig W. Clinical manifestations of reflex sympathetic dystrophy and sympathetically maintained pain. In Wall PD, Melzack R (eds). Textbook of Pain (3rd ed). Edinburgh, Churchill Livingstone, 1994, pp 685–697.
30. Ochoa JL, Verdugo R. Reflex sympathetic dystrophy: definitions and history of the ideas with critical review of human studies. In Low PA (ed). Clinical Autonomic Disorders. Boston, Little, Brown, 1993, pp 473–492.
31. Ochoa JL, Verdugo R, Campero M. Pathophysiological spectrum of organic and psychogenic disorders in neuropathic pain patients fitting the description of causalgia or reflex sympathetic dystrophy. In Gebhart GF, Hammond DL, Jensen TS (eds). Proceedings of the 7th World Congress on Pain, Progress in Pain Research and Management, vol. 2. Seattle, IASP, 1994, pp 483–494.
32. Janig W. The puzzle of "reflex sympathetic dystrophy": mechanisms, hypotheses, open questions. In Janig W, Stanton-Hicks M (eds). Reflex Sympathetic Dystrophy: A Reappraisal, Progress in Pain Research and Management, vol. 6. Seattle, IASP, 1996, p 10.
33. Gibbons J, Wilson PR. RSD score: criteria for the diagnosis of reflex sympathetic dystrophy and causalgia. Clin J Pain 8:260–263, 1992.
34. Low PA, Wilson P, Sandroni P, Willner CL, Chelimsky TC. Clinical characteristics of patients with reflex sympathetic dystrophy (sympathetically maintained pain) in the USA. In Janig W, Stanton-Hicks M (eds). Reflex Sympathetic Dystrophy: A Reappraisal, Progress in Pain Research and Management, vol. 6. Seattle, IASP, 1996, pp 49–66.
35. Mersky H, Bogduk N. Classification of Chronic Pain: Descriptions of Chronic Pain Syndromes and Definitions of Pain Terms (2nd ed). Seattle, IASP, 1994.
36. Bruehl S, Harden RN, Galer BS, et al. External validation of IASP diagnostic criteria of complex regional pain syndrome and proposed research diagnostic criteria. Pain 81:147–154, 1999.
37. Covington EC. Psychological issues in reflex sympathetic dystrophy. In Janig W, Stanton-Hicks M (eds). Progress in Pain Research and Management, vol. 6. Seattle, IASP, 1996, pp 191–215.
38. Bonica JJ. Causalgia and other reflex sympathetic dystrophies. In Bonica JJ (ed). The Management of Pain (2nd ed). Philadelphia, Lea & Febiger, 1990, pp 220–243.
39. Dondelinger R, Kurdziel JC. Percutaneous phenol neurolysis of the lumbar sympathetic chain with computed tomography control. Ann Radiol 27:376–379, 1984.
40. Wilkinson HA. Radiofrequency percutaneous upper thoracic sympathectomy: technique and review of indications. N Engl J Med 311:34–36, 1984.
41. Rauck RL, Eisenach JC, Jackson K, Young LD, Southern J. Epidural clonidine treatment for refractory reflex sympathetic dystrophy. Anesthesiology 79:1163–1169, 1993.
42. Blanchard J, Ramamurthy S, Walsh N. Intravenous regional sympatholysis: a double-blind comparison of guanethidine, reserpine, and normal saline. J Pain Symptom Management 5:357, 1990.
43. Raja SN, Treede R-D, Davis KD, Campbell JN. Systemic alpha-adrenergic blockade with phentolamine: a diagnostic test for sympathetically maintained pain, Anesthesiology 74:691–698, 1991.
44. Manart JD, Sadler RT, Schmitt EA, Rainer WG. Upper dorsal sympathectomy. Am J Surg 150:762–766, 1985.
45. Thompson JE. The diagnosis and management of posttraumatic pain syndromes (causalgia). Aust NZ J Surg 49:229–304, 1979.
46. Abram SE, Lightfoot RW. Treatment of long-standing causalgia with prazosin. Reg Anesth 6:79–81, 1981.
47. Ghostine SY, Comair YG, Turner DM, Kassell NF, Azar CG. Phenoxybenzamine in the treatment of causalgia. J Neurosurg 60:1263–1268, 1984.
48. Davis KD, Treede R-D, Raja SN, Meyer RA, Campbell JN. Topical application of clonidine relieves hyperalgesia in patients with sympathetically maintained pain. Pain 47:309–317, 1991.
49. Mellick GA, Mellick LB. Gabapentin in the management of RSD (letter). J Pain Symptom Mangement 10:265–266, 1995.
50. Wade SK. A critical review of controlled clinical trials for peripheral neuropathic pain and complex regional pain syndromes. Pain 73:123–139, 1997.
51. McFarlane BV, Wright A, Callaghan JO, Bensen HAE. Chronic neuropathic pain and its control by drugs. Pharmacol Ther 75:1–19, 1997.
52. Roberto P, Gert K, Wouter Z, Jaap JL. Treatment of reflex sympathetic dystrophy (CRPS type 1): A research synthesis of 21 randomized clinical trials. J Pain Symptom Management 21:511–526, 2001.
53. Shealy CN, Mortimer JT, Reswick JB. Electrical inhibition of pain by stimulation of the dorsal columns: preliminary clinical report. Anesth Analg 46:489–491, 1967.
54. Kumar K, Nath RK, Toth C. Spinal cord stimulation is effective in the management of reflex sympathetic dystrophy. Neurosurgery 40:503–508, 1997.
55. Barolat G. Spinal cord stimulation for chronic pain management. Arch Med Res 31:258–262, 2000.
56. Schwartzman RJ, Liv JE, Smullens SN, Hyslop T, Tahmoush AJ. Long-term outcome following sympathectomy for complex regional pain syndrome type 1 (RSD). J Neurol Sci 150:149–152, 1997.
57. Price DD, Long S, Wilsey B, Rafii A. Analysis of peak magnitude and duration of analgesia produced by local anesthetics injected into sympathetic ganglia of complex regional pain syndrome patients. Clin J Pain 14:216–226, 1998.
58. Max MB, Gilron I. Sympathetically maintained pain. Has the emperor no clothes? Neurology 52:905–907, 1999.
59. Schott GD. Interrupting the sympathetic outflow in causalgia and reflex sympathetic dystrophy. BMJ 316:792–793, 1998.
60. Nath RK, Mackinnon SE, Stelnicki E. Reflex sympathetic dystrophy. The controversy continues. Clin Plast Surg 23:435–446, 1996.
61. Kemler MA. Spinal cord stimulation in patients with chronic reflex sympathetic dystrophy. N Engl J Med 31:618–624, 2000.
62. Kumar K, Toth C, Nath RK, Laing P. Epidural spinal cord stimulation for treatment of chronic pain—some predictors of success. A 15-year experience. Surg Neurol 50:110–120; discussion 120–121, 1998.
63. Kemler MA; Barendse GAM, Van Kleef M, Oude Egbrink MGA. Pain relief in complex regional pain syndrome due to spinal cord stimulation does not depend on vasodilation. Anesthesiology 92:1653–1660, 2000.

APPENDIX A

IASP diagnostic criteria for Complex Regional Pain Syndrome:

1. The presence of an initiating noxious event or a cause of immobilization.
2. Continuing pain, allodynia, or hyperalgesia with which the pain is disproportionate to any inciting event.
3. Evidence at some time of edema, changes in skin blood flow, or abnormal sudomotor activity in the region of pain.
4. This diagnosis is excluded by the existence of conditions that would otherwise account for the degree of pain and dysfunction.

APPENDIX B

Signs of Chronic Pain Syndrome Checklist

- "Burning" pain
- Color changes
- Sweating changes
- Swelling
- Nail changes
- Hair changes
- Skin changes

Symptoms of Chronic Pain Syndrome Checklist

- Allodynia
- Hyperalgesia
- Hyperesthesia
- Temperature asymmetry

- Edema
- Tremor
- Dystonia
- Decreased range of motion
- Weakness

APPENDIX C

Proposed modified research diagnostic criteria for CRPS:

1. Continuing pain, which is disproportionate to any inciting event
2. Must report at least one symptom in each of the four following categories:

Sensory: reports of hyperesthesia

Vasomotor: reports of temperature asymmetry and/or skin color changes and/or skin color asymmetry

Sudomotor/edema: reports of edema and/or sweating changes and/or sweating asymmetry

Motor/trophic: reports of decreased range of motion and/or motor dysfunction (weakness, tremor, dystonia) and/or trophic changes (hair, nail, skin)

3. Must display at least one sign in two or more of the following categories:

Sensory: evidence of hyperalgesia (to pinprick) and/or allodynia (to light touch)

Vasomotor: evidence of temperature asymmetry and/or skin color changes and/or asymmetry

Sudomotor/edema: evidence of edema and/or sweating changes and/or sweating asymmetry

Motor/trophic: evidence of decreased range of motion and/or motor dysfunction (weakness, tremor, dystonia) and/or trophic changes (hair, nail, skin)

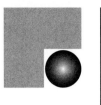

Neurosurgical Pain Therapies

Spinal Cord Stimulation for the Treatment of Chronic Pain

JOHN C. OAKLEY, MD

PAIN

"I must add, too, that the only purpose of the book is to solve the intellectual problem of suffering; for the far higher task of teaching fortitude and patience. I was never fool enough to suppose myself qualified, nor have I anything to offer my readers except my conviction that when pain is to be borne, a little courage helps more than much knowledge, a little human sympathy more than much courage, and the least tincture of the love of God more than all."[1]

C. S. Lewis

CHRONIC PAIN

"I have always been puzzled by the meaning of this phrase as distinct from intractable pain. Does it mean that there is a group of patients with tractable pains who never had access to a competent doctor? Does it mean that some patients progress through a treatable stage, which is neglected, and then later evolve into a perpetual intractable state? Or does it mean that the prolonged experience of pain can itself induce a separate and independent irreversible psychopathological state? As an outsider I read allusions to these questions but find mixed confusing answers."[2]

Patrick D. Wall

For the conscientious clinician, the question of defining chronic pain and suffering may be academic but is nonetheless faced daily. It seems that chronic or intractable pain is readily recognized but not easily defined. A little like quality. A practical definition for the interventional pain manager may be that the pain has become the disease. No longer are the acute symptoms of numbness and weakness associated with radiating pain in the extremity, having undergone the generally accepted treatment, attributed to a "curable" origin. Although the neural elements are functioning, the patient still perceives pain. For the pain manager, the first question to answer is fundamentally "Is this patient ill?" Because the dilemma of pain is that it cannot be seen or measured in any objective way, the answer to this question relies on obser-

vation of behavior and to no small amount on the medical history. Physical examination can only add information supporting the answer to the question of illness. It verifies impressions and observations already made from interview. The second question to be answered is "Can I help this patient?" and the closely related "Will this patient allow me to help?"

For the neurosurgeon who has decided to proceed with interventional management, classic pain treatment has involved ablative interventions, by nature destructive of normal neurologic tissue. Spinal cord stimulation (SCS), practically introduced in 1967 by Shealy and colleagues, was the first clinical application of electrical stimulation that reversibly modulated the function of the nervous system as a method of treating pain.[3] The introduction of this technique was prompted by the "gate-control theory" of pain, which continues, with refinements, to have a significant influence on pain research.[4] This theory postulated that stimulation of large-diameter afferent inputs to the spinal cord would result in a closing of the gate to transmission of pain-related information via small-diameter Aδ and C fibers. To test this theory, initial implant techniques placed electrodes directly on the spinal cord. Problems such as loss of stimulation due to fibrosis, cerebrospinal fluid leakage, meningitis, and neurologic damage led to the placement of stimulating leads into the epidural space.

Early in the development of SCS, the accepted mechanism of stimulation was mediated through the spinal cord dorsal columns and the technique became known as dorsal column stimulation. Later, it became obvious that while the designation was anatomically correct, it was mechanistically simplistic and the designation *spinal cord stimulation* has generally been adopted.

Throughout the 1970s, SCS was applied enthusiastically but generally uncritically. This resulted in a literature with very mixed results.[5] Due to a divergence of clinical opinion, SCS in the early to mid 1970s saw a general decline in use.[6,7] With the development of an increased understanding and consistent definitions of pain types, particularly differentiating between neuropathic and nociceptive pain, through the work of the International Association for the Study of Pain, more specific indications for the use of SCS were defined. This development, along with substantial improvements in stimulation systems leading to multiple channel and multiple contact arrays has resulted in improving outcome statistics.[8,9]

TERMINOLOGY

As SCS has become more standardized over the past three decades, certain basic terms have developed common use and definition. Through the work of the American Neuromodulation Society, a glossary of terms has been developed to assist persons just getting involved in this work. The following are terms pertinent to a discussion of spinal cord stimulation:

- **Array**. A two-dimensional arrangement of stimulating contacts either prefabricated on insulated backing as a paddle or plate, or created by insertion of percutaneous electrodes in parallel. Most commonly, and of necessity if placed percutaneously, the contacts are arranged longitudinally in columns; an array may have any number of columns. A prefabricated paddle or plate may have contacts in a diamond pattern or in rows.
- **Channel**. A pulse generator or radiofrequency receiver output, which is independent of other outputs, in particular as to amplitude (voltage or current). A true multichannel stimulator will allow simultaneous delivery of different amplitudes to different contacts. (A programmable multicontact stimulator which allows rapid sequential delivery of pulses to different contacts approaches this, but it is not, strictly speaking, a multichannel device.)
- **Contact**. An electrically conductive point or surface from which current passes into tissue. Contemporary electrode arrays have multiple contacts.
- **Electrode**. An assembly of electrically conductive contacts and wires, along with insulating spacers, catheters, and backing material. Most often used to refer to the "business end" of the assembly, where contacts deliver stimulation current to tissue. (Sometimes used to refer simply to a stimulating contact; but electrodes include insulation and other materials.)
- **Implantable Pulse Generator (IPG)**. A battery-driven power source for electrically activating a contact array(s); designed to be implanted in a subcutaneous location and not requiring an external apparatus to activate but may have an external control for off-on, amplitude, and rate control.
- **Lead**. A linear arrangement of conductors and insulators—wires and their circumferential insulation, between stimulating contacts and connectors. (Sometimes used to refer to the entire electrode, particularly if it is a percutaneous, catheter design.)
- **Paddle**. A flat, essentially two-dimensional insulated electrode or array. As it cannot be inserted percutaneously (through a needle) it is implanted in the spinal canal by laminotomy or laminectomy. Also termed a **Plate** electrode.
- **Receiver**. With regard to spinal cord stimulation, a device that is implanted in a subcutaneous location and designed to receive AM radio frequency transmissions from an external source. These transmissions are converted to an electrical signal, which activates an implanted contact array(s).

INDICATIONS AND EFFICACY

Treatment outcomes have become an important part of justifying the application of newer and more expensive technologies. SCS is no exception. The specific outcome measures applied are as varied as the groups reporting their results. Frequently, success is determined by patients' self-reports of pain reduction. Other criteria such as decreased use of healthcare resources, improved function, return to work, or closure of industrial insurance claims are reported as outcomes. Patient satisfaction is important, especially so to the treating physician, but it may not be a major concern for a third-party insurance carrier. It is estimated that 20% of patients who have repeat lumbar spine surgery return to work.[10] North and coworkers from experience at Johns Hopkins Medical Center report that 25% of patients with persisting back and leg pain following lumbar spine surgery return to work after SCS.[8] To make sense of such statistics, a number of variables need to be considered. Would any of the SCS patients have returned to work without intervention? What is the cost and effectiveness of alternative treatments? Kumar and colleagues estimate that the total per patient expense of maintaining SCS over a 5-year period ranges from $47,850 to $86,000 depending on the system and how expenses are determined.[11] The actual cost of maintaining healthcare for chronic pain patients is not well established. This compromises the ability to determine the effectiveness of a particular treatment like SCS. Bell and colleagues and Kumar and colleagues estimate that the cost of returning one person to work following implantation of a spinal cord stimulator will range from $268,000 up to $800,000.[11,12] Turk and Okifuji estimated the cost of returning one patient back to work after repeat spinal surgery as approximately $320,000.[13] At present SCS appears to be at least as cost effective as alternative medical treatments and possibly more cost effective than repeat surgery for the patient with intractable leg pain following spinal surgery.

Beginning in the early 1970s, numerous reports, predominantly case review studies, appeared in the literature.[14-63] Significant changes in equipment were made throughout the 1970s, and particularly the complication rates due to mechanical failure of the equipment changed for the better. Numerous reviews of these reports have appeared.[5,64] To summarize what has become an extensive literature, the analysis of Turner, Loeser, and Bell stands out.[5] In attempting to apply an evidence-based literature review technique, they discovered that the predominantly case review nature of the literature did not lend itself to this type of scrutiny. However, it was thought that certain conclusions could be drawn, although further, more rigorous, randomized outcome approaches should be undertaken to verify these conclusions. A total of 39 studies met the review criteria. At the average follow-up of 16 months, 59% of the patients had 50% or greater pain relief. Complications occurred in 42% of patients but were considered to be minor. The lack of randomized trials prevented any conclusion as to the effectiveness of spinal cord stimulation relative to other forms of treatment, placebo, or no treatment.

With developing pressure to produce randomized and prospective studies, preliminary results of a randomized study comparing SCS to repeat surgery for persisting leg pain following an initial spinal surgery was published by North.[65] Using the crossover from one treatment modality to the other after 6 months as the primary outcome measure, results for 27 patients showed a statistically significant advantage for SCS over repeat operation.

In a prospective, multicenter study combining 70 patients with at least 1-year follow-up, a variety of outcome measures including the average pain visual analogue scale, the McGill Pain Questionnaire, the Oswestry Disability Questionnaire, the Sickness Impact Profile, and the Beck Depression Inventory were analyzed.[66] Success of stimulation was considered achieved if 50% pain relief and patient satisfaction were reported. SCS was successful in managing the pain in 55% of the patients in whom 1-year follow-up was available. Statistically significant improvement was reported in all the outcome measures, confirming that SCS can be an effective treatment modality for the management of chronic lower extremity pain.

Ohmeiss, Rashbaum, and Bogdanffy reported a prospective study evaluating SCS in patients with intractable leg pain.[67] An isometric lift task measured lower extremity function as an attempt to identify a measurable outcome parameter. This function was demonstrated to statistically significantly improve 6 weeks after the initiation of SCS. Other outcome measures such as the Sickness Impact Profile also statistically significantly improved, confirming the results of other studies. Barolat and colleagues reported a retrospective analysis of 102 patients evaluated by extensive questionnaire and telephone interview techniques from a disinterested third party.[68] The average follow-up was 3.8 years; 21% never experienced any pain relief. Of the remaining 80, 75% were still using their stimulator. In patients experiencing a reported 75% pain relief, there was no reduction in relief over time. Patients experiencing only 50% reduction in their pain relief showed a dramatic reduction in their relief over the follow-up period. These authors thought that psychological screening contributed to a successful outcome.

Another method of analyzing the results of SCS is to evaluate results by specific syndrome. Spinal cord stimulation has been applied in a number of pain syndromes. In the world literature, the most successful application of SCS is in the relief of intractable angina pectoris.[69–80] These patients have been selected as having refractory angina pectoris and not candidates for revascularization. Stimulation appears to improve cardiac function in these patients coincident with relieving pain. Success rates between 80% and 90% have been consistently reported.[76,80] Electrodes are generally placed at the C8 to T2 level to the left of the midline with average stimulation parameters. Most notably in the European literature, peripheral vascular disease is the next most successful indication for SCS with relief of ischemic pain in the extremity reaching 70% to 80%, and limb salvage rates for extremities deemed appropriate for amputation are 60% to 70%.[81,82] Complex regional pain syndrome (CRPS) type I and II is successfully treated at an 80% to 90% rate, especially if the pain is sympathetically maintained. Neuropathic pain in the extremity, such as that found in the patient with persisting radicular pain after spinal surgery, responds at a 50% to 60% rate. While representing the most common indication for SCS in the United States, it is the least successful in the long term.[5]

The most frequent use of SCS in the United States is in the spinal disorders population and comes as a result of the prevalence of lumbar spinal surgery. There has grown a definable population of patients, estimated at 20% to 40% of those operated upon, who experience persistent or recurrent pain following intervention.[67] SCS is indicated in patients who have failed to improve with optimum medical management. Optimum medical management of this problem includes such interventions as active physical rehabilitation. Generally, a physical therapy–directed program prescribed by a physical medicine and rehabilitation physician and carried out by a licensed physical therapist may consist of strengthening and flexibility exercises, aerobic conditioning, and patient education to address lifting, posture, strengthening, and the like; neuromuscular and modality therapy may be included in this program but are not considered to constitute adequate therapy alone. Behavioral and psychological rehabilitation may also be a part of optimum management and consists of the application of pain control and stress management procedures including, but not limited to, relaxation therapy, guided imagery, cognitive restructuring, biofeedback, behavioral modification, and group or individual education. Pharmacologic management is probably the mainstay of optimum medical management and consists of the prescription of medication as required to control pain. This therapy may include narcotics, nonsteroidal anti-inflammatory drugs, antidepressants, muscle relaxants, and/or anticonvulsants as required by the patient's condition and deemed appropriate by the attending physician.

In addition to standard pain management treatments, patients may seek, within various insurance systems, relief from acupuncturists, chiropractors, and homeopaths.

It is generally after these treatments have failed that the neurosurgeon is asked to intervene with interventional pain treatments such as SCS. The criteria necessary to establish an independent neurostimulation pain program in order to offer such treatment are listed in Table 13-1. For the neurologic surgeon desiring to become active in this field, these criteria should be seriously adhered to, or, as an alternative, the surgeon should be an integral part of a total pain management team, providing the necessary resources, experience, and follow-up to ensure excellent patient management.

PATIENT SELECTION CRITERIA

Special selection criteria apply to specific pain syndromes such as angina, peripheral vascular disease, CRPS, interstitial cystitis, and peripheral neuropathic pain. These criteria are generally the diagnostic criteria applied to determine the presence of the disease or syndrome.[70,76,81,82,84,85] In these specific cases, SCS is becoming an integral part of treatment and not a last resort intervention. For the majority of neurologic surgeons, the primary indication for spinal cord stimulation will be a persisting radicular pain syndrome following primarily lumbar but also cervical spine surgery. When optimum medical management has failed to adequately restore function and relieve pain, it may be necessary to consider spinal cord stimulation to move the patient toward improved quality of life and functional ability.

● TABLE 13-1 • Physician Implanter Criteria for Experience and Training

Any physician proposing to provide management of the injured worker utilizing spinal cord stimulation should fulfill the following criteria:

I. Scientific Basis

A. Understand scientific theories behind neurostimulation;

B. Understand the role of neurostimulation in the hierarchy of pain treatment; this includes understanding alternative methods of pain control and the place of neurostimulation in the management of specific conditions;

C. Be familiar with the literature on neurostimulation.

II. Patient Selection

A. Understand the broad principles and importance of proper patient selection for interventional pain procedures; develop an in-depth understanding of specific patient selection criteria for neurostimulation including pathophysiologic diagnosis, psychological factors, and other factors important in chronic pain;

B. Know the specific pain classifications, pain patterns, and diagnoses which tend to respond to different interventional pain modalities; understand the relative indications for neurostimulation;

C. Ensure that psychological evaluation is performed to rule out psychological factors which might impede a desirable outcome if not addressed;

D. Be aware of medical, pharmacological, and technical contraindications for the use of neurostimulation;

E. Be aware of other failed therapeutic modalities, which have led to the decision to implant a neurostimulation device.

III. Patient Management

A. Prior to becoming active in neurostimulation, the physician must be aware of patient management issues, be prepared to accept the responsibility of ensuring proper patient follow-up and support services, and have personnel and facilities to provide such services;

B. Be able to provide thorough pre- and postoperative patient education, ensuring that the patient and family understand the device, its applications, and possible complications, as well as its impact on their daily lives;

C. Be able to recognize and treat immediate and delayed complications and/or designate consultants who will be available to assist in treating any complication;

D. Understand the importance of the informed consent, which must include the operative procedure, alternatives, and risks and benefits to enable the patient to make an informed choice to proceed with implant.

IV. Implant Technique

A. Understand the generally accepted surgical protocols most successfully used in implant procedures including trial screening and permanent implant;

B. Be familiar with appropriate fluoroscopic techniques and safety precautions as well as applicable licensing requirements;

C. Be able to recognize and treat possible complications or problems;

D. Know how to evaluate system efficacy and patient response to implanted systems;

E. Know how to program stimulation for optimal effect.

V. Practice Considerations

A. Establish the necessary consultative relationships to provide multidisciplinary care pre- and postimplant;

B. Be aware of appropriate protocols for prior authorization for neurostimulation and understand the economic impact of these procedures to the payor, community, the practice, and the patient;

C. Know the importance of providing after-care support services and the importance of the trained implant coordinator;

D. Understand the limitations and applications of neurostimulation systems; be able to troubleshoot system problems and otherwise manage patient and device interaction to achieve optimal patient benefit.

Patients who have undergone spine surgery who are eligible for a trial of spinal cord stimulation should have chronic, intractable back and leg(s) pain of greater than 6 months' duration. The radicular (leg) component should be more severe than the axial (back) component as estimated by the patient and confirmed by the attending physician. Axial pain is the lumbar component of pain that does not radiate to the legs. It is not restricted to an equal midline distribution over the spine.

There should be no indication for spine surgery. There is no indication for spine surgery if there is no radiographic evidence with contrast-enhanced magnetic resonance imaging or thin-cut computed tomography myelography and anteroposterior and lateral plain radiographs of a progressive deformity, a lesion concordant with the patient's pain complaint, or with progressive motor deficit. Such findings would warrant surgical consideration. Table 13-2 summarizes the accepted general inclusion and exclusion criteria for SCS intervention.

● **TABLE 13-2** • General Inclusion and Exclusion Criteria for Spinal Cord Stimulation Intervention

General inclusion criteria:
1. Appendicular pain following at least one previous spine surgery;
2. Pain of at least 6 months' duration;
3. No chronic or recurring pain complaint above the level of the T10 dermatome;
4. Leg pain which radiates below the knee greater than back pain;
5. Informed consent;
6. Clearance after psychological evaluation by a clinical psychologist. The evaluation should include at least one objective, normalized psychological test felt to be helpful in making this determination, e.g. MMPI-II; evaluation of motivation for return to work, etc.
General exclusion criteria:
1. Surgical procedure within 6 months of screening trial;
2. Evidence of an active disruptive psychiatric disorder including dissociative disorder, major affective disorder with psychotic features, active drug or alcohol abuse, personality disorders significant enough to impact the perception of pain, compliance to intervention and/or ability to evaluate treatment outcome as determined by a qualified psychological or psychiatric consult;
3. Patients younger than 18 years of age;
4. Patients who have not received an adequate course of optimum nonsurgical care;
5. Patients who have failed a previous spinal cord stimulation trial or system.

PSYCHOLOGICAL SCREENING

The usefulness of psychological screening for SCS patient selection has been controversial.[86] Some of the controversy results from a misunderstanding of the task of the psychological screening. The question asked of the evaluator is not whether the patient is a candidate for SCS. The implanting physician best answers this question based on pain type or syndrome. The appropriate question for the psychological evaluator consists of the following: "Are there any psychological, social, or support issues which might predispose to a poor outcome from SCS treatment?"[87] A number of psychological signs are of concern in regard to answering this question. An example might include motivational problems, that is, secondary gains judged to be driving pain behavior, for example, pain medications perpetuating addictive disease, abusive spouse backing off in response to a patient's pain, an employer a target of the patient's anger and being stressed by an open industrial claim, attorney discouraging return to work to maximize damages, ex-spouse delaying an effort to increase child support payments until injury recovery, or regular paycheck garnished by the state for back taxes with time loss wages exempt. Other examples might be attitudinal problems such as distrust or anger toward an employer or insurance company, no commitment to making lifestyle changes or trying pain self-management techniques, an expectation that the pain will be "fixed" by the procedure, no clear functional goal to be obtained with the procedure, or viewing the procedure as a means of validating pain or disability. A dysfunctional social history also represents a psychological concern. Here there may be work or relationship dysfunction due to chemical dependency, an abuse history with repetitive seeking of the victim role or target for anger, a multiple injury history, or catastrophic stressors

around the time of injury. A pain-prone personality is of great concern. These types are often revealed by a lack of psychological insight, a compulsion to work beyond exhaustion with unmanageably high self-expectations, a Minnesota Multiphasic Personality Inventory (MMPI) conversion "V" or passive-aggressive "V," or an MMPI chemical dependency profile. Finally, an axis I psychiatric condition such as dementia, learning disability, psychosis, major depression, panic disorder, or somatoform disorder at a disabling level or without any treatment resources or commitment, or suffering or disability from injury not being adequately differentiated from these conditions, contraindicates the use of SCS. In general, pain behavior on examination and an injury history with low or no correlation with objective findings should result in no procedure. Pain behavior on examination and an injury history with moderate or high correlation with objective findings could result in a procedure pending the satisfactory intervention of mental health treatment.

SCREENING TRIAL

While there is no literature-proven method of screening for the efficacy of spinal cord stimulation, it is generally believed that a trial of 1 week or longer of externalized lead wires utilizing a temporary external transmitter can be effective in excluding from permanent implant up to 30% of patients screened. These patients are generally excluded due to lack of pain relief with the stimulation, or to uncomfortable stimulation effects. Table 13-3 presents criteria that must apply during a screening trial of 1 week or more for the patient to be eligible to go on to permanent receiver implant.

⦿ **TABLE 13-3** • Screening Criteria to Be Met

1.	A minimum of 50% (optimum is at least 70%, see reference 80) pain reduction based on difference in VAS scores at preimplant and post-lead implant (anchors for the VAS are no pain and worst possible pain);
2.	The area of paresthesia must be concordant with the area of pain;
3.	Patient does not find the paresthesia to be undesirable;
4.	Functional improvement assessed by functional outcome evaluation as determined by each clinic, although some form of physical capacities evaluation is desirable.[62]

EQUIPMENT

The ability of SCS to modulate the nervous system is based on the delivery of electrical impulses to the spinal cord. This can be achieved by placing the active part of the SCS lead, the electrode, on the spinal cord. This was historically the earliest approach utilizing a laminectomy and durotomy. However, within a short time, about 6 weeks to 6 months, the electrodes became ineffective due to fibrosis and occasionally due to spinal cord injury. Placing the lead wire in the epidural space solved this problem. In doing so, long-term stimulation was possible without complication due to lead location. This also made the dorsal cerebrospinal fluid (CSF) space an important parameter in establishing stimulation amplitude and introduced stimulation variability with movement as a side effect.

SCS electrodes are contained within lead wires. These are manufactured in numerous configurations and are available for implantation either percutaneously or via laminotomy. The simplest form of lead contains two electrodes and allows bipolar stimulation. Lead wires progress in the number of electrodes from 4 to 8 to 16 contacts (available in laminotomy paddle or plate leads only) (Fig. 13-1). Currently available leads are generally linear arrays of either one or two columns.

A newer lead configuration deals with a transverse tripolar arrangement allowing programming across the spinal cord but must be used with a special transmitter.

Two types of power sources for producing stimulation at the electrode sites are currently manufactured. Two totally implantable battery-powered devices, similar in appearance to a cardiac pacemaker, are now available (Fig. 13-2). These devices have a finite battery lifetime of 2 to 5 years on the average, depending on stimulation parameters, before they must be replaced by a surgical procedure. An implantable pulse generator is programmed transcutaneously by using an interrogation wand attached to a programming computer. The patient may control on, off, amplitude, and rate parameters with a handheld controller. The newest version of the implantable pulse generator (IPG) allows independent control of two four-contact leads. Historically the first, and currently all other devices are powered by a radiofrequency transmitter, which is worn externally and broadcasts a signal to a subcutaneously implanted receiver connected to the lead wire (Fig. 13-3). Radiofrequency devices are programmed externally at the transmitter. Some radiofrequency devices allow the storage of multiple "programs" of electrode positive and negative combinations that the patient may select at will (patient-controlled stimulation) or which may be run in sequence independent of the patient (multiple stimulation mode).[88]

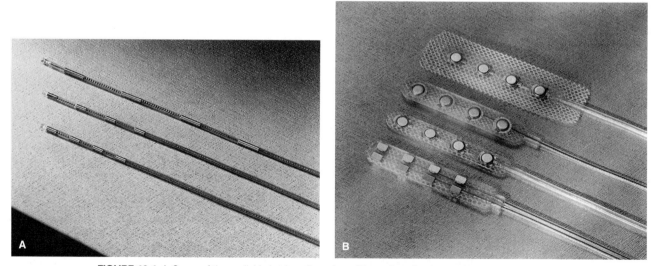

FIGURE 13-1 *A,* Some of the available lead configurations. These three leads are percutaneous electrodes. (Illustrations courtesy of Medtronic.) *B,* Four laminotomy style electrodes. The top electrode is used for peripheral nerve stimulation. (Photograph courtesy of Medtronic.)

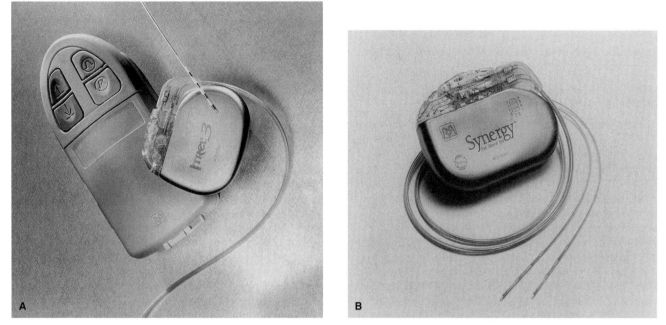

FIGURE 13-2 *A*, Medtronic implantable pulse generator, Itrel 3, and patient handheld controller "Itrel EZ." *B*, Medtronic "Synergy" implantable pulse generator allowing independent control of up to two four-contact electrode arrays.

Electrical stimulation of the nervous system may excite or inhibit neuronal action. With SCS, the active electrode that excites the desired paresthesia response is the negative electrode or cathode. The cathode depolarizes neurons within its field and the neuron becomes more active. The positive electrode or anode inhibits the neurons in its field by hyperpolarization. Hence, combinations of positive and negative electrodes are used to achieve the desired paresthesia coverage. This forms the basis for programming the stimulation

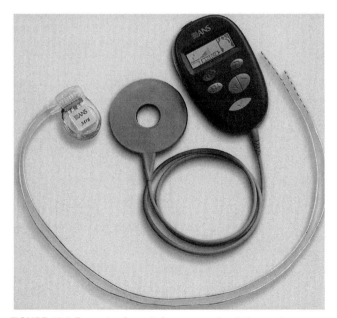

FIGURE 13-3 Example of a radiofrequency stimulation system. (Photograph courtesy of Advanced Neuromodulation Systems.)

device. There are numerous ways to approach programming and to optimize paresthesia coverage of the painful area.[88] The success of SCS at relieving pain correlates with the percentage of the painful area covered by stimulation-induced paresthesias making these techniques important for any implanter.

LEAD IMPLANT TECHNIQUES

Once a patient has been selected as a candidate for a trial of SCS, the implanting physician should be certain that the patient and the patient's support system, a spouse, family, close relative or caregiver, have been thoroughly educated concerning the intended procedure, its potential risks, and expected outcomes. Use of the intended system should not be beyond the ability of the patient to understand.

General Technical Concerns

Handling of lead wires requires special care so as not to break the lead insulation. The lead wires should not be kinked or bent or handled with sharp instruments. Rubber-shod forceps or clamps or vascular type instruments such as Debakey style forceps should be used. Sutures should not be placed directly around the lead wires; silastic or hard plastic anchors and 2–0 braided suture or larger should be used to avoid cutting the insulation. Care should be taken to plan the length of lead necessary should the system be implanted. For example, a cervical lead wire with a proposed abdominal or buttock position of the receiver or transmitter will require a longer lead wire or extension wire than normal to avoid the lead's being dislodged with flexion and extension movement. If an obstruction is encountered when moving the lead in the epidural space, do not force the lead. A guide wire technique may be tried, but it may be necessary to terminate the procedure and carefully evaluate the status of the spinal canal with regard to previously undetected stenosis or lesions.

Percutaneous Leads

A general rule is to select a target for the active electrode, the negative electrode, or cathode, based on the distribution of the patient's pain. If the predominant rhizopathy is in the S1 root, the cathode will usually give appropriate paresthesias at the T11 or T12 vertebral levels. Always bear in mind that the anatomic midline of the spinal anatomy may not correlate with the physiologic midline for the purpose of producing paresthesias, and some movement of the electrode position mediolaterally may be necessary to find the physiologic midline.

For percutaneous lead implantation, the operating room contains an operating table enabling fluoroscopic imaging. A C-arm image intensifier is used throughout the procedure to guide lead placement. If the implanter is right handed, the room is configured to allow the C-arm and video screen to be located on the patient's right side when the patient is prone. The scrub table is placed to the operator's right side. These procedures are generally performed with monitored anesthesia care under local anesthesia. The anesthesiologist is placed at the head of the table allowing enough room for the nurse or technician performing the screening trial.

Each manufacturer provides the necessary accessories with each lead that will allow either complete system implantation or placement of a tunneled electrode for screening purposes (Fig. 13-4). These accessories include a modified Tuohy needle,

a guide wire or lead blank, tunneling instrumentation, anchors, insulation boots, and hexagonal wrenches. For trial screening, disposable percutaneous extension wires are provided as well as the necessary external screening cable to allow testing.

The patient is placed prone on the operating table, prepped and draped from table to table. A chest-breast drape has a large fenestration that works particularly well for lead implantation. The vertebral interspace where the Tuohy needle will be placed in the epidural space is localized fluoroscopically. A 1- to 2-inch incision is made caudal from this point. Some clinics prefer to perform the needle placement first and confirm access to the epidural space and lead placement before making the incision. The Tuohy needle is inserted from a paraspinous approach at a 45-degree angle and directed toward the midline at the target level (Fig. 13-5). This configuration allows insertion of the electrode more parallel to the epidural space. A loss of resistance technique or "hanging drop" technique may be used to localize the epidural space. A positive contrast epidurogram may be performed if there is any question as to localization, but generally is not needed.

The electrode is then introduced through the Tuohy needle into the epidural space. The electrode is "steered" to the desired starting location using fluoroscopic guidance. The electrode is then connected to the screening cable. One end of the cable is passed over the ether screen to the implant assistant who connects it to the screening stimulator. Stimulation is then trialed. If a long eight-contact electrode is used, one method of intraoperative screening starts by stimulating the distal two electrodes, the proximal two electrodes, and two in the middle as anode-cathode bipoles. This establishes the upper middle and lower extent of the paresthesias. Adjustments to electrode positions to locate the "sweet spot" may then be made. Starting with the distal electrode negative and the proximal electrode positive and then reversing this sequence to determine the highest and lowest level of stimulation may screen four contact electrodes. The mediolateral orientation will determine the mediolateral position of the paresthesias in the extremity. Too far lateral will result in intercostal root stimulation and uncomfortable paresthesias. Perfectly midline stimulation may result in bilateral paresthesias and some interesting effects in the low back or reaching the legs if stimulating the cervical spinal cord. Occasionally, a process called "trolling" may ascertain the ideal location for the electrode. The electrode is placed higher than the expected stimulation level. The stimulator is adjusted to the perception

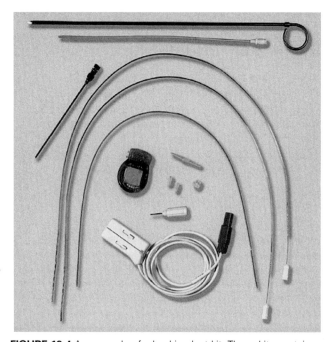

FIGURE 13-4 An example of a lead implant kit. These kits contain almost everything needed to implant the various electrodes. Each kit is specific to the electrode that it contains. Only the specific surgical instruments such as retractor, knife, cautery, and local anesthetics are required in addition. (Photograph courtesy of Advanced Neuromodulation Systems.)

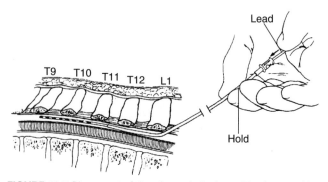

FIGURE 13-5 Placement of the electrode in the epidural space. Note the approximate 45-degree angle of the needle. (Photograph courtesy of Advanced Neuromodulation Systems.)

threshold for paresthesias and slowly pulled caudally with the patient reporting the pattern of paresthesia perception as the electrode is moved. The desired position is reached when the paresthesias "paint over" the painful areas.

When the desired electrode location has been determined, the needle is removed and the lead is anchored to the fascia by using the anchors provided with the lead. If using a silastic anchor, one method of anchoring is to place a loop through the fascia and tie the suture. The stitch is then looped around the anchor and tied again. A single loop around the anchor and fascia may loosen. Anchoring should be done only to tissue not likely to necrose or absorb. Examples of tissue to not use would be muscle or fat. The lead is then attached to a disposable percutaneous extension and sealed with a silastic boot. A subcutaneous tunnel is then fashioned to the flank using tunneling devices provided with the lead, and the disposable lead is then brought through the tunnel and externalized (Fig. 13-6A). The back incision is then closed. The externalization stab wound is dressed by placing an antiseptic patch (for example, a BioPatch, antimicrobial dressing, Johnson and Johnson, Inc., New Brunswick N.J.) around the lead and a suitable overlying dressing. The patient is now ready to undergo a screening trial.

With the conclusion of a successful screening trial the patient is returned to the operating room to implant the pulse generator or radiofrequency receiver. The intended implant site determines the patient's position. Common sites are abdominal or upper outer buttocks for the pulse generator, and supracostal or upper outer quadrant of the buttocks for the radiofrequency receiver to allow a more solid position for placing the external antenna. For abdominal or costal positions, the patient is positioned in the lateral decubitis position. For buttocks placement, the patient is prone. The previous implant site is prepped extending the preparation area to the proposed pocket site for the receiver or generator. After draping, the lead implant incision is opened and the disposable extension is cut and pulled

out from under the drape by the circulator. The back incision and electrode are then packed with an antibiotic solution–soaked sponge. Attention is turned to the pocket site. An 8- to 10-cm incision is made. Subcutaneous dissection is then used to fashion the pocket, paying attention to hemostasis. The lead wire or extension wire is then tunneled subcutaneously, connecting to the pocket. The lead or extension is then connected to the receiver or pulse generator, which is placed into the pocket, being careful to coil any excess wire behind the unit (Fig. 13-6B). The wounds are closed with an interrupted inverted absorbable stitch and dressed.

Before discharge from the clinic, the patient and a significant other are instructed in the use of the device, and if an implantable pulse generator has been used, the device is programmed. The importance of this follow-up after the procedure cannot be overemphasized. Some clinics delay programming or activating the unit until the first postoperative visit at 1 week when the patient may be more alert. This initial session of education and initiation of stimulation should not be missed to begin a successful treatment plan using stimulation.

Laminotomy Electrode Implant

The general approach to the patient is similar to that of the percutaneous lead implant. One significant difference is the level of implant. The level of lead placement may have been determined by a percutaneous screening trial, and the implanting neurosurgeon is asked to reproduce the paresthesias of the screening trial with a potentially more stable laminotomy lead. A percutaneous lead may have migrated twice, necessitating the placement of a more stable electrode.

The operating room is set up identically to that for a percutaneously implanted lead. C-arm fluoroscopy is used to guide lead orientation. The patient is placed prone on the radiolucent operating table. It is often helpful to position a pillow

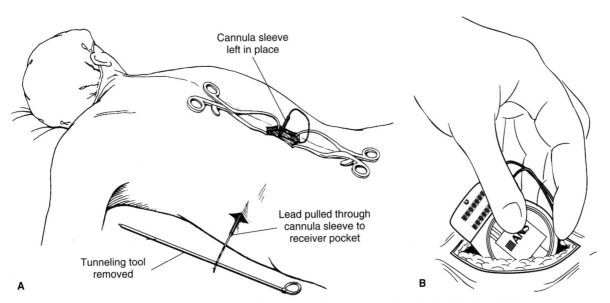

FIGURE 13-6 *A,* Tunneling the implanted lead wire to the receiver pocket site. In this case, a supracostal position. *B,* Insertion of a radiofrequency receiver into a subcutaneous pocket.

or bolster under the patient's abdomen and have the patient lie prone, not on the arms or elbows. The intended implant site is then prepped, most commonly T10 (T11 for the lower extremities), and, if the lead will be used as a screening lead, the prep site is extended laterally to the table.

A midline incision is extended caudally from the implant level for 5 to 10 cm, after anesthetizing with a long-acting local anesthetic such as bupivacaine. The muscle fascia and paraspinous muscles are blocked with the local anesthetic. When the block is established a subperiosteal dissection is performed using the electrocautery and a Cobb elevator or similar tool. After placing a self-retaining retractor in the wound, the inferior portion of the superior spinous process is resected, exposing the ligamentum flavum (Fig. 13-7A). A

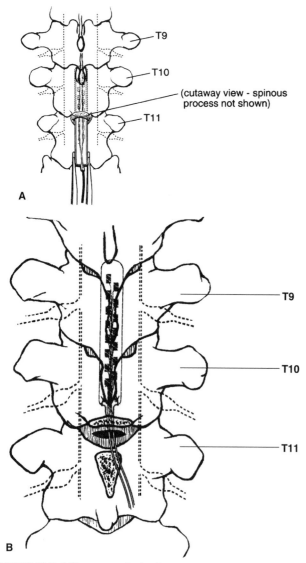

FIGURE 13-7 *A,* Placement of a laminotomy electrode through a midline opening in the ligamentum flavum after removal of the inferior portion of the cephalad spinous process. *B,* Laminotomy electrode in place having been inserted at the T10–11 interspace, a fairly standard point of entry.

window is made in the ligamentum flavum and enlarged using a 2- or 3-mm angled Kerrison rongeur. The dura is exposed and the opening widened by removing bone as necessary to allow placement of the lead. A lead blank may be advanced into the epidural space to confirm the adequacy of the exposure. The lead is then introduced into the epidural space under fluoroscopic guidance to control for side-to-side orientation (Fig. 13-7B). The electrode may be sutured to the dura with a 4–0 braided stitch if there is excessive movement. The electrode is then intraoperatively screened for appropriate paresthesia coverage as with the percutaneous lead. The position is adjusted as necessary. However, the ability to move the lead in a cephalic direction is limited, emphasizing the need for choosing the appropriate entry point or using a very large array electrode to allow electronic selection of the "sweet spot." With appropriate positioning, the wound is closed with an "O" absorbable stitch through the muscle and a second layer opposing the muscle fascia. The lead or leads are then anchored to the fascia as described for percutaneous leads. The leads may then be tunneled for a screening trial or connected to a pulse generator or radiofrequency receiver. The position of the generator or receiver pocket and its creation may be chosen as with the percutaneous leads.

COMPLICATIONS

Complications are events whose incidence may be known but whose occurrence is unanticipated. These events imply an adverse outcome but do not suggest, in and of themselves, negligence. Complications will occur but every effort should be taken to eliminate preventable errors.

Complications during the placement and management of spinal cord stimulators fall in three categories:

1. Surgical complications
2. Device-related complications
3. Stimulation-related complications

Overall complications occurred approximately 42% (20% to 75%) of the time in 13 case studies reviewed by Turner and colleagues.[5] The majority of these complications were considered to be minor and dealt with easily.

Surgical Complications

The primary surgical-related complication has been perioperative infection. This occurred in the review by Turner, Loeser, and Bell, surveying 31 studies in which complications were reported 5% of the time (range, 0% to 12%).[5] Many clinics use antibiotic prophylaxis to avoid this complication. One method is to administer a cephalosporin intravenously 1 hour before the procedure. Continuation of antibiotic coverage during the externalized screening trial is variable, and there are no specific data to suggest a "best" management technique. Biologic complications other than infection occur approximately 9% (0% to 42%) of the time. These complications include spinal fluid leakage, hemorrhage, and neurologic injury. In the large prospective study of Burchiel and colleagues, there were no infections either at lead implant or internalization.[66] In 219 cases in this study, there was one case each of cerebrospinal fluid leak and reported muscle spasm. In their review of two decades of SCS experience, North and colleagues reported no major morbidity defined as spinal cord injury, meningitis, or life-threatening infection.[9] The overall incidence of infection in this study was 5%.

Device-Related Complications

In the analysis by Turner and colleagues, stimulator complications occurred 30% of the time in 13 studies in which this could be determined.[5] The electrodes were a problem 24% of the time. Most commonly this represented migration of the electrode(s) or movement, especially side to side, with a subsequent loss of paresthesia coverage. The generator or receiver was a problem 2% of the time. In the study by Burchiel and colleagues, 12 of 219 patients required surgical procedures for revision or replacement of at least one component of the system (5%).[66] In a survey of 20 years of experience at the Johns Hopkins Hospital, North and colleagues defined electrode failure as a loss of stimulation paresthesias overlapping a patient's usual distribution of pain.[9] A Kaplan-Meier survival curve was then generated, demonstrating that multichannel devices were significantly more reliable than single-channel laminectomy or percutaneous leads. A similar analysis for discontinuation of use for all reasons again demonstrated the superiority of newer multichannel devices.

Stimulation-Induced Complications

Rarely, patients report that the stimulation paresthesias are uncomfortable or increase the underlying pain. The exact incidence is difficult to ascertain from the literature. In the study by Burchiel and colleagues, the incidence of these patient-related complications was 3% (5 of 219 patients).[66] One source of discomfort or lack of satisfaction with stimulation is posture-induced changes in paresthesia intensity. Cameron and Alo investigated stimulation thresholds as a function of posture and found that in 20 patients the threshold for paresthesia was lowest when lying, while in three patients thresholds for thoracic electrodes were lowest when sitting.[89]

Efficacy reports for spinal cord stimulation in the management of chronic pain syndromes have consistently demonstrated that 50% to 60% of patients initially receiving greater than 50% relief of pain are still using their stimulators at more than 1 year. It has been suggested that even after the 1-year period, there remains a portion of the successfully treated population who return reporting a failure of stimulation to control their pain. In a review of 126 patients (74 female) observed for longer than 2 years in the author's clinic (24 to 168 months; average, 37.8 months) reporting initially greater than 50% pain relief, 26 (20%) were documented to have discontinued the use of stimulation or requested removal of the system. A retrospective analysis was conducted to determine the reasons why such patients with long-term relief ultimately fail therapy. Diagnoses at system implant included myelographically proven arachnoiditis (61, 48%), radicular extremity pain (30, 24%), CRPS both types (8, 6%), spinal stenosis (7, 5%), peripheral neuropathy (6, 5%), peripheral vascular disease (5, 4%), and other neuropathic pain (9, 7%). All patients were implanted with four contact percutaneous or paddle electrodes (Medtronic quadripolar or Resume style electrodes).

Three reasons for failure were determined:

1. Progression of disease was determined in 12 patients (55% of failures). Seven patients were discovered to have new spine disease (32% of failures). Five patients presented with increased symptoms of peripheral neuropathy (23% of failures).
2. Tolerance, defined as continued appropriate paresthesias with loss of relief, was found in nine patients (41% of failures): five with arachnoiditis and four others including two with postherpetic neuralgia.
3. Painful hardware at the pulse generator implant site was seen in one patient (4% of failures).

Four patients, or 3% of the total, enjoyed enough resolution of their pain that they no longer required stimulation (at 58, 60, 142, 57 months of stimulation), two with arachnoiditis, and two with radicular leg pain.

APPLICATIONS OF STIMULATOR EQUIPMENT OUTSIDE THE SPINAL CORD

Electrical stimulation of the peripheral nervous system has long been used to treat specific peripheral nerve injuries.[90,91] A recent variation on this approach at the level of the nerve root has been described by Alo and colleagues.[92] The most common application of this "retrograde" technique is in the treatment of interstitial cystitis, as reported by Feler and colleagues.[84] The technique involves percutaneously or openly placing electrodes transforaminally or inferiorly in the lateral recess of the spinal canal to allow direct stimulation of individual nerve roots. In an extremity that is significantly denervated, the thresholds for paresthesia perception may be quite high and spinal cord stimulation is limited in its ability to produce the desired pattern of paresthesias without invoking uncomfortable stimulation effects in the surrounding normal tissue. This technique allows the focal production of stimulation effects in an affected nerve root distribution without undesirable side effects. For specific syndromes mediated through known nerve root innervation, such as interstitial cystitis mediated through the S2 to S4 roots, successful relief may be obtained without extraneous stimulation effects. Long-term outcomes of this technique are yet to be published, but in the lumbar region these techniques offer an alternative approach to stimulation-induced pain relief.

Weiner and colleagues have also described the use of stimulation systems in the treatment of occipital neuralgia.[85] The electrode is placed in the *subcutaneous* space inferior to the suboccipital trigger point producing the occipital headache through a slightly bent needle. The headache, if present on the operating table, will often be relieved with the onset of stimulation.

Such innovative applications of electrical stimulation using existing equipment suggest that the future of stimulation is limited only by our understanding of functional neuroanatomy and by the biomaterials necessary to access functional areas of the nervous system.

Photographs and illustrations for this chapter provided courtesy and by permission of Medtronic, Inc. and Advanced Neuromodulation Systems, Inc.

REFERENCES

1. Lewis CS. The Problem of Pain. Collier Books, New York paperback ed. 1962, pp 9,10.
2. Wall PD. Introduction to the edition after this one. *In* Wall PP, Melzack R (eds). Textbook of Pain. Philadelphia, Churchill Livingstone, 1994, pp 1, 2.
3. Shealy CN, Mortimer JT, Reswick J. Electrical inhibition of pain by stimulation of the dorsal column: Preliminary clinical reports. Anesth Analg 46:489, 1967.
4. Melzack R, Wall PD. Pain mechanisms: a new theory. Science 150:9971–9979, 1965.
5. Turner JA, Loeser JD, Bell KG. Spinal cord stimulation for chronic low back pain: A systematic synthesis. Neurosurgery 37:1088–1096, 1995.
6. Siegfried J, Lazothes Y. Long-term follow-up of dorsal column stimulation for chronic pain syndrome after multiple lumbar operations. Appl Neurophysiol 45:201, 1982.
7. Erickson DL, Long DM. Ten-year follow-up of dorsal column stimulation. *In* Bonica JJ, Lindblom U, Iggo A (eds). Advances in Pain Research and Therapy, vol. 5. New York, Raven, 1983, pp 583–589.
8. North RB, Ewend MG, Lawton MT, Piantadosi S. Spinal cord stimulation for chronic, intractable pain: Superiority of "multichannel" devices. Pain 44:119–130, 1991.
9. North RB, Kidd DH, Zahurak M, James CS, Long DM. Spinal cord stimulation for chronic, intractable pain: Two decades' experience. Neurosurgery 32:384–395, 1993.
10. North RB, Campbell JN, James CS, et al. Failed back surgery syndrome 5 year follow-up in 102 patients undergoing repeated operations. Neurosurgery 28:685–690, 1991.
11. Kumar K, Toth C, Nath RK, et al. Epidural spinal cord stimulation for treatment of chronic pain–some predictors of success. A 15-year experience. Surg Neurol 50:110–121, 1998.
12. Bell S, Bauer BL. Dorsal column stimulation (DCS): cost to benefit analysis. Acta Neurochir 52(Suppl):121–123, 1991.
13. Turk DC, Okifuji A. Treatment of chronic pain patients: clinical outcomes, cost-effectiveness, and cost-benefits of multidisciplinary pain centers. Crit Rev Phys Rehabil Med 10:181–208, 1998.
14. Blond S, Armignies P, Parker F, Dupard T, Guieu JD, Duquesnoy B, Christtiaens JL. Sciatalges chroniques par desafferentation sensitive apres chirurgie de la hernie discale lombaire: aspects cliniques et therapeutiques. Neurochirurgie 37:86–95, 1991.
15. Blume H, Richardson R, Rojas C. Epidural nerve stimulation of the lower spinal cord and cauda equina for the relief of intractable pain in failed back surgery. Appl Neurophysiol 45:456–460, 1982.
16. Broseta J, Roldan P, Gonzales-Darder J, Bordes V, Barcia-Salorio JL. Chronic epidural dorsal column stimulation in the treatment of causalgic pain. Appl Neurophysiol 45:190–194, 1982.
17. Burton C. Dorsal column stimulation: optimization of application. Surg Neurol 4:171–176, 1975.
18. Burton CV. Session on spinal cord stimulation: safety and clinical efficacy. Neurosurgery 1:164–165, 1977.
19. Clark K. Electrical stimulation of the nervous system for control of pain: University of Texas Southwestern Medical School experience. Surg Neurol 4:164–166, 1975.
20. De la Porte C, Siegfried J. Lumbosacral spinal fibrosis (spinal arachnoiditis): its diagnosis and treatment by spinal cord stimulation. Spine 8(6):593–603, 1983.
21. De la Porte C, Van de Kelft E. Spinal cord stimulation in failed back surgery syndrome. Pain 52:55–61, 1993.
22. de Vera JA, Rodriguez JL, Dominguez M, Robaina F. Spinal cord stimulation for chronic pain mainly in PVD, vasospastic disorders of the upper limbs and failed back surgery. Pain 5(Suppl):S81, 1990.
23. Demirel T, Braun W, Reimers CD. Results of spinal cord stimulation in patients suffering from chronic pain after a two year observation period. Neurochirurgia 27:47–50, 1984.
24. Devulder J, De Colvenaer L, Rolly G, Caemaert J, Calliauw L. Spinal cord stimulation and the relief of chronic non-malignant pain in 45 patients. Pain 5(Suppl):S236, 1990.
25. Devulder J, De Colvenaer L, Rolly G, Caemaert J, Calliauw L, Martens F. Spinal cord stimulation in chronic pain therapy. Clin J Pain 6:51–56, 1991.
26. Erickson DL, Long DM. Ten-year follow-up of dorsal column stimulation. *In* Bonica JJ (ed). Advances in Pain Research and Therapy. New York, Raven, 1983, pp 583–589.
27. Hoppenstein R. Electrical stimulation of the ventral and dorsal columns of the spinal cord for relief of chronic intractable pain. Surg Neurol 4:187–194, 1975.
28. Hunt WE, Goodman JH, Bingham WG. Stimulation of the dorsal spinal cord for treatment of intractable pain: a preliminary report. Surg Neurol 4:153–156, 1975.
29. Kälin M-T, Winkelmuller W. Chronic pain after multiple lumbar discectomies–significance of intermittent spinal cord stimulation. Pain 5(Suppl):S241, 1990.
30. Koeze TH, Williams AC, Reiman S. Spinal cord stimulation and the relief of chronic pain. J Neurol Neurosurg Psych 50:1424–1429, 1987.
31. Krainick JU, Thoden U. Dorsal column stimulation. *In* Wall PD, Melzack R (eds). Textbook of Pain. New York, Churchill Livingstone, 1989, pp 701–705.
32. Kumar K, Wyant GM, Ekong CEU. Epidural spinal cord stimulation for the relief of chronic pain. Pain Clin 1(2):91–99, 1986.
33. Kumar K, Nath BR, Wyant GM. Treatment of chronic pain by epidural spinal cord stimulation: a ten year experience. J Neurosurg 75:402–407, 1991.
34. Law J. Results of Treatment for Pain by Percutaneous Multicontact Stimulation of the Spinal Cord. Presented at the American Pain Society meeting, Chicago, November 11–13, 1983.
35. Leclercq T, Russo E. La stimulation epidurale dans le traitement del doleurs chroniques. Neurochirurgie 27:125–128, 1981.
36. LeDoux MS, Langford KH. Spinal cord stimulation for the failed back syndrome. Spine 18:191–194, 1993.
37. LeRoy PL. Stimulation of the spinal cord by biocompatible electrical current in the human. Appl Neurophysiol 44:187–193, 1981.
38. Long DM, Erickson DE. Stimulation of the posterior columns of the spinal cord for relief of intractable pain. Surg Neurol 4:134–141, 1975.
39. Long DM, Erickson DE, Campbell J, North R. Electrical stimulation of the spinal cord and peripheral nerves for pain control. Appl Neurophysiol 44:207–217, 1981.
40. McCarron RF, Racz G. Percutaneous Dorsal Column Stimulator Implantation for Chronic Pain Control. Presented at the North American Spine Society meeting. Banff, Alberta, Canada, June 25–28, 1987.
41. Meglio M, Cioni B, Rossi GF. Spinal cord stimulation in management of chronic pain. A 9-year experience. J Neurosurg 70:519–524, 1989.
42. Meilman PW, Leibrock LG, Leong FTL. Outcome of implanted spinal cord stimulation in the treatment of chronic pain: arachnoiditis versus single nerve root injury and mononeuropathy. Clin J Pain 5:189–193, 1989.
43. Mittal B, Thomas DGT, Walton P, Calder I. Dorsal column stimulation (DCS) in chronic pain: report of 31 cases. Ann Royal Coll Surg 69(3):104–109, 1987.
44. Nelson KD, Adams JE, Hosobuchi Y. Experience with dorsal column stimulation for relief of chronic intractable pain. Surg Neurol 4:134–141, 1975.
45. Pineda A. Dorsal column stimulation and its prospects. Surg Neurol 4:157–163, 1975.
46. Racz G, McCarron RF, Talboys P. Percutaneous dorsal column stimulator for chronic pain control. Spine 14:1–4, 1989.
47. Ray CD, Burton CV, Lifson A. Neurostimulation as used in a large clinical practice. Appl Neurophysiol 45:160–206, 1982.
48. Richardson RR, Siqueira EB, Cerullo LJ. Spinal epidural neurostimulation for treatment of acute and chronic intractable pain: initial and long term results. Neurosurgery 5:344–348, 1979.
49. Richardson DE, Shatin D. Results of Spinal Cord Stimulation for Pain Control: Long-Term Collaborative Study. Presented at the American Pain Society meeting, New Orleans, November 8–10, 1991.
50. Robb LG, Robb MP. Practical considerations in spinal cord stimulation. Pain 5(Suppl):S234, 1990.
51. Sanchez-Ledesma MJ, Garcia-March G, Diaz-Cascajo P, Gomez-Moreta J, Broseta J. Spinal cord stimulation in deafferentation pain. Stereotact Funct Neurosurg 53:40–55, 1989.
52. Shatin D, Mullett K, Hults G. Totally implantable spinal cord stimulation for chronic pain: design and efficacy. Pace 9:577–583, 1986.
53. Shealy CN. Dorsal column stimulation: optimization of application. Surg Neurol 4:142–145, 1975.
54. Shelden CH, Paul F, Jacques DB, Pudenz RH. Electrical stimulation of the nervous system. Surg Neurol 4:127–132, 1975.
55. Simpson BA. Spinal cord stimulation in 60 cases of intractable pain. J Neurol Neurosurg Psychiatry 54:196–199, 1991.
56. Spiegelmann R, Friedman WA. Spinal cord stimulation: a contemporary series. Neurosurgery 28:65–71, 1991.
57. Sweet W, Wepsic J. Stimulation of the posterior columns of the spinal cord for pain control. Clin Neurosurg 21:278–310, 1974.
58. Urban BJ, Nashold B. Percutaneous epidural stimulation of the spinal cord for relief of pain: long term results. J Neurosurg 48:323–328, 1978.

59. Vogel HP, Heppner B, Humbs N, Schramm J, Wagner C. Long-term effects of spinal cord stimulation in chronic pain syndromes. J Neurol 233:16–18, 1986.

60. Waisbrod H, Panhans C, Hansen D, Gerbershagen HU. Direct nerve stimulation for painful peripheral neuropathies. J Bone Joint Surg 67:470–473, 1985.

61. Winkelmuller W. Experience with the control of low back pain by the dorsal column stimulation (DCS) system and by the peridural electrode system (Pisces). In Hosobuchi Y, Corbin T (eds). Indications for Spinal Cord Stimulation. Amsterdam, Excerpta Medica, 1981, pp 34–41.

62. Young RF, Shende M. Dorsal column stimulation for relief of chronic intractable pain. Surg Forum 27:474–476, 1976.

63. Young RF. Evaluation of dorsal column stimulation in the treatment of chronic pain. Neurosurgery 3:373–379, 1978.

64. North RB. Spinal Cord Stimulation. In North RB, Levy RM (eds). Neurosurgical Management of Pain. New York, Springer-Verlag, 1997, pp 271–282.

65. North RB, Kidd DH, Lee MS, Piantodosi S. A prospective randomized study of spinal cord stimulation versus reoperation for failed back surgery syndrome: initial results. Stereotact Funct Neurosurg 62:267–272, 1994.

66. Burchiel KJ, Anderson CA, Brown FD, et al. Prospective, multicenter study of spinal cord stimulation for relief of chronic back and extremity pain. Spine 21:2786–2794, 1996.

67. Ohmeiss DD, Rashbaum RF, Bogdanffy GM. Prospective outcome evaluation of spinal cord stimulation in patients with intractable leg pain. Spine 21:1344–1351, 1996.

68. Barolat G, Ketcik B, He J. Long-term outcome of spinal cord stimulation for chronic pain management. Neuromodulation 1:19–29, 1998.

69. Murphy DF, Giles KE. Dorsal column stimulation for pain relief from intractable angina pectoris. Pain 28:365–368, 1987.

70. Mannheimer C, Augustinsson L-E, Carlsson C-A, Manhem K, Wilhelmsson C. Epidural spinal electrical stimulation in severe angina pectoris. Br Heart J 59:56–61, 1988.

71. Gonxalez-Darder JM, Canela P, Gonzalez-Martinez V. High cervical spinal cord stimulation for unstable angina pectoris. Stereotact Funct Neurosurg 56:20–27, 1991.

72. Sanderson JE, Brooksby P, Waterhouse D, Palmer RBG, Neubauer K. Epidural spinal electrical stimulation for severe angina: a study of its effects on symptoms, exercise tolerance and degree of ischaemia. Eur Heart J 13:628–633, 1992.

73. de Jongste M, Staal MJ. Preliminary results of a randomized study on the clinical efficacy of spinal cord stimulation for refractory severe angina pectoris. Acta Neurochir 58:161–164, 1993.

74. Mannheimer C, Eliasson T, Andersson B, Bergh C-H, Augustinsson L-E, Emanuelsson H, Waagstein F. Effects of spinal cord stimulation in angina pectoris induced by pacing and possible mechanisms of action. BMJ. 307:477–480, 1993.

75. Anderson C, Hole P, Oxhoj H. Does pain relief with spinal cord stimulation for angina conceal myocardial infarction? Br Heart J 71:419–421, 1994.

76. de Jongste MJL, Hautvast RWM, Hillege HL, Lie KI. Efficacy of spinal cord stimulation as adjuvant therapy for intractable angina pectoris: a prospective, randomized clinical study. J Am Coll Cardiol 23:1592–1597, 1994.

77. de Jongste MJL, Nagelkerke D, Hooyschuur CM, Journee HL, Meyler PWJ, Staal MJ, de Jonge P, Lie KI. Stimulation characteristics, complications, and efficacy of spinal cord stimulation systems in patients with refractory angina: a prospective feasibility study. Pacing Clin Electrophysiol 17:1751–1760, 1994.

78. de Jongste MJL, Haaksma J, Hautvast RJM, et al. Effects of spinal cord stimulation on myocardial ischaemia during daily life in patients with severe coronary artery disease. Br Heart J 71:413–418, 1994.

79. Eliasson T, Jern S, Augustinsson L-E, Mannheimer C. Safety aspects of spinal cord stimulation in severe angina pectoris. Coronary Artery Dis 5:845–850, 1994.

80. Sanderson JE, Ibrahim B, Waterhouse D, Palmer RBG. Spinal electrical stimulation for intractable angina-long-term clinical outcome and safety. Eur Heart J 15:810–814, 1994.

81. Augustinsson L-E, Holm J, Carlsson CA, Jivegard L. Epidural electrical stimulation in severe limb ischemia: evidences of pain relief, increased blood flow and a possible limb-saving effect. Ann Surg 202:104–111, 1985.

82. Claeys L, Horsch S. Epidural spinal cord stimulation (ESCS) in chronic vascular pain. In Kepplinger B, Pernak JM, Ray AL, Schmid H (eds). Pain—Clinical Aspects and Therapeutical Issues, Part II. Berlin, Verlag, 1993, pp 45–51.

83. Oakley JC, Weiner RL. Spinal cord stimulation for Complex Regional Pain Syndrome: a prospective study at two centers. Neuromodulation 2:47–50, 1999.

84. Feler CA, Whitworth LA, Brookoff D, Powell R. Recent advances: sacral nerve root stimulation using a retrograde method of lead insertion for the treatment of pelvic pain due to interstitial cystitis. Neuromodulation 2(3):211,1999.

85. Weiner R. Occipital nerve stimulation for the treatment of intractable occipital neuralgia. Neuromodulation 2(3):217,1999.

86. North RB, Kidd DH, Wimberly RL, Edwin D. Prognostic value of psychological testing in patients undergoing spinal cord stimulation: a prospective study. Neurosurgery 39:301–311, 1996.

87. Doleys DM, Olson K. Psychological assessment and intervention in implantable pain therapies. Medtronic Technical Bulletin, 1996.

88. Alo KM, Yland MJ, Kramer DL, Charnov JH, Redko V. Computer assisted and patient interactive programming of dual octode spinal cord stimulation in the treatment of chronic pain. Neuromodulation 1:30–45, 1998.

89. Cameron T, Alo KM. Effects of posture on stimulation parameters in spinal cord stimulation. Neuromodulation 1:177–183, 1998.

90. Long DM Stimulation of the peripheral nervous system for pain control. Clin Neurosurg 31:323–343, 1983.

91. Hassenbusch SJ, Stanton-Hicks M, Schoppa D, Walsh JG, Covington EC. Long-term results of peripheral nerve stimulation for reflex sympathetic dystrophy. J Neurosurg 84:415–423, 1996.

92. Alo KM, Yland MJ, Redko V. Feler C, Naumann C. Lumbar and sacral nerve root stimulation (NRS) in the treatment of chronic pain, a novel anatomic approach and neurostimulation technique. Neuromodulation 2:1, 1999.

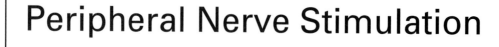

Peripheral Nerve Stimulation

SAMUEL J. HASSENBUSCH, MD, PhD

HISTORY

Electrical stimulation applied to peripheral nerves was developed first in approximately 1969.[1–2] The original electrodes often were cuff-shaped and the results were encouraging but limited.[1–3] Reports of peripheral nerve stimulation (PNS) from the 1970s and 1980s showed good long-term results and patient satisfaction, although the reports were often limited and anecdotal.[4–16]

Campbell and Long in 1976 reported on PNS applied for a variety of pain syndromes in 33 patients with 24% excellent results and 21% intermediate results.[1] In 1980, Law and colleagues reported 62% of 22 patients were using the PNS stimulators as the sole mechanism for analgesia with an average follow-up of 25 months.[17] In 1982, Nashold and colleagues reported the results in 35 patients with upper and lower extremity peripheral nerve injuries and found that 53% of those with upper extremity and 31% of those with lower extremity pain had successful results with a follow-up ranging from 4 to 9 years.[18]

Interest in the use of PNS was renewed in the late 1980s with the application of flat or oval-shaped electrode templates that contained four electrode contacts (e.g., Resume electrode, Medtronic Corporation, Minneapolis, MN).[19–21] The presence of four electrode contacts, coupled with the availability of implantable, programmable, low-voltage generators, provided greater ability to deliver consistent and evenly distributed stimulation to a peripheral nerve, although well-analyzed studies were absent.

MECHANISM

Although the mechanism of pain relief remains unclear, it appears that the peripheral stimulation might activate A-β fibers, thus providing a blocking action on nociceptive A-δ and C-fibers, probably at the dorsal horn.[22–27]

Campbell and Taub showed a loss of the A-β component of the compound action potential recording from a peripheral nerve that was stimulated transcutaneously.[28] The mechanism here might involve blockade of the peripheral axon. Further support has come from the observation that repeated electrical stimulation of peripheral nerves results in failure to excite C fibers and, to a lesser degree, A fibers.[1]

The mechanisms of action for both PNS and spinal cord stimulation (SCS) in the treatment of complex regional pain syndrome (CRPS, reflex sympathetic dystrophy) remain unclear and might be different for these two modalities. The voltage level for PNS, however, probably activates only large myelinated fibers.[29] Recordings from peripheral stimulator electrodes have shown spontaneous abnormal discharges in the affected nerve.[29] Constant peripheral stimulation might provide a consistent blockade of afferent peripheral input, allowing central processing to return to normal. Alternatively, afferent impulses from electrical stimulation of the nerve might block, at the spinal cord level, other abnormal nociceptive inputs in a gate control manner.[30]

TECHNIQUE

Peripheral nerve stimulation is usually applied via an open operation with exposure of the target nerve. The testing phase is essentially the same as the permanent phase because the permanent electrode is implanted along the side of the nerve (Figs. 14-1 and 14-2) with the temporary extension tail of the electrode protruding from a separate stab incision (Figs. 14-5, 14-7, 14-9).[31,32]

In stage I, a plate-type electrode, with a layer of free fascia covering the electrode surface, is placed in apposition to the target nerve. Target nerves are exposed surgically in the following areas: median/ulnar just proximal to the mid-humerus in the brachial groove, radial at the mid-humerus in the spiral groove, common peroneal superior to the popliteal space under the biceps femoris muscle and tendon, posterior tibial proximal to the medial malleolus of the ankle, and sciatic nerve in the gluteus or just distal to it (Figs. 14-3 through 14-9). Typically, during a 2-day screening period, stimulation parameters are adjusted and records made of pain severity, activity levels, and narcotic usage.

If the testing phase (stage I) shows at least 50% reduction in pain and objective improvement in the physical examination changes, then a permanent implanted generator or receiver is connected to the electrode in stage II. The incision is reopened, the temporary extension tail clipped off, and then a permanent extension wire and generator/receiver placed (Figs. 14-5, 14-7, 14-9). Initial stimulator settings are often a pulse rate of 75 Hz, pulse width of 210 msec,

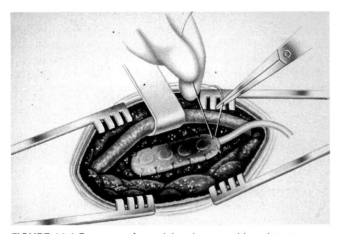

FIGURE 14-1 Exposure of a peripheral nerve with a plate-type electrode positioned along the course of the nerve. To facilitate adequate positioning of the electrode, the nerve is retracted gently away from the electrode implant site. The electrode should be secured to underlying tissues. A layer of fascia should be secured between the electrode and the peripheral nerve.

and an electrode combination with the no. 0 electrode negative and the no. 3 electrode positive. Newer plate-type electrode arrays (such as dual columns of four contacts each or two plate electrodes, one on each side of the nerve) have also been used.

Establishing an adequate pattern of stimulation is usually more difficult in patients with pain and vasomotor changes in the area of the ulnar nerve at the medial epicondyle of the elbow.

Similarly, for medial or lateral plantar nerve distribution pain, it is useful to place the electrode using local anesthesia and intravenous sedation with intraoperative testing of the electrode in different locations around the tibial nerve. Another technical point is that, for placement of the generator or receiver in the midaxillary line at the level of the nipple, tethering of the extension wire in the area of the anterior axillary fold can occur. This possibility can be eliminated by starting full abduction exercises of the arm immediately after the operation.

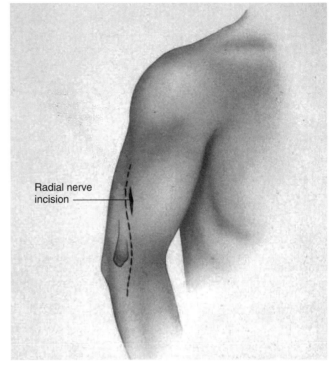

FIGURE 14-3 Location of skin incision for exposure of the radial nerve in the spiral groove in the upper arm.

OUTCOME STUDIES

With this modality, there is a paucity of published reports describing the long-term success rates, criteria for success, and technical complications. Ironically, there have been minimal recent reports in the literature of the application of PNS in non-CRPS patients.

A prospective, consecutive series by this author in 1996 described PNS in the treatment of severe reflex sympathetic dystrophy (RSD or CRPS) for patients with symptoms

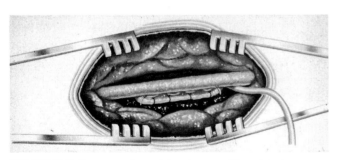

FIGURE 14-2 Exposure of a peripheral nerve with a plate-type electrode positioned adjacent to the nerve. A layer of fascia is interposed between the nerve and the stimulation electrode. The electrode should be positioned adjacent to the nerve as the nerve follows its normal course.

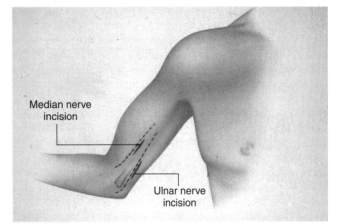

FIGURE 14-4 Location of skin incisions for exposure of median nerve in the upper arm and ulnar nerve at the elbow.

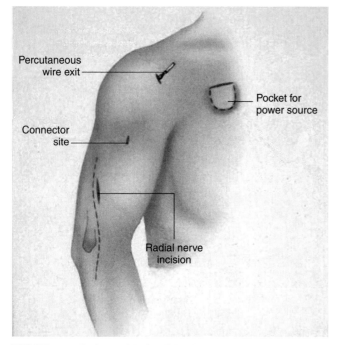

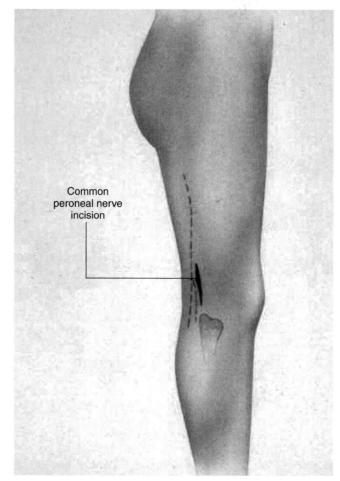

FIGURE 14-5 During a trial of peripheral nerve stimulation, a temporary percutaneous trialing wire is connected to the electrode lead, tunneled subcutaneously, and brought out through a stab incision proximal to the location of the stimulation electrode implant site. In this illustration, the electrode has been placed adjacent to the radial nerve in the spiral groove. The trialing wire is tunneled proximally, facilitating eventual connection of the electrode (via an extension wire) to a power source. The location of a power source (RF receiver or implantable pulse generator) in the infraclavicular fossa is shown.

FIGURE 14-6 Location of skin incision for exposure of common peroneal nerve.

entirely or mainly in the distribution of one major peripheral nerve.[32] Plate-type electrodes were placed surgically on affected nerves and tested for 2 to 4 days. Implanted programmable generators were placed if 50% pain reduction and objective improvement in physical changes were achieved. Patients were observed for 2 to 4 years and a disinterested third-party interviewer performed final patient evaluations (Fig. 14-10). Of 32 patients tested, 30 (94%) underwent permanent PNS placement. Long-term good or fair relief was experienced in 19 of 30 (63%) patients. Allodynic and spontaneous pain was reduced in success patients from 8.3 ± 0.3 preimplantation to 3.5 ± 0.4 (mean $\pm$ SEM) at latest follow-up ($P < .001$). Changes in vasomotor tone and patient activity levels were improved markedly but motor weakness and trophic changes were less improved. Six patients (20%) returned to part-time or full-time employment after being unemployed pre-stimulator. Initial involvement of more than one major peripheral nerve correlated with poor or no relief rating ($P < .01$).

In 1998, Calvillo and colleagues[33] reported their experience in 36 patients with advanced CRPS and treated with PNS and/or SCS. At 36 months after implantation, pain rating, using a visual analogue scale, was reduced by mean 53% and analgesic consumption reduced by 50%. Both changes were statistically significant. Of the 36 patients, 24 were treated with SCS alone, 7 with both SCS and PNS, and 5 with PNS alone.

In 2000, Ebel and colleagues[34] described six patients with CRPS who were treated with PNS with a mean follow-up of over 3 years. All patients reported good-to-excellent pain relief, defined as 75% or greater relief. These authors thought that PNS should be used in cases of mononeuropathic pain syndromes.

INDICATIONS

The best indication for peripheral nerve stimulation is where a single traumatized peripheral nerve constitutes the major source of pain.[35–37] The most common target nerves are the ulnar, median, posterior tibial, and common peroneal nerves. Less common are the radial, sciatic, and femoral nerves. This form of stimulation has also been shown to be effective for stump and phantom limb pain after amputation.[38] PNS has also been described in the treatment of severe CRPS (RSD).[2,3,20,21,29,33–34] Patients with CRPS symptoms and findings partly in the distribution of a *second* major peripheral nerve territory are more difficult to treat.

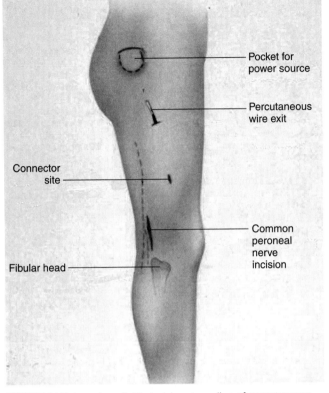

FIGURE 14-7 Location of skin incision, tunneling of percutaneous trialing wire, and power source for stimulation of common peroneal nerve.

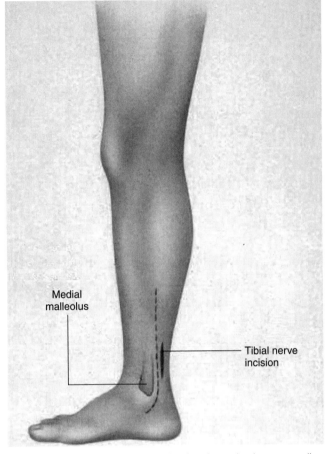

FIGURE 14-8 Location of skin incision for electrode placement adjacent to the tibial nerve.

RELATIVE ROLES OF SPINAL CORD STIMULATION AND PERIPHERAL NERVE STIMULATION

The relative roles of SCS and PNS in the treatment of patients with intractable peripheral nerve pain, especially from CRPS, remain unclear. Epidural electrode placement, especially using a percutaneously placed electrode, can result in delayed electrode movement and an inadequate stimulation pattern. With SCS, it can be difficult to match patterns of perceived electrical stimulation to some pain patterns, especially those involving only a specific part of the hand or foot. These same areas, on the other hand, often correlate well with the distribution of a major peripheral nerve and thus might favor peripheral nerve stimulation.

SCS, however, is much simpler to test with the percutaneous epidural placement of a catheter-type electrode. Severe RSD frequently will start at a focal point but then spread to involve other limbs and can become an almost systemic disease. SCS, since it provides more generalized coverage than PNS, could be more advantageous in severe RSD where symptoms have spread to other limbs. Aggressive treatment of the starting point, however, can provide permanent relief not only in the original limb but also in these secondary areas of involvement, although the mechanism for these distant effects is unclear.

CRITICAL ANALYSIS FOR USE AND FUTURE DIRECTIONS

Peripheral nerve stimulation has proven to be a good long-term treatment for patients with pain in the distribution of one major peripheral nerve. The best responses seem to be in those patients with CRPS; on an anecdotal basis the least successful seem to be those with pure sympathetic-independent ulnar neuropathy pain from multiple ulnar nerve operations at the elbow. On a technical level, improvements in electrode arrays that provide stimulation to opposing sides of a major peripheral nerve are needed for nerves such as the sciatic nerve and the posterior tibial nerve, where the peroneal and tibial nerves and the medial and lateral plantar nerves, respectively, are often already segregated in opposite halves of the nerve.

While it is difficult to do a "percutaneous trial" for PNS, there appears to be a high correlation between significant temporary pain relief with a peripheral nerve block and long-term PNS success. However, the real need in future research is a comparative study of spinal cord stimulation versus peripheral nerve stimulation for specific types of patients. At the present, the question still remains unclear about the relative roles of these two modalities.

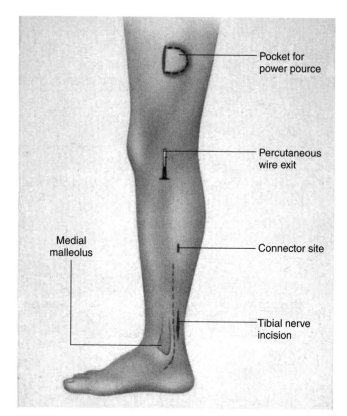

FIGURE 14-9 Location of skin incision, tunneling of percutaneous trialing wire, and power source for stimulation of tibial nerve.

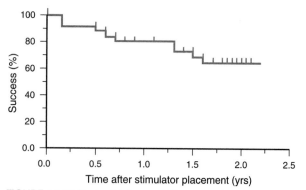

FIGURE 14-10 Kaplan-Meier graph illustrating long-term success rate in a series of patients undergoing peripheral nerve stimulation for the treatment of pain. Down-steps in the graph indicate times at which patients became treatment failures. Tick marks indicate times at which patients with good pain relief reached latest follow-up.

REFERENCES

1. Campbell JN, Long DM. Peripheral nerve stimulation in the treatment of intractable pain. J Neurosurg 45:692–699, 1976.
2. Long DM. Stimulation of the peripheral nervous system for pain control. Clin Neurosurg 31:323–343, 1983.
3. Law JD, Swett J, Kirsch WM. Retrospective analysis of 22 patients with chronic pain treated by peripheral nerve stimulation. J Neurosurg 52:482–485, 1980.
4. Picaza J, Hunter S, Cannon B. Pain suppression by peripheral nerve stimulation. Appl Neurophysiol 40:223–239, 1977.
5. Racz G, Lewis R, Heavner J, et al. Peripheral nerve stimulator implant for treatment of causalgia. In Stanton-Hicks M (ed). Pain and the Sympathetic Nervous System. Boston, Kluwer Academic, 1990, pp 225–239.
6. Campbell J, Long D. Peripheral nerve stimulation in the treatment of intractable pain. J Neurosurg 43:692–699, 1976.
7. Law J, Swett J, Kirsch W. Retrospective analysis of 22 patients with chronic pain treated by peripheral nerve stimulation. J Neurosurg 52:482–485, 1980.
8. Long DM, Erickson D, Campbell J, et al: Electrical of the spinal cord and peripheral nerves for pain control: a 10 year experience. Appl Neurophysiol 44:207–217, 1981.
9. Nashold B, Goldner J, Mullen J, et al. Long-term pain control by direct peripheral nerve stimulation. J Bone Joint Surg 64A:1–10, 1982.
10. Cauthen JC, Renner EJ. Transcutaneous and peripheral nerve stimulation for chronic pain states. Surg Neurol 4(1):102–104, 1975.
11. Clark K. Electrical stimulation of the nervous system for control of pain: University of Texas Southwestern Medical School experience. Surg Neurol 4(1):164–166, 1975.
12. Picaza JA, Cannon BW, Hunter SE, et al. Pain suppression by peripheral nerve stimulation. Part II. Observations with implanted devices. Surg Neurosurg 4(1):115–126, 1975.
13. Long DM. Electrical stimulation of the nervous system for pain control. Electroencephalog Clin Neurophysiol 34 (Suppl):343–348, 1978.
14. Nashold BS Jr, Mullen JB, Avery R. Peripheral nerve stimulation for pain relief using a multicontact electrode system. Technical note. J Neurosurg 51(6):872–873, 1979.
15. Long DM: Electrical stimulation for relief of pain from chronic nerve injury. J Neurosurg 39:718–722, 1973
16. Waisbrod H, Panhans C, Hansen D, Gerbershagen HU. Direct nerve stimulation for painful peripheral neuropathies. J Bone Joint Surgery [Br] 67:470–472, 1985
17. Law J, Swett J, Kirsch W. Retrospective analysis of 22 patients with chronic pain treated by peripheral nerve stimulation. J Neurosurg 52:482–485, 1980.
18. Nashold B, Goldner J, Mullen J, et al. Long-term pain control by direct peripheral-nerve stimulation. J Bone Joint Surg 64(A):1–10, 1982.
19. Racz GB, Browne T, Lewis R. Peripheral stimulator implant for treatment of causalgia caused by electrical burns. Tex Med 84:45–50, 1988.
20. Racz GB, Heavner JE. Comments on "A spiral nerve cuff electrode for peripheral nerve stimulation." IEEE Trans Bio Engin 36:1140–1141, 1989.
21. Racz GB, Lewis R, Heavner JE, et al. Peripheral nerve stimulator implant for treatment of causalgia. In Stanton-Hicks M, Jänig W, Boas RA (eds). Reflex Sympathetic Dystrophy. Norwell, MA, Kluwer Academic, 1990, pp 135–141.
22. Chung I, Lee K, Hori Y, et al. Factors influencing peripheral nerve stimulation produced inhibition of primate spinothalamic tract cells. Pain 19:277–293, 1984.
23. Chung J, Fang Z, Hory Y, et al. Prolonged inhibitor of primate spinothalamic tract cells by peripheral nerve stimulation. Pain 19:259–275, 1984.
24. Ignelzi R, Nyquist J. Excitability changes in peripheral nerve fibers after repetitive electrical stimulation: implications in pain modulations. J Neurosurg 51:824–833, 1979.
25. Campbell J, Taub A. Local analgesia from percutaneous electrical stimulation: a peripheral mechanism. Arch Neurol 28:347–350, 1973.
26. Wall P, Gutnick M. Ongoing activity in peripheral nerves: the physiology and pharmacology of impulses originating from a neuroma. Exp Neurol 43:580–593, 1974.
27. Meyerson B, Hakanson S. Alleviation of atypical trigeminal neuropathy by electric stimulation of the gasserian ganglion. Neurosurgery 1:59–66, 1986.
28. Campbell J, Taub A. Local analgesia from percutaneous electrical stimulation: a peripheral mechanism. Arch Neurol 28:347–350, 1973.
29. Racz GB, Lewis R, Heavner JE, et al. Peripheral nerve stimulator implant for treatment of causalgia. In Stanton-Hicks M (ed). Pain and the Sympathetic Nervous System. Norwell, MA, Kluwer Academic, 1990, pp 225–239.
30. Nam TX, Song SH, Kim YH, et al. Effect of peripheral nerve stimulation on the dorsal horn cell activity in cats with cutaneous inflammation. Yonsei Med J 33(2):109–120, 1992.
31. Urban BJ, Nashold BS Jr. Combined epidural and peripheral nerve stimulation for relief of pain: description of technique and preliminary results. J Neurosurg 57(3):365–369, 1982.

32. Hassenbusch SJ, Stanton-Hicks M, Schoppa D, et al. Long-term results of peripheral nerve stimulation of reflex sympathic dystrophy. J Neurosurg 84:415–423, 1996.

33. Calvillo O, Racz G, Didie J, et al. Neuroaugmentation in the treatment of complex regional pain syndrome of the upper extremity. Acta Orthop Belg 64(1):57–63, 1998.

34. Ebel H, Balogh A, Volz M, et al. Augmentative treatment of chronic deafferentation pain syndrome after peripheral nerve lesions. Minimally Invasive Neurosurg 43(1):44–50, 2000.

35. Shetter A, Racz G, Lewis R, et al. Peripheral nerve stimulation. *In* North R, Levy R (eds). Neurosurgical Management of Pain. New York, Springer-Verlag, 1997, pp 260–270.

36. Day M. Neuromodulation: Spinal cord and peripheral nerve stimulation. Curr Rev Pain 4:374–382, 2000.

37. Stanton-Hicks M, Salamon J. Stimulation of the central and peripheral nervous system for the control of pain. J Clin Neurophysiol 14(1):46–62, 1997.

38. Iacono RP, Linford J, Sandyk R. Pain management after lower extremity amputation. Neurosurgery 20(3):496–500, 1987.

C H A P T E R   1 5

Neuraxial Analgesic Administration

RICHARD D. PENN, MD

Intrathecal (IT) drug delivery for chronic pain should be thought of as a logical modification of systemic drug delivery. The intrathecal route has two main advantages: selective perfusion of central nervous system regions and avoidance of the blood-brain barrier. When combined with current implantable drug pump technology, a third major advance is constant drug delivery so levels of analgesia can be maintained. The major drawback is that a costly surgical procedure is involved, and patients and doctors are apprehensive about this approach. Very likely this situation will change over the next several years. The size of the drug pump will be greatly decreased. As electronic and mechanical microminiaturization techniques are applied, the current hockey puck size of the pump will shrink down to less than a quarter of the volume. If the pump reservoir is reengineered, its total space would be in the range of 20 to 30 cc. The result would be a pump size that could be readily implanted with an intrathecal catheter under local anesthesia. The operation would then become an outpatient procedure lasting 1 hour or less. Miniaturization and ease of insertion would decrease resistance to its use, and as use grows the cost per unit could be decreased. If this vision of future technical advances is correct, perhaps in 10 years, use of intrathecal medications will be seen as a simple and advantageous way to deliver medications to the nervous system and the indications for its use will greatly expand.

Another advance that is likely to occur in the next few years is the addition of patient-controlled activation (PCA) of drug delivery. Studies of postoperative pain management have clearly demonstrated that for most patients, PCA-delivered pain medicine reduces overall pain and also the amount of pain medication needed. Already a mechanical, somewhat inaccurate, implantable PCA device exists in Europe. Ideally, rather than this passive mechanical system, a handheld patient programmer could be added for the current programmable pump. Such a patient-controlled system would have limits on drug boluses and constant infusion set by the physician. Patients could learn from their own pain patterns when to give medication to avoid pain building up to high levels.

INDICATIONS

Presently, most physicians consider IT medication only when conventional oral narcotics, anticonvulsants, and antidepressants have failed or intolerable side effects have occurred. The difficult question to answer is how long does one try various oral medications before turning to another technique and what constitutes an unacceptable side effect. Oral narcotics are appropriately given for chronic pain and often work well at high dosage. However, subtle problems with cognition, alertness and mood may significantly impair many patients. When these patients are switched to IT medication and the oral medicines reduced or eliminated, they note improved mental function and less depression. Other selection criteria for intrathecal analgesic therapy include the presence of an identifiable organic etiology for the pain complaint that can not be changed by surgery, absence of significant psychological dysfunction, and a patent spinal canal.[1]

One guideline to be followed is that all patients should have a trial of IT morphine before permanent implantation of a drug pump.[1] If a patient does not get pain relief from an adequate trial of IT morphine then that patient is very unlikely to respond to a chronic infusion. Unfortunately, the converse is not always true. A positive response does not necessarily predict success with chronic infusion. In fact, depending on the study, one third to one fourth of responders to an initial trial will fail to get adequate pain relief at 12 to 18 months.[2,3] These patients may respond to other medications such as clonidine but other opiates are unlikely to be useful. Whether the loss of effect is due to true biologic tolerance or some other factors is unknown.

What type of pain responses best to IT morphine is unclear. The general maxim is that patients with chronic nociceptive pain do best and neuropathic pain is unresponsive. Clinical studies show that this is not the case. In the Winkelmuller's report, patients with neuropathic pain did as well as patients with nociceptive pain.[2] The problem may be that the classifications of pain do not provide enough clues about underlying mechanisms to predict response to a given pharmacologic agent such as morphine. The practical conclusion is that the category of pain is not as important as response to a trial of IT morphine. Many patients who could be helped will be missed if a classification of their pain as neuropathic is used to eliminate them from consideration of a trial. On the other hand, it makes little sense to treat central pain syndromes, such as post-thalamic stroke, by the intrathecal route. IT morphine will not reach areas where it is needed to have an effect. There are too few reports to know whether intraventricular infusion in such patients might be of value.

Some controversy exists about the approach to face, neck, and arm pain. IT morphine does reach the brainstem via the prepontine and ambient cisterns, and even though the concentration is reduced by three fourths from the lumbar region, it can still be very effective for facial pain.[4] Intraventricular infusion, at low dosages, may be as good or better because the periaqueductal gray region will be exposed to morphine.[5] No comparison of routes for facial pain has been done in the same study, so which technique is better is not known and local experience will vary.

INTRATHECAL MORPHINE TRIALS

As mentioned previously, before an implant it is essential to test each patient's response to morphine. Before conducting a trial, the patient's medical history and physical examination should be reviewed to confirm candidacy for IT analgesic therapy and to confirm the absence of contraindications to implantation. The nature of intraspinal drug infusion therapy, its role in pain management, and expected outcomes of treatment should be discussed thoroughly with the patient before the procedure. Patients should understand that the goal of therapy is not pain "cure" but rather pain "control." Unrealistic expectations undermine the success of the therapy and predispose to treatment failure. Patients should understand that pain may worsen (e.g., disease progression) or new pain problems may arise that might require additional treatment. These issues should be discussed before the trial because patients who are not interested in undergoing pump implantation should not undergo a trial.

A number of methods of "trialing" intrathecal analgesics have been used, including intrathecal or epidural administration, continuous or bolus administration, with or without a temporary catheter. Each approach has its own advantages and disadvantages.[1] The trialing method that most closely approximates long-term pump delivery of medication is using an intrathecal catheter going to an external pump. The dosage of IT morphine can be gradually increased over several days and the patient observed to see if oral narcotics decrease, pain score improves, and activities increase. Because the level of medication is slowly increased, the side effects of bolus administration such as vomiting, sedation, or urinary retention are less likely to occur. The drawback to the technique is the prolonged hospital stay and the chance of infection. A double bacteriostatic filter technique and tunneling the catheter may minimize the risk but not eliminate it.

A slightly less invasive trial technique is to use epidural placement of the catheter. Any bacterial contamination will be in the epidural space and meningitis is less likely. The dose of epidural morphine has to be 10 times higher than the intrathecal dose because only 10% of the epidural morphine is absorbed across the meninges; the rest goes into the systemic circulation. As with the IT catheter, continuous infusion via external pump obviates bolus doses so fewer side effects occur.

The final alternative for testing is a single bolus intrathecal dose given by lumbar puncture. This is simple, fast, and easy on the patient. If marked relief is found, this is the best method. The patient has to be warned about late side effects of bolus doses and must be observed for respiratory depression for 8 to 12 hours. However, if the patient is taking significant oral narcotics, respiratory problems are extremely rare, so under proper conditions the testing can be done on an outpatient basis. The pharmacokinetics of a bolus dose are totally different from slow continuous infusion, so estimates of an effective continuous dose are difficult to make and side effects may be exaggerated. Typically, in a patient who cannot tolerate oral narcotics because of side effects and takes only low oral doses, a $\frac{1}{4}$-mg IT bolus is safe and effective for a trial. For patients who are on high systemic doses of MS Contin® or similar potent narcotics, a 1-mg trial dose can be tried. If the patient fails to respond, the IT bolus can be doubled. Trials should be separated by at least 24 hours to avoid accumulation of drug effects. If a bolus is not effective, a catheter trial can be instituted. Because double-blind testing is not being done, the response to IT morphine should be unequivocally positive before a drug pump is implanted.

PREIMPLANT CONSIDERATIONS

If a patient meets selection criteria for implantation of an intrathecal drug administration system and has a successful response to a trial with intraspinal analgesics, pump implantation may be appropriate. Several issues should be addressed before implantation.[1] The type of infusion system to be implanted (e.g., fixed flow rate pump, programmable pump, pump size) should be determined according to the needs of the patient, the nature of available resources, and expertise of the implanting physicians and follow-up staff. The site of pump implantation should be determined well before the surgical procedure and discussed with the patient. The location of pump implantation in the abdomen may be influenced by physical characteristics such as surgical scars, colostomy, or obesity. Patient preferences for pump placement should be considered when planning the procedure (e.g., a patient who tends to sleep on the left side may want the pump implanted on the right side, automobile seatbelt use may alter pump implant site).

IMPLANTATION TECHNIQUE

The implantation technique has been described in detail.[6] Several points warrant special emphasis. Careful attention to detail is important during the implant procedure. Complications (e.g., infection) can be potentially serious and, at the very least, are costly and inconvenient to manage. Many complications of implantable drug delivery systems are related to procedural errors during implantation and can be eliminated by using careful technique.[7] Bypassing steps of the implantation procedure (e.g., catheter anchoring) to expedite system implantation can save a few minutes during the procedure but may predispose to later complications that are much more cumbersome to correct.

The infusion system may be implanted with the patient under general anesthesia, or using local anesthetic agents combined with sedation, which renders the procedure relatively safe even for medically infirm patients (e.g., late-stage cancer patients). Some implanters believe that catheter insertion is best performed with the patient awake. One approach to surgical anesthesia in awake patients is to implant the catheter under local anesthesia, then administer a spinal anesthetic through the catheter.

With the patient in the lateral decubitus position, skin is prepared with antiseptic solution and drapes are placed around the surgical sites. The Tuohy needle through which the catheter is inserted is passed into the intrathecal space at an appropriate spinal level, generally in the midlumbar region. The needle can be inserted at any level in the lumbar spine, but insertion at a midlumbar level may lessen stress placed on the catheter when the patient flexes and extends at the low back. Care should be taken that needle or catheter insertion at high lumbar levels does not injure the conus medullaris.

The needle can be inserted perpendicular to the spine, as would be done for a lumbar puncture, but a paramedian entry site with a shallow angle of approach to the spinal canal (e.g., 45 degrees) (Fig. 15-1) offers several advantages. Many physicians who implant infusion systems prefer to direct the catheter rostrally in the intrathecal space, and this is facilitated by use of a shallow-angle paramedian approach. Use of a shallow-angle paramedian approach eliminates the sharp bend the catheter would take as it exits the needle using a perpendicular approach, lessening the chance that it will be damaged or kinked at that site. Furthermore, the paramedian approach eliminates the chance that the catheter might be pinched (or fractured) between adjacent spinous processes when the patient extends at the lumbar spine, which causes compression of the spinous processes against each other. A study of catheter-related complications of intrathecal drug delivery systems revealed the highest incidence of catheter complications is associated with a straight midline insertion as opposed to paramedian insertion.[7]

For a paramedian approach, the entry site of the needle into skin is slightly lateral to the spinous processes (in approximately the same parasagittal plane as the pedicle when viewed on an anteroposterior fluoroscopic image), approximately one to two spinal levels below the interlaminar space through which the needle will be inserted. Under fluoroscopic guidance, the needle can be passed easily by aiming its tip at the base of the spinous process just above the intended interlaminar site of entry into the spinal canal. Insertion of the catheter under fluoroscopic guidance facilitates its passage in the appropriate direction and to the desired level. If the catheter must be removed for repositioning, it should not be withdrawn through the introducer needle. Withdrawal of the catheter through the needle may cause the catheter to be cut, with subsequent drug leakage at the site, or it may be sheared off completely, leaving a piece of catheter free-floating in the intrathecal or epidural space.

Catheters are placed typically in the intrathecal space but may be placed epidurally at the discretion of the implanting physician. Identification of the epidural space is accomplished using standard loss of resistance technique. Identification of the intrathecal space is confirmed typically by return of cerebrospinal fluid (CSF). If little or no CSF is returned, the patient can be placed in reverse Trendelenburg position to promote CSF accumulation in the lumbar space, or CSF may be obtained by gentle aspiration. If the catheter location cannot be ascertained, a small amount of contrast medium can be injected through the catheter to demonstrate its location. Only nonionic, low osmolar contrast medium should be injected. Intrathecal administration of ionic contrast medium has been associated with serious reactions, including seizures and death.

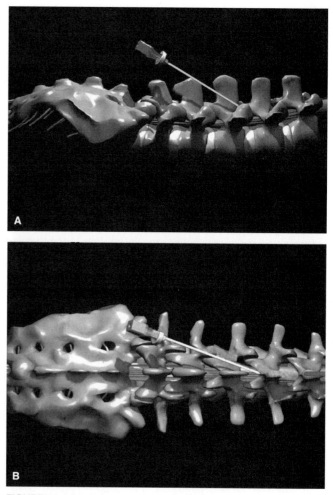

FIGURE 15-1 Paramedian approach to intrathecal catheter insertion. *A,* In the lateral projection, the needle insertion site into skin should be approximately one to two vertebral levels below the intended interlaminar puncture site. The angle of insertion should be approximately 45 degrees. *B,* In the anteroposterior projection, the needle insertion point into the skin should be approximately 1 to 2 cm off midline (overlying the pedicle as seen on a fluoroscopic image). The needle should be directed toward the midline in a trajectory that aims toward the base of the spinous process immediately above the intended interlaminar entry site.

Following insertion of the catheter, skin is incised rostral and caudal to the needle, centering the incision on the needle. The incision should extend down to the dorsal fascia or supraspinous ligament to provide a firm site for anchoring the catheter. An absorbable purse-string suture should be placed around the needle at its site of exit from the dorsal fascia and cinched down around the catheter gently after removal of the needle. This may reduce the likelihood of CSF hygroma but may increase the possibility of catheter obstruction. The catheter position can be monitored fluoroscopically during removal of the stylet and needle to ensure that the catheter is not dislodged.

An incision is made in the right or left subcostal region and a subcutaneous pocket is formed in which to place the pump. The incision should be in an area where the final location of the pump will minimize the likelihood that the device will hit the margin of the ribs rostrally or the iliac crest inferolaterally. In obese individuals, in whom skin folds may shift with changes in body position, the location of the pump pocket should be determined before surgery with the patient in a sitting or standing position. In slender individuals, the pocket can be formed immediately superficial to the external oblique fascia, and in very thin or small patients, the pump can be placed in a subfascial position. Such a placement requires more dissection and tissue damage, but helps lower the profile of the pump and is cosmetically better. In any case, the pocket should be formed no more than 1 to 2 cm below the skin surface. Deeper implantation complicates pump refilling because the access port cannot be located easily. The pump pocket should be large enough that the incision will not overlie the pump after skin closure and to minimize tension on the skin closure.

The catheter is passed around the flank from one incision to the other using a tunneling device. The pump is prepared for implantation (e.g., warming, purging, filling) according to manufacturer's recommendations. The catheter should be trimmed to appropriate length, if necessary (leaving sufficient length to coil a loop of catheter beneath the pump for "strain relief"). Flow of CSF from the catheter should be confirmed, and the catheter can be then connected to the pump. The length or volume of implanted catheter should be recorded in the patient's medical record for reference when calculating drug doses and infusion parameters. The pump is inserted into the subcutaneous pocket, taking care to place the refill port toward the skin surface, and secured to underlying tissues with nonabsorbable suture. Failure to secure the pump in its pocket can lead to pump rotation so that the access port faces inward, rendering refilling impossible. The catheter should be anchored at its site of exit from the dorsal lumbar fascia to prevent dislodgment, which is one of the most common causes of delivery system failure. Closure of the incision should be performed in multiple anatomic layers.

TYPES OF PUMPS AND CATHETER PLACEMENTS

Currently available pumps are either constant flow or programmable. The constant flow system has the advantages of simplicity and lower cost. However, in patients with pain who are likely to need frequent dose adjustments, the advantage of

programmability is considerable and makes patient management much easier. When a patient handheld programmer becomes available, the therapy will be greatly enhanced, and the programmability will be an even more desirable feature.

The catheter should be placed intrathecally, not epidurally, for several reasons: First and foremost is that most epidural medication (90% of morphine) is absorbed into the systemic circulation, with correspondingly greater likelihood of systemic side effects, so one of the key advantages of intraspinal medicine is lost. Intrathecal doses are approximately one tenth those required for epidural administration, which lessens the likelihood of systemic spread of drug (and reduces the likelihood of systemic side effects) and allows much longer intervals between pump refills. Intrathecal insertion is easier technically and catheter tip fibrosis may be less common, promoting better long-term function of the catheter. Finally, a number of water-soluble medications will not work in the epidural space because they cannot diffuse across the dura and meninges.

Controversy continues about what is the best position for the catheter tip. For water-soluble compounds such as morphine and hydromorphone, the distribution of medication along the spinal cord from a lumbar infusion site is adequate for most clinical situations. Arm and even facial pain can be treated by a lumbar intrathecal infusion. However, if a rapidly absorbed lipid-soluble agent is used (such as sufentanil), then the catheter tip must be near the site of action at the correct spinal cord level.

In general, anesthesiologists use a wider variety of medications and want the catheter to be at or near the dermatomal level of pain. Having medicine infused at the midthoracic region also decreases the total dose of medication needed and reduces symptoms from conus exposure to drug, such as bladder hypotonia. Other physicians prefer a lumbar position. Infusing the lumbar space has proven to be effective with morphine and it avoids very high local concentrations of medication in the narrow subarachnoid space in the thoracic region. A rare and dangerous complication of IT morphine infusion is the formation of a sterile granuloma at the catheter tip.[8–10] The reason for granuloma formation is not known, but high concentrations of morphine in a relatively limited area may have a role. With the catheter tip below the conus, granuloma formation may be less likely to occur and if it did it would create an equina lesion rather than direct and potentially irreversible cord damage.

Intraventricular placement of the catheter should be reserved for cases of facial pain not adequately responsive to IT morphine.[5] In these cases a reservoir alone can be used and it can be injected one to three times a day as needed. This is best for cancer pain in patients with a poor long-term prognosis. Use of a pump with an intraventicular catheter is more appropriate in patients who have a good long-term prognosis.

OUTCOMES

No large clinical trial of IT morphine for treatment of pain has been done in a blinded fashion. A randomized prospective study comparing comprehensive medical therapy (including oral narcotic agents) to intrathecal analgesic therapy for treatment of cancer pain confirms advantages of improved pain control and relief of side effects with intrathecal analgesics.[11] No randomized prospective study has been performed to evaluate the efficacy of intrathecal analgesics for noncancer pain. Historically the use of IT morphine grew out of short-term postoperative pain management and then extended treatment with external catheters. The first patients treated with an implanted pump had cancer and had failed to achieve acceptable pain relief with oral pain medications, and it was inappropriate to do comparison studies or withdraw IT morphine once it had been found to be clinically effective. When the pump was approved for IT delivery in pain patients, the drive to design blinded studies decreased. If the efficacy of IT morphine were marginal, the lack of controlled studies would be a problem. Fortunately, the studies that have been done in both cancer and noncancer patients are uniformly positive (Table 15-1).

Prospective studies as well as a large retrospective survey suggest that two-thirds to three fourths of patients will have significant sustained pain relief with IT morphine even though they failed on oral narcotics.[2,3] What is most surprising is that this holds true for both cancer-related and non–cancer-related pain. Also, neuropathic and nociceptive pain seem to respond equally well. The reason for this relatively high success rate may be that in all series, IT trials have been performed before implantation so a responsive patient population has been selected. In any case, the clinician can expect useful effects of IT morphine in a majority of implant patients, meaning that reported pain is lower, oral narcotics are decreased or stopped, and activities of daily living improve, all of which are the primary outcome measures of the reported series.

A number of important clinically relevant questions need further study. Foremost is how long IT morphine will be effective for patients with noncancer pain. Will tolerance develop in later years of treatment and will side effects eventually lead to failure? What is needed is a tracking system to follow patients for as long as they are treated to gradually accumulate data on these issues.

The current equipment available for implantation is satisfactory. The pumps have proven to be unusually reliable (less than 0.5% failure rate per year) and the improved catheters work moderately well (2% to 5% kink or dislodgment per year). New

● **TABLE 15-1** • Comments on Intrathecal Analgesia Research

References	Comments
Yaksh TL, Rudy TA. Analgesia mediated by a direct spinal action of narcotics. Science 192: 1357–1358, 1976	Early experimental paper showing effect of spinal opiates
Onofrio BM, Yaksh TL, Arnold PG. Continuous low-dose intrathecal morphine administration in the treatment of chronic pain of malignant origin. Mayo Clin Proc 56:516–520, 1981	One of the first articles on the use of an implanted pump
Penn RD, Paice JA. Chronic intrathecal morphine for intractable pain. J Neurosurg 67:182–186, 1987	Early series on intrathecal pumps for pain
Onofrio BM, Yaksh TL. Long-term pain relief produced by intrathecal morphine infusion in 53 patients. J Neurosurg 72:200–209, 1990	Another early study on intrathecal morphine
Hassenbusch SJ, Pillay PK, Magdinec M, Currie K, Bay JW, Covington EC, Tomaszewski MZ. Constant infusion of morphine for intractable cancer pain using an implanted pump. J Neurosurg 73:405–409, 1990	Another early study on intrathecal morphine
Penn RD, Paice JA. Chronic intrathecal morphine for intractable pain. J Neurosurg 67:182–186, 1987	Large retrospective survey on pumps for cancer and noncancer pain
Winkelmuller M, Winkelmuller W. Long-term effects of continuous intrathecal opioid treatment in chronic pain of nonmalignant etiology. J Neurosurg 85:458–467, 1996	Recent large retrospective series
Neuromodulation Special Issue: Intrathecal Therapy 2(2), April 1999	Reviews of IT therapy
Dougherty PM, Staats PS. Intrathecal drug therapy for chronic pain. Anesthesiology 91(6): 1891–1918, 1999	Excellent scientific review of new medications for intrathecal use (over 400 references)
Smith TJ, Staats PS, Deer T, et al. Randomized clinical trial of an implantantable drug delivery system compared with comprehensive medical management for refractory cancer pain: impact on pain, drug-related toxicity, and survival. J Clin Oncol 20(19):4040–4049, 2002	Randomized comparison of intrathecal analgesic therapy to medical management of cancer pain

improved catheters using materials other than silastic may solve some of the persistent catheter-related complications.

Chronic morphine, both systemic and IT, has a number of well-documented side effects. Neuroendocrine function is clearly affected. Most patients report a decreased libido, menses stop, and testosterone levels fall. A curious type of peripheral edema can occur which does not respond to diuretics. Occasionally, patients have myoclonic movements in their legs. Persistent nausea can be a problem. Sometimes switching to a different IT opiate may help with these side effects. Clearly, alternate medications are needed and a number of preclinical studies suggest that a wide variety of spinally active nonopiate medications can be developed in the future.[12]

The most dangerous aspects of giving medication via IT route are iatrogenic overdoses. Misprogramming, injections via the side port, and operating room medication errors can occur and have grave consequences. A large overdose of IT morphine (10 to 20 mg) leads to coma, respiratory suppression, hyperthermia, and potentially death. Less severe overdoses are relatively benign in most patients, resulting in drowsiness, sleep, and excellent pain relief.

A serious complication related to morphine delivery when the catheter tip is at the level of the spinal cord is the formation of a granuloma.[8–10] This initially causes increased pain, then progresses to motor and sensory loss and paralysis over time. The physician must be alert to this possibility and if unexplained increases in pain are reported, the patient needs to be examined for a new neurologic deficit. A granuloma can be easily detected with contrast-enhanced magnetic resonance imaging (MRI) and appropriate surgical measures taken. Because granulomas appear to be rare, routine MRI is not necessary.

An ever-present possibility with any implanted device is infection along the catheter. This usually requires removal of the system and a later reimplantation after antibiotic treatment. Meningitis is rare, because the pump reservoir outport has a bacteriostatic filter. If meningitis does occur due to seeding on the intrathecal portion of the catheter, it can be treated successfully by giving intrathecal antibiotics using the pump.

CONCLUSION

Using intrathecal medication for treating chronic pain is in its infancy. The equipment is likely to be improved to the point that a routine implant can be done as an outpatient. Many alternatives to morphine will become available and complicated polypharmacy will be used to maximize efficacy and deal with side effects. As this evolution occurs, the indications for IT pain therapy will broaden.

REFERENCES

1. Follett KA, Doleys DM. Selection of candidates for intrathecal drug administration to treat chronic pain: Considerations in pre-implantation trials. Medtronic, Inc. 2002.
2. Winkelmuller M, Winkelmuller W. Long term effect continuous intrathecal opioid treatment in chronic pain of nonmalignant etiology. J Neurosurg 85:458–467, 1996.
3. Penn RD, Paice JA. Chronic intrathecal morphine for intractable pain. J Neurosurg 67:182–186, 1987.
4. Andersen PE, Cohen JI, Everts EC, Bedder MD, Burchiel KJ. Intrathecal narcotics for relief of pain from head and neck cancer. Arch Otolaryngol Head Neck Surg 117(11):1277–1280, 1991.
5. Lazorthes YR, Sallerin BA, Verdie JC. Intracerebroventricular administration of morphine for control of irreducible cancer pain. Neurosurgery 37(3):422–428, 1995.
6. Fessler RG, Sekhar L: Placement of Morphine or Baclofen pumps: Atlas of Neurosurgical Techniques, Thieme.
7. Follett KA, Burchiel K, Deer T, DuPen S, Prager J, Turner MS, Coffey RJ. Prevention of intrathecal drug delivery catheter-related complications. Neuromodulation 6(1):32–41, 2003.
8. Blount JP, Remley KB, Yue SK, Erickson DL. Intrathecal granuloma complicating chronic spinal infusion of morphine. J Neurosurg 84:272–276, 1996.
9. Cabbell KL, Taren JA, Sagher O: Spinal cord compression by catheter granulomas in high-dose intrathecal morphine therapy: case report. Neurosurgery 45(5):1176–1181, 1998.
10. Hassenbusch S, Burchiel K, Coffet RJ, et al. Management of intrathecal catheter-tip inflammatory masses: a consensus statement. Pain Medicine 3(4):313–323, 2002.
11. Smith TJ, Staats PS, Deer T, et al. Randomized clinical trial of an implantantable drug delivery system compared with comprehensive medical management for refractory cancer pain: impact on pain, drug-related toxicity, and survival. J Clin Oncol 20(19):4040–4049, 2002.
12. Dougherty PM, Staats PS. Intrathecal drug therapy for chronic pain. Anesthesiology 91(6):1891–1918, 1999.

Intracranial Stimulation Therapies: Deep-Brain Stimulation

DONALD E. RICHARDSON, MD

Stimulation of the central nervous system to reduce pain was developed during the early 1970s following major advances in the understanding of pain pathways and the appreciation that artificial activation of specific areas in the nervous system could downregulate pain as demonstrated in the peripheral nerve by Wall and Sweet,[1] in the dorsal columns of the spinal cord by Shealey and colleagues,[2] and the demonstration of a central pain control system by Mayer and colleagues.[3]

Two major systems have been exploited for pain reduction in the central nervous system: one by Hosobuchi and colleagues[4] and the other by Akil and me.[5] These two systems will have to be discussed separately because they are based on two different mechanisms of pain modulation and have different indications and criteria for patient selection.

PHYSIOLOGY

Two systems in the central nervous system have been shown to reduce the perception of pain both in laboratory animals and in humans. The first is the large fiber or touch-proprioception system that originates in the dorsal root ganglion and ascends through the dorsal columns to synapse in the nucleus cuneatus and gracilis in the lower brainstem and ascend to the thalamus via the medial lemniscus to terminate in the posterior ventral medialis and lateralis nuclei of the thalamus. Activation of this system is analogous to electrical stimulation of the dorsal columns of the spinal cord. This system apparently has inhibitory influence on pain at each synapse in the pain pathway, producing pain reduction with what was originally called the pain gate described by Melzack and Wall.[6] Electrical stimulation of this system at multiple levels has been shown to reduce pain perception. Artificial activation of the touch-proprioception system in the brain produces contralateral paresthesia, resembling the paresthesia produced by dorsal column stimulation, and produces similar reduction in pain.

The other system that has been used for pain reduction is the endogenous opiate system, which originates in the basal hypothalamus with projection of its beta-endorphin–containing axons through the periventricular gray matter adjacent to the third ventricle to terminate in the periaqueductal gray matter, including the raphe nuclear complex and the locus ceruleus. Serotonin from the raphe nuclei, and norepinergic fibers from the locus ceruleus descend through the dorsolateral fasciculus of the spinal cord to impinge on dorsal horn cells, either directly or through an intermediate opiate neuron to inhibit pain input at the pain pathway's first synapse. Thus, electrical activation of this system produces a downregulation of noxious input to the central nervous system, although there is some evidence of effect on pain transmission at higher synaptic levels based only on clinical results.

INDICATIONS

Selection of patients for analgesic deep-brain stimulation depends on two factors: first, the location of the patient's pain, which would necessitate the stimulation of the brain itself rather than a peripheral nerve or the spinal cord; and second, the etiology of the pain.

Thus, deep-brain stimulation is primarily used for pain involving the head, neck, and cranial nerves, or pain generated within the central nervous system secondary to damage to the brain or spinal cord that is not accessible for stimulation of peripheral nerves or spinal cord. The most common indications arising from the central nervous system are central pain states such as post-traumatic brain injury, post-stroke pain, thalamic syndrome or pseudothalamic syndromes, and postoperative central pain states involving the face and neck but also including the arm, trunk, and leg.

In addition to this, pain generated in the cranial nerve sensory distribution, including anesthesia dolorosa following fifth cranial nerve section or injury; intractable dental pain; post-traumatic head and neck pain; craniocervical junction pain, such as rheumatoid arthritis; and postherpetic head and face pain, may respond to intracranial electrical stimulation.

TARGET SELECTION

Target selection is based primarily on the type of pain. The deafferentation pains, anesthesia dolorosa and post-stroke pain, are best treated by stimulation of the central nuclei of the thalamus or internal capsule.

The opiate system is usually more effective for somatically generated pain, such as temporomandibular joint pain, rheumatoid arthritic pain of the high cervical spine, postoperative pain, and mechanical pain involving the head, neck, and face. In addition, it produces bilateral pain reduction but is less effective for ipsilateral pain; the electrode should be placed on the contralateral side of the more severe pain or, if the sides are of equal intensity, on the nondominant side. Ventral posterior lateralis (VPL) and ventral posterior medialis (VPM) stimulation is limited to contralateral pain entirely.

Preoperative Preparation

It is our policy to completely withdraw patients for any type of deep brain electrode implantation from all opiate narcotics and all benzodiazepines before surgery and to have psychological testing, psychiatric evaluation, and treatment of associated emotional problems, such as depression, before surgery. We found in our early studies that external opiates will produce downregulation of the endogenous opiate system and prevent it from being adequately activated by electrical stimulation. It requires approximately 10 to 14 days for the endogenous opiate system to resume normal activity following withdrawal from long-term external opiate treatment. Therefore, we require all patients to be completely withdrawn from opiates for two weeks before surgery.[7]

Premedication with a small amount of diazepam 5 to 10 mg or promethazine 25 to 50 mg preoperatively is usually quite enough sedation for application of the stereotaxic frame and will be worn off by the time test stimulation is carried out and obviates narcotic use. If this is inadequate, intravenous propofol can be useful, but seems to have a long-lasting sedative effect. While opiate use is not as critical in stimulation of the main sensory nucleus of the thalamus, we found that patients taking large doses of opiates respond poorly to stimulation and require stimulation parameters so high that they cannot tolerate the side effects from activation of adjacent neural structures. Therefore, we follow the same detoxification procedure for anticipated sensory thalamus electrode implantation as we do for periventricular implantation.

Surgical Technique

Regardless of target site, stereotaxic head frame placement and bur hole placement are the same. The incision is made paramedian 2 to 2.5 cm lateral to the sagittal suture line (midline) and at the coronal suture line after infiltration of the scalp with local anesthetic. The bur hole is made to match the electrode locking plug provided with the electrode (Medtronic DBS Electrode Kit no. 3387-40 or no. 3389-40).[8] The dura is opened in a cruciate fashion and coagulated to make it retract and control bleeding. The cortex is coagulated and the pia mater punctured at the electrode entry site. The target area is explored with a 1 mm or smaller diameter (Radionics) ridgid electrode and test stimulation carried out.[9]

Periventricular Gray

The simplest target for placement of the deep-brain electrode is the periventricular opiate system, which is anatomically easily identified on magnetic resonance imaging (MRI) or ventriculography.

Studies carried out by myself and others indicated that stimulation of the raphe nuclear system itself produces a large number of side effects, such as severe oscillopsia from stimulation of the adjacent medial longitudinal fasciculus and a feeling of smothering or oppressiveness similar to the epigastric rising syndrome from stimulation of unknown structures in the upper brainstem. In addition to this, misplacement of electrodes posterior to the aqueduct can produce noxious side effects. Therefore, stimulation of the tract itself in the periventricular gray matter adjacent to the wall of the third ventricle is preferable. The target site is actually quite large and not difficult to approach.

The periventricular opiate system target site using the Schaltenbrand and Bailey[10] coordinate system is posterior 10 mm (from center of the anterior to posterior commissurae [ac-pc] line), lateral 4 to 5 mm (from midline), and height 0 (tip on ac-pc line) or 2 to 3 mm anterior to the posterior commissure with the tip level with the commissure if a good ac-pc line cannot be constructed on the MRI (Fig. 16-1).

Test stimulation is then carried out usually using a 250-msec pulse width, 20 to 30 hertz, up to 8 volts, or less than 10 mA. It is important to question the patient before stimulation and compare pre- and post-stimulation response. It is not uncommon for patients to have little or no pain before stimulation because the so-called "acupuncture effect" from applying the stereotaxic frame may result in significant temporary pain reduction. Manipulation or other types of stimulation of the patient's painful area may be necessary to produce enough discomfort to allow adequate testing.

A report of pain reduction and/or side effects including a feeling of warmth or coolness of the face or cheek indicates the electrode is in the proper location. Oscillopsia, which may be manifested by complaints of blurred vision, can be seen on close observation or a feeling of smothering indicates that the

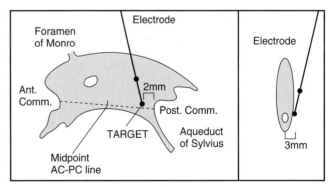

FIGURE 16-1 Target location for stimulation of the periventricular opiate system adjacent to the lateral wall of the third ventricle. The target is 10 mm posterior to the midcommissural point, or approximately 2–3 mm anterior to the posterior commissure, 4–5 mm lateral to the midline, with the electrode tip at the level of the ACPC line.

electrode is too deep (inferior). Paresthesias from stimulation are not produced by stimulation of this area and cannot be used to select the electrode placement site. Sensory paresthesia at low current levels of stimulation may indicate that the electrode may be placed too far lateral.

If good pain relief is obtained in the operating room, the electrode is locked in place for later internalization. If inadequate pain relief is obtained in the operating room, it has been our experience that no pain relief will be obtained by leaving an electrode in place for further postoperative testing unless the patient has become confused or sedated enough to interfere with adequate responses in the operating room. The results of testing in the operating room usually, quite accurately, predict the results from long-term stimulation. If inadequate results are obtained in the periaqueductal gray matter, moving on to test the VPL/VPM area is probably the next best choice.

Internal Capsule and Thalamic Sensory Nuclei Stimulation

Usually, stimulation of the main sensory nuclei in the thalamus requires more technical ingenuity and requires more extensive testing than does periventricular stimulation. Obviously, stimulation for face pain would involve stimulation of the VPM nucleus. However, in our experience and that of Hosobuchi, placement of electrodes in the sensory nuclei has produced a very localized but intense area of numbness of the hand or face due to a small lesion produced by the mechanical trauma of electrode insertion (Y. Hosobuchi, personal communication, 1976). This can be avoided by using stimulation of the internal capsule adjacent to the sensory thalamus, thus more laterally placing the electrode.

The new Medtronic (model nos. M3387 and 3389-40) DBS electrodes have a smooth exterior and a rounded tip and tend to produce less of a lesion effect than older electrodes, which required a dual insertion tool and were more likely to produce a small lesion at the time of insertion.[9] Stimulation initially for face pain would be carried out in the VPM at coordinates frontal posterior −5 to −15 mm (from midpoint of ac-pc line), lateral 12 to 18 mm (from midline), height +10 to −5 (from ac-pc line). Adjustment of the electrode position is based on the patient's response to stimulation of sensory paresthesia in the area of his or her pain. Using the Emmers and Tasker atlas[11] of the thalamus as a guide can be quite helpful, but may be difficult because it does not match the Schaltenbrand and Bailey atlas. When stimulation produces paresthesia at low voltage in the area of the patient's pain without unpleasant side effect and pain relief, the electrode is locked in place (Fig. 16-2).

Postoperative Stimulation

We found that after implantation of a deep-brain electrode, stimulation is not effective for approximately 3 to 5 days following surgery, theoretically secondary to the edema surrounding the electrode contacts and insulating it from the tissues to be activated. If adequate pain relief is obtained, internalization of the system with the Medtronic Soletra (model no. 7426) pulse generator and extension (model no. 7495)[9] is carried out. We place the connector between the

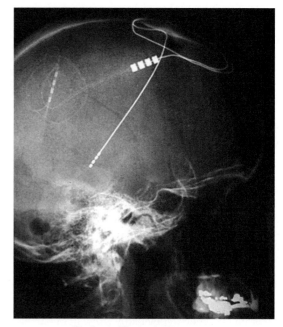

Thalamic Electrode Placement

FIGURE 16-2 Lateral skull radiograph illustrating the trajectory and location of a deep brain stimulation electrode placed in the thalamus. Also shown is a percutaneous trialing wire, connected to the implanted electrode and brought out through a separate stab incision posterior to the electrode implant site.

extension and electrode in a burred grove behind the mastoid air cells to prevent migration of the connector. The pulse generator is placed in a pocket below the clavicle and sutured to the pectoralis fascia. Care must be taken to tunnel the extension superficial to the clavicle because the brachial artery and vein and the brachial plexus are deep to the clavicle and can be easily injured.

Chronic Stimulation

Approximately 1 week following electrode implantation, testing can be started with stimulation of the target nucleus. We have found that low-frequency stimulation of the periventricular gray matter is much more effective than high-frequency stimulation; our stimulation parameters are usually between 15 and 30 Hz and at a 3- to 6-volt level with pulse durations of 250 msec. Intermittent stimulation is preferable, allowing the tissue to recover between periods of stimulation. Overstimulation in some patients has resulted in apparent fatigue of the tissue in this area and loss of effectiveness, requiring discontinuation of stimulation for 10 to 14 days to allow recovery and recapture effective pain relief. Our usual periventricular gray (PVG) stimulation is for 10 to 30 minutes of stimulation two to four times a day, which seems to be the optimum amount required. Activation of this area seems to produce a new "set point" for its activity because discontinuation of stimulation (after use for several months) requires 10 to 14 days for the pain to return to the original severity.[7] We do not allow patients to self-adjust their own stimulation voltage or parameters.

Initially L-tryptophan was used as an adjunct in stimulation of the periventricular gray matter in an attempt to increase serotonin production but it is no longer commercially available in the United States. We have found that patients over a long time do benefit from a low dose of tricyclic antidepressant such as amitriptyline at 25 to 50 mg a day to enhance activation of the periventricular gray matter.

Stimulation of the sensory nucleus or internal capsule is much more obvious and is titrated much like that with patients with spinal cord stimulation. The patient can be allowed to adjust the stimulation to his or her needs using an external voltage control device to increase stimulation when they are active and decrease stimulation when their pain is less severe. We found that it is unwise to allow patients to control pulse frequency or pulse width of stimulation because they usually will become confused and use a poor combination of parameters, tend to overstimulate, and have to be retuned after a period of rest from stimulation.

The usual parameters for sensory nucleus stimulation are lower than for periventricular stimulation and are based on threshold or perception of paresthesia and pain relief. Obviously, the contacts that produce the best stimulation in the area of the patient's pain are used. We found that the concomitant use of narcotics with deep-brain stimulation either in the periventricular area or in the internal capsule/sensory thalamus reduces the effectiveness of stimulation and we consider them contraindicated.

Complications and Side Effects

One of more obvious theoretical complications of deep brain stimulation is postoperative infection with the possibility of secondary brain abscess formation. In our hands, this has been extremely rare and in over 200 patients with deep-brain simulators in place we have had no postoperative infections and only two patients who had late infections secondary to lacerations over their electrode wiring or over the lock-down button in the bur hole. Weakness and numbness immediately following surgery is usually transient secondary to electrode placement and resolves in a few weeks. Permanent numbness secondary to thalamic nucleus damage from electrode placement was present in approximately five patients who had initial insertions with the old loop-type pull-down electrode that produced small lesions in the thalamic nuclei during insertion. This has not been seen once with the newly designed electrodes. Placement of the electrode inside the third ventricle (intraventricular electrode placement) occurred in two electrodes, one of which apparently lay against the wall of the third ventricle and good stimulation was obtained; but in the other, the electrode had to be replaced.

We had two patients who had a postoperative stroke following electrode implantation: one secondary to cortical vessel coagulation at the cortical penetration site and the other in a patient who had severe cerebral arteriosclerosis and a massive stroke on the contralateral side of the brain 3 days after electrode implantation.

Long-term Effectiveness

In our hands, 82% of patients operated on with deep-brain stimulation had initial pain relief, and in 18%, adequate stimulation could not be attained to relieve the patient's pain, either because of brain damage interfering with adequate placement or other factors not understood at the time of surgery, including poor relief despite adequate stimulation. Eighty percent of the patients had significant pain relief in the hospital; at the end of 1 year, 66% of the patients had effective pain relief. Our long-term studies reveal that the effectiveness of stimulation is maintained at approximately 60%.[12] This result is comparable to the results of Kumar and colleagues, who reported 77% good results initially and over time but had 15% screened out by initial testing.[13] Levy and colleagues reported less effectiveness initially (59%) as well as further reduction to 31% good results after 80 months.[14] We all have had poor results with paraplegic pain and anesthesia dolorosa. This may be complicated by the fact that some patients initially had trigeminal surgery for atypical face pain, not true trigeminal neuralgia. Deep-brain stimulation is contraindicated in atypical face pain because it does not respond to VPM or PVG activation.

We are in the process of a long-term follow-up study at this time.

REFERENCES

1. Wall PD, Sweet WH. Temporary abolition of pain in man. Science 155:108–109, 1967.
2. Shealy CN, Mortimer JT, Hagfors NR. Dorsal column electroanalgesia. J Neurosurg 32:560–564, 1970.
3. Mayer DJ, Wolfe TL, Akil H, et al. Analgesia resulting from electrical stimulation in the brain stem of the rat. Science 74:1351–1354, 1971.
4. Hosobuchi Y, Adams JE, Rutken B. Chronic thalamic stimulation for the relief of facial anesthesia dolorosa. Arch Neurol 9:158–161, 1973.
5. Richardson DE, Akil H. Pain reduction by electrical brain stimulation in man. Part II: Chronic self-administration in periventricular gray matter. J Neurosurg 47:184–194, 1977.
6. Melzack R, Wall PD. Pain mechanisms: a new theory. Science 150:971–979, 1965.
7. Richardson DE. Deep brain stimulation for the relief of chronic pain. Neurosurg Clin North Am 6(1):135–144, 1995.
8. Medtronic Neurological, 800 53rd Ave NE, Minneapolis, MN 55421-1200,USA.
9. Radionics Inc., 22 Terry Ave., Burlington, Massachusetts 01803-0738, USA.
10. Schaltenbrand G, Bailey P. Introduction to Stereotaxis with an Atlas of the Human Brain. New York, George Thieme Verlag, Grune and Stratton, New York USA, Vol, I, II, and III, 1959.
11. Emmers R, Tasker RR. The human somesthetic thalamus. New York, Raven, 1975, pp 1–111.
12. Richardson DE, Akil H. Long term results of periventricular gray self-stimulation. Neurosurgery 1:199–202, 1977.
13. Kumar K, Toth C, Nath RK. Deep brain stimulation for intractable pain: 15-year experience. Neurosurgery 40:736–746, 1997.
14. Levy RM, Lamb S, Adams JE. Treatment of chronic pain by deep brain stimulation: long term follow-up and review of the literature. Neurosurgery 21:885–893, 1987.

Motor Cortex Stimulation for the Treatment of Neuropathic Pain Syndromes

JEFFREY A. BROWN, MD

The development of the cortical stimulation technique is interwoven with the efforts of generations of neurosurgeons to treat chronic pain.

In the first of their classic books, White and Sweet reviewed early efforts at treatment of central pain by postcentral gyrectomy. In 1955, their review indicated that the failure rate was unacceptably high. Later, they reported on the treatment of 38 patients with central pain by postcentral gyrus removal. Although 30 of 38 patients had initial relief, 1 year after surgery only 5 of 38 continued to experience pain relief.[1] In 1971, Lende and colleagues proposed resection of the pre- and postcentral cortex for the treatment of intractable facial pain.[2] In their discussion, Lende and colleagues noted that Penfield and Jasper had elicited sensory responses upon stimulation of the precentral gyrus after removal of the corresponding portion of the adjacent postcentral gyrus. Their observations provided evidence that both the pre- and postcentral gyri are involved in the pathways that lead to the perception of neuropathic pain. Lende and colleagues treated one patient with a pontine infarct and neuropathic pain and another with postsurgical trigeminal neuropathic pain. Their follow-up periods were 20 and 30 months, respectively. In 1979, Woolsey and colleagues reviewed their treatment of two patients with phantom limb pain. In one patient, phantom pain was elicited upon stimulation of the supplementary sensory leg area. Surgical removal of this area had the immediate effect of eliminating the phantom pain. Long-term follow-up was not available.[3] Then, in 1983, Andy found that electrical stimulation of the thalamus was effective for the treatment of chronic intractable central pain of various causes.[4] Thalamic recordings revealed spontaneous focal electrical discharge patterns with low activation thresholds. By locating the optimum thalamic discharge site, the site for electrode implantation was selected for chronic stimulation. The thalamic sites that most frequently displayed the low threshold spontaneous focal discharge activity were the CM-Pf complex and related intralaminar nuclear structures. Andy hypothesized that diencephalic reverberating circuits caused pain. The applied electrical stimulation, he postulated, blocked low threshold

discharging systems.[4] Soon afterward, Hosobuchi implanted electrodes for dysesthetic chronic pain in the subcortical somatosensory region of 44 patients.[5] He reported successful pain control. Nineteen patients with dysesthetic leg pain received relief from somatosensory region stimulation.[5]

This background laid the groundwork for early work on cortical stimulation by Tsubokawa and colleagues.[6] They studied cats that had thalamic burst activity associated with deafferentation of the spinothalamic pathway. They sought a nonablative and less invasive approach to deafferentative pain than thalamic stimulation, a technique associated with significant risk of morbidity. They discovered that stimulation of the motor cortex also inhibited the thalamic burst activity. Tsubokawa and colleagues then treated seven patients with thalamic pain by chronic motor cortex stimulation using epidural plate electrodes. Excellent or good pain control was obtained in all cases. There were no documented complications or side effects. During the stimulation, regional cerebral blood flow increased to both the cortex and thalamus. Temperature in the painful skin regions increased, and there was better movement observed in the painful limbs.[6]

Two years later, Tsubokawa and colleagues elaborated on these results in a second publication.[7] Eight patients achieved excellent pain control during a 1-week test period of precentral gyrus stimulation. No benefit was observed or pain exacerbated by postcentral gyrus stimulation. The effect of precentral stimulation was unchanged in five patients (45%) during follow-up of more than 2 years. In the remaining three patients, the effect decreased gradually over several months. Pain inhibition usually occurred at intensities below the threshold for muscle contraction (pulse duration 0.1 to 0.5 msec, intensity 3 to 8 V). When pain was well controlled, the patients reported a slight tingling or mild vibration sensation during stimulation that was projected to the same area of distribution as their pain. Neither observable nor electroencephalographic seizure activity developed in these patients.[7]

From 1994 to 1997, a number of small clinical series were published reviewing the results of treatment by cortical stimulation. These studies began the development of the surgical indications for the procedure. Meyerson and colleagues emphasized that motor cortex stimulation was helpful in trigeminal neuropathy.[8] Perhaps this is because of the large area of motor cortex facial representation, making it easier to position an electrode over the appropriate site. In his series, five patients with trigeminal neuropathy had definite pain relief ranging from 60% to 90%. However, many of his patients had generalized seizures during test stimulation. None had any motor deficits after permanent implantation.[8] Katayama and colleagues extended the benefits of stimulation to patients with lateral medullary infarction. Two of their three patients reported satisfactory pain control. Pain inhibition usually occurred at intensities below the threshold for the production of muscle contraction (pulse duration, 0.1 to 0.5 msec; intensity, 3 to 8 V).[9] Migita and colleagues reviewed treatment results on a patient with neuropathic pain that extended throughout the contralateral side of his body 2 years after a putaminal hemorrhage.[10]

Magnetic coil stimulation predicted the beneficial effects of cortical stimulation. Ebel and colleagues reviewed their results from treatment of six patients using cortical stimulation for trigeminal neuropathic pain syndromes such as anesthesia dolorosa and postherpetic neuralgia.[11] In three of the six patients, good-to-excellent pain control (as measured by visual analogue scale score reduction of more than 50%) was maintained for a follow-up period of 5 months to 2 years. In the remaining three patients, the positive effect decreased over several months. In another case, a prolonged focal seizure resulting in a postictal speech arrest occurred during test stimulation. The pain inhibition appeared below the threshold for producing motor effects.[11] Rainov and colleagues treated one patient with trigeminal and a second with glossopharyngeal neuralgia.[12] Motor cortex stimulation produced long-term reduction in facial pain. It was possible to induce paresthesias and muscle movement not only contralateral to the stimulated motor cortex, but also in the ipsilateral part of the face. No stimulator-independent pain reduction resulted from long-term use of the stimulation device. During an 18-month follow-up period, a stable analgesic effect occurred. One major complication during the follow-up period was a single generalized epileptic seizure in one of the patients.[12]

Nguyen and colleagues published the first large series of patients with well-documented long-term follow-up.[13] They treated 20 patients with deafferentation pain. The central fissure was localized using stereotactic magnetic resonance imaging and the motor cortex was mapped using intraoperative somatosensory evoked potentials. Their best results were in seven patients with trigeminal neuropathic pain. These patients had definite pain relief varying between 40% and 100%. In 10 patients with central pain, a satisfactory long-lasting pain control (pain relief >40%) was obtained in 50% of cases. One patient with pain from peripheral nerve injury obtained more than 80% pain relief. Two patients had pain from spinal cord lesions. One did not respond but the other obtained an excellent long-term result. The location of the effective stimulation plots was in agreement with the somatotopic maps of the primary motor cortex. A small extradural hematoma developed in one patient and resolved spontaneously. Seizures did not occur in any of the patients. This study confirmed the value of motor cortex stimulation. It also confirmed the value of stimulation in patients with trigeminal

neuropathic pain. The next year, 1998, Katayama and colleagues reviewed their treatment of 31 patients by cortical stimulation.[14] In 48%, there was excellent or good pain control (pain reduction >60%) with follow-up of more than 2 years. Pain relief was satisfactory in 73% of patients who had mild or absent motor weakness. When motor weakness was present and moderate to severe, only 15% of the 13 patients had pain relief. When motor contractions could not be induced, only 9% of patients ($P < .01$) achieved pain relief. The authors concluded that an intact corticospinal tract neuronal system originating from the motor cortex was necessary for effective pain relief.[14]

Technical innovation has simplified the surgery. With use of neuronavigation, Krombach and colleagues identified the precentral gyrus in 23 of 23 cases in combination with somatosensory evoked potentials to identify the central sulcus using phase reversal.[15] Nguyen and colleagues also altered their technique to make use of computer-assisted imaging techniques.[13]

Using neuronavigation to facilitate location of the best site for electrode implantation, Nguyen and colleagues treated 12 patients with neuropathic facial pain.[16] Ten patients had substantial pain relief (75%). Ten of 13 patients with central pain (77%) had pain relief. The mean follow-up of these patients was longer than that in other series (27 months). Other conditions successfully treated included brachial plexus avulsion, intercostal herpes zoster, and postparaplegic pain. Nguyen and colleagues concluded that neuronavigational landmarks correlated reliably with electrophysiologic/clinical localization of the appropriate portion of the motor gyrus.[16] Bezard and colleagues, working with Nguyen and Keravel, studied the effect of cortical stimulation in three normal monkeys.[17] Using frequency and pulse duration of 40 Hz and 90 microseconds and intensity set just below the threshold for inducing muscle twitch, seizures were not induced. Increasing the stimulus intensity did induce reversible epileptic seizures; however, the threshold for this did not change even after seizures were induced.[17]

Two groups investigated the physiologic effects of stimulation on cerebral blood flow. Peyron and colleagues discussed the results from treating one patient who had a parietal infarct sparing the thalamus and a second with a mesencephalic infarction. The patient with a mesencephalic infarction and lower limb pain only benefited for 2 months. Cerebral blood flow studies with a positron emission tomography scan revealed increased flow in the ipsilateral thalamus, cingulate gyrus, orbitofrontal cortex, and brainstem. Blood flow was greater in the thalamus and brainstem in the patient with long-lasting pain relief.[18] Peyron and colleagues concluded that an intact somatosensory system is not needed for benefit to occur from cortical stimulation. Garcia-Larrea and colleagues found significant increase in regional cerebral blood flow in the lateral thalamus ipsilateral to cortical stimulation.[18] This region reflects projection from corticothalamic connections of the motor or premotor area. The blood flow increases were present, but were less evident in the anterior cingulate, insula, and upper brainstem. There was an increase in anterior cingulate regional cerebral blood flow when cortical stimulation provided good analgesia. They concluded that it is possible that stimulation influences the affective component of chronic pain through cingulate gyrus activation. Stimulation may also reduce pain by activating the brainstem periaqueductal gray area.[18] In a later paper, Garcia-Larrea and colleagues studied cerebral blood flow changes during precentral gyrus stimulation in 10 patients using positron emission tomography.[19] The most significant increases were in the ventral-lateral thalamus, but were also seen in the medial thalamus, anterior cingulate/orbitofrontal cortex, anterior insula, and upper brainstem. There were no changes in the motor regions below the stimulating electrode. Somatosensory evoked potentials did not change. They concluded that thalamic nuclei connected with motor and premotor cortex are activated by stimulation. A cascade of events in pain structures that receive afferent input from the medial thalamus, anterior cingulate, and upper brainstem then ensues. By this cingulate/orbitofrontal activation the affective component of chronic pain is modified. Brainstem descending inhibition of pain impulses, associated with attenuation of spinal reflexes, also occurs. There was no evidence that the somatosensory cortex was activated by motor cortex stimulation.[19]

There are other effects from cortical stimulation. Nguyen and colleagues treated a patient with facial pain and left arm tremor that had developed after surgical resection of an acoustic neuroma. With motor cortex stimulation, there was excellent pain relief and the tremor resolved. Adjustment of the stimulation parameters varied the benefits on both the pain and tremor. The tremor may have improved because of inhibition of subcortical structures.[20] One odd effect of stimulation was reported by Canavero, who described, in a case report, the onset of a supernumerary phantom arm during motor cortex stimulation for central pain that was a consequence of a thalamocapsular stroke.[21]

INDICATIONS

In summary, motor cortex stimulation is indicated for treatment of intractable neuropathic pain that has failed to respond to medical therapy. In neuropathic pain there is usually a delay in onset after a precipitating injury. Pain is often in the region of a sensory deficit and consists of dysesthesias (odd feelings) and paresthesias (paroxysmal shooting or stabbing pain). There is also allodynia (whereby mild stimuli are painful). Neuropathic pain is hypothesized to occur because of primary afferent or central nervous system nociceptive hypersensitivity along with a loss of central inhibitory mechanisms associated with deafferentation. Some conditions that lead to neuropathic pain include stroke, cranial nerve injury, brachial plexus avulsion, spinal cord injury, and herpes zoster infection. The most common successful application is for neuropathic facial pain, probably because of the large representation of the facial structures on the motor cortex, which makes targeting of the electrode position easier.

PREOPERATIVE EVALUATION

Patients must be candidates for general anesthesia. Because of the lengthy screening process that is done before implantation, these patients must be able to adequately communicate with healthcare personnel regarding the effectiveness of the

changes in stimulation parameters. The electrodes available are Federal Drug Administration approved for other spinal pain applications. This use represents an "off-label" application in the United States. During the initial evaluation, it is helpful to judge the nature of the patient's pain with a number of written evaluation tools. These include the McGill Pain Questionnaire and the visual analogue scale.

OPERATIVE TECHNIQUE

Before surgery, fiducial markers are fixed to the scalp on the opposite side to the site of pain encircling the expected target. A magnetic resonance image is obtained using 1-mm cuts. The data are transmitted to a neuronavigational computer workstation and the central sulcus is outlined on multiple sections. This simplifies its identification when viewing sagittal magnetic resonance images. For facial pain, the empirical target is located on the motor cortex at the level of the inferior frontal sulcus (Fig. 17-1).

Electrodes are positioned on the patient for intraoperative contralateral median nerve somatosensory evoked potentials and facial electromyographs (EMGs).

General anesthesia is induced and the patient is positioned either in a full lateral position or supine, a roll beneath the shoulder and head rotated. After induction, muscle relaxants are discontinued so that muscle movement can be monitored in response to intraoperative stimulation. Using neuronavigational guidance, the target and central sulcus are mapped onto the scalp. A linear incision or flap should be designed along the central sulcus long enough to allow a circular craniotomy opening with an approximate diameter of 5 inches.

The draping should allow a wide enough scalp exposure for the electrode wire to exit behind the ear. A diagnostic array of 20 plate electrodes will fit over the exposed dura. The array is placed in the epidural space aligned parallel to the presumed

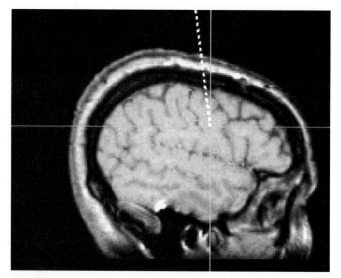

FIGURE 17-1 Simulated sagittal magnetic resonance planning image showing the target for placement of a cortical stimulating electrode at the level of the inferior frontal sulcus just posterior to the branching of the sulcus.

line of the central sulcus, covering both the regions of the pre- and postcentral gyri.

Median nerve somatosensory evoked potentials identify the N20P20 phase shift consistent with the central sulcus (Fig. 17-2). This step provides electrophysiologic confirmation of the site of the precentral gyrus in the region of the hand, located cephalad to the facial region. By using the neuronavigation, virtual reconstruction of the cortical surface and the target for electrode implantation is marked on the dura. Once the central sulcus has been identified, the facial motor region is stimulated using the grid electrodes. The contralateral face is observed for contractions and the EMG monitored for electrophysiologic confirmation of the correct site (Fig. 17-3). Contralateral facial rhythmic contractions provide the best indication of proper epidural electrode placement. When the contractions have been confirmed, the grid is removed and the implantation target site marked on the dura. A flat, four-plate electrode is positioned perpendicular to the central sulcus with the central two electrodes crossing the identified target. The electrode is sutured to the outer, periosteal layer of the dura, then its wire is brought out through a separate stab incision. The craniotomy bone flap is secured with plates.

Testing of the electrode can begin as soon as the patient is fully recovered from anesthesia and should continue for at least 3 days, or until the patient can confirm that stimulation reduces pain by at least 50%.

Permanent implantation of a pulse generator is performed during a second procedure. The generator is placed in a pocket that is created in the upper chest wall and connected to the electrode.

Therapeutic Stimulation Parameters

Stimulation is generally performed at a frequency range of 25 to 55 Hz, pulse width of 60 to 180 microseconds, and amplitude of 1.3 to 4 volts. Bipolar stimulation is used with the negative pole overlying the motor cortex and positive pole over

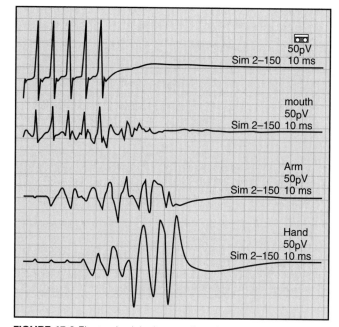

FIGURE 17-3 Electrophysiologic recording of an electromyogram. The recordings are from the buccinator muscles, muscles of the arm and of the hand. They demonstrate early movement in response to transdural stimulation of the facial motor cortex.

the sensory cortex. Pain relief is usually delayed by several minutes and may last beyond the period of stimulation. Nguyen and colleagues use a pattern consisting of 3 hours of stimulation alternating with 3 hours off.[15] Shorter periods of stimulation may also be used.

SUMMARY

The suffering inherent in neuropathic pain remains the greatest challenge to neurosurgeons focusing on the treatment of chronic pain syndromes. Its treatment by cortical stimulation has been available to patients for a decade. Technical innovations provided by the development of computer-assisted neuronavigation have simplified the operation, making it an option for many more patients at neurosurgical centers throughout the world. Because it is less invasive than deep brain electrode insertion, it has lower morbidity and is philosophically more acceptable.

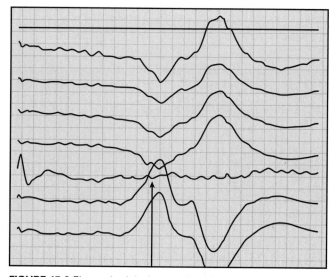

FIGURE 17-2 Electrophysiologic recording of median nerve cortical evoked potentials demonstrating the phase reversal at 20 msec from negative to positive. This reversal occurs across the central sulcus.

REFERENCES

1. White J, Sweet WH. Pain: its mechanisms and neurosurgical control. Spring Field, IL, Charles C. Thomas, 1955.
2. Lende RA, Kirsch WM, Druckman R. Relief of facial pain after combined removal of precentral and postcentral cortex. J Neurosurg 34:537–543, 1971.
3. Woolsey CN, Erickson TC, Gilson WE. Localization in somatic sensory and motor areas of human cerebral cortex as determined by direct recording of evoked potentials and electrical stimulation. J Neurosurg 51:476–506, 1979.
4. Andy OJ. Thalamic stimulation for chronic pain. Appl Neurophysiol 46:116–123, 1983.
5. Hosobuchi Y. Subcortical electrical stimulation for control of intractable pain in humans. Report of 122 cases (1970–1984). J Neurosurg 64:543–553, 1986.

6. Tsubokawa T, Katayama Y, Yamamoto T, et al. Treatment of thalamic pain by chronic motor cortex stimulation. Pacing Clin Electrophysiol 14:131–134, 1991.

7. Tsubokawa T, Katayama Y, Yamamoto T, et al. Chronic motor cortex stimulation in patients with thalamic pain. J Neurosurg 78:393–401, 1993.

8. Meyerson BA, Lindblom U, Linderoth B, et al. Motor cortex stimulation as treatment of trigeminal neuropathic pain. Acta Neurochir Suppl (Wien) 58:150–153, 1993.

9. Katayama Y, Tsubokawa T, Yamamoto T. Chronic motor cortex stimulation for central deafferentation pain: experience with bulbar pain secondary to Wallenberg syndrome. Stereotact Funct Neurosurg 62:295–299, 1994.

10. Migita K, Uozumi T, Arita K, et al. Transcranial magnetic coil stimulation of motor cortex in patients with central pain. Neurosurgery 36:1037–1039; discussion 1039–1040, 1995.

11. Ebel H, Rust D, Tronnier V, et al. Chronic precentral stimulation in trigeminal neuropathic pain. Acta Neurochir (Wien) 138:1300–1306, 1996.

12. Rainov NG, Fels C, Heidecke V, et al. Epidural electrical stimulation of the motor cortex in patients with facial neuralgia. Clin Neurol Neurosurg 99:205–209, 1997.

13. Nguyen JP, Keravel Y, Feve A, et al. Treatment of deafferentation pain by chronic stimulation of the motor cortex: report of a series of 20 cases. Acta Neurochir Suppl (Wien) 68:54–60, 1997.

14. Katayama Y, Fukaya C, Yamamoto T. Poststroke pain control by chronic motor cortex stimulation: neurological characteristics predicting a favorable response. J Neurosurg 89:585–591, 1998.

15. Krombach GA, Spetzger U, Rohde V, et al. Intraoperative localization of functional regions in the sensorimotor cortex by neuronavigation and cortical mapping. Comput Aided Surg 3:64–73, 1998.

16. Nguyen JP, Lefaucheur JP, Decq P, et al. Chronic motor cortex stimulation in the treatment of central and neuropathic pain. Correlations between clinical, electrophysiological and anatomical data. Pain 82:245–251, 1999.

17. Bezard E, Boraud T, Nguyen JP, et al. Cortical stimulation and epileptic seizure: a study of the potential risk in primates. Neurosurgery 45:346–350, 1999.

18. Garcia-Larrea L, Peyron R, Mertens P, et al. Positron emission tomography during motor cortex stimulation for pain control. Stereotact Funct Neurosurg 68:141–148, 1997.

19. Garcia-Larrea L, Peyron R, Mertens P, et al. Electrical stimulation of motor cortex for pain control: a combined PET- scan and electrophysiological study. Pain 83(Suppl):259–273, 1999.

20. Nguyen JP, Pollin B, Feve A, et al. Improvement of action tremor by chronic cortical stimulation. Mov Disord 13:84–88, 1998.

21. Canavero S, Bonicalzi V, Castellano G, et al. Painful supernumerary phantom arm following motor cortex stimulation for central poststroke pain. Case report. J Neurosurg 91:121–123, 1999.

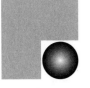

C H A P T E R   1 8

Cordotomy

DEVIN K. BINDER, MD, PhD, AND NICHOLAS M. BARBARO, MD

HISTORY

The first anterolateral cordotomy for the treatment of pain was carried out by Spiller and Martin in 1912.[1] The origin of cordotomy lay in the idea that the pain tracts in the spinal cord can be selectively interrupted. This idea was partially based on Brown-Séquard's studies of cord hemisection, although in these studies contralateral analgesia below the level of hemisection was not invariably seen. In later studies, various investigators used different-sized lesions in the anterolateral quadrant in the attempt to alleviate contralateral pain.

Although open cordotomy was effective in many patients,[2–4] the advent of percutaneous cordotomy enabled less invasive treatment. Mullan and colleagues first applied radioactive strontium-90 percutaneously to the spinal cord by the lateral approach in the C1–2 space.[5] The same investigators followed this with unilateral electrolytic lesions several years later.[6] Many technical refinements followed.[7] For example, Gildenberg and colleagues introduced impedance monitoring to detect cord penetration.[8] Onofrio developed the use of myelography for guidance.[9] Rosomoff and colleagues introduced radiofrequency cervical cordotomy,[10] based on previous work on radiofrequency lesions by Sweet and colleagues.[11] Taren, Tasker, and others refined physiologic corroboration of the target site.[12–15] More recently, Kanpolat and colleagues and others introduced computed tomography (CT)-guided percutaneous cordotomy.[16–18] CT guidance simplifies target localization and allows measurement of spinal cord diameter at the lesion site, visualization of intraoperative spinal cord deformation, and more precise localization of the electrode system in a specific part of the spinothalamic tract.[17]

Several operative approaches to percutaneous cordotomy have been described. The high cervical lateral approach in the C1–2 interspace originally described by Mullan and colleagues is most frequently used.[5] Dorsal approaches in the occipital-C1 interspace have also been described that use either the Brown-Robert-Wells[19] or Hitchcock[20] stereotactic frames. Gildenberg and colleagues described a low anterior approach to cervical cordotomy to minimize respiratory complications seen with the other techniques.[21,22]

In nearly all cases today, percutaneous cordotomy appears preferable to the open operation. The percutaneous technique is less invasive and allows intraoperative feedback from the patient with respect to lesion location and extent of pain relief. Local pathology sufficient to prevent the percutaneous procedure has not been observed,[23] although there are rare complications related to the variable dorsoventral position of the cord at the C1–2 level.[24,25] However, open cordotomy is still performed for certain patients with cancer.[26]

MECHANISM OF CORDOTOMY

The anatomic rationale for cordotomy involves interruption of pain fibers in the spinothalamic tract. Lahuerta and colleagues[27,28] studied the relationship of pain relief to specific sensory changes induced by cordotomy. The greatest deficits produced by cordotomy were sensitivity to skinfold pinch and cooling, and these had the best correlation with postoperative pain relief.

However, until relatively recently no physiologic information was available. In 1991, Di Piero and colleagues used positron emission tomography to study regional blood flow in brain areas before and after cordotomy.[29] In this study, they examined five patients with unilateral severe cancer pain before and after percutaneous, ventrolateral cervical cordotomy. They found diminished regional blood flow in the dorsal hemithalamus contralateral to the pain, which was restored to normal after cordotomy. Interestingly, there were no significant changes in prefrontal or primary somatosensory cortex, suggesting the relative importance of subcortical changes in central responses to cordotomy and chronic pain.

INDICATIONS FOR CORDOTOMY

The history of cordotomy is clouded by attempts to treat various painful conditions at a time when few options were available to treat severe focal pain. These included painful radiculopathy following spinal operations and other types of neuropathic pain. Such attempts sometimes produced additional injury to the nervous system, including the potential for painful states more severe than the original problem for which the cordotomy was used. More recently, so many medication options have become available, including intrathecal delivery, that fewer patients are considered for this technique. As Tasker notes, an entire generation of younger neurosurgeons are not familiar with these techniques.[30]

In patients being considered for cordotomy, several factors are critical. First, all noninvasive methods of pain control should have been attempted without success. Second, the patient should have no medical contraindications to surgery. Third, the pathophysiology and somatic localization of the patient's pain should be carefully considered.

Despite the long history and experience with ablative neurosurgical procedures in the treatment of pain, the indications for such procedures have narrowed dramatically over the past decade. In general, cordotomy is indicated in patients with limited life expectancy who have severe, unilateral pain. This typically includes patients with pain related to cancer. Even in this case, however, improvements in other therapies have led to a marked reduction in the use of ablative methods. Oral opioids with better absorption and fewer side effects, and transcutaneous or intrathecal routes of administration, have reduced the number of patients who are refractory to medications.[31–33] Similarly, newer agents effective against neuropathic pain have also reduced the need for ablative techniques. In spinal metastatic disease, surgical decompression and stabilization provide pain control while preventing neurologic deterioration. Vertebroplasty has taken its place as a novel minimally invasive technique for relief of pain from osteoporotic and pathologic fractures.[34]

Nevertheless, there is still a role for cordotomy and other neurodestructive procedures in the management of intractable cancer pain.[35] As Hassenbusch points out,[36] there is no consensus on the precise role of certain ablative procedures. Patients with severe intractable cancer pain and a poor prognosis represent a difficult treatment group because the severity or nature of the pain may change or increase and there may be limited survival time. In general, ablative pain procedures should be considered when the pain no longer responds to conservative treatment methods, or if the nonsurgical treatment methods have unacceptable side effects. Included in this group of avoidable side effects should be excessive sedation and memory disturbance, which frequently accompany the more commonly used medications. The goal in patients with limited life expectancy should be to improve the quality of survival, which includes improving a patient's ability to interact with others, and to reduce the amount of time spent in contact with healthcare providers. Even implanted pumps, which may reduce pain with relatively few side effects, require relatively frequent visits to the clinic for programming and refills. Ablative pain procedures can be performed percutaneously, without general anesthesia, and with brief hospitalization. When successful, the percutaneous cordotomy allows signifi-cant reduction in pain medications and reduces the need for office visits.

The pathophysiologic nature of the pain involved must be examined carefully as well. Percutaneous cordotomy is most useful for the relief of pain that depends on transmission in pain pathways of the spinal cord. Tasker has classified different pain syndromes to compare their response to cordotomy[23] (Table 18-1). In general, cordotomy is more effective for nociceptive pain (pain arising from stimulation of peripheral nociceptors) than for neuropathic pain (pain from impulses related to nerve injury or central sensitization[37,38]).[23] In 79 patients with nociceptive pain, cordotomy resulted in 70% long-term relief of pain as opposed to only 29% relief of pain in 15 patients with neuropathic pain.[23]

The anatomic localization of the pain is also important. In Tasker's experience with approximately 500 percutaneous high cervical cordotomies, persistent analgesia could be produced up to and including the C5 dermatome.[23] Unilateral pain is a much better indication than bilateral pain, because complications of bilateral cordotomies are much more severe (see subsequent section). In addition, midline trunk and perineal pain responds poorly even to bilateral cordotomy.[30]

If a neurodestructive procedure is indicated, then percutaneous high cervical cordotomy is the procedure of choice compared to other ablative procedures (Table 18-2). Percutaneous and stereotactic procedures are preferred over open procedures for their lower morbidity (pain from open laminectomy, need for general anesthesia, longer hospitalization). In addition, the radiofrequency technique of making lesions is preferred over other techniques given its reproducibility and the ability to physiologically corroborate the target site with the same equipment used for lesioning. Open cordotomy may be required in patients who are unable to lie flat on an operating table, and when pain is confined to the lower extremities.

OTHER NEUROSURGICAL OPTIONS

Other ablative procedures are generally less useful than cordotomy. Dorsal rhizotomy abolishes functions other than pain sensation, and cancer pain syndromes are not usually radicular in nature. Dorsal root entry zone lesioning is used primarily for localized neuropathic pain, such as that caused by brachial plexus avulsion.[39] High cervical stereotactic extralemniscal myelotomy is rarely used.[40,41] Medullary tractotomy (to interrupt the descending cranial nociceptive tract) is occasionally used in the case of cancers of the face or oropharynx, usually when retrogasserian trigeminal rhizotomy has failed.[26] According to one study, medial thalamotomy is relatively safe

---

● **TABLE 18-1** • Pathophysiologic Classification of Pain

Pain from stimulation of peripheral nociceptors (e.g., cancer in long bone)
Pain from direct stimulation of nerve trunks, plexuses, and roots (e.g., cancer in lumbosacral plexus, sciatica)
Pain from impulses related to neural injury (neuropathic pain syndromes, e.g., after spinal cord injury)
Pain from central reorganization (allodynia, hyperpathia in peripheral neuropathic pain syndromes, sympathetically mediated pain)

Adapted from Tasker RR. Cordotomy for pain. *In* Youmans JR (ed). Neurological Surgery. Philadelphia, WB Saunders, 1996, pp 3463–3476.

TABLE 18-2 • Neurosurgical Procedures Applicable to the Relief of Intractable Pain

Ablative Procedures	Modulatory Procedures
Dorsal rhizotomy	Morphine infusion (IT or ICV)
Dorsal root entry zone lesion	Dorsal column stimulation
Cordotomy (percutaneous or open)	Periventricular gray matter stimulation
Cervical myelotomy	Motor cortex stimulation
Medullary tractotomy	Transcutaneous electrical nerve stimulation
Mesencephalic tractotomy	
Medial thalamotomy	
Cingulotomy	

but also relatively ineffective[42]; however, the development of gamma knife thalamotomy may lead to increased adoption of this technique.[43–46] Mesencephalic tractotomy, while relatively effective, carries a higher risk of complications.[42,47–53] Bilateral radiofrequency cingulotomy has been quite useful in certain cases of chronic cancer and noncancer pain.[54–56] There are few of these types of procedures being performed in most medical centers so that training in these techniques is quite rare. In addition, as with other complicated techniques, the potential for morbidity increases as the number of cases per practitioner decreases.

OPERATIVE TECHNIQUE

This section describes the operative technique of high cervical percutaneous cordotomy in the C1–2 interspace. Other techniques described elsewhere include dorsal approaches in the occipital-C1 interspace,[19,20] the low anterior cervical approach,[21,22] and open cordotomy.[26]

Positioning

The patient is positioned supine with a special headholder. The headholder in the "OWL" cordotomy system is attached to the head of the operating table and a mechanical stage controls the electrode position. The head is placed in an anteroposterior plane with the cervical cord horizontal. The procedure can be performed with the patient lying flat on a standard operating table, but the ability to independently vary the head height improves the view obtained when intrathecal contrast material is introduced.

Anesthesia

Local anesthetic and intravenous analgesia and sedation are used. Optimal sedation allows the patient to remain still but cooperative. In patients who cannot tolerate an awake proced-

ure (e.g., children, elderly, or confused patients), percutaneous cordotomy has been performed successfully with general anesthesia.[57] Another option is open cordotomy, where direct visualization of the anterolateral spinal cord substitutes for the feedback provided by the patient during the percutaneous procedure. If percutaneous cordotomy under general anesthesia is to be used, the CT-guided technique[17] should be considered, because direct visualization of the needle in the spinal cord reduces the possibility of a misplaced lesion.

Electrode Positioning

Under fluoroscopic guidance, a true lateral image of the C1–2 interspace is obtained (Fig. 18-1). All efforts should be taken to avoid parallax in the radiographic image. This includes placing the C1–2 interspace in the direct center of the image. The spinothalamic tract is located anterior to the dentate ligament at approximately the midpoint of the anteroposterior extent of the spinal canal. A lumbar puncture needle is advanced horizontally with stylet in place, and ligamentum flavum and then dura are penetrated, with a brief twinge of pain. When cerebrospinal fluid (CSF) flows when the stylet is withdrawn, water-soluble contrast medium[58] is injected via 10-cc syringe. In the past, visualization of the spinal cord and dentate ligament was accomplished with oil-based[30] contrast medium. However, this material is no longer commercially

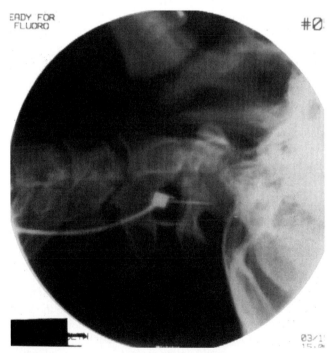

FIGURE 18-1 Fluoroscopic image obtained during percutaneous cordotomy. Spinal needle enters the C1–2 interspace and water-soluble contrast material has been injected through extension tubing. Horizontal line immediately posterior to needle tip is formed by contrast material layering over the dentate ligament. Second horizontal line is formed by the dorsal dura. Note that the region of interest is kept in the exact center of the fluoroscopy field and that the cervical spine is in a neutral position to allow contrast to layer over the dentate ligament.

available. The use of water-soluble contrast material requires that an image intensifier with the ability to store an image be used. The surgeon can use a length of intravenous extension tubing long enough to keep his hands out of the radiation field while injecting under fluoroscopy. When a sufficient amount of contrast is present in the subarachnoid space, the radiographic image can be "frozen" on the screen for review. The tip of the spinal needle should be immediately anterior to the dentate ligament. Failure to visualize the dentate ligament usually means the needle is too far posterior. It should be withdrawn and redirected slightly more anterior. The cordotomy electrode is then passed through the spinal needle and into the spinal cord. A number of electrodes are available for this purpose. These authors prefer the Levin Cordotomy Electrode (Radionics). Stimulation and lesion generation are done in monopolar fashion with the indifferent electrode consisting of a gel electrode similar to that used to ground a patient for electrocautery. As the electrode is advanced, spinal cord penetration is usually palpated, and the patient may notice slight pain. In addition, by monitoring electrical impedance, the surgeon can see a dramatic increase in impedance as the electrode leaves the spinal fluid and enters neural tissue (impedance of CSF is approximately 400 Ω, and of spinal cord 800 to 1200 Ω). Physiologic confirmation of electrode positioning is achieved via threshold electrical stimulation at 2 Hz and 100 Hz. The lower-frequency stimulation helps to avoid placement of the electrode too near the corticospinal tract. Contractions in ipsilateral neck or upper limb at low amplitudes indicate such a posteriorly placed electrode. Higher-frequency (50 to 100 Hz) stimulation should produce sensory alterations but no motor tetanization if the electrode is in good position. Patients initially report a sense of warmth at lower amplitudes, followed by burning pain at higher currents. Occasionally, it is possible to precisely select the exact portion of the spinothalamic tract to be lesioned in this manner. More typically, the patient will not be able to precisely localize the stimulation. All that is necessary for a successful cordotomy is to show that the electrode is away from the corticospinal tract and within the spinothalamic tract.

Lesion Generation

Following electrophysiologic corroboration and before making the lesion, sedation must be increased because meningeal cauterization elicits pain. The radiofrequency lesion is made by raising the temperature of the electrode tip to 60 °C for up to 60 seconds. Based on the depth of analgesia, the lesion may be enlarged further. This can be done either by increasing the temperature of the lesion, or by adjusting the electrode position. Upon completion of the lesion-making, the level of analgesia to pinprick and deep pain should extend above the level of the patient's pain. Other neurologic deficits such as Horner's syndrome, ipsilateral hypoventilation, and mild ipsilateral leg paresis should not be present and are an indication to stop the procedure.

Postoperative Care

After unilateral cordotomy, patients should be monitored for spinal headache, bladder function, respiratory function, and presence of hemiparesis.

RESULTS

It is difficult to compare published reports of outcomes following cordotomy because patient selection, outcome definition, and follow-up period all differ between studies. Nevertheless, several outcomes are clearly important following cordotomy: presence of lesion within spinothalamic tract; analgesia over area desired; and relief of pain for which the cordotomy was performed.

In the vast majority (95%) of 380 cases done by an experienced investigator, a successful lesion could be made at the first attempt.[30] On first office visit after discharge, 93% of patients demonstrated adequate analgesia. In the immediate postoperative period, 88% experienced total relief of target pain, and 94% had significant but not total relief. By latest follow-up (about 3 months), however, only 72% had total relief of pain and 84% had significant but not total relief.[30] Thus, 28% of patients in this series had at least some long-term residual pain after cordotomy. These data are similar to those of other published reports in the literature, in which there is 64% to 79% total reduction of pain and 59% to 96% partial reduction of pain following unilateral cordotomy.[59–70]

In patients with bilateral cordotomies, 71% of Tasker's series had significant bilateral pain relief.[30] Similarly, other studies reported 47% to 58% complete relief and 50% to 77% significant relief.[61,64,71] Of importance, in the relatively few patients for whom cordotomies have been done for noncancer pain, and who may be observed for years after the procedure, there appears to be a slow waning of the analgesic effect.

In addition, there appears to be an important prognostic association between reduced pinprick sensation and analgesia in the involved area postoperatively. In 1990, Lahuerta and colleagues[27] assessed sensory perception thresholds in 16 subjects who received unilateral percutaneous cervical cordotomy. In the majority of instances, they were able to confirm a relationship between deficit in pinprick sensation and pain. In a larger review in 1994 of 146 patients who underwent 181 percutaneous cervical cordotomies,[28] they found that optimum pain relief seems to be obtained only when pinprick sensation is also abolished in the affected segments. When pathologic pain was completely abolished, pinprick sensation was also abolished; but in a number of cases where pathologic pain was only partially alleviated, pinprick sensation remained intact.

The results of CT-guided cordotomy were reported in 1993 by Kanpolat and colleagues.[17] It was applied in 54 cases of intractable cancer pain. Successful pain relief was obtained in 33 of 54 cases (61%). Aside from one temporary hemiparesis and one temporary ataxia, no complications or side effects were reported.

COMPLICATIONS

The use of intraoperative electrical stimulation in an awake patient should allow the surgeon to avoid serious complications from percutaneous cordotomy. Any unusual response by the patient or lack of appropriate feedback from the patient should warn against making a lesion. Occasionally, the placement of the needle will require an inordinate amount of time, and some patients may not be able to cooperate during the all-important feedback phase of the procedure. It is far better to terminate the procedure and consider trying on a different day than to make a lesion in the wrong location.

Complications from cordotomy fall into two categories: placement or extension of the lesion into adjacent spinal regions, and addition of a lesion in a patient with preexisting neurologic impairment. Examples of the first type of complication include hemiparesis, which may be transient or permanent, or dorsal column injury. The region of the spinothalamic tract also includes descending fibers for the control of respiration (corticobulbar) and micturition. Unilateral interruption of these fibers typically does not result in measurable neurologic deficit. However, patients who may have preexisting interruption of respiratory or urinary tracts on one side, may develop new deficits as the cordotomy is performed. For example, a patient with preexisting neoplastic disease in the chest may have a paralyzed hemidiaphragm without clinical consequences. Performance of a cordotomy on the same side may produce a profound respiratory depression. Similarly, a patient with unilateral bladder denervation from preexisting pelvic pathology may become incontinent of urine as the cordotomy interrupts the tract on the second side.

Respiratory Compromise

Respiration depends on two descending pathways that activate respiratory musculature. Voluntary respiration occurs via corticospinal axons in the corticospinal tract that supply the diaphragm (C3, C4, C5) and intercostal muscles (T1–12). Involuntary respiration is mediated by the reticulospinal tract under direct control from the medullary respiratory center. Although respiratory difficulties can occur from damage to either tract, the reticulospinal tract is in anatomic proximity to the cordotomy lesion site. The reticulospinal tract (innervating ipsilateral respiratory musculature) lies just medial to the cervical fibers of the spinothalamic tract, and therefore can be easily damaged (Fig. 18-2).

While loss of one reticulospinal tract is usually well tolerated, bilateral dysfunction of reticulospinal pathways can lead to fatal failure of unconscious respiration during sleep (Ondine's curse).[72–83] In one study of 112 patients undergoing 144 cervical percutaneous cordotomies, 6 (5%) died as the result of Ondine's curse.[80] Five of six of these patients had bilateral cordotomy and the other had unilateral cordotomy with coexisting pulmonary disease.

Micturition

An accurate spinothalamic tract lesion encroaches significantly upon descending micturition pathways (see Fig. 18–2).[84] Significant worsening of bladder function was observed in 3% to 9% of patients, and transient problems were observed in 19%.[30] This rate is significantly higher with bilateral cordotomies (up to 58%) and may be permanent.

Postcordotomy Dysesthesias and Pain

Pain following cordotomy may be caused by progression of primary disease, postcordotomy dysesthesia, "mirror pain," or an unrecognized preexisting neuropathic component to

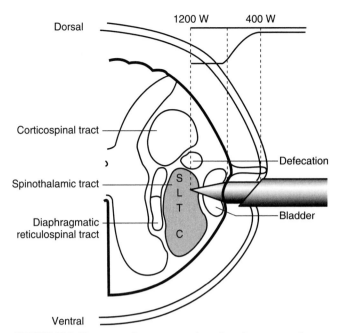

FIGURE 18-2 Diagrammatic representation of cordotomy needle inserted into the anterolateral spinal cord. Somatotopic representation of the spinothalamic tract is shown along with nearby tracts that may result in neurologic deficits if injured. (From Tasker RR. Cordotomy for pain. *In* Youmans JR (ed). Neurological Surgery. Philadelphia, WB Saunders, 1996, pp 3463–3476.)

the pain. Postcordotomy dysesthesia is a central pain syndrome due to damage to the spinothalamic tract. It may respond to medications useful in treating neuropathic pain, even if the patient's preoperative pain did not respond to such medications. Ipsilateral "mirror pain," thought to be due to unmasking of cord pathways subserving pain impulses, is seen in many patients.[61,63,85–90] A recent study of postcordotomy pain[87] found that 33 of 45 (73%) patients undergoing cordotomy for unilateral cancer pain had new pain centered on the contralateral side of the original pain in either a mirror-image location (28 patients) or more rostral (5 patients). This new mirror pain was temporary in 7 patients, weaker than the original pain in 25 patients, and as severe in 1 patient.

Hemiparesis

Transient ipsilateral paresis or ataxia may rarely occur following unilateral cordotomy. However, significant paresis or ataxia occurred in less than 10% of patients in most series.[4,30,59,65–67,70,91–93] Weakness usually affects the lower limb because the leg fibers in the corticospinal tract lie closest to the spinothalamic tract.

Bilateral cordotomies are rarely performed and may result in more profound deficits including respiratory depression and central alveolar hypoventilation (Ondine's curse, see previous discussion) requiring ventilatory support. Bilateral cordotomies can be performed more safely at thoracic levels, and patients may occasionally be suitable for unilateral percutaneous cervical and open thoracic cordotomies.

SUMMARY

In selected patients, percutaneous cordotomy can be quite effective in relieving nociceptive pain, in particular cancer pain below the C5 dermatome. It is most useful in unilateral pain, although it can be performed bilaterally with increased risk. One important benefit of cordotomy may be to allow patients with chronic pain to be weaned off high-dose narcotic infusions, thereby minimizing medication side effects and improving activity level. The current role for ablative as well as augmentative neurosurgical procedures in cancer pain and other pain syndromes remains to be better defined by well-designed clinical studies.

REFERENCES

1. Spiller WG, Martin E. The treatment of persistent pain of organic origin in the lower part of the body by division of the anterolateral column of the spinal cord. JAMA 58:1489–1490, 1912.
2. Stookey B. Chordotomy of the second cervical segment for relief from pain due to recurrent carcinoma of the breast. Arch Neurol Psychiatry 26:443, 1931.
3. Nathan PW. Cordotomy and neurosurgical history. J Neurosurg 83:764–765, 1995.
4. Nathan PW. Results of antero-lateral cordotomy for pain in cancer. J Neurol Neurosurg Psychiatry 26:353–362, 1963.
5. Mullan S, Harper PV, Hekmatpanah J, Torres H, Dobben G. Percutaneous interruption of spinal-pain tracts by means of a strontium-90 needle. J Neurosurg 20:931–939, 1963.
6. Mullan S, Hekmatpanah J, Dobben G, Beckman F. Percutaneous, intramedullary cordotomy utilizing the unipolar anodal electrolytic system. J Neurosurg 22:548–553, 1965.
7. Sweet WH. Recent observations pertinent to improving anterolateral cordotomy. Clin Neurosurg 23:80–95, 1976.
8. Gildenberg PL, Zanes C, Flitter M, Lin PM, Lautsch EV, Truex RC. Impedance measuring device for detection of penetration of the spinal cord in anterior percutaneous cervical cordotomy: technical note. J Neurosurg 30:87–92, 1969.
9. Onofrio BM. Cervical spinal cord and dentate delineation in percutaneous radiofrequency cordotomy at the level of the first to second cervical vertebrae. Surg Gynecol Obstet 133:30–34, 1971.
10. Rosomoff HL, Brown CJ, Sheptak P. Percutaneous radiofrequency cervical cordotomy: technique. J Neurosurg 23:639–644, 1965.
11. Sweet WH, Mark VH, Hamlin H. Radiofrequency lesions in the central nervous system of man and cat: including case reports of eight bulbar pain-tract interruptions. J Neurosurg 17:213–225, 1960.
12. Tasker RR, Organ LW, Smith KC. Physiological guidelines for the localization of lesions by percutaneous cordotomy. Acta Neurochir (Wien) 21 (Suppl):111–117, 1974.
13. Tasker RR, Organ LW. Percutaneous cordotomy: physiological identification of target site. Confin Neurol 35:110–117, 1973.
14. Taren JA. Physiologic corroboration in stereotaxic high cervical cordotomy. Confin Neurol 33:285–290, 1971.
15. Taren JA, Davis R, Crosby EC. Target physiologic corroboration in stereotaxic cervical cordotomy. J Neurosurg 30:569–584, 1969.
16. Fenstermaker RA, Sternau LL, Takaoka Y. CT-assisted percutaneous anterior cordotomy: technical note. Surg Neurol 43:147–149; discussion 149–150, 1995.
17. Kanpolat Y, Akyar S, Caglar S, Unlu A, Bilgic S. CT-guided percutaneous selective cordotomy. Acta Neurochir (Wien) 123:92–96, 1993.
18. Kanpolat Y, Deda H, Akyar S, Bilgic S. CT-guided percutaneous cordotomy. Acta Neurochir Suppl (Wien) 46:67–68, 1989.
19. Crue BL, Todd EM, Carregal EJ. Posterior approach for high cervical percutaneous radiofrequency cordotomy. Confin Neurol 30:41–52, 1968.
20. Hitchcock ER. An apparatus for stereotactic spinal surgery: a preliminary report. J Neurosurg 31:386–392, 1969.
21. Gildenberg PL, Lin PM, Polakoff PP, Flitter MA. Anterior percutaneous cervical cordotomy: determination of target point and calculation of angle of insertion: technical note. J Neurosurg 28:173–177, 1968.
22. Lin PM, Gildenberg PL, Polakoff PP. An anterior approach to percutaneous lower cervical cordotomy. J Neurosurg 25:553–560, 1966.
23. Tasker RR. Cordotomy for pain. In Youmans JR (ed). Neurological Surgery. Philadelphia, WB Saunders, 1996, pp 3463–3476.
24. Voris HC. Variations in the spinothalamic tract in man. J Neurosurg 14:55–60, 1957.
25. Voris HC. Ipsilateral sensory loss following cordotomy: report of a case. Arch Neurol Psychiatry 65:95–96, 1957.
26. Poletti CE. Open cordotomy and medullary tractotomy. In Wilkins RH, Rengachary SS (eds). Neurosurgery. New York, McGraw-Hill, 1996, pp 2430–2443.
27. Lahuerta J, Bowsher D, Campbell J, Lipton S. Clinical and instrumental evaluation of sensory function before and after percutaneous anterolateral cordotomy at cervical level in man. Pain 42:23–30, 1990.
28. Lahuerta J, Bowsher D, Lipton S, Buxton PH. Percutaneous cervical cordotomy: a review of 181 operations on 146 patients with a study on the location of "pain fibers" in the C-2 spinal cord segment of 29 cases. J Neurosurg 80:975–985, 1994.
29. Di Piero V, Jones AK, Iannotti F, Powell M, Perani D, Lenzi GL, Frackowiak RS. Chronic pain: a PET study of the central effects of percutaneous high cervical cordotomy. Pain 46:9–12, 1991.
30. Tasker RR. Percutaneous cordotomy. In Wilkins RH, Rengachary SS (eds). Neurosurgery. New York, McGraw-Hill, 1996, pp 2423–2429.
31. Gilmer-Hill HS, Boggan JE, Smith KA, Wagner FC, Jr. Intrathecal morphine delivered via subcutaneous pump for intractable cancer pain: a review of the literature. Surg Neurol 51:12–15, 1999.
32. Hassenbusch SJ, Pillay PK, Magdinec M, Currie K, Bay JW, Covington EC, Tomaszewski MZ. Constant infusion of morphine for intractable cancer pain using an implanted pump. J Neurosurg 73:405–409, 1990.
33. Penn RD, Paice JA, Gottschalk W, Ivankovich AD. Cancer pain relief using chronic morphine infusion. Early experience with a programmable implanted drug pump. J Neurosurg 61:302–306, 1984.
34. Barr JD, Barr MS, Lemley TJ, McCann RM. Percutaneous vertebroplasty for pain relief and spinal stabilization. Spine 25:923–928, 2000.
35. Fenstermaker RA. Neurosurgical invasive techniques for cancer pain: a pain specialist's view. Curr Rev Pain 3:190–197, 1999.
36. Hassenbusch SJ. Surgical management of cancer pain. Neurosurg Clin North Am 6:127–134, 1995.
37. Woolf CJ, Salter MW. Neuronal plasticity: increasing the gain in pain. Science 288:1765–1769, 2000.
38. Mannion RJ, Woolf CJ. Pain mechanisms and management: a central perspective. Clin J Pain 16:S144–S156, 2000.
39. Nashold BS, Ostdahl RH. Dorsal root entry zone lesions for pain relief. J Neurosurg 51:59–69, 1979.
40. Hitchcock ER. Stereotactic cervical myelotomy. J Neurol Neurosurg Psychiatry 33:224–230, 1970.
41. Schvarcz JR. Stereotactic extralemniscal myelotomy. J Neurol Neurosurg Psychiatry 39:53–57, 1976.
42. Frank F, Fabrizi AP, Gaist G, Weigel K, Mundinger F. Stereotactic mesencephalotomy versus multiple thalamotomies in the treatment of chronic cancer pain syndromes. Appl Neurophysiol 50:314–318, 1987.
43. Young RF, Jacques DS, Rand RW, Copcutt BC, Vermeulen SS, Posewitz AE. Technique of stereotactic medial thalamotomy with the Leksell Gamma Knife for treatment of chronic pain. Neurol Res 17:59–65, 1995.
44. Leksell L, Meyerson BA, Forster DM. Radiosurgical thalamotomy for intractable pain. Confin Neurol 34:264, 1972.
45. Young RF, Jacques DS, Rand RW, Copcutt BR. Medial thalamotomy with the Leksell gamma knife for treatment of chronic pain. Acta Neurochir Suppl (Wien) 62:105–110, 1994.
46. Young RF, Vermeulen SS, Grimm P, Posewitz AE, Jacques DB, Rand RW, Copcutt BG. Gamma Knife thalamotomy for the treatment of persistent pain. Stereotact Funct Neurosurg 64 (Suppl 1):172–181, 1995.
47. Whisler WW, Voris HC. Mesencephalotomy for intractable pain due to malignant disease. Appl Neurophysiol 41:52–56, 1978.
48. Tasker RR. Mesencephalotomy for cancer pain. J Neurosurg 1992;76:1052–1053.
49. Amano K, Kawamura H, Tanikawa T, Kawabatake H, Iseki H, Taira T. Stereotactic mesencephalotomy for pain relief. A plea for stereotactic surgery. Stereotact Funct Neurosurg 59:25–32, 1992.
50. Bosch DA. Stereotactic rostral mesencephalotomy in cancer pain and deafferentation pain. A series of 40 cases with follow-up results. J Neurosurg 75:747–751, 1991.
51. Shieff C, Nashold BS Jr. Stereotactic mesencephalotomy. Neurosurg Clin North Am 1:825–839, 1990.
52. Shieff C, Nashold BS Jr. Thalamic pain and stereotactic mesencephalotomy. Acta Neurochir Suppl (Wien) 42:239–242, 1998.
53. Frank F, Tognetti F, Gaist G, Frank G, Galassi E, Sturiale C. Stereotaxic rostral mesencephalotomy in treatment of malignant faciothoraco-

brachial pain syndromes. A survey of 14 treated patients. J Neurosurg 56:807–811, 1992.

54. Wilkinson HA, Davidson KM, Davidson RI. Bilateral anterior cingulotomy for chronic noncancer pain. Neurosurgery 45:1129–1136, 1999.

55. Hassenbusch SJ, Pillay PK, Barnett GH. Radiofrequency cingulotomy for intractable cancer pain using stereotaxis guided by magnetic resonance imaging. Neurosurgery 27:220–223, 1990.

56. Pillay PK, Hassenbusch SJ. Bilateral MRI-guided stereotactic cingulotomy for intractable pain. Stereotact Funct Neurosurg 59:33–38, 1992.

57. Izumi J, Hirose Y, Yazaki T. Percutaneous trigeminal rhizotomy and percutaneous cordotomy under general anesthesia. Stereotact Funct Neurosurg 59:62–68, 1992.

58. Krol G, Arbit E. Percutaneous lateral cervical cordotomy: target localization with water-soluble contrast medium. J Neurosurg 79:390–392, 1993.

59. Ischia S, Luzzani A, Ischia A, Pacini L. Role of unilateral percutaneous cervical cordotomy in the treatment of neoplastic vertebral pain. Pain 19:123–131, 1984.

60. Amano K, Kawamura H, Tanikawa T, Kawabatake H, Iseki H, Iwata Y, Taira T. Bilateral versus unilateral percutaneous high cervical cordotomy as a surgical method of pain relief. Acta Neurochir Suppl (Wien) 52:143–145, 1991.

61. Sanders M, Zuurmond W. Safety of unilateral and bilateral percutaneous cervical cordotomy in 80 terminally ill cancer patients. J Clin Oncol 13:1509–1512, 1995.

62. Ischia S, Luzzani A, Ischia A, Magon F, Toscano D. Subarachnoid neurolytic block (L5-S1) and unilateral percutaneous cervical cordotomy in the treatment of pain secondary to pelvic malignant disease. Pain 20:139–149, 1984.

63. Ischia S, Ischia A, Luzzani A, Toscano D, Steele A. Results up to death in the treatment of persistent cervico-thoracic (Pancoast) and thoracic malignant pain by unilateral percutaneous cervical cordotomy. Pain 21:339–355, 1985.

64. Ischia S, Luzzani A, Ischia A, Maffezzoli G. Bilateral percutaneous cervical cordotomy: immediate and long-term results in 36 patients with neoplastic disease. J Neurol Neurosurg Psychiatry 47:141–147, 1984.

65. Meglio M, Cioni B. The role of percutaneous cordotomy in the treatment of chronic cancer pain. Acta Neurochir (Wien) 59:111–121, 1981.

66. Lahuerta J, Lipton S, Wells JC. Percutaneous cervical cordotomy: results and complications in a recent series of 100 patients. Ann R Coll Surg Engl 67:41–44, 1985.

67. Kühner A. Percutaneous cordotomy: actual situation in pain surgery. Anesth Analg (Paris) 38:357–359, 1981.

68. Lipton S. Percutaneous cervical cordotomy. Acta Anaesthesiol Belg 32:81–85, 1981.

69. Stuart G, Cramond T. Role of percutaneous cervical cordotomy for pain of malignant origin. Med J Aust 158:667–670, 1993.

70. Siegfried J, Kühner A, Sturm V. Neurosurgical treatment of cancer pain: recent results. Cancer Res 89:148–156, 1984.

71. Rosomoff HL. Bilateral percutaneous cervical radiofrequency cordotomy. J Neurosurg 31:41–46, 1969.

72. Krieger AJ, Rosomoff HL. Sleep-induced apnea. Part 1: A respiratory and autonomic dysfunction syndrome following bilateral percutaneous cervical cordotomy. J Neurosurg 40:168–180, 1974.

73. Chevrolet JC, Reverdin A, Suter PM, Tschopp JM, Junod AF. Ventilatory dysfunction resulting from bilateral anterolateral high cervical cordotomy: dual beneficial effect of aminophylline. Chest 84:112–115, 1983.

74. Bohmfalk GL. Respiratory failure after cordotomy. South Med J 80:537, 1987.

75. Belmusto L, Brown E, Owens G. Clinical observations on respiratory and vasomotor disturbances as related to cervical cordotomies. J Neurosurg 20:225, 1963.

76. Fox JL. Localization of the respiratory motor pathway in the upper cervical spinal cord following percutaneous cordotomy. Neurology 19:1115–1118, 1969.

77. Hitchcock ER, Leece B. Somatotopic representation of the respiratory pathways in the cervical cord of man. J Neurosurg 27:320–329, 1967.

78. Mullan S, Hosobuchi Y. Respiratory hazards of high cervical percutaneous cordotomy. J Neurosurg 28:291–297, 1968.

79. Nathan PW. The descending respiratory pathway in man. J Neurol Neurosurg Psychiatry 26:487–499, 1963.

80. Tranmer BI, Tucker WS, Bilbao JM. Sleep apnea following percutaneous cervical cordotomy. Can J Neurol Sci 14:262–267, 1987.

81. Polatty RC, Cooper KR. Respiratory failure after percutaneous cordotomy. South Med J 79:897–899, 1986.

82. Rosomoff HL, Krieger AJ, Kuperman AS. Effects of percutaneous cervical cordotomy on pulmonary function. J Neurosurg 31:620–627, 1969.

83. Tenicela R, Rosomoff HL, Feist J, Safar P. Pulmonary function following percutaneous cervical cordotomy. Anesthesiology 29:7–16, 1968.

84. Nathan PW, Smith MC. The centrifugal pathway for micturition within the spinal cord. J Neurol Neurosurg Psychiatry 21:177, 1958.

85. Bowsher D. Contralateral mirror-image pain following anterolateral cordotomy. Pain 33:63–65, 1988.

86. Ischia S, Ischia A. A mechanism of new pain following cordotomy. Pain 32:383–384, 1988.

87. Nagaro T, Adachi N, Tabo E, Kimura S, Arai T, Dote K. New pain following cordotomy: clinical features, mechanisms, and clinical importance. J Neurosurg 95:425–431, 2001.

88. Nagaro T, Amakawa K, Arai T, Ochi G. Ipsilateral referral of pain following cordotomy. Pain 55:275–276, 1993.

89. Nagaro T, Kimura S, Arai T. A mechanism of new pain following cordotomy: reference of sensation. Pain 30:89–91, 1987.

90. Nagaro T, Amakawa K, Kimura S, Arai T. Reference of pain following percutaneous cervical cordotomy. Pain 53:205–211, 1993.

91. Lipton S. Percutaneous cervical cordotomy and the injection of the pituitary with alcohol. Anaesthesia 33:953–957, 1978.

92. Grote W, Roosen K, Bock WJ. High cervical percutaneous cordotomy in intractable pain. Neurochirurgia (Stuttg) 21:209–212, 1978.

93. O'Connell JEA. Anterolateral cordotomy for intractable pain in carcinoma of the rectum. Proc R Soc Med 62:31–33, 1969.

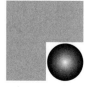

Spinal Ablative Therapies: Myelotomy

KENNETH A. FOLLETT, MD, PhD

The origin of spinal ablative procedures for pain control dates back at least 100 years. Spiller[1] reported in 1905 that tuberculous granulomas in the anterolateral portion of the spinal canal caused unilateral sensory loss. He proposed on the basis of this observation that surgical section of the pain transmission fibers in the anterolateral quadrant of the spinal cord (lateral spinothalamic tract) might be effective for the relief of pain. In 1912, Spiller and Martin[2] reported pain relief in a patient who underwent anterolateral cordotomy. Subsequent to that time, anterolateral cordotomy has become recognized as an effective procedure for the neurosurgical treatment of intractable pain, especially when pain is limited to one side of the body below midcervical levels. Treatment of bilateral pain by anterolateral cordotomy is complicated by a significant incidence of unacceptable side effects. Potential complications include sleep apnea (associated with bilateral high cervical anterolateral cordotomies), permanent hypotension, weakness (up to 40%), bladder or bowel dysfunction (incidences ranging from 15% to 90%), sexual dysfunction, and relatively little success in treating midline pain (e.g., visceral abdominal and pelvic pain).

Commissural myelotomy was introduced to overcome some of the limitations of bilateral cordotomies for the treatment of bilateral pain syndromes. The anatomic and physiologic rationale for commissural myelotomy is well understood: second-order spinothalamic tract fibers, which are the target of anterolateral cordotomy, originate in the spinal cord dorsal horn, cross in the anterior commissure of the spinal cord, then ascend in the anterolateral quadrant of the spinal cord. Based on this knowledge, it becomes apparent that the clinical effects of bilateral anterolateral cordotomy might be achieved with a lesion of the anterior commissure, which would transect spinothalamic tract fibers from both sides as they decussate in the midline. In 1927, Armour[3] reported the use of commissurotomy to treat bilateral pain distributed over several spinal levels. Since then, several variations of commissural myelotomy have evolved as our understanding of the anatomy and physiology of spinal nociceptive pathways has matured.[4,5] In addition to classical commissurotomy, pain relief can be achieved with central myelotomy (extralemniscal myelotomy),[6–9] limited midline myelotomy,[10,11] and punctate midline myelotomy.[12–15] Compared to

bilateral anterolateral cordotomy, myelotomy has the benefit of a single procedure to treat bilateral pain, and it is more effective for midline abdominal and pelvic pain. It may have a lower incidence of complications, especially dysfunction of bladder and bowel. The primary indication for myelotomy is for the treatment of pain of the abdomen, pelvis, perineum, sacrum, and legs arising from cancer.

Commissural myelotomy is performed at least three spinal segments above the dermatomal level of pain to take into account the fact that afferent nociceptive fibers entering the spinal cord may ascend ipsilaterally several spinal segments before termination in the spinal cord dorsal horn. Careful attention must be paid to identifying the midline of the spinal cord. Midline can be identified by locating the dorsal root entry zones bilaterally and determining the midpoint between them, or by identifying the midline septum of the spinal cord. Careful inspection of the region of the midline of the spinal cord typically reveals small diameter blood vessels penetrating into the parenchyma. Intraoperative magnification (e.g., operating microscope) facilitates identification of the midline. The midline incision should extend to the depth of the anterior median sulcus, usually approximately 6 to 7 mm (Fig. 19-1). The length of the myelotomy should vary according to the extent of pain, and may range from approximately 2.5 to 10 cm or more to cover the spinal segmental levels over which pain is distributed. The lesion is generally accomplished using a small dissector or blade but use of laser has been described.[16]

In the early postoperative period, pain relief is achieved in more than 90% of patients undergoing commissural myelotomy. Long-term pain relief diminishes but remains in approximately 50% to 60% of patients.[5,17] As with other types of ablative techniques for pain control, nociceptive pain responds more consistently than neuropathic pain. Sensory loss is inconsistent except for the occurrence of girdle hypalgesia in the dermatomes innervated by the transected fibers.[5,17] Morbidity and mortality are relatively low.[5,17] Mortality has been reported in up to 14% of cases but contemporary series typically report mortality rates of 0%. Leg weakness may occur, with an incidence ranging from 0% to 44%. Bladder and bowel dysfunction has been described in 0% to 11% of patients.[5] As with anterolateral cordotomy, postoperative dysesthesias may occur. Dysesthetic pain, which may be radicular and/or nonradicular in distribution, has been reported to occur in 0% to 27% of patients.

Commissural myelotomy can provide good pain relief but the clinical benefit cannot always be reconciled with the anatomic lesion, especially the depth of the lesion into the spinal cord. It was noted in clinical series that the degree of postoperative sensory loss did not always correlate with the degree of pain relief,[10,11,18] and postmortem studies revealed that pain relief was sometimes achieved even though the surgical lesion did not extend to or through the anterior commissure.[17] Furthermore, Hitchcock[6] described widespread analgesia resulting from a midline C1 lesion. These observations led to speculation that an extralemniscal pain pathway might exist in the central portion of the spinal cord[7,10,11] and that pain relief after anterior commissurotomy was actually due to lesioning of this extralemniscal pathway rather than lesioning of the anterior commissure. Such a pathway would provide a target for lesioning that could produce a wide region of pain relief with a simple, restricted lesion with minimal risk of neurologic complication.

Hitchcock[6] and Schvarcz[7] described "stereotactic extralemniscal myelotomy," a technique that supported the idea of a midline, pericentral pain pathway. This technique is not used commonly despite its refinement by Kanpolat and colleagues,[8,9] who have championed the use of computed tomography (CT) guidance for stereotactic pain-relieving procedures. Stereotactic extralemniscal myelotomy is performed using local anesthesia. With the patient in the prone position, the lesion needle is inserted into the spinal cord at the occipito-atlantal level under CT guidance. Intraoperative stimulation is used to confirm proper electrode placement following which the radiofrequency (RF) lesion is placed. Special RF electrodes have been developed for this procedure.[19]

Based on the observations described previously, and the theorized presence of a midline pericentral pain pathway, Gildenberg[10] and colleagues[11] proposed limited midline myelotomy for the treatment of bilateral lower body pain. This procedure is similar to the stereotactic central cervicomedullary myelotomy described by Hitchcock[6] and Schvarcz[7] in that it is characterized by the disruption of central spinal fibers over a limited distance, generally less than one spinal segmental level. The limited midline myelotomy is performed generally at the T9 or T10 level for treatment of pelvic pain. The midline is identified and pia is incised over a distance of 1 to 2 mm in the midline. A blunt instrument is inserted into the midline to a depth of approximately 5 to 6 mm (see Fig. 19-1). As the instrument is inserted, the surgeon may feel resistance from the central canal ependyma or the pia-arachnoid of the anterior median sulcus. The instrument is then swept longitudinally over a distance of 3 to 7 mm.[12] The procedure may result in lesioning of the anterior commissure but its primary purpose is to disrupt a pericentral pain pathway rather than the anterior commissure.

Within the past several years, animal studies have confirmed the presence of a visceral nociceptive pathway ascending in the medial aspect of the dorsal columns.[20] The relief of visceral pain by commissural myelotomy and limited midline myelotomy may be related to disruption of this medial dorsal column visceral pain pathway rather than disruption of anterior commissure fibers. Identification of this midline visceral pain pathway led to the development of "punctate midline myelotomy,"[12] which has been used by several groups for the treatment of intractable cancer-related pain.[12–15] In contrast to classical myelotomy or limited midline myelotomy, punctate midline myelotomy is intended to disrupt only the visceral pain pathway located along the mesial aspects of the dorsal columns (Fig. 19-2). Punctate midline myelotomy is usually performed at the level of T8 or T10 for abdominal or pelvic pain but has been performed as high as the T1 level for treatment of pain related to stomach cancer.[15] The midline of the spinal cord is identified by visual inspection. The original procedure was described as insertion of a 16-gauge needle 5 mm into the cord twice at the midline, with the bevel of the

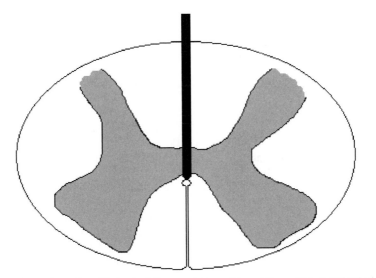

FIGURE 19-1 Commissural and limited midline myelotomy. The midline of the dorsal spinal cord is identified. A pial incision is made and a dissector is inserted to a depth of 5 to 6 mm, then swept longitudinally. The tip of the dissector should extend through the anterior commissure but not into the ventral spinal sulcus.

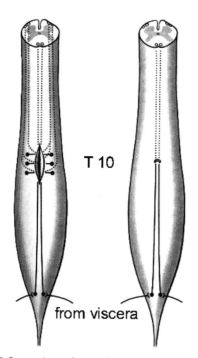

FIGURE 19-2 Comparison of commissural and limited midline myelotomy (*left*) and punctate midline myelotomy (*right*). In commissural myelotomy, spinothalamic fibers decussating in the anterior commissure are transected. In the process, fibers ascending in the midline visceral pain pathway would also be lesioned. In contrast, punctate midline myelotomy disrupts only the midline visceral pain pathway without lesioning spinothalamic tract fibers. (From Nauta HJ, Hewitt E, Westlund KN, Willis WD. Surgical interruption of a midline dorsal column visceral pain pathway. Case report and review of the literature. J Neurosurg 86:541, 1997, with permission.)

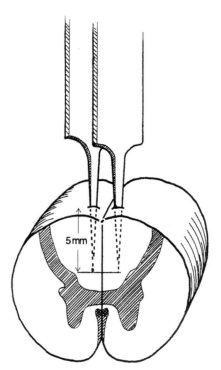

FIGURE 19-3 Modified technique of punctate midline myelotomy. A fine forceps is used to disrupt tissue extending 1 mm to each side of the midline, to a depth of 5 mm. (From Nauta HJ, Soukup VM, Fabian RH, et al. Punctate midline myelotomy for the relief of visceral cancer pain. J Neurosurg (Spine 2) 92:127, 2000, with permission.)

needle pointing laterally in opposite directions in the two passes.[12] The cord is cut approximately 1 mm away from the midline. There is no sagittal movement.[12] More recently, Nauta and colleagues[14] have described lesioning with forceps rather than needle to minimize the potential for bleeding within the spinal cord. In this modification, the midline tissue, extending 1 mm to either side, is crushed between the blades of a small forceps inserted 5 mm into the cord (Fig. 19-3). Punctate midline myelotomy might lend itself to a percutaneous approach; however, caution is advised due to the possibility of injury to the midline dorsal spinal vein and to the possibility that the pia-arachnoid of the posterior spinal sulcus might cause the needle to veer laterally, resulting in injury to the dorsal columns.[12]

The number of patients reported in contemporary series of limited midline myelotomy and punctate myelotomy is relatively small. The success rate of limited midline myelotomy is comparable to that of commissural myelotomy with more than 70% of patients obtaining pain relief, but neurological complications occur less frequently than they do with commissural myelotomy.[11] Only a handful of patients undergoing punctate midline myelotomy have been reported in the literature.[12–15] Approximately 60% of patients have good or excellent pain relief, and another 35% have fair pain relief, with follow-up periods extending months to several years. Complete failure of pain relief is unusual. Neurologic deficits caused by the procedure are unusual, although transient paresthesias have been reported in a few patients,[15] and dorsal column dysfunction may occur, presumably if the lesion extends too far laterally.[15]

A major advantage of limited midline myelotomy and punctate midline myelotomy over commissural myelotomy is the much more limited laminectomy required to perform the procedure. It is not clear, however, whether relief of leg pain is comparable to that achieved with commissural myelotomy, since the putative target of limited midline myelotomy and punctate midline myelotomy is a visceral pain pathway that may not be involved in the transmission of nociceptive information from the extremities. The use of limited midline myelotomy for the treatment of visceral pain plus cordotomy for the treatment of extremity pain has been described.[11]

The advent of intrathecal analgesic therapy has had a profound effect on the frequency with which ablative neurosurgical therapies must be employed for the treatment of pain. Myelotomy is nearly a lost art within the discipline of neurosurgery. However, it still has a role in the treatment of intractable pain in a select group of patients. Among these are those individuals who have failed therapy with intraspinal analgesics or for whom it is not possible to treat with intraspinal analgesics.[21] While intraspinal analgesic therapy has the advantages of being nondestructive and adjustable, it has disadvantages of significantly greater cost and mandates regular patient follow-up with a care provider for refilling of the infusion pump. In contrast, ablative procedures such as myelotomy may provide acceptable pain relief, especially for patients with limited expected survival, in a one-step procedure that does not require regular follow-up or long-term maintenance, and which is less costly than implanted pain therapy devices. As with all treatments for intractable pain, therapy for each patient must be individualized according to the patient and the resources available. For some patients, myelotomy will be an acceptable means of providing pain relief.

REFERENCES

1. Spiller WG. The location within the spinal cord of the fibers for temperature and pain sensations. J Nerv Ment Dis 32:318–320, 1905.
2. Spiller WG, Martin E. The treatment of persistent pain of organic origin in the lower part of the body by division of the anterolateral column of the spinal cord. JAMA 58:1489–1490, 1912.
3. Armour D. Surgery of the spinal cord and its membranes. Lancet 1:691–697, 1927.
4. Gybels J. Commissural myelotomy revisited. Pain 70:1–2, 1997.
5. Van Roost D, Gybels J. Myelotomies for chronic pain. Acta Neurochir 46 (Suppl):69–72, 1989.
6. Hitchcock E. Stereotactic cervical myelotomy. J Neurol Neurosurg Psychiatry 33:224–230, 1970.
7. Schvarcz JR. Stereotactic extralemniscal myelotomy. J Neurol Neurosurg Psychiatry 39:53–57, 1976.
8. Kanpolat Y, Atalag M, Deda H, Siva A. CT guided extralemniscal myelotomy. Acta Neurochir (Wein) 91:151–152, 1988.
9. Kanpolat Y, Caglar S, Akyar S, Temiz C. CT-guided pain procedures for intractable pain in malignancy. Acta Neurochir 64 (Suppl):88–91, 1995.
10. Gildenberg PL. Myelotomy and percutaneous cervical cordotomy for the treatment of cancer pain. Appl Neurophysiol 47:208–215, 1984.
11. Gildenberg PL, Hirshberg RM. Limited midline myelotomy for the treatment of intractable cancer pain. J Neurol Neurosurg Psychiatry 47:94–96, 1984.
12. Nauta HJ, Hewitt E, Westlund KN, Willis WD. Surgical interruption of a midline dorsal column visceral pain pathway. Case report and review of the literature. J Neurosurg 86:538–542, 1997.
13. Becker R, Sure U, Bertalanffy. Punctate midline myelotomy. A new approach in the management of visceral pain. Acta Neurochir (Wein) 141:881–883, 1999.
14. Nauta HJ, Soukup VM, Fabian RH, et al. Punctate midline myelotomy for the relief of visceral cancer pain. J Neurosurg (Spine 2) 92:125–130, 2000.
15. Kim YS, Kwon SJ. High thoracic midline dorsal column myelotomy for severe visceral pain due to advanced stomach cancer. Neurosurgery 46:85–92, 2000.
16. Fink RA. Neurosurgical treatment of nonmalignant intractable rectal pain: Microsurgical commissural myelotomy with the carbon dioxide laser. Neurosurgery 14:64–65, 1984.
17. Goedhart ZD, Francaviglia N, Feirabend HKP, Voogd J. Technical pitfalls in median commissural myelotomy for malignant sacral pain. Appl Neurophysiol 47:216–222, 1984.
18. Cook AW, Nathan PW, Smith MC. Sensory consequences of commissural myelotomy. A challenge to traditional anatomical concepts. Brain 107:547–568, 1984.
19. Kanpolat Y, Cosman ER. Special radiofrequency electrode system for computed tomography-guided pain-relieving procedures. Neurosurgery 38:600–603, 1996.
20. Al-Chaer ED, Lawand NB, Westlund KN, et al. Visceral nociceptive input into the ventral posterolateral nucleus of the thalamus: A new function for the dorsal column pathway. J Neurophysiol 76:2661–2674, 1996.
21. Watling, CJ, Payne R, Allen RR, Hassenbusch S. Commissural myelotomy for intractable cancer pain: Report of two cases. Clin J Pain 12:151–156, 1996.

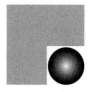

C H A P T E R   2 0

Dorsal Root Entry Zone Lesions

MARC P. SINDOU, MD, DSc, AND PATRICK MERTENS, MD, PhD

In the 1960s, a large number of neurophysiologic investigations proved that the dorsal horn was the first and an important level of modulation for pain sensation. In 1972 the Gate Control Theory[1] drew our attention to the dorsal root entry zone (DREZ) as a possible target for pain surgery.[2] Therefore, we undertook anatomic studies and preliminary surgical trials in the human DREZ to determine whether a destructive procedure at this level was feasible.[2,3]

Our first attempt at surgery occurred in March 1972 at the Neurological Institute Pierre Wertheimer in Lyon, on a patient with painful Pancoast-Tobias syndrome. The microsurgical techniques were used to perform a destructive lesion in the ventrolateral region of the DREZ. Several other patients with cancer pain were operated on the same year. Because the first results in malignancies were encouraging, within the next 2 years we attempted the procedure in patients with neuropathic pain syndromes, namely those associated with paraplegia in December 1972, amputation in July 1973, and brachial plexus avulsion in January 1974. Soon after (September 1974) Nashold and his group at Duke University started to develop DREZ lesions using radiofrequency (RF) thermocoagulation as the lesion-maker, in the substantia gelatinosa of the dorsal horn[4] and later in the whole DREZ,[5] especially for pain due to brachial plexus avulsion. Lately, DREZ procedures were performed in the United States with the use of the laser by Levy and colleagues[6] and Powers and colleagues,[7] and in Moscow with an ultrasound probe by Kandel and colleagues[8] and Dreval[9] for pain caused by brachial plexus avulsion.

ANATOMIC-PHYSIOLOGIC RATIONALE AND TECHNICAL DESCRIPTIONS OF DORSAL ROOT ENTRY ZONE LESIONS

In our medical thesis we defined the DREZ as an entity including the (1-mm) central portion of the dorsal rootlet, the most medial part of the tract of Lissauer, and the most dorsal layers (I to V) of the dorsal horn, where the afferent fibers synapse with the cells of the spino-reticulo-thalamic pathways (Fig. 20-1).

Each dorsal root divides into 4 to 10 rootlets according to metameres, and of 0.25 to 1.50 mm in diameter according to levels.[10,11] As shown in reference 2, each rootlet can be considered an anatomic-functional entity, that is, a root in mini-

ature. Anatomic studies[2,3] revealed the existence in each dorsal rootlet and in the corresponding DREZ, of a spatial segregation of afferent fibers according to their size and destination, the fine fibers regrouping in the lateral region of the DREZ (Fig. 20-2). The tract of Lissauer (TL), which is situated dorsolateral to the dorsal horn, consists of: 1) a medial part that the small afferents enter and where they trifurcate to reach the dorsal horn, either directly or through (a few metameres) ascending or descending pathways. This part transmits the excitatory effects of each dorsal root to the adjacent segments[12,13]; and 2) a lateral part through which a large number of longitudinal endogenous propriospinal fibers interconnect different levels of the substantia gelatinosa (SG). This latter part conveys the inhibitory influences of the SG into the neighboring metameres.[13] Most of the fine nociceptive afferents enter the dorsal horn through the TL medial part and then the dorsal aspect of the SG. Ramon and Cajal's recurrent collateral vessels of the large lemniscal fibers[14] enter the dorsal horn through the ventromedial aspect of SG.[15] Because the dendrites of the spino-reticulo-thalamic (SRT) cells make synaptic connections with the primary afferent fibers inside the SG layers, the SG exerts a segmental modulating effect on the nociceptive input. When the large lemniscal afferents in peripheral nerves or dorsal roots are altered, there is a reduction in the inhibitory control of the dorsal horn.[16] This situation may result in excessive firing of the dorsal horn neurons. This phenomenon, thought to be at the origin of deafferentation pain, has been identified in patients with electrophysiologic recordings[17–19] and reproduced in animal experiments.[20,21]

There are several different options for performing DREZ lesions. Our favorite is the microsurgical technique; we call it microsurgical DREZotomy (MDT).

Microsurgical Dorsal Root Entry Zone–otomy (Micro DREZotomy)

The procedure consists of a longitudinal incision of the dorsolateral sulcus, ventrolaterally at the entrance of the rootlets into the sulcus and then of microbipolar coagulations performed continuously—in a dotted manner—inside the sulcus, down to the apex of the dorsal horn, along all the spinal cord segments selected for surgery. The lesion, which penetrates the lateral part of the DREZ and the medial part of TL, extends down to the apex of the dorsal horn (Fig. 20-3), which can be recognized by its brown-grey color. The average lesion is 2 to 3 mm deep and is made in the axis of the dorsal horn, that is, at a

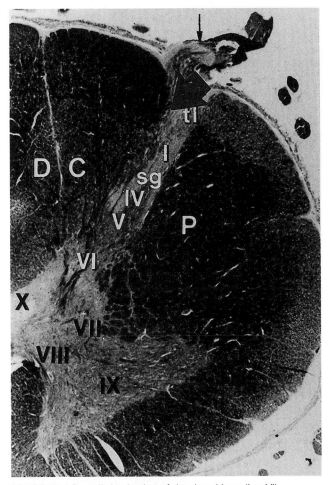

FIGURE 20-1 Rexed's lamination of the dorsal horn (I to VI). Transverse hemisection of the spinal cord at the lower cervical level with myelin stained by luxol-fuschine, showing the myelinated rootlet afferents that reach the dorsal column (*DC*). The nonmyelinated fibers enter the dorsal horn (substantia gelatinosa = *sg*) through the tract of Lissauer (*TL*). *P*: pyramidal tract. The small arrow designates the pial ring which is the junction between the central and the peripheral segment of the dorsal rootlet (diameter: 1 mm). The *black large arrowhead* shows the direction of the MDT target.

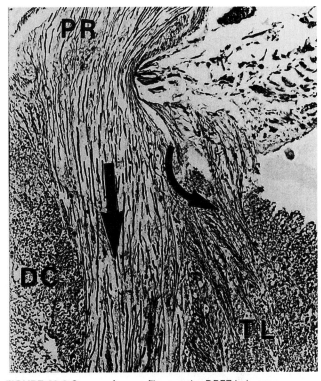

FIGURE 20-2 Course of nerve fibers at the DREZ in human. Example of a cervical rootlet; longitudinal section of the rootlet in its central segment after crossing the pial ring (*PR*) and at its entry into the spinal cord. Axons stained by the Bodian method. The large afferent fibers (*straight large arrow*) are grouped medially to enter the dorsal column (*DC*). The small fibers (*thin curved arrow*) are regrouped laterally to enter the tract of Lissauer (*TL*).

30-degree angle medially and ventrally for the cervical, 35 degrees for the thoracic, and 45 degrees for the lumbar and sacral segments of the spinal cord (Fig. 20-4). The procedure is presumed to preferentially destroy the nociceptive fibers grouped in the lateral bundle of the dorsal rootlets, as well as the excitatory medial part of the TL. The upper layers of the dorsal horn are also destroyed if microbipolar coagulations are made inside the dorsal horn. The procedure is presumed to preserve at least partially the inhibitory structures of the DREZ (i.e., the lemniscal fibers reaching the dorsal column, as well as their recurrent collateral branches to the dorsal horn and the SG propriospinal interconnecting fibers running through the lateral part of the TL). This method was conceived with a view to preventing complete abolition of tactile and proprioceptive sensations and avoiding deafferentation phenomena[22] (Fig. 20-5). Working in the DREZ requires knowledge of the morphologic anatomy of dorsal roots, according to the spinal level. Details have been given in previous publications.[10,11,23,24]

With regard to the surgical technique, the procedure is performed with the patient under general anaesthesia, but with only an initial short-lasting curarization to allow intraoperative observation of motor responses to bipolar electrical stimulation of the nerve roots. Stimulated ventral roots have a motor threshold at least three times lower than the dorsal roots. Standard microsurgical techniques are used with ×10 to ×25 magnification.

For operative procedure at the cervical level, the prone position with the head and neck flexed in the "Concorde" position has the advantage of avoiding brain collapse–caused cerebrospinal fluid (CSF) depletion. The head is fixed with a threepin head holder. The level of laminectomy is determined after identification of the prominent spinous process of C2 by palpation. A hemilaminectomy, generally from C4 to C7, with preservation of the spinous processes, allows sufficient exposure to the posterolateral aspect of the cervical spinal cord segments that correspond to the upper limb innervation, that is, the rootlets of C5 to Th1 (Th2). After the dura and the arachnoid are opened longitudinally, the exposed roots and rootlets are dissected free by separation of the tiny arachnoid filaments that bind them to each other, to the arachnoid sheath, and to the spinal cord pia mater. The radicular vessels are preserved. Each ventral and dorsal root from C4 to T1 is electrically stimulated at the level of its corresponding foramen to identify precisely its muscular innervation and its functional value. Responses are in the diaphragm for C4 (the response is palpable below the lower ribs), in the shoulder abductors for C5, in the elbow flexors for C6, in the elbow and wrist extensors for C7, and in the muscles of the hand for C8 and T1.

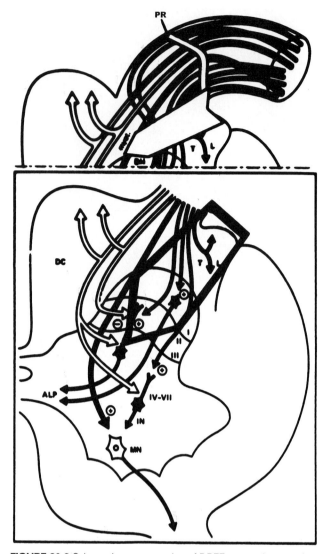

FIGURE 20-3 Schematic representation of DREZ area and target of Micro-DREZotomy. *Upper part:* each rootlet can be divided, thanks to the transition of its glial support, into a peripheral and a central segment. The transition between the two segments is at the pial ring (*PR*), which is located approximately 1 mm outside the penetration of the rootlet into the dorsolateral sulcus. Peripherally, the fibers are mixed together. As they approach PR, the fine fibers, which are considered nociceptive, move toward the rootlet surfaces. In the central segment, they group in the ventrolateral portion of the DREZ, to enter the dorsal horn through the tract of Lissauer (*TL*). The large myotatic fibers (*myot*) are situated in the middle of the DREZ, whereas the large lemniscal fibers are located dorsomedially to reach the dorsal column (*DC*). *Lower part:* schematic data on DH circuitry. Note the monosynaptic excitatory arc reflex, the lemniscal influence on a DH cell and an interneuron (*IN*), the fine fiber excitatory input onto DH cells, and the IN, the origins in layer I and layers IV to VII of the anterolateral pathways (*ALP*), and the projection of the IN onto the motoneuron (*MN*). Rexed's laminae are marked from I to VII . MDT (*arrowhead*) cuts most of the fine and myotatic fibers and enters the medial (excitatory) portion of TL and the apex of the dorsal horn. It should preserve most lemniscal presynaptic fibers, the lateral (inhibitory) portion of TL and most of the DH.

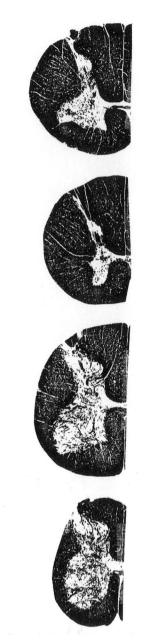

FIGURE 20-4 Variations of shape, width, and depth of the DREZ area, according to the spinal cord level (from *top to bottom:* cervical n. 7, thoracic n. 5, lumbar n. 4, sacral n. 3). The axis of the dorsal horn in relation to the sagittal plan crossing the dorso-lateral sulcus will condition the angulation of the DREZotomy. According to 82 measurements performed by Young (personal communication, 1991), the mean DREZ angle is 30 degrees at C6, 26 degrees at T4, 37 degrees at T12, and 36 degrees at L3. The site and extent of the DREZ lesion will also be conditioned by the shape, width, and depth of Lissauer tract and dorsal horn. Note how, at the thoracic level, Lissauer's tract is narrow and dorsal horn deep. So, it is easy to understand that DREZ lesions especially at this level can be dangerous for the corticospinal tract and the dorsal column.

Microsurgical lesions are performed at the selected levels, that is, those that correspond to the pain territory. The technique is summarized and illustrated in Figure 20-6. The incision is made with a microknife. Then microcoagulations are made in a "chain" (i.e., dotted) manner. Each microcoagulation is performed—under direct magnified vision—by short (a few seconds), low intensity, bipolar electrocoagulation with a special sharp bipolar forceps incremented at every milimeter. Depth and extent of the lesion depend on the degree of the desired therapeutic effect and the preoperative sensory status of the patient.

If the laxity of the root is sufficient, the incision is performed continuously in the dorsolateral sulcus, ventrolaterally along all of the rootlets of the targeted root, thus

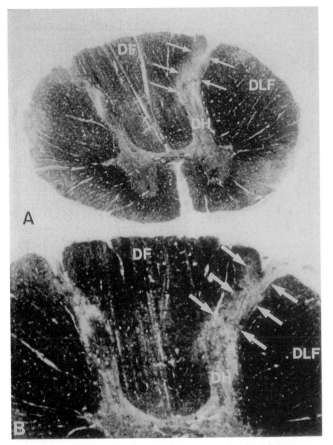

FIGURE 20-5 Postmortem histopathologic examination of the spinal cord after microsurgical DREZotomy Transverse section of the spinal cord at the lower cervical level (C7/C8), with myelin stained by luxol-fuschine, in two different patients who died 3 months (A) and 45 days (B) after a microsurgical DREZotomy procedure performed for an advanced Pancoast syndrome on left side in both patients. DF, dorsal funiculus; DLF, dorsal lateral funiculus; DH, dorsal horn. Notice the postoperative changes in the dorsal root entry and the uppermost layers of the dorsal horn, on left side, between white arrows.

accomplishing a sulcotomy (myelotomy). If not, a partial ventrolateral section is made successively on each rootlet of the root, after the surgeon had isolated each one by separation of the tiny arachnoid membranes that hold them together.

For pain due to brachial plexus avulsion, after incision of the dorsolateral sulcus, dotted microcoagulations inside the dorsal horn down to approximately the fifth layer (i.e., at least 3 mm in depth from the surface of the cord) are performed with the sharp graduated bipolar forceps, at the level of the avulsed roots (Fig. 20-7). Selective ventrolateral DREZ lesions are extended to the root remaining above and below. In brachial plexus avulsion, dissection of the spinal cord is sometimes difficult to achieve safely, because of scar tissue adhering to the cord. Atrophy and/or gliotic changes at the level of the avulsed roots can make identification of the dorsolateral sulcus hazardous. In such cases, it is necessary to start from the remaining roots, above and below. The presence of tiny radicular vessels that enter the cord may help determine the site of the sulcus. Yellow areas corresponding to old hemorrhages on the surface of the cord and/or microcavities in the depth of the sulcus and/or gliotic tissue within the dorsal horn provide some guidance for tracing the sulcomyelotomy. When the dorsolateral sulcus is difficult to find,

intraoperative monitoring of the dorsal column somatosensory evoked potentials (SEPs) evoked by stimulation of the tibial nerve is especially helpful.

For operative procedures at the lumbosacral level, the patient is positioned prone on thoracic and iliac supports, and the head placed 20 cm lower than the level of the surgical wound to minimize the intraoperative loss of CSF. The desired vertebral level is identified by palpation of the spinous processes or, if this is difficult, with lateral radiography including the S1 vertebra. Interspinous levels identified by a needle can then be marked with methylene blue. A laminectomy—either bilateral or unilateral, according to pain topography—from Th11 to L1 (or L2) is performed. The dura and arachnoid are opened longitudinally and the filum terminale is isolated. Identification of roots is then performed with electrical stimulation.

The roots L1 and L2 are easily identified at their penetration into their respective dural sheaths. Stimulation of L2 produces a response of the iliopsoas and adductor muscles. Identification of L3 to L5 is difficult for many reasons:

1. The exit through their respective dural sheaths is caudal to the exposure.
2. The dorsal rootlets enter the DREZ along an uninterrupted line.
3. The ventral roots are hidden in front of the dentate ligament.
4. The motor responses in the leg to stimulation of the roots are difficult to observe intraoperatively, because of the patient's prone position.

Stimulation of L3 produces a preferential response in the adductors and quadriceps, of L4 in quadriceps, and of L5 in the anterior tibialis. Stimulation of the S1 dorsal root produces a motor response of the gastrocnemius-soleus group that can be confirmed later, by repeatedly checking the Achilles ankle reflex before, during, and after MDT at this level. Stimulation of the S2 to S4 dorsal roots (or better, directly, the corresponding spinal cord segments) can be assessed by recordings of the motor vesical/anal response by use of cystomanometry/rectomanometry/electromyography of the anal sphincter (or simply for the later with a finger into the rectum). Because neurophysiologic investigations are time-consuming to perform in the operative room, we have found that measurements at the conus medullaris can be sufficient in the patients who already have severe preoperative impairment of their vesicoanal functions. These measurements, based on human postmortem anatomical studies, have shown that the landmark between the S1 and S2 segments is situated around 30 mm above the exit from the conus of the tiny coccygeal root.[2]

Microsurgical DREZotomy at the lumbar-sacral levels has the same principles as the ones at the cervical level. The technique is summarized and illustrated in Figure 20-8. At the lumbosacral level, MDT is difficult and possibly dangerous because of the rich vasculature of the conus. The posterolateral spinal artery courses along the posterolateral sulcus. Its diameter is between 0.1 and 0.5 mm and it is fed by the posterior radicular arteries and joins caudally with the descending anterior branch of the Adamkiewicz artery through the conus medullaris anastomotic loop of Lazorthes. This artery has to be preserved by being freed from the sulcus.

Intraoperative neurophysiologic monitoring, especially of SSEPs at the surface of the exposed spinal cord,[25–27] can be an

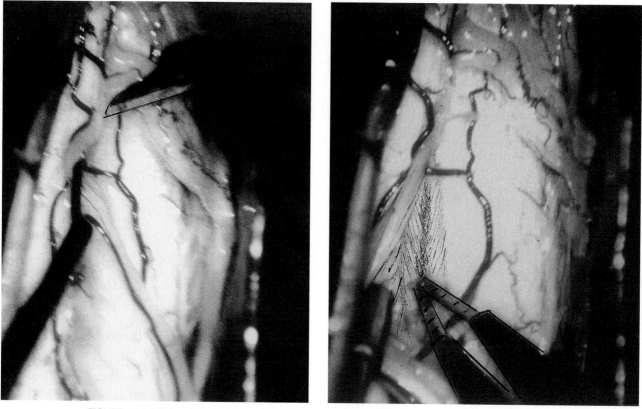

FIGURE 20-6 MDT technique at the cervical level. Exposure of the right dorsolateral aspect of the cervical cord at C6. *Left:* The rootlets of the selected dorsal root(s) are displaced dorsally and medially with a hook (or a microsucker) to obtain access to the ventrolateral aspect of the DREZ in the dorsolateral sulcus. Then, an incision, 2 mm in depth, at 30 degrees ventrally and medially, is made with a microknife in the lateral border of the dorsolateral sulcus. *Right:* Microcoagulations are then performed, down to the apex of the dorsal horn, in a dotted manner, using a sharp graduated bipolar microforceps.

aid to surgery. Recordings of dorsal root presynaptic potentials and dorsal horn postsynaptic potentials can be useful for identification of the spinal cord segments. As a matter of fact, potentials have a maximal intensity in C6 to C7, and C8, for stimulation of the median, and ulnar nerve, respectively, and in L5 to S2, and S2 to S4, for stimulation of the tibial nerve, and the dorsal nerve of the penis (or clitoris), respectively.

Recordings of surface spinal cord SEPs can also be helpful to monitor the surgical lesion itself: The dorsal column potentials can be monitored for checking the integrity of the ascending dorsal column fibers, especially when the dorsolateral sulcus is not clearly marked (as is common in [brachial] root avulsion); the dorsal horn potentials can be monitored to follow the extent of MDT, particulary when good sensory functions are present before surgery (see legend of Fig. 20-9).

In addition (at present time—more for research than for strictly monitoring), unitary spikes generated in the dorsal horn neurons can be recorded during DREZotomy to evidence abnormal activites. This may help identify the surgical target and better understand the electrophysiologic mechanisms underlying painful phenomena. With that purpose, our group in Lyon developed special simplified floating microelectrodes, at first of the Merril and Ainsworth's type,[18] later of an original design, that is, a double microelectrode with a better ability to distinguish spikes from artifacts.[19,28] These unitary electrophysiologic recordings can be correlated

to microdialysis studies that we are developing in parallel during MDT procedures.[29]

Radiofrequency Thermocoagulation Procedure

In 1976 Nashold and his group published a method using RF thermocoagulation to destroy hyperactive neurons in the substantia gelatinosa[4] and in 1979 in the whole DREZ region.[5] In 1981,[30] the technique was modified to produce less extensive lesioning, so that the risk of encroachment of the neighboring corticospinal tract and dorsal column is minimized. With the modified technique, the lesion is made with a 0.5-mm insulated stainless steel electrode, with a tapered noninsulated 2-mm tip, designed and manufactured by Radionics Inc. For treatment of pain after brachial plexus avulsion, the electrode penetrates the dorsolateral sulcus to a depth of 2 mm at an angle of 25 to 45 degrees in the lateral-medial direction. A series of RF coagulations are made under a current of 35 to 40 mA (not over 75 °C) for 10–15 seconds. The RF lesions are spaced at 2- to 3-mm intervals along the longitudinal extent of the dorsolateral sulcus. The lesion observed under magnification is seen as a circular whitened area that extends 1 to 2 mm beyond the tip of the electrode. Nashold emphasizes on the interest of impedance measurements.[31] Before and after each lesion, the impedance has to be measured. It is usually less than 1200 ohms in damaged spinal cord. The authors state that as the transition from

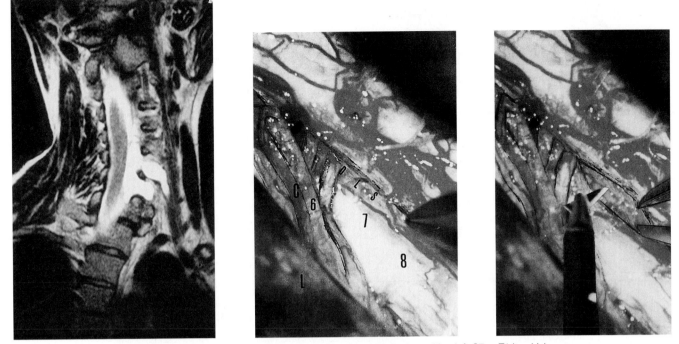

FIGURE 20-7 MDT technique in brachial plexus avulsion. *Left:* Patient with a left C7 to T1 brachial plexus avulsion. Magnetic resonance image shows pseudo-meningocoeles on the left side at the lower cervical spine. *Middle:* Operative view showing, on left side (*L*), a C6 dorsal root remaining intact, and avulsion of dorsal rootlets at the C7 and C8 levels. Dorsolateral sulcus (*DLS*). *Right:* Operative view showing MDT procedure on avulsed spinal root levels: incision with a microknife of the dorsolateral sulcus and dotted microcoagulations inside the sulcus with a sharp bipolar microforceps.

injured parenchyma into more normal tissue is made, impedance readings should increase and eventually reach normal levels of 1500 ohms. The authors use these numbers as a guide to stop the lesion-making at the desired end.

Dorsal Root Entry Zone Procedure with the Laser Beam

Levy and colleagues in 1983[6] and Powers and colleagues in 1984[7] advocated CO_2 and argon laser, respectively, as lesion-maker. According to the description of Levy and colleagues, the pulse duration of the CO_2 laser is 0.1 sec and the power is adjusted to approximately 20 W, so that one or two single pulses create a 2-mm depression at a 45-degree angle in the DREZ. The lesions are probed with a microinstrument marked at 1-mm increments to ensure that the depth of the lesions (1 to 2 mm) is adequate. Intraoperative observations in humans and experimental studies comparing DREZ lesions performed with RF thermocoagulation to those made with various laser beams found that the laser lesions were generally more circumscribed and less variable.[32] However, Walker and colleagues reported on the danger of creating extensive damage and syrinx cavities with the laser (CO_2).[33] In a well-documented study evaluating the effects in dog spinal cord of DREZ lesions with RF or CO_2 (or YAG laser), Young found that the size and extent of the lesion related primarily to the magnitude of power used to make the lesion (Young RF, Foley K, Chambi IV, Rand RW. Personal communication, 1988). They showed that, provided the procedures are performed with proper parameters, the lesions could be successfully localized to the DREZ, including layers I to VI of the dorsal horn, and spare the dorsal column and the corticospinal tract,

using any of the three techniques. The main difference was that with laser the lesion was shaped like the letter "V," with the maximum width at the surface, while with RF it was more spherical. In both methods, in chronic animals, the same glial reactions were observed. In a series of patients, Young made a comparative analysis of RF and CO_2 laser procedures.[34] With RF, 39 of the 58 patients (67%) reported good results (pain regressed by 50% or more), and good results were reported in 9 of 20 patients (45%) with the CO_2 laser. Postoperative complications with RF were noted in 26%, and with CO_2 laser in 15%.

Ultrasonic Dorsal Root Entry Zone Procedure

This procedure was developed by Kandel and Dreval[8,9] in Moscow. It has been mostly used for pain due to brachial plexus avulsion. According to the description given by Dreval, the technique consists of a continuous longitudinal opening of the dorsolateral sulcus at the level of the avulsed roots to the depth of the microcavities and the changed spongy cord tissue. At the same time, ultrasonic destruction of the pathologic tissues is made. The lesion is strictly in the projection of the dorsolateral sulcus at an angle of 25 degrees medially and ventrally. The depth of the microcavities is the main criterion of the depth of the lesioning. After ultrasonic DREZsulcomyelotomy, the grey color of the dorsal horn is well seen in the depth of the opened dorsolateral sulcus. The vessels crossing the sulcus are kept intact. The ultrasonic lesions are produced at a working frequency of 44 kHz, and the amplitude of ultrasonic oscillation is 15 to 50 mcm. The lesions are placed in a "dotted" manner along the sulcus.

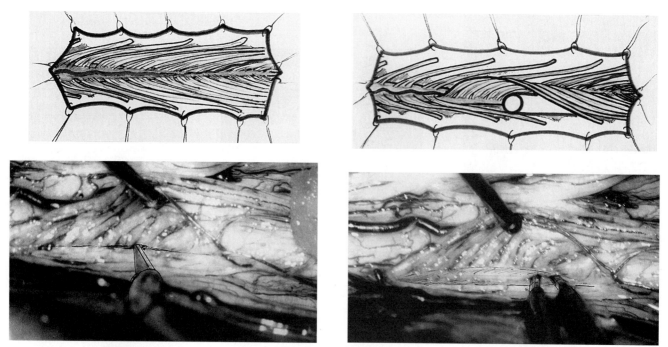

FIGURE 20-8 MDT technique at the lumbosacral level. *Top (drawings)*: Exposure of the conus medullaris through a T11 to L1 laminectomy and approach of the left dorsolateral sulcus. For doing so, the rootlets of the selected lumbosacral dorsal roots are displaced dorsally and medially to obtain proper access to ventrolateral aspect of the DREZ. *Bottom (operative view, left side)*: The rootlets of the selected dorsal roots are retracted dorsomedially and held with a (specially designed) ball-tip microsucker, used as a small hook, to gain access to the ventrolateral part of the DREZ. After division of the fine arachnoidal filaments sticking the rootlets together with the pia mater with curved sharp microscissors (not shown), the main arteries running along the dorsolateral sulcus are dissected and preserved, while the smaller ones are coagulated with a sharp bipolar microforceps (not shown). Then, a continuous incision is performed using a microknife, made with a small piece of razor blade inserted within the striated jaws of a curved razorblade holder. The cut is, on average, at a 45-degree angle and to a depth of 2 mm. *Bottom (operative view, right side)*: The surgical lesion is completed by performing microcoagulations under direct magnified vision, at a low intensity, inside the posterolateral sulcomyelotomy down to the apex of the dorsal horn. These microcoagulations are made all along the segment of the cord selected to be operated on by means of the special sharp bipolar forceps, insulated except at the tip over 5 mm and graduated every millimeter.

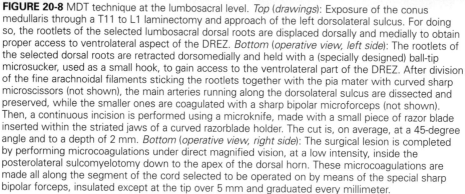

FIGURE 20-9 Effects of MDT on somatosensory evoked potentials recorded on the spinal cord surface (i.e., the evoked electrospinogram). Effects of MDT on the evoked electrospinogram (EESG) in two different patients, one operated on at the cervical level (left recordings), the other at the lumbosacral level (right recordings). Recordings from the surface of the dorsal column, medially to the DREZ at the C7 cervical (Ce) and the L5 lumbosacral (LS) segments, ipsilateral to the stimulation of the median and the tibial nerve, respectively, before (A and C) and after (B and D) MDT. The inital positive event P9 (for cervical) (P17 for lumbosacral) corresponds to the farfield compound potential originating in the proximal part of the brachial (lumbosacral) plexus. The small and sharp negative peaks N11 (N21) correspond to nearfield presynaptic successive axonal events, probably generated in the proximal portion of the dorsal root, the dorsal funiculus and the large diameter afferent collaterals to the dorsal horn. After MDT, all of these presynaptic potentials remain unchanged. The larger slow negative wave N13 (N24) corresponds to the postsynaptic activation of the dorsal horn by group I and II peripheral afferent fibers of the median (tibial) nerves. They are diminished after MDT (in the order of two thirds). The later negative slow wave N2 (just visible in the cervical recording) corresponds to postsynaptic dorsal horn activity consecutive to the activation of group II and III afferent fibers. N2 is suppressed after MDT.

CRITERIA FOR INDICATIONS (WITH ILLUSTRATIVE RESULTS)

Cancer Pain

Good candidates are patients with long life expectancies and sufficiently good general conditions to safely undergo open surgery under general anesthesia who have topographically limited pain caused by well-localized lesions. These criteria restrict indications of MDT to a limited number of patients with cancer. Thoracic apex syndrome (i.e., the Pancoast syndrome) is a good indication for MDT.[35] The procedure is generally performed from C7 to T2. For more extended cervicothoracic cancers, high cervical anterolateral cordotomy or spinothalamic tractomy are preferable. Other good indications for MDT are represented by algias caused by circumscribed invasions of the thorax or the abdomen wall, or of the perineal floor, and also pain due to limited neoplastic involvement of lumbar-sacral roots and/or plexuses. Because extensive DREZ operations at the lumbar and/or sacral segments would inevitably result in leg hypotonia and/or sphincter disturbances, for pain below the waist in patients who can walk, the procedure is indicated only if limited. Intrathecal morphine is the technique of choice for advanced widespread pelvic cancers. In our series, a good result (withdrawal of narcotics) was obtained with MDT in 87% of the 46 patients operated on at the cervical or the cervico-thoracic level, and in 78% of the 35 patients who underwent surgery at the lumbar and/or sacral levels for well-localized cancers. Survival time ranged from 1 month to 4 years (13 months on average). Postoperative infection occurred in two cases, and in two patients surgery was considered to have precipitated death.

Pain after Brachial Plexus Avulsion

All the authors experienced in DREZ procedures, whatever their technical modality may be, agree to consider DREZ operations effective for pain developing after brachial plexus avulsion. For us, the DREZ lesion must not be limited to the avulsed segments, but has to be extended to the adjacent remaining roots, especially if their level is included in the painful territory. Our results with the microsurgical DREZotomy technique in patients observed for longer than 1 year are summarized in Table 20-1. The long-term results in our series are concordant with those of the literature series. The group of Duke University has reported a success rate of 54% in a series of 39 patients operated on with the RF thermocoagulation technique.[36] The Queen Square group in London in their series of 44 cases treated also with thermocoagulation, obtained a 68% success rate.[37,38] Rath and colleagues in Germany reported a 61% rate of success in their 13 cases also treated with RF thermocoagulation.[39] Dreval reported a 87% succes rate in 127 patients in whom the DREZ lesions were performed using a special small ultrasonic probe.[39] Analysis of literature concerning postoperative complications with RF or laser DREZ procedures for brachial plexus avulsion revealed corticospinal and/or dorsal column deficits (more or less severe), in 0% to 10% of patients with the laser and in up to 50% with the RF technique according to the reviewed series.[9,40]

Pain Due to Spinal Cord and/or Cauda Equina Lesions

Most patients who underwent DREZ surgery for spinal cord or cauda equina lesions corresponded to spine injuries, as well in our series as in those reported in the literature.[39,41-44] Nashold's group has analysed in details his results in several publications.[41,42] Our results have been studied recently; they are summarized in Table 20-2.[45] Because in our series a majority of the traumatic cases did not have a complete anatomic treatment of their vertebral fracture(s) at the time of the injury, MDT was preceded by a long dissection of the dura from the surrounding epidural fibrosis, a delicate freeing of the cord and of the roots from adhesive arachnoiditis, and an eventual desincarceration of the neural structures from residual bone fragments occupying the subdural space. This preparatory approach was performed in approximately half of the patients as the first step of a whole operation. In the other half, because the approach was particularly long and bloody—especially when metallic rods had to be removed—it was the first part of a two-staged operation, the second one being done approximately 2 weeks later. As shown in Table 20-2, our experience is that MDT performed for pain associated with spinal cord lesions was only effective in patients whose pain had a "radiculo-metameric" distribution, that is, the pain corresponding to the level and extent of the spinal cord lesion. We called this pain *segmental* pain. On the contrary, pain in the territory below the lesion, especially the one in the perineosacral area, was not favorably influenced even when DREZ surgery was performed at the lower medullary segments.

Therefore, MDT must be reserved for pain syndromes that are related to the injured medullary segments and the adjacent ones if modified by consecutive pathological processes (cavitation, gliosis, arachnoiditis); the procedure has to be performed at the corresponding segmental levels (Fig. 20-10). In patients with incomplete paraplegia, DREZ lesions have to be performed not too deeply to avoid additional neurologic deficits. On the contrary, in patients with complete motor and sensory deficits below the lesion, MDT can be done extensively on the selected segments. The best indications for DREZ surgery are the same as those for cordectomy, that is, the traumatic lesions of the spine below T10 (conus medullaris), especially when pain is located in the legs rather than in the totally anesthetic perineum.

Pain caused by lesions of cauda equina can also be favorably influenced by MDT performed at the corresponding spinal cord segments.

Pain Due to Peripheral Nerve Lesions

When pain due to peripheral nerve injury is not relieved by transcutaneous neurostimulation or spinal cord stimulation, MDT may be considered. According to our experience—which consists of 48 cases operated on—MDT may only be effective when the predominant component of pain is of the paroxysmal type (electrical flashing pain) and/or corresponds to allodynia (hyperalgesia). Good results can also be achieved in disabling post-traumatic causalgic syndromes with severe hyperpathia; generally, the vasomotor disturbances are also favorably influenced. In patients without significant neurologic deficits, DREZ lesion must not be too extensive in length and depth so that the tactile and proprioceptive sensory capacities be at least partially retained, and uncomfortable paresthesias avoided.

● **TABLE 20-1** • Results of MDT for Pain due to Brachial Plexus Avulsion

I. Results on Pain (55 patients)

No. of Patients	Follow-up	Total Pain Relief (=No Medical Treatment)	Pain Controlled with Additional Medications (but No Opiods)	Failures
55	On discharge	54 (98%)		1 (2%)
55	At 1 y	39 (71%)	13 (23.6%)	3 (5.4%)
		94.6%		
55	>1 y (Average: 6 y)	21 (38%)	17 (31%)	17 (31%)
		69%		

II. Complications and Side-Effects (55 patients)

Mortality: nil

Local complications
– Cerebrospinal fluid fistula: one (transient)
– Meningitis: one (cured by antibiotics)

Neurologic complications
– Ataxia in homolateral lower limb
  mild: 4; severe: 2
– Motor deficit in homolateral limb
  mild: 1
– Urogenital disturbances: 1

Neurologic side effects
– Decrease in sensation in homolateral upper thorax
  mild: 5; marked: 1
– Dysesthesias in homolateral upper limb
  mild: 2
– New Sensory deficit in homolateral upper limb
  mild: 3; marked: 2

After limb amputation, two main types of pain that may co-exist can be encountered: pain in the phantom limb and pain in the stump. If spinal cord stimulation fails, DREZ surgery may be considered. Phantom limb pain is generally well relieved when rootlets are avulsed. Pain in the stump is inconstantly influenced; better results are obtained when stump pain is of the paroxysmal and/or allodynic type. The non-painful phantom phenomenum is generally not totally suppressed by DREZ surgery, at least in our experience using the MDT procedure.

A DREZ operation of the microsurgical type may be also considered for severe occipital neuralgia or unbearable latero-cervical pain. Surgery is performed at the C2 to C3 medullary segments. At this level, the procedure is quite easy through a C2 hemilaminectomy. The effect on pain in our three such patients was good. In the series of 11 cases published by Dubuisson, the effects of the operation were also good.[46]

Postherpetic Pain

Results of surgery in the DREZ for postherpetic pain have been reported by a few groups.[39,47] In our experience of MDT for postherpetic neuralgias in 10 cases, only superficial pain located in the affected dermatome(s) was significantly improved, especially when of the allodynic type. The permanent (burning and/or aching) deep component was unrelieved; it can even be aggravated, the patient complaining of additional constrictive sensations after surgery. Before deciding on DREZ surgery in patients with postherpetic neuralgia, one must be very cautious. Although no deaths or postoperative neurologic complications occurred in this group in our series, we think it is necessary to stress the possible vital risks in these patients; as a matter of fact, most are elderly and psychologically impaired. Besides, when the thoracic spinal cord is the target, because at this particular level the dorsal horn is very narrow and deeply situated, as shown in Figure 20-4, encroachment of the corticospinal tract laterally and of the dorsal column medially may occur. Whatever the topographic level of the pain may be, the exact clinical identification of the root(s) corresponding to the herpetic lesions is difficult. At surgery, the observation of atrophy and a greyish color in the concerned root(s) is very helpful.

Hyperspastic States with Pain

Because muscular tone was diminished in the operated territories after MDT performed for treatment of pain,[2,23] the procedure was applied as early as 1973 for harmful spasticity.[24,48–51] The antispastic effects can be explained by the interruption of the afferent components of the myotatic

● **T A B L E 2 0 - 2** • Results of MDT for Pain Due to Spinal Cord or Cauda Equina Injuries in 44 Patients

Site of the Causative Lesion (Total No. of Patients)	No. of Pts Observed More Than 1 yr ---------------- Extreme Follow-up in Mo (Average Follow-up in y)	Type of Pain	Level of MDT Upper Segment ↕ Lower Segment (According to Patients)	Result on Pain after 1 y Follow-up		
				Good (>75%)	Fair (75%≥ −≥25%)	Poor (<25%)
Conus medullaris (25)	17 ---------------- 12–240 m (6 y)	Segmental	Th12 ± 3 ↕ L4 ± 3	14 (82%)	1	2
Cauda Equina (4)	3 ---------------- 60–135 m (7 y)	Segmental	L3 ± 2 ↕ L5 ± 1	1 (33%)	1	1
Thoracic cord (8)	5 ---------------- 12–180 m (6 y)	Segmental	Corresp Thor. Segm	2 (40%)	1	1
Thoracic cord (4)	2 ---------------- 12–108 m (5 y)	Below lesion	L3 ± 1 ↕ S4 ± 2	0 (0%)	1	1
Cervical cord (3)	3 ---------------- 15–180 m (9 y)	Below lesion	L2 ± 1 ↕ S2 ± 1	0 (0%)	2	1
Overall results						
1) Total segmental (37)	25 patients (6 y)	Segmental	Corresponding segmental	17 (68%)		
2) Total below lesion (7)	5 patients (7 y)	Below lesion	Lumbosacral	0 (0%)		

(monosynaptic) and the nociceptive (polysynaptic) reflexes, which would deprive the somatosensory relays of the dorsal horn from most of its excitatory inputs.

Forty-two patients, mostly hemiplegic, underwent MDT at the cervical level for hyperspasticity in the upper limb, and 121 patients underwent MDT at the lumbosacral level for excessive spasticity complicating severe paraplegic states such as those observed in advanced multiple sclerosis. For the upper limb, MDT was performed from C5 to T1 segments. In paraplegic patients, MDT was performed bilaterally from L2 down to S2, and additionally down to S5 when there was an hyperactive neurogenic bladder with urine leakage around the catheter or unvoluntary micturation in between intermittent catheterization.

Twenty-nine of the 42 patients with harmful spasticity in the upper limb had permanent associated pain. Seventy-five of the 121 paraplegic patients suffered from pain mostly due to spasms and/or contractures.

Results on hyperspasticity (with follow-up ranging from 2 to 20 years; average, 8 years) are detailed elsewhere.[50–53]

Only a brief summary will be given here. For paraplegic patients, a useful effect on lower limbs (i.e., a lasting decrease in tone allowing easy passive mobilization) was obtained in 87% of the patients. For most hemiplegic patients, the effect on upper limb was significant and lasting only at the level of the shoulder and elbow, allowing reappearance of voluntary movements (when hidden behind hypertonia before surgery). The effect was much less beneficial at the level of the wrist and fingers, so that additional peripheral neurotomies and orthopedic surgery were often required.

Concerning sensory functions, MDT constantly produced a decrease in sensation in the operated territories, when present preoperatively: mild in 40%, marked in 40%, and severe in 20%. When present, pain was relieved in 88% in both groups.

From this experience, indications for hyperspasticity can be summarized as follows: (1) The hyperspastic hemiplegic upper limb can benefit from MDT, predominantly for shoulder and elbow functions. Wrist and fingers are much less favorably influenced, especially if there are irreducible contractures and

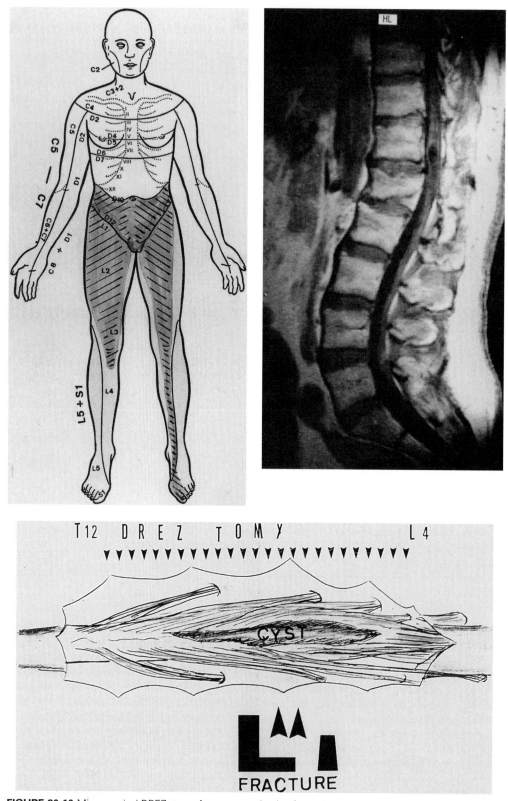

FIGURE 20-10 Microsurgical DREZotomy for segmental pain after spinal cord injury in a paraplegic patient after spinal cord injury due to L1 fracture with "segmental" pain in both legs. *Upper left:* Segmental pain represented by hatched areas. *Upper right:* Corresponding magnetic resonance image showing conus medullaris contusion at the level of T12 to L1 vertebral bodies. *Lower:* Drawing illustrating intraoperative findings: necrotic cyst and gliosis in the segments of the conus medullaris corresponding to the vertebral fracture (L1 level). Microsurgical DREZotomy was performed on both sides in the T12 to L4 spinal cord segments.

deformities in flexion and no motor function in the extensors. So, MDT is particularly indicated when there is an important excess of spasticity in the proximal muscles. (2) For lower limbs, because MDT has generally a dramatic effect on tone, indications must be restricted to paraplegic patients with severe disability, who are unable to walk, especially if uncomfortable in wheelchair, and/or exposed to pressure sores in bed. Of course, indications for MDT are reinforced if additional pain is present, the more so as it is due to spasms, contractures, and/or neurotrophic disturbances.

CONCLUSIONS

After a total experience of 390 cases operated on since 1972 for severe chronic pain, we conclude that indications are:

1. Cancer pain that is limited in extent (such as in Pancoast-Tobias syndrome).

2. Persistent neuropathic pain that is due to:
   - Brachial plexus injuries, especially those with avulsion
   - Spinal cord lesions, especially the pain corresponding to segmental lesions. Pain below the lesion is not favorably influenced. Segmental pain caused by lesions in the conus medullaris or the cauda equina is generally well relieved.
   - Peripheral nerve injuries, amputation, or herpes zoster, when the predominant component of pain is of the paroxysmal type and/or corresponds to provoked allodynia/hyperalgesia.

3. Disabling hyperspasticity with pain.

Of course, surgery in the DREZ must be considered within the frame of all the methods belonging to the armamentarium of pain surgery. Figure 20-11 summarizes our present process of decision making for neuropathic pain of peripheral nerve, dorsal root, and spinal cord origin. Supraspinal pain, especially central pain after stroke, can be treated—now—by Precentral (motor) Control Stimulation.[54,55]

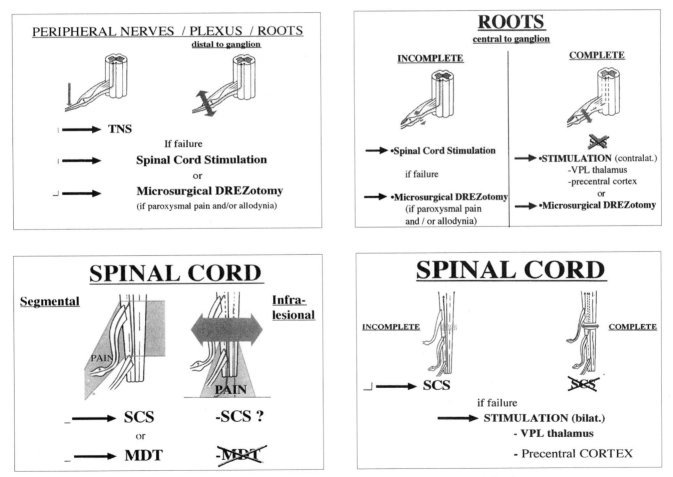

FIGURE 20-11 Algorithms for neuropathic pain, originating from lesions of: (1) peripheral nerves, plexus, roots distal to ganglion (*upper left*); (2) roots central to ganglion (*upper right*), (3) spinal cord: incomplete and complete. Treatment for the segmental (*lower left*) and the infralesional components of the pain is different, as shown in the drawing (*lower right*).

REFERENCES

1. Melzach R, Wall PD. Pain mechanism. A new theory. Science 150:971–979, 1965.
2. Sindou M. Study of the dorsal root entry zone. The selective micro DREZotomy for pain surgery. Lyon, University Medical Thesis Press, 1972.
3. Sindou M, Quoex C, Baleydier C. Fiber organization at the posterior spinal cord-rootlet junction in man. J Comp Neurol 153:15–26, 1974.
4. Nashold BS, Urban B, Zorub DS. Phantom pain relief by focal destruction of substantia gelatinosa of Rolando. In Bonica JJ, Albe-Fessard D (eds). Advances in Pain Research and Therapy, vol. 1. New York, Raven, 1976, pp 959–963.
5. Nashold BS, Ostdahl PH. Dorsal root entry zone lesions for pain relief. J Neurosurg 51:59–69, 1979.
6. Levy WJ, Nutkiewicz A, Ditmore M, Watts C. Laser induced dorsal root entry zone lesions for pain control. Report of three cases. J Neurosurg 59:884–886, 1983.
7. Powers SK, Adams JE, Edwards SB, Boggan JE, Hosobuchi Y. Pain relief from dorsal root entry zone lesions made with argon and cardon dioxide microsurgical lasers. J Neurosurg 61:841–847, 1984.
8. Kandel EL, Ogleznev KJA, Dreval ON. Destruction of posterior root entry zone as a method for treating chronic pain in traumatic injury to the brachial plexus. Vopr Neurochir 6:20–27, 1987.
9. Dreval ON. Ultrasonic DREZ-operations for treatment of pain due to brachial plexus avulsion. Acta Neurochir 122:76–81, 1993.
10. Sindou M, Fischer G, Mansuy L. Posterior spinal rhizotomy and selective posterior rhizidiotomy. In Krayenbühl H, Maspes PE, Sweet WH (eds). Progress in Neurological Surgery, vol 7. Basel, Karger, 1976, pp 201–250.
11. Sindou M, Goutelle A. Surgical posterior rhizotomies for the treatment of pain. In Krayenbül HH (ed). Advances and Technical Standards in Neurosurgery, vol. 10. Vienna, Springer-Verlag, 1983, pp 147–185.
12. Rand R. Further observations on Lissauer's tractolysis. Neurochirurgica 3:151–168, 1960.
13. Denny-Brown D, Kirk EJ, Yanagisawa N. The tract of Lissauer in relation to sensory transmission in the dorsal horn of spinal cord in the macaque monkey. J Comp Neurol 151:175–200, 1973.
14. Ramon y, Cajal S. Histologie du Système Nerveux. Vol. 1. Paris, Maloine, 1901, p 986.
15. Szentagothai J. Neuronal and synaptic arrangement in the substantia gelatinosa. J Comp Neurol 122:219–239, 1964.
16. Wall PD. Presynaptic control of impulses at the first central synapse in the cutaneous pathway. In Eccles JC, Schadé JP (eds). Physiology of Spinal Neurons. Amsterdam, Elsevier, 1964, pp 92–118.
17. Loeser JD, Ward AA Jr, White LE Jr. Chronic deafferentation of human spinal cord neurons. J Neurosurg 29:48–50, 1968.
18. Jeanmonod D, Sindou M, Magnin M, Baudet M. Intra-operative unit recordings in the human dorsal horn with a simplified floating microelectrode. Electroencephalogr Clin Neurophysiol 72:450–454, 1989.
19. Guenot M, Hupe JM, Mertens P, Ainsworth A, Bullier J, Sindou M. A new type of microelectrode for obtaining unitary recordings in the human spinal cord. J Neurosurg (Spine) 91:25–32, 1999.
20. Loeser JD, Ward AA Jr, White LE Jr. Some effects of deafferentation of neurons. J Neurosurg 17:629–636, 1967.
21. Albe-Fessard D, Lombard MC: Use of an animal model to evaluate the origin of and protection against deafferentation pain. In Bonica JJ, Liebeskind JC, Albe-Fessard DG, et al (eds). Pain Research Therapy, vol 5. New York, Raven, 1983, pp 691–700.
22. Jeanmonod D, Sindou M. Somatosensory function following dorsal root entry zone lesions in patients with neurogenic pain or spasticity. J Neurosurg 74:916–932, 1991.
23. Sindou M, Fischer G, Goutelle A, Mansuy L. La radicellotomie postérieure sélective. Premiers résultats dans la chirurgie de la douleur. Neurochirurgie 20:391–408, 1974.
24. Sindou M, Fischer G, Goutelle A, Schott B, Mansuy L. La radicellotomie postérieure sélective dans le traitement des spasticités. Rev Neurol 130:201–215, 1974.
25. Jeanmonod D, Sindou M, Mauguière F. The human cervical and lumbo-sacral evoked electrospinogram. Data from intra-operative spinal cord surface recordings. Electroencephalogr Clin Neurophysiol 80:477–489, 1991.
26. Turano G, Sindou M, Mauguière F. SCEP monitoring during spinal surgery for pain and spasticity. In Dimitrijevic MR, Halter JA (eds). Atlas of Human Spinal Cord Evoked Potentials. Boston, Butterworth-Heinemann, 1995.
27. Sindou M, Turano G, Pantieri R, Mertens P, Mauguière F. Intraoperative monitoring of spinal cord SEPs, during microsurgical DREZotomy (MDT) for pain, spasticity and hyperactive bladder. Stereotact Funct Neurosurg 62:164–170, 1994.
28. Guenot M, Hupe J.M, Mertens P, Mauguière F, Bullier J, Sindou M. Microelectrode recordings during microsurgical DREZotomy. Stereotact Funct Neurosurg 67:1–2, 1996–1997.
29. Mertens P, Ghaemmaghami C, Perret-Liaudet A, Guenot M, Sindou M, Renaud B. In vivo amino-acids concentrations in human dorsal horn studied by microdialysis during DREZotomy. Methodology and preliminary results. Stereotact Funct Neurosurg 67:1–2, 1996–1997.
30. Nashold BS. Modification of DREZ lesion technique (letter). J Neurosurg 55:1012, 1981.
31. Nashold JRB, Nashold DS. Microsurgical DREZotomy in treatment of deafferentation pain. In Schmidek HH, Sweet WH (eds). Operative Neurosurgical Techniques (3rd ed). Philadelphia, WB Saunders, 1995, pp 1623–1636.
32. Levy WJ, Gallo C, Watts C. Comparison of laser and radiofrequency dorsal root entry zone lesions in cats. Neurosurgery 16:327–330, 1985.
33. Walker JS, Ovelmen-Levitt J, Bullard DE, Nashold BS. Dorsal root entry zone lesions using a CO2 laser in cats with neurophysiologic and histologic assessment. Neurosurgery 15:265, 1984.
34. Young RF: Clinical experience with radio-frequency and laser DREZ lesions. J Neurosurg 72:715–720, 1990.
35. Sindou M, Lapras C. Neurosurgical treatment of pain in the Pancoast-Tobias syndrome. Selective posterior rhizotomy and open antero-lateral C2-cordotomy. In Bonica JJ, Ventafrida V, Pagni CA (eds). Advances in Pain Research and Therapy, vol. 4. New York, Raven, New York, 1982, pp 199–209.
36. Friedman AH, Nashold BS, Bronec PR. Dorsal root entry zone lesions for the treatment of brachial plexus avulsion injuries: a follow-up study. J Neurosurg 22:369–373, 1988.
37. Thomas DGT, Jones ST. Dorsal root entry zone lesions in brachial plexus avulsion. Neurosurgery 15:966–968, 1984.
38. Thomas DGT, Kitchen ND. Long-term follow-up of dorsal root entry zone lesions in brachial plexus avulsion. J Neurol Neurosurg Psychiatry 57:737–738, 1994.
39. Rath SA, Braun V, Soliman N, Antoniadis G, Richter MP. Results of DREZ-coagulations for pain related to plexus lesions, spinal cord injuries and post-herpetic neuralgia. Acta Neurochir 138:364–369, 1996.
40. Sindou M, Daher A. Spinal cord ablation procedures for pain. In Dubner A, Gebbart GF, Bond MR (eds). Proceedings of the Fifth World Congress on Pain. Amsterdam, Elsevier, 1988, pp 477–495.
41. Nashold BS, Bullitt E. DREZ-lesions to control central pain in paraplegics. J Neurosurg 55:414–419, 1981.
42. Sampson JH, Cashman RE, Nashold BS, Friedman AH. Dorsal root entry zone lesions for intractable pain after lesions to the conus medullaris and cauda equina. J Neurosurg 37:412–417, 1972.
43. Sindou M. Microsurgical DREZotomy (MDT) for pain, spasticity and hyperactive bladder: a 20 year experience. Acta Neurochir 137:1–5, 1995.
44. Spaic M, Petkovic S, Tadic R, Minic L. Drez-surgery on conus medullaris (after failed implantation of vascular omental graft) for treating chronic pain due to spine (gunshot) injuries. Acta Neurochir 141:1309–1312, 1999.
45. Sindou M, Mertens P, Wael M. Microsurgical DREZotomy for pain due to spinal cord and/or cauda equina injuries. Long-term results in a series of 44 patients. Pain 92:159–171, 2001.
46. Dubuisson D. Treatment of occipital neuralgia by partial posterior rhizotomy at C1–3. J Neurosurg 82:581–586, 1995.
47. Friedman AH, Nashold BS, Ovelmen-Levitt J. Drez-lesions for the treatment of post-herpetic neuralgia. J Neurosurg 60:1258–1261, 1984.
48. Sindou M, Millet MF, Mortamais J, Eyssette M. Results of selective posterior rhizotomy in the treatment of painful and spastic paraplegia secondary to multiple sclerosis. Appl Neurophysiol 45:335–340, 1982.
49. Sindou M, Abdennebi B, Sharkey P. Microsurgical selective procedures in the peripheral nerves and the posterior root-spinal cord junction for spasticity. Appl Neurophysiol 48:97–104, 1985.
50. Sindou M, Mifsud JJ, Boisson D, Goutelle A. Selective posterior rhizotomy in the dorsal root entry zone for treatment of hyperspasticity and pain in the hemiplegic upper limb. Neurosurgery 18:587–595, 1986.
51. Sindou M, Jeanmonod D. Microsurgical DREZ-tomy for the treatment of spasticity and pain in the lower limbs. Neurosurgery 24:655–670, 1989.
52. Sindou M, Jeanmonod D, Mertens P. Surgery in the DREZ: microsurgical DREZotomy for treatment of spasticity. In Sindou M, Abbott R, Keravel Y (eds). Neurosurgery for Spasticity. Berlin, Springer Verlag, 1991, pp 165–182.
53. Decq P, Mertens P. La neurochirurgie de la spasticité. 49:133–416, 2003.
54. Tsubokawa T, Katayama Y, Yamamoto T, Hirayama T, Koyama S. Chronic motor cortex stimulation for the treatment of central pain. Acta Neurochir Suppl (Wien) 1991a; 52:137–139.
55. Mertens P, Nuti C, Sindou M. Precentral cortex stimulation for the treatment of central neuropathic pain. Stereot Funct Neurosurg 73:122–125, 1999.

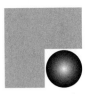

C H A P T E R   2 1

Brainstem Ablative Procedures

JOHN P. GORECKI, MD, AND KENNETH M. LITTLE, MD

Ablative procedures are normally performed only for nociceptive or cancer-related pain. Midbrain tractotomy (MBT) and nucleus caudalis dorsal root entry zone lesion (DREZ; NCD) are procedures that take advantage of brainstem anatomy. The spinothalamic tract, within the midbrain, is uniquely located so that fiber tracts representing the contralateral face and body are in close association. The nucleus caudalis and the descending trigeminal tract are involved with the dissociated perception of pain and temperature. The nucleus caudalis is histologically indistinguishable from the DREZ in the upper cervical cord. Both MBT and NCD involve permanent destruction of second-order neurons within the brainstem. MBT results in the destruction of axons within the spinothalamic and quintothalamic tracts in addition to adjacent peri-aqueductal neurons. NCD results in the destruction of neurons within the nucleus caudalis and the adjacent axons within the descending trigeminal tract. While ablative procedures should be limited to cancer pain, NCD as well as spinal cord DREZ procedures are major exceptions to this rule. In this chapter, the indications, techniques, outcomes, and complications for MBT and NCD are reviewed.

MIDBRAIN TRACTOTOMY

Indications

MBT is the procedure of choice for cancer-related pain that extends above the C5 dermatome. MBT is especially effective for pain associated with head and neck cancer. MBT is most commonly performed for unilateral pain, but MBT can safely be performed bilaterally. MBT avoids the risk of respiratory depression that is a potential complication of bilateral cordotomy. Most patients achieve excellent permanent pain control.

Compared to intraspinal narcotic analgesia, MBT achieves more satisfactory relief for cancer-related pain extending above C5.[1] A retrospective review of 27 patients who underwent MBT showed that all but 1 patient achieved immediate relief, and 85% were relieved of pain until death.[2] The same authors reported 40 MBTs performed on 38 cancer patients and found that 35 patients were pain free until death.[3]

Tasker reviewed 33 cancer patients who underwent 39 MBT procedures and found that 74% were pain free until death.[4] Beauvillain and colleagues reported excellent pain relief in 10 of 11 patients treated with MBT.[5] Frank and colleagues treated 109 patients with cancer, and 83.5% were pain free until death, which occurred up to 7 months later.[6–8] Frank and colleagues found MBT was more effective than thalamotomy in a retrospective comparison.[6]

Surgical Technique

MBT is performed under local anesthesia. Stereotactic localization is accomplished with magnetic resonance imaging. Axial imaging is supplemented with coronal imaging. The target is located in an axial plane between the superior and inferior colliculi. The target is in line with the aqueduct. The target is 5 to 10 mm from the midline contralateral to the pain. The following structures are easily identified on magnetic resonance imaging and help to localize the lesion site: aqueduct of Sylvius, red nucleus, posterior commisure, quadrigeminal plate, and peri-aqueductal gray matter. The entry point through the skull is a twist drill hole located 15 mm from the midline and anterior to the coronal suture. The sagittal angle for the penetrating trajectory is 30 degrees anterior from vertical. The lesion is made with a thalamotomy electrode. The electrode has a diameter of 1.2 mm and an exposed lesioning tip that is 3 mm long. Lesions are made for 60 seconds at a temperature of 80 °C. Producing lesions at a new but adjacent position sequentially enlarges the entire lesion. The end point is the absence of spontaneous or induced pain and dense dissociated analgesia in the contralateral hemi-body and face. One to three lesions are common.

Stimulation is used to confirm the target location. At the perfect target, stimulation at a frequency of 100 Hz results in a well-localized sensation of pain or temperature in the contralateral face and body with a very low threshold. A low threshold is less than 0.3 V. Other responses to stimulation result from activation of structures located near the spinothalamic tract (STT) in the midbrain. The dorsal columns terminate in the nucleus cuneatus and gracilis, which project to the medial lemniscus. The medial lemniscus is ventral and adjacent to the STT. Stimulation of the medial lemniscus also results in contralateral paresthesia but does not normally include sensation in the face. The paresthesia that results from lemniscal stimulation is less discrete than the sensation produced by stimulation of the STT. Stimulation close to the inferior colliculus results in auditory hallucinations that are time-locked to the stimulus. Five hertz stimulation results in a faster clicking than 2 Hz stimulation; 100 Hz stimulation results in the perception of buzzing. A lesion in this location results in hearing loss. Stimulation close to the superior colliculus results in version of the eyes. Stimulation close to the medial longitudinal fasciculus or the third or fourth nerve nuclei results in diplopia. Stimulation within the peri-aqueductal gray matter results in an indescribable sensation. Sometimes patients report fear; they may report an odd sensation rising out of the stomach. There is often an alerting response to stimulation of the peri-aqueductal gray matter with wide opening of the eyes sometimes associated with mastication.

Following surgery, the patient is watched closely for several hours. The blood pressure is monitored closely and aggressively maintained in the normal range. In our experience, hypertension is associated with an increased incidence of hemorrhage. Steroids are not routinely administered.

Complications

The general risks of MBT are the same as those for all stereotactic procedures and include hemorrhage, stroke, infection, drug reactions, wound problems, and death. Complications specific to MBT relate to injury of structures adjacent to the target. Failure of pain relief is uncommon. Hearing loss was more common with open MBT, when lesions were made more caudally. Lesions made during open MBT were closer to the inferior colliculus. Transient contralateral visual field defects due to traction on Meyer's loops during elevation of the temporal lobe was a relatively common complication following open MBT. Lesions that include the medial lemniscus result in contralateral loss of light touch and position. Lemniscal lesions might result in unpleasant paresthesia and may be the source of post-tractotomy dysesthesia. The incidence of post-tractotomy dysesthesia is difficult to quantify. Post-tractotomy dysesthesia may be more common after open procedures. McKenzie in fact abandoned open MBT quickly, stating that the incidence of dysesthesia was 50%.[9] The quoted incidence of induced dysesthesia following cordotomy is 4.3% and following stereotactic MBT is 8.5%.[10] Diplopia is a relatively common complication of MBT. Diplopia results from injury of the ocular nuclei, the medial longitudinal fasciculus, or the superior colliculus. Diplopia is surprisingly well tolerated. Many patients do not volunteer the presence of diplopia and some only respond positively to direct, leading questions specifying blurred or double images. Patching of one eye immediately corrects the problem. There is significant recovery over time. More than 50% of patients experience diplopia following MBT at least transiently. Placing the lesion more caudally[11] reduces the incidence of diplopia; however, the risk of hearing loss is greater for a lesion in this position. A depressed level of consciousness can occur following MBT. This has occurred one time at our institution. Excessive ablation of the peri-aqueductal reticular activating system or placement of the lesion too caudal, close to the pons, may account for this complication.

NUCLEUS CAUDALIS DREZ

Indications

NCD is the same as spinal DREZ, except for the fact that NCD is performed in the medulla and the cervico-medullary junction. NCD is physiologically similar to descending trigeminal tractotomy and trigeminal nucleotomy. These three procedures achieve dense analgesia, while avoiding anesthesia, in the ipsilateral face in the distribution of cranial nerves V, VII, IX, and X. It is easiest to achieve dense analgesia in the first trigeminal division, and most difficult in the teeth and central portion of the mouth. The corneal reflex is preserved following these procedures. The risk of producing anesthesia dolorosa with these procedures is significantly lower than that with more peripheral denervating operations. NCD can safely be performed bilaterally. Although NCD has been used to effectively treat cancer-related facial pain, NCD is a major open microsurgical procedure that should be reserved for patients with a relatively long life expectancy. As described previously, MBT is a very effective alternative for patients with pain in the face due to malignancy. Nociceptive type pain syndromes with intermittent or induced pain respond particularly well to NCD. NCD is especially useful in the management of pain in the eye or first trigeminal division because NCD avoids the risk of corneal anesthesia and anesthesia dolorosa.

NCD has been used for each of the following: trigeminal neuralgia that is refractory to the more common surgical interventions, post-traumatic pain either from accident or surgery, postherpetic neuralgia, pain from a tumor involving the fifth cranial nerve, central pain following stroke, cluster headache, and multiple sclerosis. The short-term efficacy for postherpetic pain is satisfying while the long-term benefit is quite variable. There are few alternative interventions available for patients with postherpetic neuralgia. There are unconfirmed reports of good outcome for cluster headache and migraine. In our experience, intermittent-induced pain is more responsive to NCD than spontaneous steady pain, but we have seen a number of modest successes for atypical facial pain. It is more useful to classify the patients by type of pain rather than disease etiology.[12,13]

We retrospectively reviewed 113 NCD operations performed at Duke since 1982. The surgical technique was the same for 58 patients operated upon after 1990; 51 of those patients were interviewed. The follow-up period was more than 2 years. At the time, patients were not being selected based on the presence of intermittent-induced pain. The severity of the pain was documented using a verbal pain score ranging from 0 to 10. The mean preoperative pain score was 9 with a range of 6 to 10 and the mean postoperative pain score fell to 5.2. All 58 patients were taking narcotic analgesic agents every day before surgery. Following NCD, only 19 of 51 (37%) were still using any narcotics. Based upon a subjective quality of life score, 16 patients were significantly improved, 6 somewhat improved, 16 no different, and 13 were worse following NCD.[12,13]

Surgical Technique

NCD is an open microsurgical procedure performed under general anesthesia. Muscle relaxation is allowed to wear off during the case in order to allow electromyography (EMG) recording. Patients are placed in the prone position with the head secured with Mayfield pin fixation. The incision is midline over the occiput and upper neck because dissection is easiest in the midline. The muscles are stripped away from the occipital bone, arch of C1, and the lamina of C2. A craniectomy is performed eccentric to the painful side and the arch of C1 is removed on the same side. The dura is opened in a Y shape or in a curved line so as to expose the cerebellar tonsils, the obex, the posterior inferior cerebellar artery (PICA), the ipsilateral vertebral artery, the sensory rootlets of C2, the motor rootlets of C1, and the rootlets of the 11th cranial nerve. There usually are no sensory rootlets for C1.

The descending trigeminal tract and the nucleus caudalis is then mapped by recording trigeminal somatosensory evoked potentials (TSSEP) through a bipolar electrode inserted systematically in a line along the lateral margin of the dorsal column extending cephalad from the rootlets of C2. The stimulus is applied peripherally through bipolar electrodes in proximity to the supraorbital, infraorbital, and mental nerves. The location for the maximum amplitude response for each trigeminal division is identified. Somatosensory evoked potentials (SSEP) are recorded with an electrode placed into the dorsal column and stimulating the ipsilateral median nerve. As the electrode in the dorsal column is marched laterally, a point is reached where the amplitude suddenly drops or the evoked potential can no longer be recorded. This occurs at the lateral margin of the dorsal column where the descending trigeminal tract is located. Marking this point accurately reduces the chances of inadvertently lesioning the dorsal column. Once the site to lesion is selected, the El-Naggar/Nashold electrode is used to penetrate the cord. The lesion site is selected by identifying the location of maximum amplitude TSSEP corresponding to the trigeminal division or divisions involved with pain. The lesion site is further modified by identifying a site that is lateral to the border of the dorsal column as defined both visually and by the absence of median nerve SSEP. The El-Naggar/Nashold electrode consists of two electrodes, each of different length that both incorporate insulation on the proximal part of the active electrode that penetrates the brainstem. The purpose of the insulation is to avoid coagulation of the spinocerebellar tract, which overlies the nucleus caudalis. The longer electrode is used cephalad to the C1 rootlets and the shorter electrode is used caudal to the C1 rootlets. The nucleus caudalis is larger in the more cephalad position and the pyramidal tract is immediately deep to the nucleus caudalis closer to C2. Immediately before lesioning, stimulation is carried out through the monopolar El-Naggar/Nashold electrode. The stimulus is a square wave with 0.1-msec duration and a frequency of 2 Hz that is ramped up in amplitude. If a time-locked EMG response in the arm or leg is induced by stimulation at a threshold below 1 V, a lesion is *not* created at this location. The assumption is that the electrode is too close to the corticospinal tract. Sometimes switching from the longer to the shorter electrode corrects this problem. We are working on methods to identify the spinocerebellar tract electrically. It is possible to record over the surface of the cerebellum while stimulating the location of the spinocerebellar tract. The line for potential lesions extends over a length of 16 to 20 mm cephalad to the sensory rootlets of C2 and lies just lateral to the dorsal column or cuneate nucleus. The rootlets of cranial nerve XI mark the lateral border for a potential lesion. Lesions are made with radiofrequency current so that the tissue temperature is raised to 80 °C for 15 seconds.

The trigeminal nerve is the main sensory nerve for the face and head. Cell bodies of trigeminal primary sensory neurons are located within the gasserian ganglion and the mesencephalic nucleus. The gasserian ganglion corresponds anatomically to segmental dorsal root ganglia. Cranial nerves VII, IX, and X in addition to the upper cervical sensory branches also transmit sensation for the head and face. The nuclei of the trigeminal nerve include the motor nucleus of V, the chief sensory nucleus, the mesencephalic nucleus, and the nucleus of the spinal tract. The nucleus of the spinal tract is located in the medulla. The nucleus of the spinal tract is divided into three parts[14]: pars caudalis, pars interpolaris (or oralis), and pars rostralis. The histology of the nucleus of the trigeminal tract and the gray matter of the dorsal horn of the upper cervical cord is identical. The nucleus caudalis is considered to be a rostral extension of the dorsal horn of the spinal cord. The nucleus of the spinal tract receives input from the descending trigeminal tract, which is comprised of fibers transmitting pain and nociceptive signals originating from cranial nerves V, VII, IX, and X. Some of the fibers in the spinal tract mingle within Lissauer's zone in the uppermost three segments of the cervical cord. Nociceptive fibers terminate in the nucleus caudalis within the medulla. Somatotopic organization is described within the descending trigeminal tract and the nucleus caudalis. Two different patterns describe this segmental organization of sensory representation. The first is a pattern of concentric rings that have been compared to "onion skin rings." Sensation from the middle portion of the face immediately surrounding the mouth is represented at more rostral levels within the medulla. The difficulty in achieving dense analgesia close to the midline of the face with nucleotomy or tractotomy supports this theoretical pattern. When nucleotomy is performed at more caudal levels within the medulla, preservation of pain appreciation occurs in the midline of the face. The second pattern is based on the segmental trigeminal divisions. Fibers that originate in the first trigeminal division reach a more caudal level within the nucleus caudalis and descending tract than do fibers that originate in the third division.

Direct sensory evoked potential recording performed during surgery confirms this anatomy. Observations following nucleotomy or tractotomy also confirm that dense analgesia is much easier to achieve in the first trigeminal division than in the third division. The third division of the trigeminal nerve is not represented as far caudal in the medulla. Based on trigeminal divisions, segmentation is also present from medial to lateral within the medulla. At the most medial aspect of the descending tract, immediately adjacent to the dorsal column are fibers from cranial nerves VII, IX, and X. Just lateral to these are fibers from the third trigeminal division. Fibers from the first trigeminal division are located most lateral within the descending tract, farthest from the dorsal columns, and closer to the motor roots of the vagus and spinal accessory nerve. As a result, the lesion must be made close to the dorsal column and relatively rostral in the medulla to achieve dense analgesia that includes the third trigeminal division. Lesions in this location are associated with a risk of proprioceptive deficits from undesired injury to the dorsal column.

Complications

Not all patients obtain satisfactory pain relief. The pain relief that is achieved is not always maintained long term, although most of the recurrences occur within the first year.

Sjoqvist described the most common complication following descending tractotomy as ataxia, implicating injury to the spinocerebellar tract and restiform body.[15] Ataxia is the most common complication following NCD. The complication usually affects the ipsilateral arm, but sometimes the leg is also affected resulting in gait impairment. The patient may report inability to use the affected arm. This complaint is often out of proportion to the physical findings, especially if the patient has completed a course of physical therapy. Patients may report significant disability even though the residual symptoms are only subjective. Deficits that may be identified include: ataxia, past pointing, loss of two-point discrimination, and weakness. Modest weakness is often present as the patient is emerging from anesthesia that resolves completely. We place all patients on high doses of systemic steroids. This complication results from injury to the spinocerebellar tract. Less commonly injured adjacent tracts include the cuneate tract and nucleus as well as the pyramidal tract.

In an effort to reduce the risk of ataxia, NCD has been modified three times. The addition of proximal insulation to the electrode was the first modification. The second modification was the introduction of electrodes with two different lengths for lesions of different parts of the nucleus. The Nashold/El-Naggar electrode also includes a bend in the electrode to make placement of lesions physically more accurate. Furthermore, precise and rigid electrophysiologic monitoring is now used. In the earliest reports of NCD, the incidence of ataxia was 90%.[16] With the use of the Nashold/El-Naggar electrode, the incidence of ataxia was reported to be 33%.[17]

NCD was performed in 113 patients at Duke. In these patients, there were no episodes reported of serious wound complication, cerebrospinal fluid leak, infection, or death. Out of the 58 patients treated with the Nashold/El-Naggar electrode system, 29 (50%) reported no untoward effect at all. Reported complications included ataxia in 21 (36%), hemiparesis in 1, aseptic meningitis in 1, retinal artery thrombosis in 1, hearing loss in 2, neck pain in 1, "turtle neck" tightness of the neck in 3, vertigo in 1, suicide in 1, and a suicide attempt in 1. The suicide and attempted suicide occurred in patients who did not experience any pain relief. The suicide attests to the severity of the underlying pain. Patients who experienced complications but also enjoyed pain relief were willing to repeat the operation expecting the same outcome. This patient population suffered greatly before surgery.

SUMMARY

Although ablative procedures should normally be reserved for pain associated with cancer, NCD is useful for certain cases of pain in the face due to benign pathology. NCD is especially useful for pain involving the first trigeminal division. NCD will not result in corneal anesthesia and avoids the risk of anesthesia dolorosa. NCD is most useful for intermittent, induced, or nociceptive pain. NCD is effective at least in the short term for postherpetic neuralgia and the long-term outcome remains to be defined. NCD can be used to salvage patients with trigeminal neuralgia in whom surgical intervention fails, especially when the pain involves the first division. NCD is more effective when there is less preoperative deafferentation; therefore, it should be considered before condemning a patient to anesthesia dolorosa with multiple denervating operations. The value of NCD for cluster headache is promising but awaits confirmation and long-term follow-up. Intermittent and induced pain that is caused by previous injury to the face and nerve or previous surgical trauma responds to NCD. NCD is useful for a number of patients with atypical facial pain, especially when the pain is intermittent or at least has a component that is induced. Central pain following stroke only responds to a limited degree to NCD.

Midbrain tractotomy is clearly the procedure of choice for unilateral pain due to cancer that extends above the C5 dermatome. MBT is an excellent procedure for pain due to head and neck cancer. MBT is more appropriate than NCD in patients debilitated by cancer with pain in the face. MBT is less invasive and can also treat pain in the body. Both operations can be done safely for bilateral pain.

ACKNOWLEDGMENT

The author would like to acknowledge that support was obtained for this work from the Durham Veterans Administration Medical Center.

REFERENCES

1. Blond S, Assaker R, Meynadier J, Merienne L. La tractotomie pedonculaire sterotaxique: sa place dans le traitement des alties cervico-faciales neoplastiques. Agressologie 29:77–80, 1988.
2. Voris HC, Whistler WW. Results of stereotactic surgery for intractable pain. Confin Neurol 37:86–96, 1975.
3. Whistler WW, Voris HC. Mesencephalotomy for intractable pain due to malignant disease. Appl Neurophysiol 41:52–56, 1978.
4. Tasker RR. Neurological concepts of pain management in head and neck cancer. Can J Otolaryngol 4:480–484, 1975.
5. Beauvillain de Montreuil C, Lajat Y, Resche F. Use of stereotactic neurosurgery in the treatment of pain in the cervicofacial cancers. Ann Otolaryngol Chir Cervicofaciale 100:181–186, 1983.
6. Frank F, Fabrizi AP, Gaist G. Stereotactic mesencephalotomy versus multiple thalamotomies in the treatment of chronic cancer pain syndromes. Appl Neurophysiol 50:314–318, 1987.
7. Frank F, Frank G, Gaist G. Rostral Stereotactic mesencephalotomy in treatment of cancer pain: a survey of 40 treated patients. Acta Neurochir 33(Suppl):437–443, 1984.
8. Frank F, Tognetti F, Gaist G. Stereotactic mesencephalotomy in treatment of malignant facialbrachial pain syndromes: a survey of 14 treated patients. J Neurosurg 56:807–811, 1982.
9. McKenzie KG. Trigeminal tractotomy. Clin Neurosurg 2:50–70, 1955.
10. Gorecki JP. Stereotactic midbrain tractotomy. In Gildenberg PL, Tasker RR, Franklin PO (eds). Textbook of Stereotactic Functional Neurosurgery. New York, McGraw-Hill, 1997, pp 1651–1661.
11. Amano K, Kawamura H, Tanikawa T. Long term follow up study of rostral mesencephalac reticulotomy for pain relief: report of 34 cases. Appl Neurophysiol 49:105–111, 1986.
12. Gorecki JP. Dorsal root entry zone and brainstem ablative procedures. In Hunt Batjer H, Loftus, CM (eds). Textbook of Neurological Surgery. New York, Lippincott-Raven, 1999.
13. Gorecki JP, Nashold BS. The Duke experience with the nucleus caudalis DREZ operation. Acta Neurochir 64(Suppl):128–131, 1995.

14. Olszewski J. On the anatomical and functional organization of the spinal trigeminal nucleus. J Comp Neurol 92:401–413, 1950.

15. Sjoqvist O. Studies on pain conduction in the trigeminal nerves: A contribution to the surgical treatment of facial pain. Acta Psychiatry Neurol 17(Suppl):1–139, 1938.

16. Young JN, Nashold BS Jr, Cosman ER. A new insulated caudalis nucleus DREZ electrode. Technical note. J Neurosurg 70:283–284, 1989.

17. Nashold BS Jr, El-Naggar AO, Ovelmen-Levitt J, Abdul-Hak M. A new design of radiofrequency lesion electrodes for use in the caudalis nucleus DREZ operation. J Neurosurg 80:1116–1120, 1994.

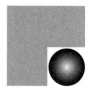

Intracranial Ablative Procedures

R.R. TASKER, MD, FRCSC

The concept that pain was conducted cephalad over specific Cartesian pathways, confirmed by the demonstration by Spiller and Martin[1] that open cordotomy could relieve pain, led naturally to attempts to interrupt pain pathways intracranially. Chapter 21 discusses mesencephalic tractotomy. The introduction of the stereotactic technique by Spiegel and Wycis[2] allowed various authors to carry this concept one step further[3–5] when they attempted to relieve pain by making lesions in the specific relay nucleus of the thalamus, called Hassler's nucleus ventrocaudalis (Vc).[6,7]

ANATOMIC AND PHYSIOLOGIC CONSIDERATIONS

Even at that time it was realized, as has been mentioned under mesencephalic tractotomy, that pain-conducting pathways could be divided into two portions: one paucisynaptic rapidly conducting, mostly contralateral and somatotopographically organized; the other multisynaptic, bilateral, slowly conducting, nonsomatotopographically organized, sometimes referred to as the neo- and paleospinothalamic pathways, respectively; doubtless the situation is more complex as reviewed in Chapters 2 and 3. Initially, the neo-spinothalamic pathway was seen as traversing the brainstem via the mesencephalic and pontine spinothalamic tract to relay in Vc and then to project to specific somatosensory cortex along with non–pain-conducting fibers. Whereas anatomic and physiologic studies in man supported this concept, it has always proven difficult to follow and recognize pain and temperature pathways through the thalamus and cerebral cortex in animals or man.[8,9] In the operating room, pain and temperature responding neurons have been identified in Vc[8,9] and spinothalamic tract can be recognized by stimulation[10] through the induction of contralateral somatotopographically organized sensations such as warmth, cold, and pain. Hassler identified a specific subnucleus of Vc that he considered specifically related to pain transmission named nucleus ventralis caudalis parvocellularis (Vcpc)[11] lying posteroinferiorly to the main body of Vc. However, it has never been clear to this author what the role of this structure really is, an issue that has become even more complex with the recognition of other pain-related nuclei in the area, most notably nucleus

submedius discovered by Craig and colleagues.[12] The concept of the neospinothalamic tract is even more puzzling when it is realized that only a few fibers of this pathway have been recognized as passing rostral to mesencephalon in man.

The paleospinothalamic tract is thought to carry non-somatotopographically organized fibers associated with pain ascending from the spinal cord. It lies medial to spinothalamic tract in the mesencephalon and lateral to the periaqueductal grey (PAG) whence it ascends to relay in the reticular formation on route to thalamus. Its thalamic relay nuclei have been difficult to identify, many structures having been implicated such as pulvinar, centrum medianum, dorsomedian, parafascicular, and centrolateral nuclei as well as the internal thalamic lamina. A dichotomy sprang up early in the history of pain physiology that this medial pathway, which probably also passes to hypothalamus, mediates the suffering aspect of pain in contrast to the discriminative activity mediated by the neospinothalamic tract. However, the medial pathway has been difficult to study in animals or man so that our understanding of it is less clear than one would like. In my experience, stimulation of this tract in conscious man elicits no perceptible effect, and lesions within it cause no identifiable sensory loss.[10] Only occasionally have microelectrode recordings in man identified pain sensitive neurons within it.[13]

The advent of functional imaging studies has complemented traditional anatomic and physiologic studies,[14–19] implicating thalamus, somatosensory cortex (SI, SII), insula, and anterior cingulate cortex in pain processing. Imaging studies in the cingulate cortex are supported by the demonstration of pain-related neurons in that structure.[20] The current concept of the pain-related cingulate cortex is that it consists of at least two parts: a rostral area (area 24) and a caudal area, with differing functions[19,21] receiving projections, perhaps with a predominance in the nondominant hemisphere, from the ventrocaudal portion of dorsomedian nucleus of the thalamus. The rostral area may be involved with pain processing with responses contralateral to the stimuli and proportional to its intensity. Rostral to this area again is cortex concerned with attention getting, possibly in supplementary motor cortex bilaterally. The caudal part of the anterior cingulate gyrus may be more involved with affective and evaluative function. Thus, the anterior cingulate cortex is part of the medial pain-processing system whose interruption might be expected to benefit pain sufferers.

In summary then, we have the classical fast-conducting paucisynaptic largely contralaterally distributed spinothalamic tract, lesioning of which produces dissociated sensory loss traceable in man from spinal cord through mesencephalic and pontine spinothalamic tract to Vcpc, and in a poorly understood manner on from there through Vc to somatosensory cortex. Obviously, it would be postulated that sectioning this system should affect chronic pain. On the other hand, we have a diffuse, multisynaptic, slowly conducting, bilaterally distributed pathway accompanying spinothalamic tract to the brainstem, then passing on to reticular formation and to the medial thalamic nuclei, perhaps to dorsomedian nucleus particularly, and on from there to hypothalamus and cingulate cortex. Although sectioning this pathway produces no clinically detectable sensory loss, it has been postulated that such lesioning should reduce chronic pain.

With these thoughts in mind, mesencephalic tractotomy (see Chapter 21) aimed at one or both structures has been carried out, and lesions have been performed both in Vc[3–5,22–26] and in Vcpc[10,11,27–29] and in various medial thalamic nuclei,[3,4,10,13,22–26,30,31] hypothalamus,[30–36] and cingulum.[37–40] Just as in the case of mesencephalotomy where many contemporary authors think that lesioning the nonspecific portion is more effective than that of the neospinothalamic tract, Mark and his colleagues as well as others[22–26] showed early on that medial thalamotomy was more effective for pain relief than Vc thalamotomy; lesioning Vc also resulted in an unacceptable incidence of dysesthesia.

A different strategy in treating chronic pain caused by cancer is hormonal intervention through hypophysectomy. Open hypophysectomy was originally used in an attempt to control hormonally dependent carcinoma of the breast that had spread beyond the scope of local therapy.[41–43] When successful, hypophysectomy appeared beneficial also for the control of the associated pain and similar results were seen in carcinoma of the prostate gland. But open hypophysectomy was a major undertaking in these sick patients so that the use of stereotactic implantation of radioactive seeds and radiofrequency lesion making were explored in an attempt to secure the same benefits with less surgical impact. A surprising development was the demonstration that alcohol injection into the pituitary gland could control the pain of hormonally dependent and also non–hormonally dependent cancer,[44–46] a technique especially popularized by Moricca. There followed a vigorous use of this technique to treat cancer pain that was not amenable to local or less invasive therapy by transnasal freehand injection of ethanol into the pituitary gland. The procedure has also been done stereotactically with reduction of complications such as postoperative cerebrospinal fluid leakage.[47] No matter by which approach, the mechanism of the pain relief is unclear not being due to associated hormonal manipulation, hypothalamic involvement, or levels of endorphin in the patient's blood or cerebrospinal fluid.[48–50]

INDICATIONS FOR INTRACRANIAL ABLATIVE PROCEDURES

This chapter will deal with medial thalamotomy, hypophysectomy, and cingulotomy. Neurosurgical intervention is indicated only after all noninvasive measures have failed, and

intracranial ablative procedures only after more peripheral procedures and modulatory treatment such as drug infusion or chronic stimulation are considered unsuitable. Generally, deep brain stimulation in PVG has been used infrequently to treat pain in cancer patients because of limited life expectancy, although Meyerson and colleagues[51] have successfully used manual stimulation of such electrodes transcutaneously, obviating the cost of the implant without the expected risk of infection. Obvious contraindications such as cognitive disorders and bleeding diatheses have to be taken into account.

At this point, the thought will run through the minds of many neurosurgeons, based on their experience, personal communications with colleagues, and on the growing familiarity with chronic stimulating and drug infusion techniques, as to whether there still remain any indications for supraspinal destructive lesions for the relief of pain. Gybels and Nuttin[52] sent questionnaires on the subject to 215 members of the European Society for Stereotactic and Functional Neurosurgery in 1994. Only 54 were returned documenting 63 such procedures done during 1993 for cancer pain and 51 for neuropathic pain compared with 836 spinal procedures in the same period. Thus, in practice, the indications appear limited and these will be considered separately for nociceptive, usually cancer, and neuropathic pain.

Nociceptive Pain

The evidence seems convincing that nociceptive pain is dependent upon transmission of signals in pain pathways, interruption of which has a reasonable chance of ameliorating the pain. For that reason, intracranial ablative surgery is indicated only when pain tract interruption at the cord level or even more distally, such as percutaneous cordotomy, myelotomy, or neurectomy, are not feasible or when pain is very diffuse, located in the head, or above the C5 dermatome, where it is not amenable to cordotomy.

It also may be indicated in patients in whom spinal destructive surgery carries an unusually high risk of, particularly, respiratory complications. Gybels and Sweet concluded that the risks of failure and of complications are significantly greater for intracranial ablative procedures than for more peripheral ones, so that the former should be reserved for patients with cancer pain in the head and neck and for certain other select cases.[38] They also add "Appropriately placed and circumscribed frontal lobe lesions may be gratifyingly beneficial." Life expectancy must be appropriate for the procedure being considered, greater than 5 months for central ablative procedures according to Gybels.[53] Beyond these issues, it is my opinion that, before considering supraspinal destructive procedures, the diagnosis should be clear and the underlying pathophysiology appropriate to the procedure proposed. Finally, the cost effectiveness of the operation must be considered in the sense of likelihood of pain relief diminished by expected complications.

The indications are similar for the three procedures to be discussed, there being no comparative studies of which the author is aware. It would seem that hypophysectomy might be preferable in hormone-dependent cancer pain and cingulotomy where the affective aspect of the pain is striking. Frank and colleagues compared medial thalamotomy with mesencephalic tractotomy concluding that the former achieves a

57.9% incidence of pain relief, the latter 83.5%; for mesencephalic tractotomy the mortality was 1.8% for medial thalamotomy 0% and the morbidity 10.1% compared with usually transient cognitive problems after thalamotomy.[54]

Neuropathic Pain

I do not believe that the evidence supports the dependence of the steady burning dysesthetic, the most common element of neuropathic, including central, pain on transmission in pain pathways. Hence, the notion of its relief by interrupting pain conduction at any level including supraspinal ones seems ill-founded.[55] However, not all neuropathic pain syndromes consist of a steady burning causalgic dysesthetic element; after injury to the conus medullaris and cauda equina region, for example, lancinating pain shooting distally from the somatotopographic level of the lesion especially into the legs can be a prominent feature, and this pain responds well to interruption of pain pathways cephalad to the causative lesion as does allodynia and hyperpathia associated with peripheral and cord lesions. This interruption can be accomplished by cordotomy, cordectomy, and the dorsal root entry zone (DREZ) procedure.[56] With these excellent options, there is no need to consider supraspinal destructive procedures for these types of pain associated with peripheral or cord lesions. There is also some evidence that mesencephalic tractotomy can alleviate the lancinating pain caused by supraspinal lesions,[57] and very limited personal experience suggests that destructive supraspinal surgery in general may relieve lancinating pain and allodynia and hyperpathia associated with central lesions.[58] In my opinion, the steady dysesthetic causalgic element is best treated by a chronic stimulation technique that induces paresthesia in the area of the pain.

MEDIAL THALAMOTOMY

Technique

Medial thalamotomy is always performed stereotactically, the details varying only with respect to the target chosen. In contemporary practice, the target is usually the internal thalamic lamina though more recent information would recommend the ventrocaudal portion of dorsomedian nucleus. Another commonly used target is the central lateral nucleus,[13,19,21,30,31,54] and although seldom used, pulvinarotomy is another alternative.[59–63]

My stereotactic technique has been described elsewhere.[64] Under local anesthetic a suitable stereotactic frame is applied to the patient's head and either magnetic resonance imaging (MRI; preferably) or computed tomography (CT) is done to determine the stereotactic coordinates of the anterior and posterior commissures. A computer program is then used to redraw the sagittal diagrams from the Schaltenbrand and Wahren brain atlas[7] with the same length of anterior commissure-posterior commissure line as that of the patient that has just been determined from the brain scan. The computer program rules the diagrams in a millimeter grid corresponding to the millimeter scales of the stereotactic frame. The desired target is selected on the appropriate sagittal diagram and its

stereotactic coordinates are read off. By setting these on the stereotactic frame, a probe introduced into the brain through either a twist drill or a bur hole will arrive at the chosen target. However, there is some variability in arrangement of structures from one brain to another and it is usually desirable to confirm a probe's position in the correct target before proceeding to make a destructive lesion. Unfortunately, stimulation usually evokes no response in the medial thalamic nuclei and it is difficult to record identifiable neurons with a microelectrode there. As a result, one must depend solely on anatomic or indirect physiologic localization. The latter can be accomplished by verifying the position of the medial border of Vc and then extrapolating the expected position of the selected medial thalamic nucleus. This can be done by stimulation at approximately 12 mm from the midline producing threshold paresthesias usually in the face or mouth with less than 0.5 V with a 0.5-mm electrode tip stimulated bipolar against a 1.1-mm ring separated by 0.5 mm from the pole. This equipment is available from DIROS Technology, Toronto. Or else microelectrode recording can be done to identify medial Vc, locating neurons with receptive fields in the lips or face. Once the target site has been identified, usually a radiofrequency lesion is made with a 1.1-mm diameter electrode with a 3-mm bare tip and a suitable generator such as the OWL System available from DIROS Technology. Usually, large lesions are required—60 seconds at 90 °C—and possibly multiple clustered lesions. The patient usually experiences nothing during stimulation or lesion making and demonstrates no neurologic deficit postoperatively. Nevertheless, serial neurologic monitoring should be done during lesion making and postoperatively to avoid inadvertent damage to neighboring structures and postoperative complications. A plain CT scan of the head in the postoperative period can rule out a developing hematoma, and a postoperative MRI can be used to confirm lesion localization.

Although most destructive thalamotomies are done with radiofrequency current, there is growing experience with radiosurgery with equipment such as the Leksell gamma knife.[65–68]

Outcome

My reviews have always suggested that outcome is much better (46% to 85% useful pain relief) after medial thalamotomy for cancer pain than it is for neuropathic pain (22% to 32%)[69,70] (Table 22-1). Pagni concluded after a thorough literature review that thalamotomy was " . . . only exceptionally indicated in cases of pain of non-malignant origin . . ." noting the usually small series reported.[71] However, complications were few consisting of, usually, transient confusion with very rare mortality and usually transient neurological complication, affecting 4% to 21% in the series in Table 22-1. The higher complication rate after combined medial and lateral thalamic lesions reflects the higher risks of lateral thalamic (Vc) lesioning.

Most of the larger series reported in Table 22-1 are old, so the recent work of Jeanmonod and colleagues is interesting.[72,73] In the first paper, 67% pain relief was reported in 69 cases of central pain—twice as good as in many published series. In the second paper, 54 medial thalamotomies were performed for neuropathic pain and 24 for central pain, half of

● **TABLE 22-1** • Medial Thalamotomy for Chronic Pain

| Lesion Site | Pain Type | | | | | |
| | Neuropathic | | | Nociceptive | | |
	No. of Cases	Significant Pain Relief (%)	Complications (%)	No. of Cases	Significant Pain Relief (%)	Complications (%)
Medial and lateral thalamus	56	32	32	31	77	32
Medial thalamus uni- or bilateral	47	29	4–21	175	46	7
Pulvinar uni- or bilateral	18	22	5	26	88	21

the latter caused by cord, half by brain lesions. Fifty percent to 100% reduction in pain level was achieved in 71% of those patients who had neuropathic pain of peripheral origin and 60% of those with central pain. Ninety-one percent developed no somatosensory deficits as expected and it is stated that 47% of patients showed improved somatosensory function postoperatively. In 9%, lesions extended too for laterally usually causing only slight to moderate or transient neurologic deficits. Their more detailed observations were interesting, although 92% of patients suffered from steady, 72% intermittent, and 52% evoked pains (allodynia and/or hyperpathia) preoperatively; of the patients enjoying partial pain relief, 81% still suffered from residual steady pain, but only 39% from residual intermittent pain, and 13% from residual evoked pain; 57% reported persisting isolated steady pain. These data suggest that medial thalamotomy may be more effective for intermittent and evoked pain than for steady pain.

RADIOTHALAMOTOMY

Medial thalamotomy is an ideal operation to be performed by radiosurgery because the target is large, devoid of important specific contents, and incapable of readily performed physiologic corroboration in the first place. Young and colleagues reported 24 gamma knife thalamotomies, 27% of which totally abolished the patients' pain at follow-up, 33% achieved over 50% relief.[68] In an earlier report on 10 cases of neuropathic pain, 30% enjoyed excellent and 40% good pain relief without complications.[67]

CINGULUMOTOMY

Technique

This procedure can be done freehold or stereotactically; I prefer the latter approach.[74–76] The technique is the same as in medial thalamotomy except for the target selection. The cingulum bundle and the cortex can be visualized and directly targeted from the MRI and the cingulum cortex can be also identified by microelectrode recording.[20] The aim is to destroy the cingulum bundle and overlying cingulate cortex bilaterally. MRI is used to identify the midline of the brain and the rostral tip of the lateral ventricles. The roof of the latter is then identified on each side 2.5 cm caudal to the anterior tip. Symmetric radiofrequency lesions are usually made to the maximum output of the generator (90 °C for 60 seconds using a 1.1 mm diameter electrode with a 5-mm bare tip available from DIROS Technology). The lesions are usually made 7 mm from the midline with the lesions' periphery extending to the ventricular roof. Following the deeper lesion, the electrode is withdrawn 5 mm and lesioning repeated using the same parameters making a stacked lesion 5 to 10 mm in diameter and 10 to 20 mm in length. As with medial thalamotomy, there is usually no clinically detectable effect from the lesions made.

Outcome

Cingulotomies were most often done originally for the relief of psychiatric illness with casual observations on accompanying pain relief. However, with the contemporary interest in the involvement of the cingulate cortex in pain processing the focus has changed. Ballantine and colleagues carried out bilateral cingulumotomy in 139 patients for relief of chronic pain between 1964 and 1987.[74] Of the 35 cases with terminal cancer, 57% of those who survived up to 3 months enjoyed moderate to complete pain relief; only 2 of the 10 who survived longer continued to receive benefit. Of 95 patients who had pain not due to cancer, 61 of whom suffered "failed back" pain, 26% had complete or marked sustained relief while 36% enjoyed moderate relief. Pillay and Hassenbusch reported 40% excellent and 20% good results in 10 patients; eight of whom had cancer pain and two neuropathic pain.[75] It is interesting that Gybels thought that Ballantine's lesions shown in MRI lay rostral to area 24.[58] Wilkinson and colleagues provided a current review of 28 cingulumotomies in 23 patients (5 repeated) all of whom were dependent on narcotics based on questionnaires returned by 18 of the patients; 2 died of intercurrent problems.[76] The majority of these patients suffered from failed back pain or adhesive arachnoiditis. Seventy-two percent reported improvement, 55% were able to discontinue narcotics, and 56% judged the operation beneficial; 28% returned to their usual activities. However, seizures developed in 39%, but there were no deaths. There was one case of brain abscess and neurologic problems developed in four other patients. Optimum pain relief was delayed 4 to 6 months and Wilkinson's follow-up was 1 to 15 years (average, 7.7 years). Results were described as stable over the longer follow-up periods.

HYPOPHYSECTOMY

Hypophysectomy to relieve chronic pain is now nearly always done by intrasellar injection of alcohol. Although usually used to relieve pain caused by cancer, there are reports of relief of neuropathic pain as well. Although relief is perhaps greater in cases of pain caused by hormonally dependent cancer, relief also occurs in non–hormone-dependent disease.

Technique

An 18-gauge 15-cm spinal needle is tapped transnasally through the floor of the sphenoid using image intensification and then hammered into the sella in the midline 2 mm inferior to its anterior rim. It is directed onward toward the superior posterior portion of the sella where 1 to 2 mL of absolute alcohol is injected in 0.1-mL aliquots every minute while neurologic status is monitored. The needle is then withdrawn until its tip is halfway between the initial site and the sellar floor and a second similar injection made. Further withdrawal through 50% of the remaining intrasellar distance is then followed by a third injection—the total volume injected ranging from 1 to 5 mL. The procedure can also be done stereotactically.[77]

Outcome

Pain relief is usually short-term, lasting less than 3 to 4 months. In patients with hormone-dependent cancer, 41% to 95% report relief, while 69% of patients with non–hormone-dependent cancer do so.[47,77] The review by Gybels and Sweet suggested that 67% to 84% of patients probably enjoyed short-term relief.[38] Complications include a 2% to 6.5% mortality, a 5% to 60% incidence of diabetes insipidus, a 3% to 20% rate of cerebrospinal fluid rhinorrhea, a 2% to 10% incidence of visual and oculomotor palsies, and 0.3% to 1% incidence of meningitis; the stereotactic technique[47] reduces the incidence of CSF leak.

REFERENCES

1. Spiller WG, Martin E. The treatment of persistent pain of organic origin in the lower part of the body by division of the anterolateral column of the spinal cord. JAMA 58:1489–1490, 1912.
2. Spiegel EA, Wycis HT. Pallidothalamotomy in chorea. Presented at the Philadelphia Neurological Society, April 22, 1949.
3. Hécaen H, Talairach J, David M, Dell MB. Coagulations limitées du thalamus dans les algies du syndrome thalamique. Rev Neurol 81:917–931, 1949.
4. Monnier M, Fischer R. Stimulation électrique et coagulation thérapeutique du thalamus chez l'homme (Névralgies faciales). Confin Neurol 11:282–286, 1951.
5. Hassler R. Riechert Klinische und anatomische Befunde der stereotaktischen Schmerzoperationen im Thalamus. Archiv Psychiatr Nervenkrankheiten 200:93–122, 1959.
6. Schaltenbrand G, Bailey P. Introduction to Stereotaxis with an Atlas of the Human Brain. Stuttgart, Thieme, 1959.
7. Schaltenbrand G, Wahren W. Atlas for Stereotaxy of the Human Brain (2nd ed). Stuttgart, Thieme, 1977.
8. Lenz FA, Gracely RH, Rowland LH, et al. A population of cells in human thalamic principal sensory nucleus respond to painful mechanical stimuli. Neurosci Lett 18:46–50, 1984.
9. Davis KD, Lozano AM, Manduch M, et al. Thalamic relay site for cold perception in humans. J Neurophysiol 81:1970–1973, 1999.
10. Tasker RR, Organ IW, Hawrylyshyn PA. The Thalamus and Midbrain of Man. A Physiological Atlas Using Electrical Stimulation. Springfield, Ill, Charles C Thomas, 1982.
11. Hassler R. The division of pain conduction into systems of pain and pain awareness. In Janzen R, Keidel WD, Herz A, Steichele C (eds). Pain: Basic Principles – Pharmacology – Therapy. Stuttgart, Thieme, 1972, pp 98–112.
12. Craig AD, Bushnell MC, Zhang E-T, et al. A thalamic nucleus specific for pain and temperature sensation. Nature 372:770–773, 1994.
13. Sano K, Yoshioka M, Sekino H. Functional organization of the internal medullary lamina in man. Confin Neurol 32:374–380, 1970.
14. Talbot JD, Marrett S, Evans AC, et al. Multiple representations of pain in human cerebral cortex. Science 251:1355–1358, 1991.
15. Rainville P, Duncan GH, Price DD, et al. Pain affect encoded in human anterior cingulate but not somatosensory cortex. Science 277:968–971, 1997.
16. Davis KD, Wood ML, Crawley AP, et al. MRI of human somatosensory and cingulate cortex during painful electrical nerve stimulation. Neuroreport 7:321–325, 1995.
17. Davis KD, Taub E, Duffner F, et al. Activation of the anterior cingulate cortex by thalamic stimulation in patients with chronic pain: a positron emission tomography study. J Neurosurg 92:64–69, 2000.
18. Davis KD, Taylor SJ, Crawley AP, et al. Functional MRI of pain and attention-related activations in the human cingulate cortex. J Neurophysiol 77:3370–3380, 1997.
19. Ingvar M, Hsieh J-C. The image of pain. In Wall PD, Melzack R (eds). Textbook of Pain (4th ed). Edinburgh, Churchill Livingstone, 1999, pp 215–233.
20. Hutchison WD, Davis KD, Lozano AM, et al. Pain-related neurons in the human cingulate cortex. Nat Neurosci 2:403–405, 1999.
21. Craig AD, Dostrovsky JO. Medulla to thalamus. In Wall PD, Melzack R (eds). Textbook of Pain (4th ed). Edinburgh, Churchill Livingstone, 1999, pp 183–214.
22. Ervin FR, Mark VH. Stereotactic thalamotomy in the human. Physiologic observations on the human thalamus. Arch Neurol 3:368–380, 1960.
23. Mark VH, Ervin FR. Role of the thalamotomy in treatment of chronic severe pain. Postgrad Med 37:563–571, 1965.
24. Mark VH, Ervin FR, Hackett TP. Clinical aspects of stereotactic thalamotomy in the human. The treatment of chronic severe pain. Arch Neurol 3:351–367, 1960.
25. Mark VH, Ervin FR, Yakovlev PI. Correlation of pain relief, sensory loss, and anatomical lesion sites in pain patients treated by stereotactic thalamotomy. Trans Am Neurol Assoc 86:86–90, 1961.
26. Mark VH, Ervin FR, Yakovlev PI. Stereotactic thalamotomy. III. The verification of anatomical lesion sites in the human thalamus. Arch Neurol 8:78–88, 1963.
27. Halliday AM, Logue V. Painful sensations evoked by electrical stimulation in the thalamus. In Somjen GG (ed). Neurophysiology Studied in Man. Amsterdam, Excerpta Medica, 1972, pp 221–230.
28. Siegfried J, Krayenbühl H. Clinical experience with the treatment of intractable pain. In Janzen R, Keidel WD, Herz A, Steichele C (eds). Pain: Basic Principles – Pharmacology – Therapy. Thieme, Stuttgart, 1972, pp 202–204.
29. Hitchcock ER, Teixeira MJA. A comparison of results from center-median and basal thalamotomies for pain. Surg Neurol 15:341–351, 1981.
30. Sano K. Intralaminar thalamotomy (thalamolaminotomy) and posterior hypothalamotomy in the treatment of intractable pain. In Krayenbühl H, Maspes PE, Sweet WH (eds). Progress in Neurological Surgery, vol. 8. Karger, Basel, 1977, pp 50–103.
31. Sano K. Stereotaxic thalamolaminotomy and posteromedial hypothalamotomy for the relief of pain. In Bonica JJ, Ventrafridda V (eds). Advances in Pain Research and Therapy, vol. 2. New York, Raven, 1979, pp 475–485.
32. Fairman D. Hypothalamotomy as a new perspective for alleviation of intractable pain and regression of metastatic malignant tumours. In Fusek I, Kunc Z (eds). Present Limits of Neurosurgery. Prague, Avicenum, 1972, pp 525–528.
33. Fairman D. Stereotactic hypothalamotomy for the alleviation of pain in malignant disease. J Surg Oncol 5:79–84, 1973.
34. Fairman D. Neurophysiological bases for the hypothalamic lesion and stimulation by chronic implanted electrodes for the relief of intractable pain in cancer. In Bonica JJ, Albe-Fessard D (eds). Advances in Pain Research and Therapy, vol 1. New York, Raven, 1976, pp 843–847.

35. Mayanagi Y, Sano K. Posteromedial hypothalamotomy for behavioural disturbances and intractable pain. *In* Lunsford LD (ed). Modern Stereotactic Neurosurgery. Boston, Martinus Nijhoff, pp 377–388, 1978.

36. Mayanagi Y, Hori T, Sano K. The posteromedial hypothalamus and pain behaviour with special reference to endocrinological findings. Appl Neurophysiol 41:223–231, 1978.

37. Foltz EL, White IE. Pain "relief" by frontal cingulotomy. J Neurosurg 19:89–100, 1962.

38. Gybels JM, Sweet WH. Neurological treatment of persistent pain. Physiological and pathological mechanisms of human pain. *In* Gildenberg PL (ed). Pain and Headache, vol 11. Karger, Basel, 1989, pp 141–145.

39. Bouckoms AJ. Limbic surgery for pain. *In* Wall PD, Melzack R (eds). Textbook of Pain (3rd ed). Edinburgh, Churchill Livingstone, 1994, pp 1171–1187.

40. Ballantine HT, Cosgrove R, Giriunas I. Surgical treatment of intractable psychiatric illness and chronic pain by stereotactic cingulotomy. *In* Schmidek H, Sweet W (eds). Operative Neurosurgical Techniques: Indications, Methods and Results (3rd ed). Philadelphia, WB Saunders, 1995, pp 1423–1430.

41. Luft R, Olivecrona H. Experiences with hypophysectomy in man. J Neurosurg 10:301–316, 1953.

42. Perrault M, LeBeau J, Klotz B, et al. L'hypophysectomie totale dans le traitement du cancer du sein; premier cas français; avenir de la methode. Therapie 7:290–300, 1952.

43. Tindall GT, Christy JH, Nixon DW, et al. Trans-sphenoidal hypophysectomy for pain of disseminated carcinoma of the breast and prostate gland. *In* Lee JF (ed). Pain Management. Baltimore, Williams and Wilkins, 1977, pp 172–185.

44. Greco T, Sbaragli F, Cammilli L. L'alcolizzazione della ipofisi per via transfenoidale nella terapia di particoloari tumori maligni. Settim Med 45:355–356, 1957.

45. Moricca G. Chemical hypophysectomy for cancer pain. *In* Bonica JJ (ed). Advances in Neurology, vol. 4. New York, Raven, 1974, pp 707–714.

46. Moricca G. Neuroadenolysis for diffuse unbearable cancer pain. *In* Bonica JJ, Albe-Fessard DD (eds). Advances in Pain Research and Therapy, vol. 1. New York, Raven, 1976, pp 863–866.

47. Levin AB. Stereotactic chemical hypophysectomy. *In* Lunsford LD (ed). Modern Stereotactic Neurosurgery. Boston, Martinus Nijhoff, 1988, pp 365–375.

48. Takeda F, Fujii T, Uki J, et al. Cancer pain relief and tumour regression by means of pituitary neuroadenolysis and surgical hypophysectomy. Neurol Med Chir (Tokyo) 23:41, 1983.

49. Takeda F, Uki J, Fujii T, et al. Pituitary neuroadenolysis to relieve cancer pain: observations of spread of ethanol instilled into the sella turcica and subsequent changes of the hypothalamo-pituitary axis at autopsy. Neurol Med Chir (Tokyo) 23:50, 1983.

50. Capper SJ, Conlon JM Lahuerta J, et al. Peptide concentration in the CSF following injection of alcohol into the pituitary gland. Pain 2(Suppl): S316, 1984.

51. Meyerson BA, Boethius I, Carlsson AM. Percutaneous central gray stimulation for cancer pain. Appl Neurophysiol 41:57–65, 1978.

52. Gybels JM, Nuttin B. Are there still indications for destructive neurosurgery at supra- spinal levels for the relief of painful syndromes? *In* Besson JM, Guilbaud G, Ollat H (eds). Forebrain Areas Involved in Pain Processing. Paris, John Libbey Eurotext, 1995, pp 253–259.

53. Gybels JM. Indications for the use of neurosurgical techniques in pain control. *In* Bond MR, Charlton JE, Woolf J (eds). Proceedings of the Sixth World Congress on Pain. Amsterdam, Elsevier, 1991, pp 475–482.

54. Frank F, Fabrizi AP, Gaist G, et al. Stereotactic lesions in the treatment of chronic cancer pain syndromes: mesenencephalotomy or multiple thalamotomies. Appl Neurophysiol 50:314–318, 1987.

55. Tasker RR, Dostrovsky JO. Deafferentation and central pain. *In* Wall PD, Melzack R (eds). Textbook of Pain (2nd ed). Edinburgh, Churchill Livingstone, 1989, pp 154–180.

56. Tasker RR, DeCarvalho GTC, Dolan EJ. Intractable pain of spinal cord origin: clinical features and implications for surgery. Neurosurgery 77:373–378, 1992.

57. Nashold BS Jr, Wilson WP. Central pain: observations in man with chronic implanted electrodes in the midbrain tegmentum. Confin Neurol 27:30–44, 1966.

58. Gybels JM, Tasker RR. Central neurosurgery *In* Wall PD, Melzack R (eds). Textbook of Pain (4th ed). Edinburgh, Churchill Livingstone, 1999, pp 1307–1339.

59. Fraioli B, Guidetti B. Effect of stereotactic lesions of the pulvinar and lateralis posterior nucleus on intractable pain and dyskinetic syndromes of man. Appl Neurophysiol 38:23–30, 1975.

60. Mayanagi Y, Bouchard G. Evaluation of stereotactic thalamotomies for pain relief with reference to pulvinar intervention. Appl Neurophysiol 39:154–157, 1976–1977.

61. Laitinen L. Anterior pulvinotomy in the treatment of intractable pain. Acta Neurochir 24(Suppl):223–225, 1977.

62. Yoshii N, Mizokami T, Ushikubo T, et al. Longterm follow-up study after pulvinotomy for intractable pain. Appl Neurophysiol 43:128–132, 1980.

63. Yoshii N, Mizokami T, Usikubo Y. Postmortem study of stereotactic pulvinarotomy for relief of intractable pain. Stereotact Funct Neurosurg 54:55–103, 1990.

64. Tasker RR, Dostrovsky JO. Invasive lesioning of the central nervous system for functional disorders. *In* Eben A II, Maciunas RJ (eds). Advanced Neurosurgical Navigation. New York, Thieme, 1999, pp 483–506.

65. Leksell L, Meyerson BA, Forster DMC. Radiosurgical thalamotomy for intractable pain. Confin Neurol 34:264, 1972.

66. Steiner L, Forster D, Leksell L, et al. Gammathalamotomy in intractable pain. Acta Neurochir 52:173–184, 1980.

67. Young RF, Jacques DS, Rand RW, et al. Medial thalamotomy with the Leksell gamma knife for treatment of chronic pain. Acta Neurochir 62(Suppl):105–110, 1994.

68. Young RF, Jacques DS, Rand RW, et al. Technique of stereotactic medial thalamotomy with the Leksell gamma knife for treatment of chronic pain. Neurol Res 17(1):59–65, 1995.

69. Tasker RR. Pain. Thalamic procedures. *In* Schaltenbrand G, Walker AE (eds). Textbook of Stereotaxy of the Human Brain. Thieme, Stuttgart, 1982, pp 484–497.

70. Gybels JM, Kupers R, Nuttin B. Therapeutic stereotactic procedures on the thalamus for pain. Acta Neurochir 124(1):19–22, 1993.

71. Pagni CA Central Pain. A Neurosurgical Challenge. Turino, Minerva Medica, 1998, pp 137–142.

72. Jeanmonod D, Magnin M, Morel A. Chronic neurogenic pain and the medial thalamotomy. Schweizerische Rundschau Med Praxis 83(23): 702–707, 1994.

73. Jeanmonod D, Magnin M, Morel A. A thalamic concept of neurogenic pain. *In* Gebhart GF, Hammond DL, Jensen TS (eds). Proceedings of the 7th World Congress on Pain. Progress in Pain Research Management, vol 2. Seattle, IASP, 1994, pp 767–787.

74. Ballantine HT, Bouckoms AJ, Thomas EK, et al. Treatment of psychiatric illness by stereotactic cingulotomy. Biol Psychiatry 22:807–819, 1987.

75. Pillay PK, Hassenbusch SJ. Bilateral MRI-guided stereotactic cingulotomy for intractable pain. Stereotact Funct Neurosurg 59:33–38, 1992.

76. Wilkinson HA, Davidson KM, Davidson RI. Bilateral anterior cingulotomy for chronic noncancer pain. Neurosurgery 45:1129–1136, 1999.

77. Levin AB. Hypophysectomy in the treatment of cancer pain. *In* Arbit E (ed). Management of Cancer-related Pain. Mt Kisko, Futura, 1993, pp 281–295.

Peripheral Ablative Techniques

RICHARD K. OSENBACH, MD

Destructive neurosurgical techniques have a long and rich history. These procedures have been used for many years, primarily for the treatment of cancer pain, and to a lesser extent for nonmalignant pain syndromes. However, with the evolution of intrathecal (IT) opiates, there has been a radical trend away from the use of ablative procedures. This is rather unfortunate because some of these techniques can be very effective in properly selected patients.

There are both advantages and disadvantages to destructive pain procedures. On the negative side, destructive procedures are obviously irreversible and carry the risk of neurologic morbidity. Also, the analgesic efficacy of most destructive procedures cannot be tested with the degree of certainty that is present with augmentative procedures such as electrical stimulation and/or spinal drug infusion. On the other hand, many of these techniques can be performed as a single stage procedure that can produce immediate analgesia. Indeed, an effective ablative procedure often allows the patient more freedom because it can often eliminate the requirement of continuous interactions with healthcare providers that is necessary in the case of spinal drug pumps that require periodic refilling and sometimes frequent reprogramming to achieve effective pain control. Moreover, the overall cost of ablative procedures is probably less because the high costs of an implant are avoided. Consequently, I believe, along with other neurosurgeons who are familiar with these techniques, that they should continue to play an important role in the management of patients with chronic intractable pain.

The purpose of this chapter is to review the pertinent anatomy, indications, techniques, and outcome for a number of peripheral ablative procedures including peripheral neurectomy, dorsal rhizotomy, dorsal root ganglionectomy, sympathectomy, and spinal facet denervation.

PERIPHERAL NEURECTOMY

Pathophysiology of Peripheral Nerve Pain

Pain is a common symptom of many peripheral nerve injuries and diseases of peripheral nerve. Peripheral nerve injury pain is classically associated with traumatic injury to a pure sensory or mixed nerve. However, there are numerous pathologic conditions that are associated with peripheral nerve pain including mononeuropathies (e.g., diabetic and rheumatoid mononeuropathy), entrapment syndromes, brachial or lumbar plexitis, as well as a range of painful polyneuropathies. Injuries to a major nerve may lead to the devastating pain syndrome known as causalgia while relatively minor extremity trauma may lead to a similar syndrome such as so-called "reflex sympathetic dystrophy" (RSD). In both of these conditions, the generation and maintenance of pain in some cases is believed to involve the sympathetic nervous system.

Peripheral nerve injury results in two types of pain; pain at the site of injury and pain that is remote from the site of injury. Pain experienced at the primary site of injury is related to activation of nociceptive nerve endings in the region. In addition, many patients experience pain *within* the distribution of the nerve but remote from the site of injury (e.g., meralgia paresthetica). The pain that develops remote from the site of injury is associated with intrinsic nerve damage and is *not* related to activation of nociceptors in the region in which the pain is felt. This is an important concept to understand when making rational treatment decisions that might offer effective pain relief.

Several pathophysiologic mechanisms have been proposed to explain nerve injury pain including sensitization of peripheral nerve terminals, abnormalities within primary afferent fibers, abnormal electrical communication between adjacent axons, and pathophysiologic alterations in the dorsal horn of the spinal cord.[1,2]

Sensitization of peripheral terminals may occur as part of the normal response to inflammation and/or injury. Chemical mediators that sensitize nerve endings may be liberated in response to tissue damage or secondary to antidromically conducted electrical impulses. This mechanism may be relevant in sympathetically maintained pain (SMP) syndromes, such as RSD or causalgia, in which there is some evidence that sympathetic efferent activity may be capable of sensitizing somatic afferent fibers. However, the precise role of peripheral sensitization in the generation of neuropathic pain in general is not entirely clear. Indeed, a number of observations seem to be in opposition to this mechanism. First, although inflammatory processes produce sensitization of nerve terminals, modalities effective in treating the inflammatory process are ineffective in relieving the pain. Second, total denervation is capable of inactivating this mechanism, yet is incapable of eliminating the pain. Lastly, nerve injury pain is not uniformly associated with symptoms or physical signs suggestive of hypersensitivity.

A second hypothesis is centered on the notion that injury to a nerve converts a passive conducting axon into a source of abnormal electrical impulses, either spontaneous or evoked by a variety of chemical or mechanical stimuli. Much work has revolved around the role of neuromas in the generation of pain and it has been shown that all neuromas are electrically active. In fact, abnormal single-unit discharges have actually been recorded from the parent nerves of patients with neuromas or other painful neuropathies. This electrical activity within a neuroma is believed to be related to the sprouting of unmyelinated or lightly myelinated fibers that are unusually sensitive to mechanical and/or chemical stimuli. Indeed, neuromas seem to be exquisitely sensitive to adrenergic agonists that have been shown to augment electrical activity within the neuroma. This may explain the extreme pain experienced if local anesthetic containing epinephrine is infiltrated around a neuroma as well as the resolution of pain through the use of sympathetic blockade. It is widely recognized that resection of a painful neuroma can often result in elimination of pain.

Although much attention is focused on neuromas, it is clear that neuroma formation is not necessary to produce abnormal activity within a peripheral nerve. Minor inflammation may lead to ectopic foci in afferent fibers, thereby transforming peripheral nerves into impulse generators. However, even in the absence of spontaneous hyperactivity, axons may nevertheless play a role in peripheral nerve pain as a result of afterdischarges. This is a situation in which a single electrical impulse results in a large number of discharges from the pathologic region of the axon. Also, peripheral injury can lead to abnormal electrical activity in the dorsal root ganglion (DRG). Although this phenomenon has not been described in humans, it may in part explain the ineffectiveness of dorsal rhizotomy in relieving pain in this condition.

A third interesting hypothesis to explain peripheral nerve pain is the development of abnormal electrical connections at sites of axonal damage or demyelination. Indeed, studies have demonstrated electrical junctions between adjacent axons in neuromas and segments of degenerating or regenerating nerve. These so-called ephaptic connections may lead to "cross-talk" or short-circuiting between axons. This phenomenon appears to affect fibers of quite disparate diameters. Consequently, activation of a low threshold receptor might lead to propagation of an action potential not only in its own axon but also in a high threshold nociceptive afferent fiber with the result that a normally innocuous stimulus is reported as being painful.

Lastly, peripheral nerve pain may occur due to central changes within the dorsal horn of the spinal cord or even more rostral structures. It is known that afferent discharges in the dorsal horn are able to influence the activity of adjacent neurons, a phenomenon known as the dorsal root reflex. It has been speculated that peripheral nerve damage may alter the magnitude of the dorsal root reflex and in some way produce pain, although this issue has not been resolved. Alternatively, peripheral injury may result in an abrupt unmasking of previously silent or ineffective synapses. In the weeks following nerve injury, fiber sprouting is known to occur in the dorsal horn. This may result in the development of unusual sensory fields and/or loss of sensory modality specificity that may contribute to the development of neuropathic pain. Finally, it is well known that dorsal horn neurons develop spontaneous hyperactivity following removal of afferent input that persists for long periods and may be one of the causes of pain after peripheral nerve injury. It is also conceivable that neurons within the dorsal horn may be hypersensitive to endogenous neurotransmitters that are normally present such as substance P and glutamate.

Indications for Peripheral Neurectomy

Painful nerve injuries can be complex problems that demand commitment and perseverance from the treating physician. The initial goal is to define the pain syndrome as specifically as possible with avoidance of grouping patients into inaccurate general diagnostic categories such as RSD, causalgia, and the like. Conservative nonsurgical therapy of peripheral neuropathic pain has met with limited success. Nonetheless, treatment using non-narcotic analgesics, tricyclic antidepressants, anti-epileptic medications, and sodium channel blockers (mexiletine) does cause adequate pain relief in some patients and should be attempted before surgical intervention. Other conservative nonpharmacologic modalities may also be tried, including local or regional anesthetic blocks, acupuncture, biofeedback, and so on; however, no single approach has uniformly been successful.

Assuming all appropriate conservative measures have been exhausted and neuropsychologic testing reveals no major contraindication, surgical therapy may be considered. Before proceeding with surgery, repetitive nerve blocks should be performed. Because injured nerves and neuromas express adrenoreceptors, activation of which produces an algesic response, local anesthetic blocks should be performed *without* epinephrine. *Complete* relief of pain by a properly performed nerve block should prompt consideration toward a peripheral surgical intervention. In general, the block should be repeated at least one time to ensure that the initial response was not a false-positive response due to placebo effect. Other factors that seem to have positive predictive value for pain relief with peripheral neurectomy include pain secondary to traumatic nerve injury, pain limited to the territory of a *single* nerve, and the presence of a Tinel's sign. However, even with pain relief from local anesthetic blockade and adherence to the latter criteria, the success rate for surgical excision of a painful neuroma may not be more than 50% to 60%.[3]

An important concept in the treatment of nerve injury pain is *prevention* of neuroma formation. To this end, nerve repair should play a prominent role in patients with peripheral nerve injury. Indeed, nerve repair with either primary anastomosis or interposition grafts represents the best option for preventing neuroma formation and secondary pain in critical nerves. In patients in whom nerve repair is not an option (e.g., postamputation stump neuroma), or in cases that involve noncritical pure sensory nerves, peripheral neurectomy is a reasonable alternative. The following pure sensory nerves are amenable to neurectomy: greater/lesser occipital, superficial radial sensory, medial antebrachial cutaneous, ilioinguinal, iliohypogastric, lateral femoral cutaneous, sural, and saphenous. Peripheral neurectomy may also be applied to peripheral branches of the trigeminal system including the supraorbital/supratrochlear nerves, infraorbital nerve, and even the inferior alveolar nerve. Peripheral trigeminal neurectomy may be indicated in selected patients with trigeminal neuralgia who are too ill to undergo other procedures, and in selected patients with trigeminal neuropathic pain related to traumatic nerve injury.[4]

Peripheral neurectomy is generally a straightforward operation. The primary requirement is a thorough knowledge of the anatomy of the involved nerve. There have been numerous ingenious methods devised for preventing axonal regeneration and neuroma formation, but none have proven to be uniformly effective. My technique of peripheral neurectomy is to doubly ligate the proximal nerve stump and cauterize the intervening epineurium in an effort to prevent or confine the growth of regenerating axons. The proximal stump is then buried deep into the adjacent muscle where it is not subject to repetitive mechanical trauma. Implantation of the cut end of a nerve into muscle seems to result in less production of connective tissue and a reduction in the regenerative capacity possibly related to the microenvironment of the cut nerve end. Alternatively, the proximal nerve stump can be placed into bone, which also limits mechanical trauma and limits neuroma formation. In the case of a neuroma, a 4- to 5-cm segment of normal nerve proximal and distal to the neuroma is isolated and removed. The proximal end is then implanted as described previously.

SYMPATHECTOMY

Indications

Sympathectomy has been in use since the late 1800s and has been performed for a variety of conditions. Presently, the most common indication for sympathectomy is symptomatic hyperhidrosis. As far as a primary treatment for pain is concerned, the major indication for sympathectomy is for the treatment of SMP. SMP is most often associated with the group of painful disorders know as complex regional pain syndrome (CRPS), type I (reflex sympathetic dystrophy) and type II (causalgia). However, not all patients with CRPS display SMP. While many patients with CRPS I or II may have a component of SMP, there is usually also one or more components of sympathetically independent pain (SIP) that will clearly not respond to sympatholysis.

Generally, sympathectomy may be indicated for patients with a component of SMP who respond favorably to temporary chemical sympathetic blockade. It is generally better suited for SMP involving the upper extremity. Customarily, at least in my opinion, several successful sympathetic blocks should be performed in which the patient obtains either complete or nearly complete pain relief before considering a surgical sympathectomy.

Selective sympathetic ganglion block can be accomplished through local anesthetic injection of the stellate ganglion (head, neck, and upper extremity), lumbar sympathetic chain (lower extremity), or celiac plexus (abdomen).[5] The diagnostic utility of chemical sympathetic blockade depends on the ability to selectively interrupt sympathetic activity while leaving somatic pathways undisturbed. Therefore, it is necessary to perform careful sensory testing to conclude that pain relief is not in part related to a subtle somatosensory block, thereby producing a false-positive result. There are no accepted standards to judge the adequacy of sympathetic blockade.[5] Observation of Horner's syndrome indicates interruption of the sympathetic fibers to the head but does not ensure blockade of sympathetic efferent fibers to the upper extremity. Generally, effective upper extremity blockade is indicated by a temperature increase of 1.0 °C to 3.0 °C, although this method may be ineffective if the initial skin temperature is warm. Other techniques include microneurography, which is invasive and requires sophisticated equipment, and measurement of skin blood flow using laser Doppler flowmetry.

There are a number of problems in interpreting efficacy studies of regional sympathetic blockade for CRPS. First, the success rate of actually achieving a complete selective sympathetic block is not known.[5] Second, no randomized placebo-controlled trials have been published. Finally, the specificity of sympathetic blockade is not known. In other words, inadvertent blockade of somatic nerve fibers from diffusion of local anesthetic may produce pain relief and lead to a false-positive result. Unfortunately, the specificity of chemical sympathetic blockade and its ability to predict the response to permanent surgical sympathectomy is less than ideal. However, despite its limitations, sympathetic blockade is still an important adjunct in the treatment of CRPS, especially before pursuing surgical sympathectomy as a viable treatment option.

Upper Thoracic Sympathectomy

Anatomy

The sympathetic innervation of the upper extremity is supplied by preganglionic fibers that originate from the intermediolateral cell column. The second-order sympathetic efferent fibers exit the spinal cord in the ventral roots of T2 to T10, enter the sympathetic chain via the white rami, and synapse in the paravertebral sympathetic ganglia. Postganglionic sympathetic efferent fibers leave stellate and middle cervical ganglia and join the C5 through T1 roots, although the majority of the fibers travel with the C7 to T1 roots. According to this schema, resection of the T2 ganglia is usually sufficient to produce near-complete sympathetic denervation of the upper extremity. Pupillary fibers originate from T1 and pass through the stellate ganglion to synapse in superior cervical ganglion. If stellate resection is required, Horner's syndrome is likely to occur. This can sometimes be avoided by resecting only the lower one half of the stellate ganglion.

Various alternative efferent pathways have also been described, including extraganglionic sympathetic pathways, origin of fibers from the C8 and T1 roots, and intermediate ganglia in the spinal roots of C8 to T2. In most cases, it would appear that these pathways are probably not clinically significant and resection of the T2 ganglion is adequate for near complete sympatholysis to the arm. Previously, preganglionic sympathectomy (resection of ventral roots, white rami, and sympathetic chain with preservation of the ganglia) was considered preferable to a postganglionic sympathectomy. The rationale for this was that preservation of the ganglia might prevent "hypersensitivity" of target organs to circulating catecholamines. It is now believed that this phenomenon either does not occur at all or is of minimal clinical significance.

Dorsal Interscapular Approach

T2 sympathetic ganglionectomy can be performed through either a midline incision (bilateral) or a curvilinear paramedian incision (unilateral).[6–8] The spinous process of T2 is an important landmark because it sits adjacent to the T3 lamina and head of the third rib. Upon completion of the initial exposure, a Kerrison punch or rongeur is used to remove the transverse process of T3 and medial portion of the third rib. The underlying pleura can be adherent and should be carefully dissected to avoid a tear. The T2 nerve root is identified and as it is followed distally, the communicating rami and sympathetic ganglion are seen. The communicating rami along with the sympathetic chain above and below the ganglion are clipped and resected in order to prevent regeneration. The tissue is sent for pathologic examination to confirm that ganglionic tissue has been removed. If the T3 ganglion can be visualized and is readily accessible, it may also be removed.

The most frequent complications of this approach are pneumothorax and intercostal neuralgia. In the event the pleura is violated, a red rubber catheter may be inserted in the pleural space until the fascia is closed. Once an airtight closure has been achieved, gentle suction is applied to the catheter as it is withdrawn while the patient is simultaneously being ventilated with positive pressure. A postoperative chest radiograph should be obtained, and if a significant pneumothorax is present, tube thoracostomy may be necessary.

Transaxillary Approach

The transaxillary approach is often preferred by thoracic and vascular surgeons and is generally performed unilaterally.[6] Although bilateral operations can be done, they are customarily staged several weeks apart. The operation is performed through an intercostal approach between the third and fourth ribs, with temporary deflation of the lung. The apex of the lung can then be compressed and displaced to visualize the sympathetic chain, which lies alongside the vertebra beneath the pleura. The third through fifth sympathetic ganglia are easily removed through this approach. Access to T2 can at times be difficult. The T2 ganglion may lie above the pleural reflection, and dissection may be necessary. In obese patients, the ganglia may be hidden in the paravertebral extrapleural adipose tissue. Caution must be exercised to avoid damage to the azygous veins or thoracic duct. The major complications of the transaxillary approach include pneumothorax, pleuritic chest pain, and empyema.

Supraclavicular Approach

The thoracic sympathetic chain may also be exposed through a supraclavicular approach.[6] An incision is made about one finger breadth above and parallel to the clavicle. The clavicular head of the sternocleidomastoid muscle is divided to gain sufficient medial exposure. The phrenic nerve is identified running in a medial direction on top the anterior scalene muscle. The phrenic nerve and anterior scalene muscle may be retracted laterally as a unit or the nerve can be separately retracted and the scalene muscle divided. The lower element of the brachial plexus will be evident exiting between the anterior and middle scalene muscles. The key to finding the stellate ganglion is to identify the subclavian artery posterior to the anterior scalene muscle. The artery should be followed medially to the origin of the vertebral artery. At this point, the vertebral artery is surrounded by fibers from the upper portion of the cervicothoracic sympathetic chain. The stellate ganglion is formed by fusion of the inferior cervical ganglion and the most superior or even first several thoracic ganglia. While applying gentle traction to the stellate ganglion, the sympathetic chain can be followed inferiorly and the sympathetic ganglia and their thoracic root contributions are divided as they are encountered. The T2 ganglion can usually be reached, but access to T3 may be substantially more difficult, especially in obese patients.

Percutaneous Radiofrequency Sympathectomy

Percutaneous radiofrequency (RF) sympathectomy was introduced in 1979 as a quick and easy method for sympathetic denervation of the upper extremity. Several modifications of the technique over the past two decades have resulted in improved immediate as well as long-term results. The indications are identical to those for both open and endoscopic procedures. The operation can be performed on a same-day outpatient basis under neuroleptic analgesia. The operation has been described in detail by Wilkinson, who developed the procedure.[7,9] Briefly, the patient is positioned prone and C-arm fluoroscopy is used to direct and position two 18-gauge RF TIC needle electrodes (Radionics, Burlington, MA) in the vicinity of the T2 and T3 sympathetic ganglia. The center of the ganglion is usually located lateral to the midline along the dorsal half of the vertebral body. Once the electrodes have been satisfactorily positioned, intraoperative stimulation is performed to confirm proper electrode placement. The lesion is made for 180 seconds at 90 °C; the effectiveness of the lesion is judged by monitoring finger plethysmography and/or cutaneous temperature. A successful lesion is indicated by observing a significant widening of the pulse amplitude from the plethysmographic tracing and/or an increase in skin temperature of more than 2 °C. Two additional lesions are made 10 to 15 mm rostral and caudal to the first lesion to ensure complete destruction of the entire fusiform-shaped ganglion and minimize the chance of recurrence.

The advantages of the percutaneous RF technique include avoidance of general anesthesia, the ease of performing bilateral procedures, and the ability to tailor the procedure based on physiologic monitoring. Moreover, the procedure can be easily repeated with good results. The most common complications include pneumothorax and intercostal neuralgia, which is usually transient.

Video-Assisted Thoracoscopic Sympathectomy

The transthoracic endoscopic approach was initially described in the mid-1950s and then reintroduced nearly a quarter century later.[8,10] The evolution of contemporary video-assisted endoscopic techniques and refinement of endoscopic instrumentation made video-assisted thoracoscopic sympathectomy (VATS) a relatively easy and safe procedure.

VATS is performed through an intercostal approach with deflation of the ipsilateral lung. Generally three, but occasionally two ports are used for introduction of a video camera and the various instruments that are used. The endoscope port is placed in the midaxillary line through the third or fourth intercostal space and the instrument ports are placed in the fifth or sixth intercostal space. The lung is manually retracted and the appropriate anatomic landmarks are identified. The sympathetic chain is identified beneath the pleura lying alongside the lateral portion of the vertebral body coursing over the head of each rib. A segment of the sympathetic chain and the associated ganglia are excised. At a minimum, the T2 ganglion is resected, but for a complete denervation of the upper extremity, the sympathetic chain extending from just below the stellate ganglion to T4 should be excised. At the conclusion of the procedure, the lung is reinflated and a chest tube placed. A postoperative radiograph should be obtained to ensure proper inflation of the lung. The most common complication of VATS is persistent pneumothorax. Some patients will complain of local pain at the portal sites, but this is usually rather self-limited and customarily resolves without any specific treatment.

Splanchnicectomy

Visceral afferent fibers have been described that carry nociceptive information from internal organs such as the heart, pancreas, kidneys, and other organs. Pathologic processes that involve the pancreas such as carcinoma and chronic pancreatitis can be a source of intractable pain. Visceral afferent fibers from the pancreas travel exclusively through the splanchnic chain and enter the spinal cord primarily through the greater splanchnic nerve (GSN) via the celiac ganglion. In addition to bilateral innervation through the GSN (T4 to T9), visceral nociceptive afferents may also travel with the lesser splanchnic nerves (LSNs), the least splanchnic nerves, and perhaps even from lower portions of the thoracic ganglia and upper lumbar chains. The deep, diffuse, aching pain associated with pancreatic carcinoma or chronic pancreatitis in particular suggests involvement of visceral afferent fibers, while radicular pain implies involvement of somatic afferent fibers. The source of pain can often be determined through the use of temporary splanchnic block. In the event that temporary splanchnic blockade produces significant pain relief, the splanchnicectomy can be considered. A bilateral operation is usually required to achieve adequate pain relief and involves removal of the T9 to T12 thoracic ganglia along with the GSN, LSN, and least splanchnic nerves.[6]

Splanchnicectomy is performed with the patient positioned prone on a spinal frame or padded chest rolls.[6] The incision is localized approximately four finger-breadths lateral to spinous process overlying 11th rib and the dissection is performed to expose the 11th rib. The periosteum over the rib is carefully stripped with an elevator, the pleura separated, and the lateral 4 to 6 cm of rib removed. The pleura is then dissected from the remaining medial rib surface and the undersurface of the adjacent ribs to expose the lateral surface of the adjacent vertebra (T10 to T12). The remaining medial portion of 11th rib is removed and the pleura protected beneath moist laparotomy sponges. Intercostal veins should be controlled with metallic clips and/or bipolar cautery. Resection of the splanchnic nerves, the T9 to T12 sympathetic ganglia, and their communicating rami is then performed.

Lumbar Sympathectomy

The sympathetic efferent outflow to the lower extremity originates from lower thoracic cord and then passes through the lumbar ganglia whose efferent fibers leave the spinal canal with the ventral roots of L1 and L2. Customarily, resection of the L2 and L3 sympathetic ganglia should be sufficient to produce relatively complete sympatholysis in the lower extremity. Some sympathetic efferents may originate in L2 or L3 and then course caudally through the sympathetic chain and exit with postganglionic rami of the L4 and L5 roots. Consequently, some authors have advocated additional resection of L4 and L5 ganglia to improve long-term results.

Lumbar sympathectomy is performed through a muscle-splitting transverse flank incision extending from beneath the costal margin to the lower quadrant.[6] The peritoneum and renal fascia are dissected free of the quadratus lumborum and iliac muscles using blunt finger dissection, and the dissection is then carried medially over the anterior surface of the psoas muscle. The sympathetic chain should be encountered between the psoas muscle and the vertebral column. Although lumbar sympathectomy is a relatively straightforward operation, there are a number of pitfalls that must be avoided. The ureter should be identified and retracted medially with the kidney; the vena cava or aorta must be carefully preserved at the extremes of the dissection. Also, care must be exercised not to injure somatic nerves passing through the psoas and quadratus lumborum muscles. It must also be recognized that in males, bilateral sympathectomy is often accompanied by sexual dysfunction.

Results of Sympathectomy for Pain

A survey of the literature over the past decade regarding the effectiveness of surgical sympathectomy for CRPS indicates variable rates of success ranging from 65% to 100%. For the most part, this is consistent with the older literature. On average, "long-term" successful outcomes have been reported in 70% to 85% of cases. In general, upper thoracic sympathectomy is more effective in alleviating upper extremity pain than is lumbar sympathectomy in relieving lower extremity pain. There does not appear to be any major difference in outcomes based on surgical approach. Indeed, although less invasive, the results of VATS is similar to those of open procedures. It has been suggested that an important factor in determining the success of surgical sympathectomy is related to the duration of symptoms before sympathectomy. In a study of 21 patients with CRPS type I who were observed from 4 months to 12 years, 95% of patients who underwent sympathectomy within 1 year of injury achieved a good result.[11] Similarly, Schwartzmann and colleagues reported long-term pain relief (follow-up 36 to 68 months) for patients with CRPS type I who underwent sympathectomy within 12 months.[12] In contrast, only 44% of patients operated on after 12 months had the same success. On the other hand, there are studies that have concluded that timing of surgery has no effect on outcome. Unfortunately, my experience with surgical sympathectomy has been less positive than some of the outstanding results reported in the literature. Despite preoperative positive responses to chemical sympathetic blockade, pain relief exceeding 1 year has been the exception rather than the rule.

There may be one or more explanations for failed surgical sympathectomy. First, the diagnosis may have been incorrect, leading to poor patient selection. The difficulty with patient selection based on the response for sympathetic blockade has already been mentioned. There is a high placebo response rate among patients with chronic pain in general and CRPS in particular. Therefore, multiple blocks that produce unequivocal pain relief for the duration of the anesthetic block are essential. Another reason for failure is inadequate resection of the sympathetic chain. Consequently, to maximize the chance for success, it is imperative to completely interrupt all sympathetic outflow to the involved extremity. Recurrent pain following an initial successful result may result from regeneration of the sympathetic chain, which is well known to occur. Lastly, there are reports of cross communication of the sympathetic system, more common in the lumbar region, where anatomic studies have shown crossover fibers in nearly 30% of specimens. As a result, some patients may develop recurrent pain due to contralateral sympathetic reinnervation of the affected extremity following an ipsilateral sympathectomy.

DORSAL RHIZOTOMY AND DORSAL ROOT GANGLIONECTOMY

Dorsal Rhizotomy

The application of *dorsal rhizotomy* for the relief of pain is based on the law of Bell and Magendie, which states that afferent or sensory input to the central nervous system is segregated in the dorsal roots and that efferent or motor fibers are located in the ventral roots. It would therefore intuitively seem that selective destruction of the dorsal roots should eliminate the entry of segmental nociceptive information that normally would enter the spinal dorsal horn at these levels. Unfortunately, the results of dorsal rhizotomy have been variable at best and often unrewarding. Two factors likely contribute to the poor outcomes associated with dorsal rhizotomy. First, dorsal rhizotomy depends on denervation of the area from which the pain is believed to be generated. However, the ability to completely denervate a particular region with this procedure is limited by the high degree of sensory innervation between adjacent dermatomes. In other words, complete denervation of a single thoracic dermatome requires that afferent input be interrupted *at least* two dermatomal levels above and below the dermatome of interest. Secondly, a substantial body of literature now exists that indicates that as many as 30% of nociceptive afferent fibers enter the spinal cord through the ventral root. Consequently, dorsal rhizotomy fails to completely interrupt the nociceptive afferent input. In animal studies, it has been shown that removal of the DRG leads to degeneration of most of these small unmyelinated high threshold fibers that enter through the ventral root, and horseradish peroxidase–labeling studies have confirmed the origin of these fibers to be the DRG.

Notwithstanding, dorsal rhizotomy may have limited applicability, especially in the treatment of cancer pain in which

the tumor has not spread into an extensive area.[13] Pain from deep and extensive facial cancer can sometimes be effectively treated by rhizotomy. In such cases, it is necessary to cut the trigeminal nerve, nervus intermedius, glossopharyngeal nerve, and upper third of the vagus, combined with dorsal rhizotomy from C1 (if present) through C4. Rhizotomy from C8 to T4 may be used for pain produced by tumors in the upper thoracic and lower cervical region that are limited in size (e.g., Pancoast tumor) and that involve the brachial plexus to such an extent that there is irreversible lack of function in the upper extremity. For more extensive tumors where rhizotomy is required at more rostral levels, a useless, nonfunctional extremity is an absolute prerequisite. Bilateral dorsal rhizotomy has proven effective for pain related to pelvic cancer when the tumor involves the more caudal sacral levels (S2 or S3 and below). Sacrococcygeal rhizotomy may also be useful for perineal pain related to cancer. However, bilateral sacral rhizotomy is contraindicated in patients with normal bladder and bowel control.

Not unlike other destructive pain procedures, the application of dorsal rhizotomy in patients with nonmalignant pain is more problematic and demands even more prudent judgment.[13] Rhizotomy has no role in the treatment of spontaneous steady pain and in fact leads to further deafferentation. However, rhizotomy may have a role in relieving hyperpathia limited to a radicular distribution, particularly if the pain is relieved by local anesthetic block as described previously.

Rhizotomy has been used for pain in the occipital and upper cervical regions with variable degrees of success. Rhizotomy has also been used for traumatic arm pain, nerve roots trapped in thoracic fractures, and in highly selected cases of pain generated from the lumbar region. It is my opinion that, due to its limited success and risk of morbidity, rhizotomy essentially has no role in the treatment of lumbar pain syndromes such as failed back syndrome, adhesive arachnoiditis, and the like.

Dorsal Root Ganglionectomy

Based on the observations above and the large number of failures with dorsal rhizotomy, *dorsal root ganglionectomy* is now generally the preferred technique that is expected to produce the best results.[14] Dorsal root ganglionectomy offers several other advantages over intradural dorsal rhizotomy. Ganglionectomy obviates a laminectomy and an intradural exposure and therefore reduces the anesthetic time to which a debilitated patient must be exposed. It also significantly reduces the risk of cerebrospinal fluid leak. Additionally, each DRG is associated with its corresponding neural foramen making localization somewhat easier.

Dorsal root ganglionectomy may be indicated for pain of peripheral origin involving the neck, trunk, or abdomen. It is *contraindicated* for extremity pain since the extent of denervation required to produce the desired effect would result in near complete loss of tactile and proprioceptive function, thereby rendering the extremity useless. Therefore, the procedure can be applied to the following roots: C1 to C4, T1 to T12, and L1 to L2.[14] Although dorsal root ganglionectomy is infrequently performed, it is indicated and has been effective in a selected number of pain conditions. Before surgery, selective nerve root blocks that result in 100% pain relief may *suggest* but not unequivocally prove that ganglionectomy may be effective. On the other hand, failure to derive any pain relief from local anesthetic blockade may indicate that there is a central component to the pain that will not be helped by ganglionectomy.

Dorsal root ganglionectomy may be effective in the following conditions: intractable occipital neuralgia that has not responded to electrical stimulation (either occipital nerve stimulation or high cervical [C1 to C2] SCS), or peripheral neurectomy; post-thoracotomy or postlaparotomy pain; chest wall pain related to pleural-based malignant tumor invasion; and perineal pain secondary to pelvic malignancy. In patients with perineal pain, bilateral interruption of the sacral roots is necessary. Because this may produce a sensory neurogenic bladder, bilateral ganglionectomy should be limited to patients who have either already lost control of urinary and rectal sphincter function or patients who have undergone colostomy and urinary diversion. For patients with preserved sphincter function, midline myelotomy may be a reasonable alternative.

Results of Dorsal Rhizotomy and Dorsal Root Ganglionectomy

The success of dorsal rhizotomy for either benign or malignant pain depends on several factors including extent of tissue involvement, the degree of success in denervating the painful area, and the relative contributions of peripheral and central pain mechanisms. Rhizotomy may be very effective in the short term; however, the long-term failure rate is high. The overall success rate for patients with cancer pain is 25% to 72%.[13] The very best results have been achieved in patients with pain secondary to pelvic tumors. For nonmalignant pain, rhizotomy appears most effective for nontraumatic pain in the cervical region, and least effective for pain related to peripheral nerve injury such as post-thoracotomy or post-laparotomy pain.

The results of dorsal root ganglionectomy vary.[14–17] Immediate and short-term pain relief is often dramatic but is often not durable over long periods. Lozano and colleagues reported a 90% improvement in pain in 19 (49%) out of 39 patients who underwent microsurgical ganglionectomy for chronic refractory occipital pain.[15] Young reported the results of ganglionectomy in 56 patients, most of whom had thoracic pain.[14] Initial pain relief was achieved in 83% of patients, but on long-term follow-up only 68% of patients continued to report a 50% reduction in baseline pain accompanied by reduction in analgesics and improvement in function. More recently, Wilkinson and colleagues published their results of ganglionectomy in 19 patients who presented with radicular or segmental pain related to injury of a specific nerve or plexus.[16] The average preoperative analogue (0 to 10) pain score was 9.6. Patients were considered candidates for ganglionectomy if they achieved at least temporary pain relief from a diagnostic selective nerve root block. At 6-month follow-up, the average analogue pain score was 4.5, and 74% of patients reported at least a 50% reduction in their baseline pain. These results were sustained in at least 13 patients who were available for follow-up at 1 year. An often-quoted study by North and colleagues in which dorsal root ganglionectomy

was performed in a small group of patients with failed back syndrome reported a 50% or greater reduction in pain in only 2 of 13 patients observed for 2 years.[17]

FACET RHIZOTOMY

Chronic lower back pain (LBP) represents one if not the most common clinical problem for which patients seek medical attention. Chronic LBP has a lifetime prevalence of more than 60% and LBP affects anywhere between 35% to 79% of persons at some point during their lifetimes. Chronic LBP incapacitates up to 20% of workers for prolonged periods (>4 weeks) and accounts for around 40% of all worker's compensation claims. The total annual cost of caring for patients with LBP totaled $24 billion in 1990 and the current cost is undoubtedly considerably higher.

The zygapophyseal joint has long been considered to be a potential source of pain, particularly in the lumbar spine.[18] Lumbar facet syndrome was first described in the early 1930s, consisting of LBP with or without sciatic pain occurring suddenly following a twisting or rotatory strain of the lumbosacral region. Injection of hypertonic saline either in the region of the facet or into the joint proper has been shown to reproduce the type of pain generally associated with facet syndrome. Moreover, intra-articular injection of local anesthetics was shown to relieve the pain. Surgical approaches to sever the sensory nerve supply to the facet were subsequently developed. Later, based on an improved understanding of facet joint anatomy and innervation, less invasive percutaneous techniques evolved.

Lumbar Facet Joint Anatomy

The lumbar facets are paired diarthrodial synovial joints formed by the inferior and superior articular processes of the vertebra above and below, respectively. The facet joints are complex structures that display distinct patterns depending on the region of the spine. The synovium is covered by the facet capsule superiorly, inferiorly, and posteriorly. Ventrally, the facet joint is in direct contact with ligamentum flavum; immediately anterior is the epidural space along with the dural sleeve of the nerve root. The upper lumbar facets have a primary sagittal orientation that becomes slightly more oblique as one moves caudally.

The rather poor localization of facet joint pain can be attributed to the extensive overlap of sensory innervation of the facet.[18] The sensory innervation of the facet joint is provided by the posterior ramus of the spinal nerve. The anterior and posterior rami diverge at the intervertebral foramen, and the posterior ramus passes dorsally and caudally through a foramen in the intertransverse ligament. Approximately 5 mm distal to its origin, the posterior ramus divides into medial, lateral, and intermediate branches. The medial branch in turn divides into two branches that supply the lower portion of the facet joint at the same level and the upper portion of the facet below. Therefore, each facet receives dual innervation from two posterior primary rami; one branch from the nerve at the same level, and a branch from the nerve above. The location of the medial branch and its division vary between the lumbar, thoracic, and cervical regions. In the lumbar spine, the medial branch of the posterior primary ramus runs in a groove on the superior articular process and lies in direct contact with the junction of the base of the superior articular process with the transverse process. In addition to supplying the facet, each medial branch supplies several paraspinal muscles along with ligaments and periosteum of the neural arch.

In summary, each facet joint has dual innervation and each segmental nerve supplies two facet joints, plus the adjacent soft tissues. Consequently, complete interruption of the sensory supply to a given facet joint requires denervation at two segmental levels, at and above the level of the involved joint.

Cervical Facet Innervation

Innervation of the cervical facets differs from the lumbar region in that the medial branches primarily supply the facet joints with limited innervation of the posterior cervical musculature.[18] The facets at C3 to C4 through C7 to T1 are supplied by the medial branch at the same level and the level above. The medial branches curve dorsal and medial to wrap around the waist of each articular pillar, lie 5 to 7 mm caudal to the tip of the superior articular process, and are bound to the periosteum by the fascia and tendons of the semispinalis capitis. Rostral and caudal branches supply the joint above and below, respectively. From a lateral view, the medial branch passes through the centroid of the articular pillar.

The C2 to C3 joint is predominantly supplied by the dorsal ramus of C3 and to a far lesser extent by C2. The dorsal ramus of C3 divides into a deep branch that runs inferiorly to innervate the C3 to C4 facet joint and into superficial branch, also known as the third occipital nerve. The latter passes dorsally and medially around the superior articular process of C3, crosses the C2 to C3 facet joint just below or across the joint margin. The dorsal branch of C3 is also the only cervical dorsal ramus caudal to C2 that has a cutaneous distribution. The occipitoatlantal (O to C1) and C1 to C2 joints receive their innervation from the ventral rami of first and second cervical nerves. From a practical standpoint, local anesthetic blockade of the third occipital nerve will effectively denervate the C2 to C3 facet joint. However, because the O to C1 and C1 to C2 joints are innervated by fibers from the ventral roots, the only effective method of blocking these joints is by intra-articular injection.

Pathophysiology

Reduction in disk hydration and subsequent degeneration leads to narrowing of the disk space. Segmental reduction in disk space height can lead to abnormal stress on the facet joint with subluxation and nerve root impingement. The initial events may produce irritation and inflammation of the facet capsule that can result in reflex spasm of the paraspinal muscles. As further degeneration occurs, the abnormal motion leads to secondary osteophyte formation and further exacerbation of symptoms.[18,19]

Despite a relatively large body of literature and scientific research, the concept of the facet as a distinct pain generator is still not universally accepted. Proponents of the facet as a source of nociception point to the presence of a variety of algesic substances that have been identified in facet synovium and facet capsule neurons including substance P, calcitonin gene–related peptide, and vasoactive intestinal peptide. Several types of articular receptors that mediate nociception have been identified including slow-conducting, high threshold mechanosensitive units. It has also been shown that the medial branch transmits nociceptive as well as proprioceptive signals from the facet. Lastly, chronic inflammation may lead to accumulation of intra-articular fluid that can not only distend the facet capsule but also stimulate the densely innervated synovium resulting in pain.[18,19]

Clinical Diagnosis of Facet Syndrome

Unfortunately, the clinical findings of facet joint syndrome are nonspecific. Indeed, there is no anatomic, physiologic, histopathologic, or diagnostic imaging standard to identify the facet as a pain generator. The greatest challenge is in selecting patients with symptomatic facet pathology and identifying the appropriate facet(s) as the pain generator. Facet syndrome is usually a diagnosis of exclusion based on reproduction of pain with facet arthrography and by reduction in pain by intra-articular local anesthetic blockade or extra-articular blockade of the two medial branches supplying the facet.

Lumbar facet syndrome is most commonly characterized by unilateral or bilateral pain in the lower back, with or without radiation.[18,19] The pain may begin without provocation or in some cases may occur suddenly following a twisting or bending motion. The pain is most often described as a deep, dull, aching sensation that is poorly localized. In contrast to discogenic pain, that secondary to facet arthropathy is usually not severely aggravated by sitting or with Valsalva maneuver. Referred pain is common and may be felt in the buttocks, groin, hip, and posterior thigh. However, pain referred to the coccygeal area is unlikely due to facet pathology. Because of the proximity of the facet joint to the spinal nerve root and the existence of dermatomes, myotomes, and sclerotomes, it is possible for facet arthropathy to sometimes produce radicular symptoms.

Physical examination commonly demonstrates tenderness over the facet joints associated with spasm of the paraspinous muscles. Classical teaching is that facet pain is exacerbated by extension and/or lateral bending as opposed to flexion, although this is quite nonspecific. In the absence of nerve root compression, straight-leg raising is usually negative for sciatic symptoms. Some patients may demonstrate mechanical hyperalgesia of the skin overlying the involved facets.[18,19]

In the presence of the appropriate clinical symptoms and signs, the diagnosis of facet arthropathy is most often confirmed through the application of diagnostic medial branch or intra-articular facet blocks. Unfortunately, specificity of diagnostic facet blocks is far less than ideal, which limits their prognostic value. It is also impossible to determine whether complete blockade of the facet has been achieved because there is no cutaneous innervation that corresponds to the facet. Remember that the ventral border of the facet joint communicates with the epidural space. Therefore, intra-articular injection of too large a volume of local anesthetic can result in spread to the epidural space or intervertebral foramen and interrupt nociceptive impulses from sites other than the facet, thereby producing a false-positive result. Also recall that the medial branch supplies muscles as well as the ligament and periosteum of the neural arch, also limiting specificity. Because intra-articular block corresponds somewhat poorly with RF denervation, medial branch blockade is the preferred method.

Lumbar and Cervical Facet Block

Lumbar medial branch block is performed with the patient prone using C-arm fluoroscopy.[20] A skin wheal is raised 5 cm lateral to the midline and a 22-gauge, 3.5-inch spinal needle is introduced and directed toward the most superomedial point at which the transverse process joins the superior articular facet. Reproduction of concordant pain with introduction of the needle lends further support that the facet joint may be the pain generator. Once contact with the bone is made, the needle is withdrawn slightly. After confirmation of needle placement using bi-plane fluoroscopy and aspiration is negative for blood or cerebrospinal fluid, 1 cc of 0.5% bupivacaine is injected and the needle withdrawn. The L5 medial branch may be blocked at the groove between the ala and superior articular process of the sacrum. For intra-articular block, the C-arm is positioned with a 45-degree oblique view. An entry point is marked on the skin and infiltrated with local anesthetic. A 22-gauge, 3.5-inch spinal needle is then advanced into the joint using a trajectory parallel to the X-ray beam. A volume of 1 cc of local anesthetic is then instilled. It is important that small amounts of local anesthetic be used because volumes in excess of 2 cc will rupture the capsule and spill over into the epidural space.

Cervical medial branch block is performed with the patient prone.[21] The C-arm is positioned for a posteroanterior view to identify the articular pillars. A 22-gauge needle is directed toward the centrum of the articular pillar until bony contact is made. Again, 1 cc of local anesthetic is delivered after aspiration is negative for blood or cerebrospinal fluid. For a variety of reasons, intra-articular injection is discouraged in the cervical region. The joint space is very small and narrow and the epidural space is immediately medial, and the vertebral artery immediately lateral to the joint. Therefore, there is a greater risk of direct injection of anesthetic into the cerebral circulation or direct blockade of the cervical nerve roots.

Facet Joint Denervation

Medial branch denervation can be accomplished using either RF ablation or cryoneurolysis.[19] The targets are localized using the identical anatomic principles used for diagnostic blockade of the facets. The RF technique uses an RF lesion generator designed for the following: (1) impedance measurement; (2) temperature; (3) measurement of voltage, current, and power output; and (4) nerve stimulation. An insulated temperature-monitoring electrode with an exposed active tip is advanced into the groove where the upper portion of the transverse process joins the superior articular facet. Electrical impedance is measured to confirm continuity of the electrical circuit. Once the electrode is positioned properly, electrical stimulation with voltage monitoring is performed to determine the relative proximity of the electrode to the segmental spinal nerve. Stimulation at 50 Hz and 2 Hz is performed to elicit sensory and motor responses, respectively. If the electrode is too close to the nerve, the response thresholds will be under 1 V. In fact, if the electrode is in contact with the nerve, the discharge threshold will be as low as 0.25 V.

However, if the electrode is at least 1 cm away from the spinal nerve, the discharge threshold will be 2 volts or greater, indicating that it is safe to make a lesion.

The RF lesion develops radially around the end of the exposed electrode tip in an oblate spheroid shape; it does not extend beyond the tip of the electrode.[22] The size of the lesion depends on several factors including the length and diameter of the active electrode tip, temperature, and to some extent lesion time. The initial signs of coagulation occur around 62 °C and maximal lesion size is achieved by maintaining the target temperature for 20 to 40 seconds. A variety of electrodes with varying diameters and exposed tip lengths have been used.[18,22] Lesion temperatures varying between 65 °C and 90 °C for periods of 90 seconds have been used.

Facet denervation may also be performed using cryoablation.[19] The advantage of cryoneurolysis is that although freezing has been shown to cause nerve damage with loss of function, regeneration without neuroma formation almost always occurs. Histologic analysis has shown that cryolysis results in wallerian degeneration, but the perineurium and epineurium remain intact. Cryolysis probes function according to the Joule-Thompson effect; that is, a gas under pressure which is emitted through a small orifice will expand which produces cooling. Cryolysis probes are constructed of stainless steel with a coaxial design, and are either hemispherical in shape or in the shape of a needle bevel. The hemispherical tip produces a circular lesion centered around the tip while the bevel design creates a lesion proximal to the tip. Some of the larger probes also are capable of monitoring temperature and providing electrical stimulation.

Results of Facet Denervation

Most reports in the literature regarding lumbar RF facet rhizotomy with at least 2-year follow-up report relatively similar rates of success, ranging between 35% to 45%.[23,24] It has been suggested by some authors that facet denervation is less effective in patients who have had lumbar spine surgery while others have found that success rates are not appreciably different in patients who have had prior surgery. Lord and colleagues performed a randomized double-blinded study of facet denervation in 24 patients with cervical facet pain following motor vehicle accident.[25] Patient selection was based on confirmation of cervical facet syndrome using double-blinded, placebo-controlled diagnostic facet blocks. The outcome was measured as the period of time required for the pain to return to 50% of the pre-procedural level. Patients who underwent RF denervation had a median duration of pain relief of 263 days compared to 8 days in the control group. Another study performed in patients with whiplash injury who underwent cervical facet denervation, demonstrated a significant reduction in cervical pain and associated psychological distress as measured by the standardized valid instruments such as the McGill Pain Questionnaire.[26]

SUMMARY

All of the procedures reviewed have a definite place in the treatment of patients with chronic intractable pain. These procedures all have their specific indications and contraindications and an understanding of the role of each is essential for their proper application. However, in the end, probably the most important aspect is careful patient selection. Consequently, if one proceeds with a careful and thoughtful approach, it is possible to provide a significant degree of pain relief to a large number of patients who suffer from a variety of chronic intractable pain problems.

REFERENCES

1. Burchiel K, Israel Z. Surgical treatment of painful peripheral nerve injuries. *In* Burchiel K (ed). Surgical Management of Pain. New York, Thieme, 2002, pp 654–665.
2. Loeser J. Peripheral nerve disorders. *In* Bonica JJ (ed). The Management of Pain (2nd ed). Philadelphia, Lea and Febiger, 1990, pp 211–219.
3. Burchiel K, Johans T, Ochoa J. Surgical treatment of post-traumatic neuromas. J Neurosurg 78:714–719, 1993.
4. Osenbach R. Peripheral trigeminal neurectomy. *In* Burchiel K (ed). Surgical Management of Pain. New York, Thieme, 2002, pp 728–740.
5. Hogan Q, Abram S. Neural blockade for diagnosis and prognosis. Anesthesiology 86:216–241, 1997.
6. Hardy R, Bay J: Surgery of the sympathetic nervous system. *In* Schmidek H, Sweet W (eds). Operative Neurosurgical Techniques: Indications, Methods, and Results (2nd ed). Orlando, Grune & Stratton, 1988, pp 1271–1280.
7. Wilkinson HA: Sympathectomy for pain. *In* Youmans JR (ed). Neurological Surgery (4th ed). Philadelphia, WB Saunders, 1996, pp 3489–3499.
8. Kim K, DeSalles A, Johnson J, Ahn S. Sympathectomy: open and thoracoscopic. *In* Burchiel K (ed). Surgical Management of Pain, New York, Thieme, 2002, pp 688–700.
9. Wilkinson HA. Percutaneous radiofrequency upper thoracic sympathectomy. Neurosurgery 38:715–725, 1996.
10. Johnson J, Obasi C, Hahn M, Glatleider P: Endoscopic thoracic sympathectomy. J Neurosurg 91:90–97, 1999.
11. AbuRahma A, Robinson P, Powell M, et al. Sympathectomy for reflex sympathetic dystrophy: factors affecting outcome. Ann Vasc Surg 8:372–379, 1994.
12. Schwartzman R, Liu J, Smullens S, et al. Long-term outcome following sympathectomy for complex regional pain syndrome type I (RSD). J Neurol Sci 150:149–152, 1997.
13. Harris AB. Dorsal rhizotomy for pain relief. *In* Wilkins R, Rengechary S (eds). Neurosurgery. New York, McGraw-Hill, pp 4029–4033, 1985.
14. Young RF. Dorsal rhizotomy and dorsal root ganglionectomy. *In* Youmans JR (ed). Neurological Surgery (4th ed). Philadelphia, WB Saunders, 1996, pp 3442–3451.
15. Lozano A, Vandelinden G, Bachoo R, et al. Microsurgical C-2 ganglionectomy for chronic intractable occipital pain. J Neurosurg 89:359–365, 1998.
16. Wilkinson H, Chan A. Sensory ganglionectomy: theory, technical results, and clinical experience. J Neurosurg 95:61–66, 2001.
17. North R, Kidd D, Campbell J, et al. Dorsal root ganglionectomy for failed back surgery syndrome: a 5-year follow-up study. J Neurosurg 74:236–242, 1991.
18. Gray D, Bajwa Z, Warfield C. Facet block and neurolysis. *In* Waldman S (ed). Interventional Pain Management (2nd ed). Philadelphia, WB Saunders, 2001, pp 446–484.
19. Panchal S, Belzberg A. Facet blocks and denervations. *In* Burchiel K (ed). Surgical Management of Pain. New York, Thieme, 2002, pp 666–676.
20. Waldman S. Lumbar facet block: medial branch technique. *In* Waldman S. Atlas of Interventional Pain Management. Philadelphia, WB Saunders, 1998, pp 300–303.
21. Waldman S. Cervical facet block: medial branch technique. *In* Waldman S. Atlas of Interventional Pain Management. Philadelphia, WB Saunders, 1998, pp 113–116.
22. Bogduk N, Macintosh J, Marsland A. Technical limitations to the efficacy of radiofrequency neurotomy for spinal pain. Neurosurgery 20:529–535, 1987.
23. Goupille P, Cotty P, Fouquet B, et al. Denervation of the posterior lumbar vertebral apophyses by thermocoagulation in low back pain: results of the treatment of 103 patients. Revue du Rheumatisme, Edition French 60:791–796, 1993.
24. North R, Han M, Zahurak M, et al. Radiofrequency lumbar facet denervation: analysis of prognostic factors. Pain 57:77–83, 1994.
25. Lord S, Barnsley L, Wallis B, et al. Percutaneous neurotomy for chronic cervical zygapophyseal-joint pain. N Engl J Med 335:1721–1726, 1996.
26. Wallis B, Lord S, Bogduk N. Resolution of psychological distress of whiplash patients following treatment by radiofrequency neurotomy: a randomized, double-blinded, placebo-controlled trial. Pain 73:15–22, 1997.

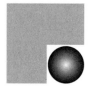

Trigeminal Neuralgia— Peripheral Neurectomy

HAROLD A. WILKINSON, MD, PhD

RATIONALE

As its name describes, the trigeminal nerve has three divisions that exit the skull and traverse rather easily accessible peripheral courses to innervate the face and mouth. It is now generally recognized that a common cause of trigeminal neuralgia is neurovascular compression of the trigeminal nerve not peripherally but near the brainstem. This seems to cause ephaptic transmission or "short circuiting" of electrical impulses. Thus, tactile impulses, or other impulses initiated by innocuous stimuli, may be rerouted at the point of compressive injury to enter pain transmission pathways and registered as painful experiences. Surgically decompressing the point of neurovascular injury to correct the abnormality has proven to be highly effective in clinical application. Unfortunately, neurovascular decompression requires craniotomy under general anesthesia; operating in a narrow space adjacent to the cerebellum, brainstem, and acoustic nerve; and manipulating posterior fossa vessels. Consequently, this represents a significant neurosurgical intervention with the potential for brainstem infarction, unilateral deafness, or other serious complications.

An alternative approach to reducing the painful ephaptic transmission is to reduce the number or intensity of electrical impulses that arise peripherally to be rerouted at the point of neurovascular injury. One cardinal clinical feature of trigeminal neuralgia is that the neuralgic pains can be, and commonly are, "triggered" by tactile or other facial cutaneous or dental stimuli. Neuralgic pains, usually in the same trigeminal division, can be initiated from the triggering area by touching the skin or facial hair, chewing or talking, or even by a gust of wind. Reducing cutaneous or dental sensitivity to tactile stimuli in the zone of triggering should reduce both the spontaneous and the induced neuralgic pains. Complete anesthesia of the area is not necessary to achieve useful or even complete relief of the neuralgia. Because the three peripheral trigeminal divisions are relatively easily accessible by needle insertion or surgical incision, peripheral interruption or neurectomy should offer a much simpler treatment alternative than craniotomy. This simplicity is especially attractive because trigeminal neuralgia commonly develops after the age of 50 or 60 years, and many patients do not "escape" from pharmacologic control of their neuralgia to become candidates for surgical intervention until they are quite elderly and often frail.

INDICATIONS AND PATIENT SELECTION

If the goal of peripheral intervention is to reduce both spontaneous pain and triggering of pain by interrupting sensory input from a single trigeminal division, it follows that the optimum patients for peripheral branch denervation are those with single division pain and trigger zones. As is true of all of the invasive treatments for trigeminal neuralgia, it is reasonable to consider patients as candidates for peripheral denervation surgery when their trigeminal pain is intolerably severe and no longer can be controlled pharmacologically or when unacceptable side effects, such as drowsiness or ataxia, occur.

Because there are now several effective invasive techniques for surgical treatment of trigeminal neuralgia, it is my practice to give patients, along with a discussion in the office, a written sheet describing each of the surgical alternatives. The sheet contrasts the major surgical options (peripheral needle or surgical denervation, gasserian ganglion glycerol or Renografin injection, gasserian ganglion balloon compression, gasserian ganglion radiofrequency lesioning, posterior fossa exploration for neurovascular decompression or subtotal trigeminal nerve sectioning, and trigeminal nerve radiosurgery) in terms of surgical complexity and risk, type of anesthesia required, degree and extent of sensory loss to be expected, likely effectiveness in terms of the initial percentage and mean or average duration of relief, and risks of complications (including anesthesia dolorosa, which has been reported following radiofrequency lesioning and radiation surgery, deafness, or stroke).

Peripheral denervation surgery provides a less surgically stressful alternative than craniotomy, which can be especially important for patients who are elderly or have other illnesses. Peripheral denervation can be achieved with even less surgical stress by needle insertion and injection of alcohol or, preferably, phenol, which requires only local anesthesia, than by open surgical peripheral denervation. An additional and important value of the peripheral needle denervation procedures is that they can be accomplished in the office or outpatient clinic, so a patient may return home after his or her first visit to the neurosurgeon with pain relief and need not wait for a surgical procedure to be scheduled in an operating room or special procedures suite. These procedures produce sensory loss over a limited portion of the face, but most patients tolerate this sensory loss quite well. Furthermore, the sensory loss is rarely permanent, at least following needle peripheral neurectomy, and pain relief often persists well after reasonably normal sensory perception returns.

Patients whose pain and trigger zones involve two adjacent trigeminal divisions also can be offered peripheral denervation procedures with a reasonable chance of pain relief with relatively limited surgical stress. Peripheral denervation in two adjacent divisions does leave a larger area of the face partially or totally insensate, and the larger area can be disturbing—especially to older patients. Peripherally denervating an additional trigeminal division, however, becomes especially attractive to the patient who has already achieved lasting pain relief in a single division following peripheral denervation in that division, and is especially attractive if pain relief persists in that division despite return of partial or nearly normal sensation in that division.

OPERATIVE TECHNIQUES

Needle Techniques for Peripheral Trigeminal Denervation

Figure 24-1 illustrates the most common sites for needle insertion for peripheral trigeminal denervation. These are usually done, and are usually extremely well tolerated by patients, in an office or outpatient setting with strictly local anesthesia. Light systemic sedation, anxiolytics, or anodynes can be given if patients are extremely anxious or uncooperative—but if good surgical technique is used, this should rarely be necessary. The cutaneous (or mucosal) insertion site is prepared with alcohol or an alternative antiseptic. The bony anatomic landmark (see below) is identified by palpation and a skin wheal is raised, usually with a 25- or 27-gauge needle (a 1.5-inch needle will be needed for the percutaneous approach to the mandibular nerve to anesthetize the full length of the needle tract). The anesthetizing needle is slowly advanced to the target nerve while injecting small increments of anesthetic, usually no more than 1 mL being required for first and second division injections, though as much as 2 or 3 mL may be required for third division mandibular nerve injection. The anesthetic injected is usually 1% lidocaine without epinephrine, but 2% lidocaine or a mixture with bupivacaine can also be used (the latter being my preference).

The neurolytic solution used is generally either absolute alcohol or 10% phenol in glycerol—the latter is my strong preference. For many years alcohol was the recommended solution. It has several disadvantages, however. Alcohol is quite painful if it reaches tissues that have not been completely anesthetized, and its low viscosity can result in its tracking back along the needle into the skin and spreading laterally and

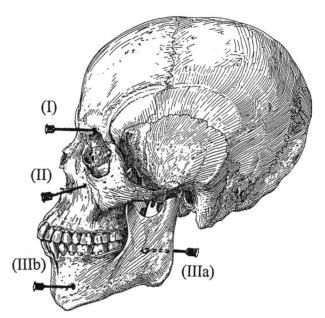

FIGURE 24-1 Four common sites for peripheral trigeminal nerve branch neurolytic injections are illustrated. *I,* First division injections are usually made into the supraorbital nerve as it passes through the supraorbital bony notch in the medial aspect of the superior orbital rim. *II,* Second division injections are made into the infraorbital nerve in the infraorbital canal below the orbit. *IIIa,* Mandibular nerve injection is the most useful type of third division chemical neurolysis. Depicted is the percutaneous approach to the mandibular nerve as it enters the mandibular canal on the medial aspect of the jaw. A transoral approach to this site is more popular with dentists and oral surgeons. *IIIb,* Mental nerve injections are useful only for those patients with trigger zones in this portion of the face.

at times seemingly capriciously into unwanted areas of the face. Alcohol destroys tissue, so that if it reaches the skin or spreads laterally it can produce cosmetically unacceptable tissue destruction and deformity. In contrast, phenol in glycerol seems to be less painful when injected, and its high viscosity makes spread into surrounding tissues or backward into the skin much less likely. I have never encountered unsightly tissue destruction. However, the high viscosity does mean that a 22-gauge needle must be used to inject this solution. Fardy and colleagues demonstrated that injections of glycerol alone, without phenol, were ineffective.[1] Radiofrequency lesioning and cryotherapy have been reported for peripheral trigeminal branch denervation, but are more technically complex than phenol injection and have never been widely used. Following injection, firm pressure is held by the patient with a small, dry cotton gauze for several minutes before a small adhesive bandage is applied (except not following intraoral mandibular nerve injection).

Following needle denervation procedures, I instruct my patients not to discontinue their antineuralgia medications for at least the first 2 weeks, although higher doses that cause unpleasant side effects may be reduced. If good pain relief is achieved, antineuralgia medications can then be slowly tapered and discontinued.

First division injections are most commonly done into the supraorbital nerve branch, but at times the cutaneous trigger zone may be within the territory of the more lateral supratrochlear nerve branch. The position of the supraorbital nerve can easily be ascertained by palpating the bony notch in the medial supraorbital rim. Localizing the supratrochlear nerve branch is usually less precise and requires careful and incremental anesthetic injection until an appropriate area of sensory loss is obtained above the lateral aspect of the orbit. The skin wheal for needle insertion is made below the eyebrow. The needle should be inserted into the supraorbital notch or just below the lateral orbital rim, but care must be taken not to insert deep enough that the injected sclerosing solution enters the orbit. The volume of solutions injected rarely needs to exceed 1.0 or 1.5 mL of anesthetic and 0.5 to 1.0 mL of 10% phenol in glycerol.

Second division injections are made into the infraorbital nerve as it exits the infraorbital canal in the cheek. The bony infraorbital canal can usually be palpated approximately 1 to 2 cm caudal to the lower orbital bony rim. The infraorbital canal courses in a slightly rostrocaudal and medial to lateral direction, so it is helpful to angle the needle accordingly. The needle should be inserted a few millimeters into the canal, after thoroughly anesthetizing the nerve. Penetrating too deeply can enter the maxillary sinus so that little of the sclerosing solution remains in contact with the nerve. As in first division injections, the volume of solutions injected rarely needs to exceed 1.0 or 1.5 mL of anesthetic and 0.5 to 1.0 mL of 10% phenol in glycerol.

Third division injections can be made into the mandibular nerve as it enters the medial aspect of the jaw or into its terminal mental branch as it exits the mental foramen below the lower lip. Third division trigger zones seem to be more common along the lower dental ridge than trigger zones confined to the small mental nerve territory of the lower lip and adjacent skin, so mental nerve branch injections are less commonly helpful than are mandibular nerve injections. Injections into the mandibular nerve distal to its lingual branch spare the patient numbness of the side of the tongue, which is often quite annoying and can interfere with movement of food around the mouth. Dentists and oral surgeons are quite familiar with the intraoral technique of mandibular nerve injection, but I prefer to avoid working inside the mouth (especially in elderly and sometimes not fully cooperative patients) and generally use a retromandibular percutaneous approach. For this approach, a skin wheal is made 1 to 2 cm behind the jaw and just below the mastoid process. A 1.5-inch 22-gauge needle, which I usually bend at the hub for convenience, is directed (with incremental anesthetic injection) under the jaw to a point nearly in the center of the vertical ramus, or slightly proximal thereto, and adjacent to the bone. Needle insertion should elicit tingling paresthesias into the jaw and mental area, and these areas should promptly become numb after injection of a small amount of anesthetic at this location. Once the nerve has been located, from 1.0 to 1.5 mL of 10% phenol in glycerol are injected. Fluoroscopic or radiographic monitoring could be used, but is rarely necessary. Injections into the mental branch begin with placement of a skin wheal 1.5 cm below the vermilion border of the lower lip and 2.0 cm lateral to the midline of the jaw. With additional anesthetic injection, the needle is used to probe for the small mental canal, but this is at times difficult to locate. Once the nerve has been anesthetized, injection of 0.5 to 0.75 mL of phenol in glycerol should suffice.

Open Surgical Techniques for Peripheral Trigeminal Denervation

Open surgical trigeminal branch or peripheral denervation (Fig. 24-2) may be done with local anesthesia and supplemental intravenous sedation and analgesia. However, it is usually more satisfactory to use light general anesthesia with either orotracheal intubation or a "deep pharyngeal mask" anesthetic technique. Skin incision sites are prepared antiseptically with alcohol or other standard solutions, while the transmucosal incision sites for infraorbital or mental nerve denervation are prepared either with antiseptics or an antibiotic solution. Injecting the nerve with a local anesthetic lessens the dependence on systemic anesthesia. Once the nerve is identified, it is grasped in a hemostat, sectioned distally (for first and second division and mental branch procedures) or proximally (for the mandibular nerve), then the nerve is twisted around a rotated hemostat and avulsed. Cutaneous incisions are closed with absorbable subcutaneous sutures and fine subcuticular sutures, with or without Steristrips. Mucosal incisions are closed with fine catgut sutures, which usually fall out within 1 to 2 weeks without the need for removal by the surgeon. As is true following needle denervation procedures, I instruct my patients not to discontinue their antineuralgia medications for at least the first 2 weeks, although higher doses that have been causing

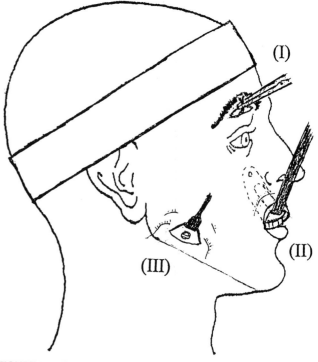

FIGURE 24-2 The three most common open surgical approaches for peripheral trigeminal nerve branch resection and avulsion are illustrated. *I*, An incision below the eyebrow and centered over the supraorbital notch allows resection/avulsion of the supraorbital nerve. *II*, An incision through the apex of the mucosal fold beneath the upper lip allows access to the maxillary bone. A short dissection in this plane exposes the infraorbital nerve as it exits from the infraorbital canal. *III*, A small incision below the angle of the jaw is moved upward to center over the ramus of the jaw. Here an opening is drilled in the cortical surface of the bone to expose the neural canal. Once the canal has been opened the nerve is transected and avulsed.

unpleasant side effects may be reduced. If good pain relief is achieved, antineuralgia medications can then be slowly tapered and discontinued.

First division peripheral trigeminal denervation surgery can be aimed at the supraorbital nerve, the supratrochlear nerve, or both. It is best not to shave the eyebrow, because regrowth cannot be guaranteed. A 1.0- to 1.5-cm transverse skin incision is made below the eyebrow centered over the supraorbital bony notch and, if needed, over the expected location of the supratrochlear branch laterally along the superior orbital rim. The nerve branch is identified, sectioned distally, and avulsed. A small collodion or adhesive bandage is applied once suture closure has been completed.

Second division peripheral trigeminal denervation surgery is aimed at the infraorbital nerve as it exits through the infraorbital canal. The upper lip is elevated and a transverse 2.0 to 2.5 cm incision is made through the mucosa at its apex. The surface of the maxillary bone is exposed and blunt dissection is used to elevate skin and soft tissues to a depth of 1.0 to 2.0 cm to expose the mouth of the infraorbital canal and its adjacent bony rim. The nerve is identified, sectioned distally, and avulsed with a rotated hemostat. The mucosal incision is closed with fine absorbable sutures, but no surgical dressing is applied to the incision line. Moderate pressure can be applied to the cheek with a gauze pad or small water bag for several minutes to an hour or so, especially if there has been troublesome operative site bleeding.

Third division peripheral trigeminal denervation surgery can be aimed at the terminal mental branch, but is most often and most effectively aimed at the mandibular nerve within its osseous canal in the jaw. The mental nerve is approached in a manner quite similar to that described previously for the approach to the infraorbital nerve, except that the incision is made under the lower lip at the mucosal apex. To approach the mandibular nerve, a horizontal or slightly curved 2.0- to 2.5-cm skin incision is made just below the angle of the jaw. The skin incision is pulled upward until it is centered over the midportion of the horizontal ramus of the jaw where it joins the vertical ramus. The periosteum is incised and a 1.0-cm circle of bone is exposed. A high-speed drill, preferably with a diamond bur, is used to create a 5.0- to 7.0-mm round or elliptical opening through the cortical bone to expose the denser lining of the neural canal within the cancellous bone of the jaw. The neural canal is opened; then the nerve is elevated, sectioned proximally, and avulsed. The bone dust generated by the drill can be packed into the canal to occlude it. Some surgeons occlude the canal with bone wax, and others have even advocated inserting a small wooden splinter to occlude the canal. Subcutaneous and subcuticular sutures are placed, then a small collodion or adhesive bandage is applied.

OUTCOMES

Most of the published outcome data for needle techniques used to create peripheral trigeminal denervation date from the time when alcohol was the predominantly used agent. My published data with phenol in glycerol injections is one of the few publications regarding the use of that neurolytic agent for this purpose.[2] In that series, 87% of injections brought marked or total relief initially. The median duration of relief was 9 months, but of those injections that provided initial relief, 37% still provided relief after 1 year and 30% after 2 years. For those patients who had received two or more injections into the same peripheral site, 39% were still pain free for a minimum of 2 years following their last injection. Most of the patients whose pain recurred after a number of months or years of relief requested a repeat procedure, rather than undergoing a gasserian ganglion procedure or open surgery. The reasons cited for choosing a repeat needle procedure were the possibility of achieving immediate pain relief at the time of their office visit with a neurosurgeon, the relative simplicity and the benign nature of the procedure, and the fact that the procedure could be repeated if necessary—often with even better or more long-lasting results than following a single injection. There were no serious complications and even elderly patients (the median patient age was 74 years) tolerated the procedure quite well in an office setting. There were a few instances of minor and annoying formications or paresthesias, which often had preceded the phenol in glycerol injections, but dysesthetic pain or anesthesia dolorosa did not develop. Facial sensory loss usually cleared within 6 months, even though pain relief often persisted, and the limited area of facial sensory loss was well tolerated by patients—even though some found that numbness of the lower lip was annoying and caused them to worry that they might be drooling.

The best modern publication of the outcome following open surgical peripheral trigeminal branch resection is that of Murali and Rovit.[3] Seventy-two percent of their patients had developed recurrent pain after previous radiofrequency gangliolysis, and 40% of their patients were aged between 80 and 94 years. All of their patients reported "excellent" or "good" pain relief, 50% having undergone surgical denervation in two adjacent trigeminal divisions. After a mean follow-up time of 24 months, 15% experienced a return of pain in the same division, and all of these underwent a successful repeated neurectomy. Five percent of their patients complained of dysesthesiae, but the authors stated that their patients, "preferred this inconvenience to the pain they had previously experienced." There were no major complications.

Earlier reports of the outcomes following peripheral branch open surgical neurectomy also documented good outcomes. For example, Fremont and Millac in 1981 reported 77% long-term pain relief.[4] Quinn in 1965 reported median pain-free intervals of 24 to 38 months.[5] Grantham and Segerberg in 1952 reported an average pain-free period of more than 33 months.[6]

REFERENCES

1. Fardy MJ, Zakrezewska HM, Patton DW. Peripheral surgical techniques for the management of trigeminal neuralgia—alcohol and glycerol injections. Acta Neurochir 129:181–184, 1994.
2. Wilkinson HA. Trigeminal nerve peripheral branch phenol/glycerol injections for tic douloureux. J Neurosurg 19:828–832, 1999.
3. Murali R, Rovit RL. Are peripheral neurectomies of value in the treatment of trigeminal neuralgia? An analysis of new cases and cases involving previous radiofrequency gasserian thermocoagulation. J Neurosurg 85:435–437, 1996.
4. Fremont AJ, Millac P. The place of peripheral neurectomy in the management of trigeminal neuralgia. Postgrad Med J 57:75–76, 1981.
5. Quinn JH. Repetitive peripheral neurectomies for neuralgia of second and third divisions of trigeminal nerve. J Oral Surg 23:600–608, 1965.
6. Grantham EG, Segerberg LH. An evaluation of palliative surgical procedures in trigeminal neuralgia. J Neurosurg 9:390–394, 1952.

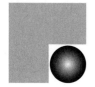

C H A P T E R 2 5

Trigeminal Neuralgia— Percutaneous Trigeminal Nerve Compression

JEFFREY A. BROWN, MD

This chapter discusses the use of percutaneous balloon compression for the treatment of trigeminal neuralgia. It begins with a brief history of the events leading to the development of the technique, then outlines the indications for this type of surgery followed by a description of the technique. Next, the morbidity associated with the procedure is examined. Finally, I review my results with use of the balloon compression technique and its merits compared to those of other percutaneous procedures.

BACKGROUND

In the 1950s, Taarnhoj, Shelden, and Pudenz thought that decompressing the ganglion or peripheral divisions would be effective for treating trigeminal neuralgia. Analysis of their results showed that patients with some numbness after surgery had better results than those without trigeminal injury. They realized that they could treat trigeminal neuralgia by exposing the ganglion with a middle fossa craniectomy and compressing it.[1–4] John Mullan later developed a percutaneous approach for compression. I modified this technique to achieve more consistent results.[5]

INDICATIONS FOR SURGERY

Balloon compression is indicated as a choice of treatment for trigeminal neuralgia or for trigeminal neuralgia associated with multiple sclerosis for which medical therapy has ceased to be effective, or has produced undesirable side effects. Also, patients must be candidates for a brief general anesthetic and should understand and accept that compression is an ablative procedure and will cause facial numbness.

OPERATIVE TECHNIQUES

Balloon compression is performed either using volume control or volume combined with pressure control. Volume measurement alone is straightforward and was the original

technique described by Mullan and Lichtor.[6] The incidence of severe numbness was higher in the earlier series of patients when this technique was used. This higher incidence was a consequence of a longer compression time and the need of the surgeon to develop judgement regarding the volume of inflation required for effective treatment. Volume is only one of the variables affecting the total energy used to compress the retrogasserian myelinated fibers. To further standardize the technique, it is beneficial to add pressure control and a fixed compression interval.[7]

BEFORE SURGERY

Preoperative magnetic resonance images of the brain focusing on the trigeminal nerve at the pontine level are useful. If obvious vascular compression is present, this aids in confirming the diagnosis of trigeminal neuralgia. An electrocardiogram identifies patients at risk for intraoperative arrhythmias during the few seconds of pacing that may be needed when bradycardia occurs. To date, no arrhythmias have been reported. For patients taking warfarin anticoagulation for cardiac or cerebrovascular conditions, a judgement must be made regarding when to discontinue the anticoagulant and when to restart treatment. Patients with a known history of "cold sores" may be treated preoperatively with acyclovir; however, this is not effective after outbreak of the painful mouth sores that commonly appear after surgical manipulation of the trigeminal system.

ANESTHESIA

Before surgery, intramuscular atropine need not be given. Atropine blocks the trigeminal depressor response that occurs in two thirds of patients. The depressor response is an excellent indicator of nerve compression. There is no morbidity from this bradycardia and it is helpful to know that the balloon is compressing the nerve.

General anesthesia is induced with propofol and maintained with isoflurane. After induction, the anesthesiologist positions an external pacemaker on the patient's chest. The anesthetist must confirm that the pacemaker is set at an energy level sufficient to allow transcutaneous capture of paced beats. The external pacer is set to automatically trigger at 45 beats per minute. When triggered, it will respond immediately, more rapidly than the anesthesiologist can by injecting atropine intravenously. Also, atropine may have a prolonged tachycardia associated with its injection. Esophageal pacemakers are not automatically triggered nor do they automatically stop when the bradycardia ceases, which complicates the role of the anesthesiologist.

The depressor response consists of initial bradycardia. It differs from a pressor response (tachycardia and hypertension) seen during thermal rhizotomy, most likely because compression selectively injures myelinated fibers, whereas thermal rhizotomy also injures unmyelinated fibers.

Reflex tachycardia and hypertension often occur after the pacemaker is triggered. The hypertension can be significant and is usually controlled by increasing the depth of anesthesia.

POSITIONING

The neck remains in a neutral position with a soft support. The mean age of the population under treatment is 65 years and therefore exhibits a higher incidence of cervical spondylosis than that found in the general population. Under these circumstances, neck extension may be either impossible or not well tolerated. By obtaining multiplanar views and leaving the head in this neutral position, the risk of discomfort or injury from neck manipulation during anesthesia should be lower.

EQUIPMENT PLACEMENT AND DRAPING

The radiology suite setup is diagrammed (Fig. 25-1). Imaging monitors are positioned toward the foot of the table. The surgeon should learn to control the joystick that alters the table and imaging unit positions. If he does, the operation will proceed more efficiently. The anesthesiologist's equipment is placed below the patient's waistline to accommodate the movements of the imaging unit when a lateral view is obtained. A long plastic connection to the endotracheal tube

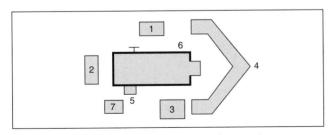

FIGURE 25-1 Diagrammatic representation of the equipment position when balloon compression is performed in the radiology suite for treatment of trigeminal neuralgia on the right side: (1) Equipment table; (2) external pacemaker; (3) anesthesiology equipment; (4) imaging unit; (5) digital monitor; (6) surgeon; (7) imaging screen.

keeps the area near the head free of encumbrances during movement of the imaging unit. The digital pressure monitor is located opposite the surgeon (Merit Medical, Salt Lake City, Utah). The patient's eyes are lubricated and taped shut. Towels drape off the sterile face and there is a long drape over the neck and chest. The balloon catheter and insufflation syringe can be placed on this sterile field.

INTRAOPERATIVE IMAGING

The more sophisticated the imaging techniques used, the easier it is to insert the cannula. Most often the best imaging is available in a radiology suite rather than the traditional neurosurgical operating room. Three views are used: modified submental, modified anteroposterior (AP), and a lateral view.

For the modified submental view, the imaging unit is set at an angle of approximately 25 to 30 degrees above horizontal while the head is set in an anatomically neutral position. The imaging unit is then angled 15 degrees toward the operative side. The foramen ovale is visualized medial to the mandible, lateral to the maxillary sinus and above the petrous bone. With this image, the cannula can safely be directed to the foramen ovale.

A modified A-P view is obtained with the imaging unit after the cannula is positioned at the foramen, the blunt obturator removed, and the guiding stylet is inserted. Center the petrous bone in the ipsilateral orbit. A medial dip in the petrous ridge identifies the entrance to Meckel's cave. It is the groove through which the trigeminal nerve passes into the cave. The guiding stylet and the balloon catheter tip are directed to the center of this dip at the edge of the petrous bone. This modified A-P view is very important to achieve selective injury of the trigeminal nerve.

For a true lateral view, the imaging unit is angled perpendicular to the plane of the head. Align the petrous bones. In this way, the position of the balloon catheter is best determined.

OPERATIVE PROCEDURE (PRESSURE MONITORING TECHNIQUE)

The cannula entry point varies depending on the division targeted. For first division trigeminal pain, the entry point should be several millimeters more than the standard 2.5 cm distance from the angle of the lip. This angle directs the balloon tip more toward the medial portion of the entrance to Meckel's cave nearer the ophthalmic fibers. For jaw pain, the entry point should be closer to the angle of the lip. This angle directs the balloon toward the more lateral portion of the entrance, so that it compresses the mandibular fibers first.

A kit is available (Cook, Bloomington, Indiana) that includes the cannula insertion system. A second kit (Merit Medical, Salt Lake City, Utah) contains the insufflation syringe. This disposable syringe has a pressure transducer attached to it. The syringe will be connected to a digital pressure monitor that is calibrated to measure pressure in tenths of an atmosphere (75 mm Hg). Using the included 18-gauge needle, fill the insufflation syringe with 10 cc of 180 mg% water-soluble iodine dye. Nick the skin with a no. 11 blade.

The obturator has a 45-degree sharp edge and is used to penetrate the skin at the cheek. Identify the foramen ovale with a modified submental view. Replace the sharp obturator with a blunt obturator. Angle the cannula parallel to the x-ray beam of the image intensifier and direct it to the center of the foramen ovale. As the foramen is engaged, the depressor response will often briefly occur. The intensifier image, the tactile feedback, and the presence of a depressor response all confirm that the cannula is at the foramen ovale. It should not penetrate beyond it. A lateral image will now show that the cannula tip is at the base of the middle fossa. Remove the blunt obturator and insert a straight guiding stylet. Hold the cannula in position with one hand while doing this step. There may be some venous bleeding from the epidural venous complex if the cannula is not firmly set in the foramen.

Following insertion of the guiding stylet, obtain an AP view. Position the tip of guiding stylet at the dip in the petrous bone that demarcates the entrance to Meckel's cave. For a third division trigger to the pain, direct the stylet to the lateral porous; for second division pain, to the center. If the patient has first division pain, the cannula should enter from a slightly more lateral approach and a curved guiding stylet directed to the medial porous. The entrance to Meckel's cave is usually 17 to 22 mm beyond the foramen ovale. When the curved stylet slides through the cannula, the curve should point caudally. When it passes beyond the cannula, rotate it so that it points superomedially. This protects the stylet from perforating the dura. The guiding stylet creates a path for the catheter to follow. If the stylet were to penetrate the dura, the balloon could be inflated in the subdural space of the temporal lobe and would not compress the nerve. No injury to the temporal lobe has been reported from balloon compression.

Once the track is created, remove the stylet. Advance the 4-F balloon catheter to the same location at the edge of the petrous bone. Lateral and modified AP views confirm the catheter location. The catheter has an inner thin wire that identifies the catheter position on the image intensifier. The balloon lifts the inelastic dura off the ganglion when it is inflated. Because the dura is elastic, the compression pressure on the ganglion is not enough to give long-term pain relief. At the entrance to Meckel's cave, however, the balloon compresses the retrogasserian fibers against the firm edge of the dura and petrous ridge where the dura splits and allows the nerve to pass into Meckel's cave. When the balloon inflates within the porous, the characteristic "pear" shape occurs. If the catheter tip is distal to the porous, then the numbness created will be less and will be limited to mandibular fibers. If the balloon only compresses the ganglion, then it is not possible to generate sufficient pressure. Instead, the balloon merely elevates the dura off the ganglion when it inflates. If the balloon slips into the posterior fossa, no harm occurs, but the operation will not be successful because the nerve will not be compressed.

For second or third division trigeminal pain, the balloon catheter is properly positioned when the catheter stylet is seen to "hug" the petrous bone. It lies parallel to it, its end just beyond the radiographic clival line as seen on the lateral view. For first division pain, the balloon catheter tip lies medially in the porous trigeminus as seen on the anterior posterior view and more superiorly above the petrous bone on the lateral view. The "pear" shape appearance of the inflated balloon is

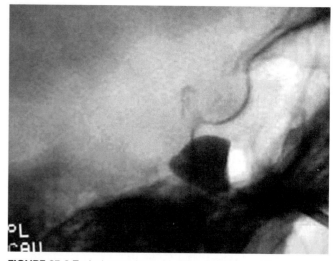

FIGURE 25-2 Typical pear shape of distended balloon. The narrow tip of the balloon indicates inflation at the entrance to Meckel's cave where the trigeminal retrogasserian fibers may be adequately compressed.

seen on the lateral view, showing that it is compressing the retrogasserian trigeminal fibers on the petrous ridge (Fig. 25-2).

Inflate with 0.75 to 1 cc of radio-opaque dye by using the insufflator with attached pressure transducer (Merit Medical, Salt Lake City, Utah). The goal is to achieve an intraluminal balloon pressure of 1.2 to 1.4 atm. Overinflation can lead to more severe numbness or even a temporary seventh cranial nerve palsy. Leave the balloon inflated for 1 minute, or up to $1\frac{1}{2}$ minutes if there have been multiple postoperative recurrences of pain and more numbness is sought.

After deflation remove the balloon and catheter and compress the entrance site against the maxilla for 5 minutes to stop any periosteal venous bleeding. Blood-tinged cerebrospinal fluid will drip through the cannula if the balloon catheter is removed without the cannula. The presence of cerebrospinal fluid does not correlate with success of the procedure. It only indicates that the subarachnoid space has been opened.

VOLUME-CONTROLLED APPROACH

With this technique, inflate the balloon with a 1-mL tuberculin syringe (included in the cannula kit) to a volume of 0.75 to 1 cc. Connect a three-way stopcock to the catheter and use it to maintain the balloon volume once set. Judge variations in inflation volume by the extent to which the pear shape appears on the image intensifier. Correlating the degree of numbness with the appearance of the balloon during compression requires experience

RESULTS

One hundred eighty-three patients were treated over 14 years and evaluated with a mean follow-up of $4\frac{1}{2}$ years. There was initial success in 93%. Subjective numbness was present after surgery in 61%: mild in 80% and moderate in 14%. In 6% it was severe, but these were patients treated early in the series, before pressure was monitored. Masseter/pterygoid muscle weakness was present in 19% and the corneal reflex was absent in one patient. There was no anesthesia dolorosa.

Recurrence overall was 25%, with a rate of 12% in the last 2 years and with an initial success rate of 95% in those patients. There was numbness in 50% and temporary muscle weakness in 26%. A pear shape was present during compression in 74%. Of patients who underwent a repeat balloon compression after pain recurrence, pain was relieved in 68%. Many series have been reported over the past two decades with similar results.[8–10]

Morbidity

Sensory Loss

Compression does not selectively impair Aδ and C fibers. It only injures myelin. The corneal reflex is selectively preserved because of this preservation of the small myelinated and unmyelinated fibers. Because the blink reflex is mediated by these fibers, there is less risk of corneal injury.

If there is little postoperative sensory loss, the risk of early recurrence increases. A previously ineffective dose of carbamazepine may now relieve pain, however. The pain may persist for several days, then resolve. At first, patients may find their numbness uncomfortable, but they soon adjust to it. It is important that the surgeon be very supportive of the patient while they make this adjustment. It is equally important that the surgeon carefully identify any patients who may be intolerant of the numbness before surgery. The numbness, which consists of an objective decreased sensitivity to touch (hypoesthesia) and a decreased sensitivity to pain (hypalgesia), does improve over 3 to 6 months. The pain does not automatically return once the symptoms disappear, nor does its persistence guarantee that there will not be a recurrence. However, pain relief generally persists long after the return of good sensation apparently because subjectively adequate sensation does not require that the nerve be intact.

Jaw Weakness

Motor weakness of the ipsilateral temporal and masseter muscles occurs more often with balloon compression than with thermal rhizotomy or glycerol injection. It resolves after 3 months, although it may take up to 1 year. The temporomandibular joint may ache because of the muscular imbalance. Treat this ache with oral anti-inflammatory medication until the masseter/pterygoid weakness resolves.

Abnormal Sensations

Early in the series, compression was maintained for up to 6 minutes. Dysesthesias were more common. Such dysesthesias usually consist of a pins and needles sensation (paresthesias), an odd water dripping perception, a worm crawling feeling, tightness, or a mild burning sensation. More recently, with measurement of the compression pressure, no such effects have been observed.

Recurrence

Most recurrences appear within the first 2 years. Kaplan-Meyer survival curves show that there is a steady, but slow, continuing recurrence up to the 10th year, when it is approximately 30%.[11] After recurrence, the patient may be treated with carbamazepine. It provides satisfactory relief at a tolerably low dose. If carbamazepine fails, balloon compression may be repeated. Most patients choose another compression, again tolerating the subsequent mild numbness. The repeat procedure is not technically more difficult, but statistically the success rate is lower if repeat compression is required. This is likely a consequence of the inclusion in this group of patients with intractable pain from severe nerve root entry zone compression. Repeated recurrences after balloon compression should suggest that microvascular decompression is needed.

Multiple Sclerosis

In patients with multiple sclerosis, the recurrence rate is approximately 50%. These patients may need several compressions over their lifetime. It is better to injure the nerve less by compression, accepting the higher recurrence rate, but preventing the incidence of dysesthesias for which they are at a higher risk.

Bilateral Procedures

The procedure may be performed bilaterally, although to date it has not been reported to have been done at the same surgery. If substantial residual numbness is present on the first side and numbness on the other side is added, the patient may experience some subjective difficulty in chewing. Patients with multiple sclerosis are particularly susceptible to bilateral pain. They tolerate a staged bilateral procedure.

Other Complications

Since 1983, numerous series, comprising over 800 patients worldwide, treated by balloon compression have been reported. These studies have recognized the following additional but rare complications.[5,6,11–13]

In one case, a patient died after a subarachnoid hemorrhage, later complicated by the onset of hydrocephalus requiring multiple shunt procedures and leading to a shunt infection. The sharp needle used to guide the catheter insertion in this case was inserted beyond the foramen ovale. In another case, a carotid-cavernous fistula was created. A sharp needle lacerated the carotid artery. A sharp needle should not be used in this operation. Several instances of very small arteriovenous fistulae have been reported. By using only a blunt cannula that is inserted no farther than the foramen, the risk for any of these vascular complications is minimized. When a no. 3 Fogarty catheter was used, instead of the larger no. 4 size, a high recurrence rate was reported. Corneal anesthesia can happen, but by using pressure control, the risk can be considerably reduced.[14] Other investigators have reported performing the procedure with the patient under local and intravenous anesthesia, using similar anesthetic techniques to those used during thermal rhizotomy. Diplopia of very short duration has been observed. Pressure monitoring should limit this risk.

Mechanism of Effectiveness

Histologic investigation of the nature of the injury induced in the trigeminal nerve indicates that balloon compression selectively injures the myelin present in large myelinated fibers.[15] These are the fibers that mediate light touch. Compression selectively preserves the small unmyelinated fibers that mediate pain and temperature sensation. It does not injure the axons themselves. This is different from the selective injury thought to occur with thermal injury. Balloon compression reduces the sensory neuronal input, thus, in essence, turning off the trigger to the neuropathic trigeminal pain.

SUMMARY

It has been 20 years since the technique of percutaneous trigeminal compression was first performed. Through use, the technique has evolved and proven to be an effective, relatively trouble-free method of relieving trigeminal neuralgia pain. Its results are similar to those seen with thermal rhizotomy, glycerol rhizolysis, and microvascular decompression. It is a simpler procedure to learn than other ablative procedures because it is performed while the patient is under general anesthesia. It is pain free for the patient. Selective nerve injury is possible. Compression is especially indicated for first-division pain because of the low risk of corneal anesthesia (when pressure is monitored). Although percutaneous compression does not address the cause of the neuropathic pain, as does microvascular decompression, it is less invasive.

Balloon compression due to its simple and cost-effective qualities is an ideal method for the treatment of trigeminal neuralgia.

REFERENCES

1. Graf CJ. Trigeminal compression for tic douloureux: an evaluation. J Neurosurg 20:1029–1032, 1963.
2. Shelden CH. Compression procedure for trigeminal neuralgia. J Neurosurg 25:374–381, 1966.
3. Shelden CH, Pudenz RH, Freshwater DB. Compression rather than decompression for trigeminal neuralgia. J Neurosurg 12:123–126, 1955.
4. Taarnhoj P. Decompression of the trigeminal root and the posterior part of the ganglion as treatment in trigeminal neuralgia. Preliminary communication. J Neurosurg 9:288–290, 1952.
5. Brown JA. Direct carotid cavernous fistula after trigeminal balloon microcompression gangliolysis: case report [letter; comment]. Neurosurgery 40:886, 1997.
6. Mullan S, Lichtor T. Percutaneous microcompression of the trigeminal ganglion for trigeminal neuralgia. J Neurosurg 59:1007–1012, 1983.
7. Brown JA, McDaniel MD, Weaver MT. Percutaneous trigeminal nerve compression for treatment of trigeminal neuralgia: results in 50 patients. Neurosurgery 32:570–573, 1993.
8. Correa CF, Teixeira MJ. Balloon compression of the Gasserian ganglion for the treatment of trigeminal neuralgia. Stereotact Funct Neurosurg 71:83–89, 1998.
9. Barker FG 2nd, Jannetta PJ, Babu RP, et al. Long-term outcome after operation for trigeminal neuralgia in patients with posterior fossa tumors. J Neurosurg 84:818–825, 1996.
10. Taha JM, Tew JM Jr. Comparison of surgical treatments for trigeminal neuralgia: reevaluation of radiofrequency rhizotomy [see comments]. Neurosurgery 38:865–871, 1996.
11. Lichtor T, Mullan JF. A 10-year follow-up review of percutaneous microcompression of the trigeminal ganglion. J Neurosurg 72:49–54X, 1990.
12. Fraioli B, Esposito V, Guidetti B. Treatment of trigeminal neuralgia by thermocoagulation, glycerolization and percutaneous compression of the gasserian ganglion and/or retrogasserian rootlets: long term results and therapeutic protocol. Neurosurgery 24:239–245, 1989.
13. Revuelta R, Nathal E, Balderamma J, et al. External carotid artery fistual due to microcompression of the gasserian ganglion for relief of trigeminal neuralgia: case report. J Neurosurg 78:499–500, 1993.
14. Cruccu G, Inghilleri M, Fraioli B. Neurophysiologic assessment of trigeminal function after surgery for trigeminal neuralgia. Neurology 37:631–638, 1987.
15. Brown JA, Hoeflinger B, Long PB, et al. Axon and ganglion cell injury in rabbits after percutaneous trigeminal balloon compression. Neurosurgery 38:993–1003, 1996.

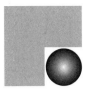

C H A P T E R 2 6

Trigeminal Neuralgia—Percutaneous Glycerol Rhizotomy

TODD P. THOMPSON, MD, AND L. DADE LUNSFORD, MD

For the 15,000 patients diagnosed with trigeminal neuralgia each year, there are fortunately a number of successful medical and surgical management strategies. Surgical treatments include microvascular decompression (MVD), balloon compression, percutaneous radiofrequency rhizotomy, percutaneous retrogasserian glycerol rhizotomy (PRGR), and radiosurgery. We use MVD, radiosurgery, and percutaneous procedures at our institution. The selected procedure depends on the patient's condition, previous interventions, and the patient's personal preferences. The surgical treatment goal for tic douloureux is pain relief while minimizing facial sensory loss.

Successful PRGR includes proper patient selection, positioning, anesthesia, imaging, trajectory planning, and glycerol administration. By adhering to a standardized technique, the risk of associated complications is reduced. In this chapter, we review our treatment algorithm for the management of trigeminal neuralgia and the specifics of PRGR. The technique described here has been used successfully at our institution since 1981.

DEFINITION AND NATURAL HISTORY

Trigeminal neuralgia is an intermittent, lancinating pain in one or more divisions of the trigeminal nerve. Characteristically, trigeminal neuralgia has an acute, memorable onset with periods of exacerbation and remission. Trigeminal neuralgia is triggered by light touch, or pressure, facial sensory stimulation. Typical exacerbating triggers described by patients include brushing the teeth, chewing, cold wind, shaving, and talking. Typical trigeminal neuralgia tends to respond favorably to treatment with carbamazepine. With time, the pain becomes more intense, and the periods of remission fewer and of shorter duration. While the rate of progression is variable, symptoms often progress.

Various causes of trigeminal neuralgia have been recognized. In many patients, trigeminal neuralgia is caused by vascular compression of the trigeminal nerve, most often by a branch of the superior cerebellar artery.[1] It is postulated that with the development of atherosclerosis, the intracranial arteries elongate and become more tortuous, compressing the

trigeminal nerve. Segmental demyelination has been shown in the trigeminal nerve. The demyelinating fibers are thought to be responsible for the paroxysmal pain. In patients with multiple sclerosis, a demyelinating plaque at the root entry zone may lead to development of typical trigeminal neuralgia.

INCIDENCE AND ETIOLOGY

The annual incidence of trigeminal neuralgia is estimated as 4 per 100,000 people,[2] affecting men more often than women (1.2:1). Trigeminal neuralgia is usually unilateral, but may be bilateral. Trigeminal neuralgia will develop in up to 2% of patients with multiple sclerosis (MS). Of the patients with bilateral trigeminal neuralgia, 18% have MS.[3] Trigeminal neuralgia usually affects adults older than 40 years of age, but may affect even children.[4]

MEDICAL TREATMENT

The first-line therapy of trigeminal neuralgia is medical management with carbamazepine. Many patients achieve long-term relief from medical management alone. Although many other oral agents have been tried, we are not aware of any other drug with an equivalent efficacy. Additional medications that also may provide relief include phenytoin, baclofen, gabapentin, and clonazepam. When medical management fails due to a lack of efficacy or side effects, surgical options may be considered.

SURGICAL OPTIONS AND PATIENT SELECTION

There is no absolute guideline for selecting the best procedure for patients. Patient selection and procedure selection consider the patient's medical condition, previous procedures, and the patient's willingness to accept the associated risks and

219

benefits of each procedure. The currently available surgical options include microvascular decompression, percutaneous retrogasserian glycerol rhizotomy, radiofrequency rhizotomy, balloon compression, partial neurolysis, and gamma knife radiosurgery. While the scope of this chapter does not permit a detailed discussion of each procedure, patient selection, positioning, anesthesia, and targeting are similar for each of the percutaneous techniques (Table 26-1).

Surgical candidates, those who have failed medical therapy, fall into one of three groups: idiopathic trigeminal neuralgia, MS with associated trigeminal neuralgia, or trigeminal neuralgia secondary to a skull base or posterior fossa mass. Tumor resection may be desirable in such patients. If a craniotomy fails to relieve the symptoms, patients may be considered for PRGR. Patients with unresectable brain tumors may also be considered for PRGR. Patients with MS-associated trigeminal neuralgia are not considered for microvascular decompression because the outcomes have not been favorable. PRGR is recommended as an adjunct surgical option for multiple sclerosis patients.[5]

Patients with idiopathic trigeminal neuralgia, likely due to a microvascular compression syndrome, are candidates for a number of procedures. For idiopathic trigeminal neuralgia in older patients (>65 years old), or those with complicating medical conditions, PRGR is often recommended. Patients with idiopathic trigeminal neuralgia who undergo microvascular decompression and do not obtain relief of symptoms are candidates for PRGR. Patients with all causes of trigeminal neuralgia who obtain symptomatic relief with PRGR but subsequently suffer a recurrence are considered for repeat PRGR.

The addition of the gamma knife to the surgical armamentarium has made the decision algorithm slightly more sophisticated. Of the patients listed previously as potential candidates for PRGR, gamma knife radiosurgery also is available. The gamma knife is also a valid option for many patients who might otherwise elect to undergo microvascular decompression.

● TABLE 26-2 • Treatment of Trigeminal Neuralgia at the University of Pittsburgh		
PRGR	936	20.4%
Microvascular decompression	3392	73.9%
Gamma knife radiosurgery, since 1992	264	5.7%

In our current treatment algorithm, patients who fail to obtain relief of symptoms with either gamma knife or PRGR are considered for the other procedure.

As a tertiary neurosurgical referral center, we offer percutaneous rhizotomy, microvascular decompression, and radiosurgery options to patients. Over the past 25 years, the surgical management of trigeminal neuralgia cases has included over 930 glycerol rhizotomies (Table 26-2).

HISTORY

Jefferson first reported the injection of phenol mixed with glycerol into the trigeminal ganglion for the ablation of trigeminal neuralgia in 1963.[6] Although this was the first report of the neurolytic effects of phenol for trigeminal neuralgia, he was unaware that glycerol alone might be a sufficient treatment without producing extensive facial deafferentation. This discovery occurred serendipitously by Håkanson, who injected a mixture of glycerin and tantalum into the trigeminal cistern to provide a radiographic marker for subsequent gamma knife radiosurgery. To his surprise, 96% of his patients obtained relief of their pain before the radiosurgical procedure was performed.[7,8] Håkanson later reported the use of water-soluble iodine contrast material to radiographically define the trigeminal cistern.[7]

After a fellowship at the Karolinska Institute observing Håkanson, the senior author (LDL) performed the first percutaneous retrogasserian glycerol rhizotomy at the University of Pittsburgh in 1981. Since that time, PRGR has been the preferred procedure over radiofrequency rhizotomy, given its high efficacy and low rate of complications. The original procedure as described by Håkanson has been modified by some, but we continue to use Håkanson's technique because it is based on a sound foundation of anatomic definition. The procedure continues to provide consistent results.[9–13]

MECHANISM OF ACTION

Glycerol is a weak alcohol that injures both myelinated and unmyelinated axons when injected into the nerve.[14,15] Glycerol is actually a native constituent of human plasma, but the highly viscous 99.9% anhydrous form used in the operating room has a potent neurolytic potential. In animal models, direct injection of the sciatic nerve destroyed myelinated axons, and caused wallerian degeneration.[16] Other authors have reported nonselective fiber destruction with topical application or direct injection

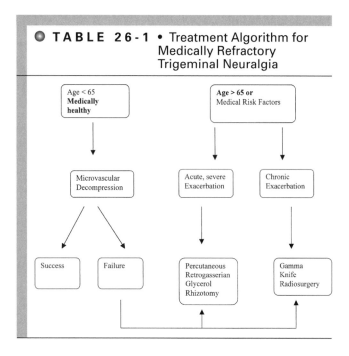

● TABLE 26-1 • Treatment Algorithm for Medically Refractory Trigeminal Neuralgia

of glycerol into the nerve.[17] We performed a series of experiments monitoring the trigeminal evoked potentials in 22 patients before and after PRGR.[18] Sensory thresholds (as measured with trigeminal evoked potentials stimulating the maxillary gums) differed significantly between the normal and affected side both before and after rhizotomy. After glycerol, the threshold improved, suggesting that glycerol inactivated the abnormally functioning, already damaged pool of myelinated neurons that are implicated in the pathogenesis of trigeminal neuralgia.

TECHNIQUE

The initial technique described by Håkanson remains the benchmark for our procedure. The procedure is performed in the operating room, with the availability of anesthesia support and a skilled fluoroscopy technician.

Preoperative Evaluation

Between 1981 and 1985, we obtained a complete preoperative skull radiograph series including a submental vertex view as part of the preoperative evaluation. Although the size and appearance of the foramen ovale was useful to predict the success and ease of accessing the cistern with a transovale trajectory, the skull series was not cost effective. Currently, the only preoperative image obtained is a gadolinium-enhanced magnetic resonance image to rule out a posterior fossa mass, vascular lesion, skull base tumor, or sinus disease. The age-appropriate medical workup is obtained to assess cardiovascular risks.

Positioning

Patients are positioned supine, on an electric operating room table with the neck supported by a horseshoe adapter to the Mayfield head holder. It is important to position the horseshoe at the cervical-occipital junction to provide head stability without interfering with fluoroscopic imaging. Positioning should allow the use of anterior-posterior and lateral fluoroscopy in both the horizontal and semisitting positions. The feet are supported by an adjustable platform to prevent the patient from sliding as the table is angulated to the sitting position. The patient's hands must be secured along the side of the table to prevent unintentional hand grasping movements during the procedure, while under mild sedation.

Initially, patients are supine, with anteroposterior fluoroscopy alignment. With needle advancement, alternating lateral and direct anterior-posterior views are used. After the needle is advanced through the foramen ovale, the stylet is removed to check for the spontaneous drainage of cerebrospinal fluid. The patient is then elevated to the sitting position for the injection of a nonionic water-soluble iodine contrast agent. After cerebrospinal fluid (CSF) is visualized, contrast material injection confirms correct needle placement and the cistern volume is determined. The patient is returned to the supine position for approximately 2 to 3 minutes to allow the contrast agent to drain from the cistern. The patient is finally returned to the sitting position for injection of anhydrous glycerol. The semisitting position is maintained while transferring the patient to the postoperative stretcher and for approximately 2 hours postoperatively to prevent the early drainage of glycerol into the posterior fossa.

Anesthesia

Successful PRGR requires skilled anesthesia assistance. Although general anesthesia has been required in less than 1% of cases, careful anesthetic management and monitoring is necessary for pain control, patient apprehension reduction, and cardiovascular responses. Patients are monitored with an automatic blood pressure cuff, electrocardiography, and pulse oximetry. A nasal oxygen cannula is applied at the start of the procedure and taped to the forehead. Because the procedure does not require verbal feedback from the patient, adequate intravenous sedation may be given to the patient to alleviate anxiety and minimize discomfort. As the needle enters the foramen ovale, patients may experience brief but significant facial discomfort. Oversedation will necessitate transient mask ventilation and interrupt the procedure. Ideally, patients are lightly sedated until the needle approaches the foramen ovale, and then the depth of anesthesia is increased. The skin at the entry site is initially anesthetized with 1% lidocaine using a 25-gauge needle. A longer needle is then used to inject 1% lidocaine near the pterygoid process. Sedation is achieved with small doses of preoperative midazolam followed by a brief bolus of Brevital® or a short infusion of propofol during the procedure. Propofol allows excellent control of analgesia and level of consciousness with rapid postoperative clearance.

In addition to analgesic and anxiolytic concerns, the anesthesiologist must be prepared for potential cardiovascular responses, including either vasovagal responses or hypertension with penetration of the foramen ovale or the injection of glycerol. Approximately 20% of the patients have cardiovascular responses. Up to 15% of patients, most often younger men, may have a vasovagal response associated with penetration of the foramen ovale or injection of the glycerol. A vasovagal response is predictable in anxious patients who report cranial nerve V1 pain upon the injection of glycerol. The anesthesiologist should be prepared to administer an intravenous anticholinergic with the first signs of bradycardia. One anxious physician-patient suffered cardiac arrest after penetration of the foramen ovale, but was successfully resuscitated with a precordial thump and the rapid administration of intravenous atropine. A normal cardiac rhythm and blood pressure were restored within 30 seconds and the procedure was completed successfully. There has been one perioperative death in a 77-year-old patient without a history of cardiac problems. With the injection of glycerol, she complained of substernal tightness and left arm pain. Pain was associated with transient electrocardiogram S-T elevations that subsided within 15 minutes. However, in the recovery room 20 minutes later, the patient had a sudden cardiac arrest from which she could not be resuscitated.

Hypertensive episodes occur in approximately 10% of patients with needle placement or the injection of glycerol and must be treated intraoperatively. We will not begin the procedure until the blood pressure is less than 150/90 mm Hg. Hypertension may be due to anxiety, discomfort, or the omission of routine antihypertensive agents the morning of surgery. In addition to the cardiac concerns associated with hypertension, it may increase the possibility of a submaxillary hematoma. All antiplatelet agents should be discontinued 1 week before surgery.

Landmarks, Trajectory, and Imaging

With the patient positioned and intravenous sedation initiated, the ipsilateral lower face is prepared with isopropyl alcohol. An entry site is marked 2.5 cm lateral to the lateral canthus of the mouth, with the mouth slightly open. Trajectory lines are marked from this point to the midpupil, defining the (X) coordinate. The needle is directed toward a point 2.5 cm anterior to the tragus, defining the anterior posterior (Y) coordinate and the superior-inferior (Z) coordinate of the foramen ovale (Figs. 26-1 and 26-2).

Lidocaine is injected at the entry site with a 25-gauge needle. A longer 22-gauge needle is used to infiltrate the area near the pterygoid fossa. A 22-gauge spinal needle is inserted from the entry site, along the trajectory lines, with an unsterile finger in the oral cavity to ensure that the needle remains submucosal. The correct trajectory will guide the needle to the superior-inferior and anterior-posterior coordinates of the foramen ovale. Accurate needle placement is confirmed with both anteroposterior (AP) and lateral fluoroscopic images.

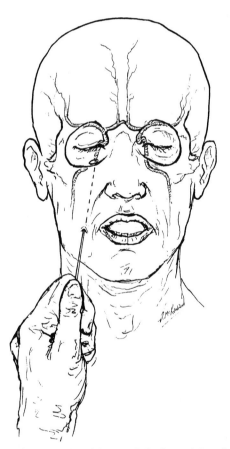

FIGURE 26-1 The entry site of the needle is shown 2.5 cm lateral to the corner of the mouth. The trajectory is toward the medial pupil, defining the left right coordinate of the foramen ovale, and 2.5 cm anterior to the tragus, defining the anterior-posterior coordinate.

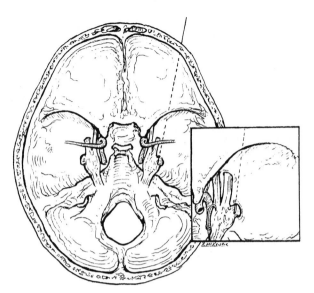

FIGURE 26-2 An intracranial view shows the needle passing through the foramen ovale into the trigeminal cistern. The proximity of the target to the internal carotid artery, the cavernous sinus, and the temporal lobe can be appreciated from this vantage.

The procedure begins with a true AP projection, aligned so that the petrous ridge appears at the level of the inferior orbital rim. In this projection, appropriate needle placement will be confirmed when the needle is inserted at the point visualized as the junction of the inferior orbital rim and medial orbital rim (Fig. 26-3). Although some surgeons use a submentovertex view to visualize the foramen, we found that the hyperextension associated with this image is often difficult for elderly patients, and the foramen ovale is usually identified on the correct AP projection. We have occasionally used an oblique view as described by Apfelbaum in some patients, but find its routine use cumbersome and unnecessary.[19] The lateral position is used to confirm appropriate needle placement and to visualize the volume and size of the cistern. The true lateral projection requires alignment of both internal auditory canals and both sphenoid ridges (Fig. 26-3).

With the needle appropriately positioned, the stylet is removed to check for the spontaneous flow of CSF. Unfortunately, CSF does not ensure cisternal placement. CSF may also be obtained from inadvertent subtemporal placement of the needle (Fig. 26-4). The flow of CSF may vary, depending on the size of the cistern. On occasion, CSF may not be obtained despite accurate placement; however, the absence of CSF reduces the likelihood of a successful result.

With presumed localization of the cistern, the patient is elevated to the semisitting position and the neck is slightly flexed. A 1-mL syringe is used to inject 0.1 to 0.5 mL of contrast material with live lateral fluoroscopic imaging. Contrast fluid is injected until the cistern fills and contrast fluid overflows into the posterior fossa, estimating the volume of the retrogasserian cistern. In our early experience with 376 patients, cistern volume varied from 0.15 to 0.5 mL (average, 0.25 mL). The volume of glycerol injected should be significantly less than the maximal cistern volume and adjusted according to the distribution of the patient's symptoms.

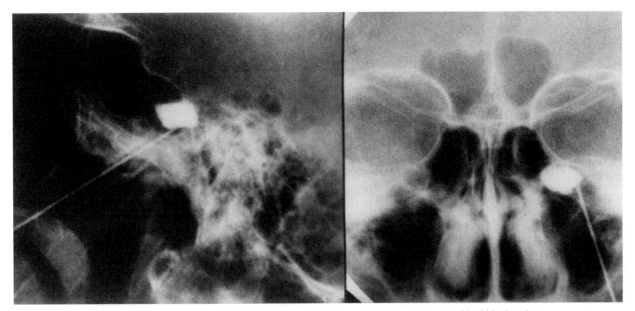

FIGURE 26-3 Intraoperative lateral and AP fluoroscopy demonstrates contrast material within the trigeminal cistern. In the AP view, the cistern is visualized at the junction of the inferior and medial orbital rims.

Håkanson originally proposed that the dose of glycerol injected could be adjusted to affect selective divisions of the trigeminal nerve.[8] The trigeminal nerve is oriented within the cistern with cranial nerve V3 fibers located most laterally and inferiorly. Cranial nerve V1 fibers are located most medial and superior within the cistern. To selectively treat trigeminal neuralgia of cranial nerves V2 and V3, we fill approximately two thirds of the cistern, based on the initial volume calculation obtained with contrast injection. The volume of the spinal needle (0.05 mL for a 20-gauge needle) should be considered.

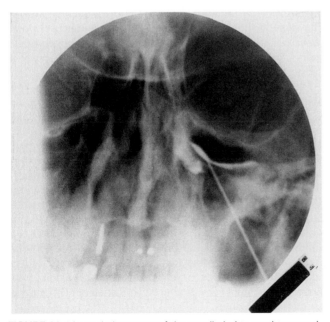

FIGURE 26-4 Lateral placement of the needle led to a subtemporal injection of contrast dye. The dye is visualized as a thin horizontal layer in the temporal fossa.

As done by Håkanson, selective cranial nerve V1 trigeminal neuralgia is treated by leaving a small volume of contrast material in the cistern before injecting the glycerol. Because contrast material is more dense than glycerol, the lower cistern, and lower divisions of the trigeminal nerve, receive less glycerol. The selective distribution of glycerol within the cistern improves the safety and precision of the procedure, resulting in no significant sensory loss in the unaffected divisions (Fig. 26-5).

Glycerol mixed with sterile tantalum dust is injected with the patient in the semisitting position. Originally proposed by Håkanson, the permanent cistern marking with tantalum has proved advantageous, especially in those patients undergoing repeated procedures (Fig. 26-6). During injection of glycerol, approximately 25% of patients have ipsilateral, periorbital cranial nerve V1 pain thought to be related to the distension of the cistern dura that is innervated by cranial nerve V1 fibers. Less than 20% of patients experience intraoperative paresthesias or dysesthesias. Although Arias reported that the incremental injection of small volumes of glycerol can be used to monitor physiologically the production of a trigeminal lesion, we have not found this to be reliable.[9]

At the completion of the procedure, the needle is removed, and a bandage is applied to the cheek. The patient is kept in the semisitting position for 2 hours and observed in the postanesthesia recovery room for 1 to 2 hours. Patients generally stay overnight in the hospital and are discharged the following morning.

Complications and Avoidance

Intraoperative complications include hematoma formation, inability to access the trigeminal cistern, and bradycardia. Hematoma formation is usually due to perforation of a branch of the maxillary artery. In addition to the postoperative appearance and discomfort associated with a large hematoma, intraoperative

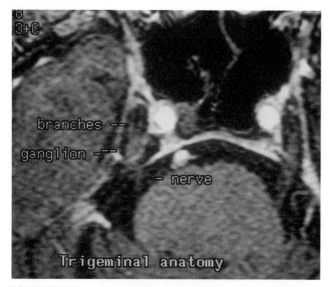

FIGURE 26-5 An axial magnetic resonance image at the level of the pons shows the trigeminal nerve, the ganglion, and the divisions.

hematoma formation can interfere with needle trajectory, and invariably interrupts the procedure. When the procedure is aborted due to a hematoma, we wait 3 to 4 weeks before attempting it again. The risk of facial hematomas may be minimized by accurate planning, few adjustments of the trajectory, control of hypertension, and discontinuance of antiplatelet agents for 1 week. Postoperative hematoma care includes a cold compress and elevation of the head to reduce associated edema.

With entry of the foramen ovale, a prominent trigeminal-vagal reflex may be elicited, causing significant transient bradycardia. For this reason, the anesthesiologist must be aware of the possibility, and have atropine prepared and immediately available. On rare occasions, the trigeminal cistern cannot be entered. More often, it is difficult to visualize, or CSF is not obtained when the imaging strongly suggests

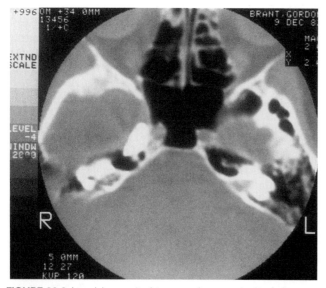

FIGURE 26-6 An axial computed tomography scan obtained after glycerol rhizotomy reveals tantalum within the right trigeminal cistern.

that the needle is appropriately positioned. CSF is not always visualized, especially with repeat procedures. When the surgeon is confident that the needle is accurately positioned and CSF is not obtained, it is reasonable to attempt a small injection of contrast agent to visualize the cistern. With continued difficulty accessing the foramen, an oblique submental vertex fluoroscopy view, along the needle trajectory, may help to visualize the foramen ovale.

Even when CSF drains spontaneously from the needle, it does not ensure that the needle is positioned within the cistern. It is possible to place the needle through the thin floor of the temporal fossa, just lateral to the foramen ovale, and obtain subtemporal CSF. Errant needle placement is important to identify before glycerol injection to avoid the risk of temporal lobe injury and associated seizures.

Posterior fossa injury may occur when glycerol escapes the trigeminal cistern and drains into the posterior fossa. Deafness has been reported as a complication of PRGR, likely due to this mechanism. The risk of posterior fossa injury must be controlled by limiting the volume of glycerol injected to less than the maximal volume of the trigeminal cistern (as evaluated with contrast injection), and by maintaining the patient in an upright position for 2 to 3 hours postoperatively. The inadvertent deep injection of bupivacaine for diagnostic purposes can lead to ipsilateral sixth cranial nerve paresis as an initial sign of overflow into the posterior fossa. With further injection, brainstem anesthesia will mimic sudden death. This complication is fortunately reversible with immediate intubation, ventilation, and cardiac support while the Marcaine wears off.

Perioperative complications include meningitis, sensory loss, anesthesia dolorosa, posterior fossa injury, and persistent pain. Although the risk of postoperative infection is small, patients are observed overnight. Postoperative fever, malaise, or meningismus may dictate a longer period of observation and evaluation. The risk of meningitis is minimized with careful attention to sterile technique. In passing the needle from the skin toward the pterygoid process, the surgeon places one finger inside the mouth to detect violation of the oral mucosa. The surgeon should not apply pressure to the mucosa, which pushes it into the trajectory of the needle. The surgeon must apply clean gloves after this maneuver or any other break in the sterile field.

Facial sensory loss occurs in an estimated 30% to 76% of patients after PRGR.[20,21] The major effects seem to be due to large fiber injury. In our series, sensation was evaluated preoperatively and then 24 hours and 6 weeks postoperatively. A distinct decrease in sensation was detected in less than 30% of patients, some of whom had undergone a variety of surgical procedures. The risk of sensory loss increases to 50% with second procedures and is as high as 70% with a third procedure. Even so, the degree of sensory loss usually can be confined to the trigeminal distributions affected with pain. Patients with a significant loss of sensation or a diminished corneal reflex should be observed for keratitis. For many patients, sensory loss is an acceptable deficit given relief from intolerable paroxysmal pain. Anesthesia dolorosa is a rare but potentially devastating complication of all trigeminal neurolytic procedures.

Before discharge, patients are reminded that they may have a reactivation of herpes simplex virus (HSV, cold sores), particularly if they have a history of herpes. Reactivation of HSV, likely due to irritation of the trigeminal nerve, cannot be prevented. Patients with a particularly strong history of HSV may be given a prescription for oral acyclovir.

REPORTED SUCCESS

The long-term efficacy of PRGR has been documented by a number of surgeons.[9–13,21] Early results from our institution reported a 67% to 76% complete relief of pain, with an additional 16% to 23% of patients achieving pain relief with medication. Eight percent to 10% had inadequate relief of pain, usually associated with poor demonstration of the trigeminal cistern intraoperatively.

In our series of patients documenting the long-term results, follow-up ranged from 6 months to 7.5 years. During this interval, 376 patients had a total of 466 PRGR procedures: 301 patients had one operation, 56 patients had two operations, 15 patients had three operations, and 4 patients had staged bilateral procedures for bilateral trigeminal neuralgia. Given the nature of referrals to our center, approximately half of these patients had undergone one or more surgical procedures including microvascular decompression, radiofrequency rhizotomy, or peripheral neurectomy. Sixteen procedures were initially aborted due to an inability to visualize the cistern or to enter the foramen ovale. Six of these patients had successful procedures performed later.

Inadequate pain relief cannot be evaluated completely in the first 24 postoperative hours. While many patients report that they are pain free on arrival to the recovery room, some patients do not achieve maximal pain relief for several days. Of the patients obtaining pain relief, 90% were relieved within 7 to 10 days of the procedure. Half of these patients had pain relief within 24 hours postoperatively. In patients with a normal trigeminal cistern visualized intraoperatively, almost 95% obtained initial complete success.

Positive intraoperative prognostic factors include easy penetration of the foramen ovale, free flow of CSF, normal appearance of the trigeminal cistern with contrast injection, free flow of CSF and contrast medium after cisternography, ipsilateral retro-orbital cranial nerve V1 pain with glycerol injection, and a normal appearance of the trigeminal cistern after the procedure. In patients for whom all of these conditions were met, our success rate was approximately 99%. The most important predictor of success was the normal anatomic appearance of the trigeminal cistern.

The episodic nature of trigeminal neuralgia requires that patients be observed over time. Additionally, some patients will describe an increased severity of pain or a dull aching facial pain in the immediate postoperative period, likely due to irritation of the trigeminal nerve fibers. This is not indicative of success or failure. Some patients have a superimposed myofascial pain syndrome from jaw muscle disease. This aching discomfort takes time and/or physical therapy to resolve.

The incomplete relief of pain is usually due to technical difficulties during the procedure. Possible confounding variables include variations in cistern anatomy, previous surgery, subdural injection of contrast material and/or glycerol, insufficient volume of injection, and escape of glycerol from the cistern earlier than desired for maximal benefit. In particular,

successful procedures can fail due to a 1 to 2 mm withdrawal of the needle under the weight of the cheek. As a consequence, glycerol can be injected into the subdural space. We attempt to minimize this risk by mixing tantalum powder with the glycerol, allowing it to be visualized with fluoroscopy at the time of injection. A second probable and preventable source of failure may occur as patients are transferred to the recovery room stretcher. If they extend their neck, glycerol may escape the cistern and drain into the posterior fossa.

Recurrent pain after initial pain relief is initially treated with medicines. If medical management fails to control the pain, repeat procedures may be considered once or twice. Patients in whom recurrent pain develops after three successful procedures are considered for radiofrequency rhizotomy, or more often, gamma knife radiosurgery.

CONTRAINDICATIONS

Contraindications to PRGR include uncontrolled hypertension, cardiovascular instability, bleeding diathesis, and a preexisting diagnosis of anesthesia dolorosa or atypical trigeminal neuralgia.

SUMMARY

While trigeminal neuralgia remains a relatively common neurosurgical disease, a number of successful interventions are now available. Among the earliest options, percutaneous retrogasserian glycerol rhizotomy remains a useful tool. The procedure is minimally invasive but not noninvasive, has a high success rate and acceptable complications. The neurosurgeon undertaking PRGR must use the history and physical examination to confirm the diagnosis, exercise their understanding of the anatomy, and collaborate effectively with anesthesiologists and the fluoroscopic technician.

REFERENCES

1. Jannetta PJ. Arterial compression of the trigeminal nerve at the pons in patients with trigeminal neuralgia. J Neurosurg 26:159–162, 1967.
2. Wepsic JG. Tic douloureaux: etiology, refined treatment. N Engl J Med 288:680–681, 1973.
3. Brisman R. Bilateral trigeminal neuralgia. J Neurosurg 67:44–48, 1987.
4. Resnick DK, Levy EI, Jannetta PJ. Microvascular decompression for pediatric onset trigeminal neuralgia. Neurosurgery 43(4):804–807, 1998.
5. Kondziolka D, Lunsford LD, Bissonette DJ. Long-term results after glycerol rhizotomy for multiple sclerosis-related trigeminal neuralgia. Can J Neurol Sci 21(2):137–140, 1994.
6. Jefferson A. Trigeminal root and gangliion injection using phenol in glycerin for the relief of trigeminal neuralgia. J Neurol Neurosurg Psychiatry 26:345–352, 1963.
7. Håkanson S. Transoval trigeminal cisternography. Surg Neurol 10:137–144, 1978.
8. Håkanson S. Trigeminal neuralgia treated by the injection of glycerol into the trigeminal cistern. Neurosurgery 9:68–646, 1981.
9. Arias MJ. Percutaneous retrogasserian glycerol rhizotomies for trigeminal neuralgia. A prospective study of 100 cases. J Neurosurg 65:32–36, 1986.
10. Beck DW, Olson JJ, Urig ES. Percutaneous retrogasserian glycerol rhizotomies for treatment of trigminal neuralgia. J Neurosurg 65:28–31, 1986.

11. Burchiel KS. Percutaneous retrogasserian glycerol rhizolysis in the management of trigeminal neuralgia. J Neurosurg 69:361–366, 1988.

12. Dieckmann G, Veras G, Sogabe K. Retrogasserian glycerol injection in percutaneous stimulation in the treatment of typical and atypical trigeminal pain. Neurol Res 9:48–49, 1987.

13. Young RI. Glycerol rhizolysis for treatment of trigeminal neuralgia. J Neurosurg 69:39–45, 1988.

14. Lunsford LD, Bennett MH, Martinez AJ. Experimental trigeminal glycerol injection. Electrophysiologic and morphologic effects. Arch Neurol 42(2):146–149, 1985.

15. Burchiel KS, Russel LC. Glycerol neurolysis: neurophysiological effects of topical glycerol application on cat saphenous nerve. J Neurosurg 63:784–788, 1985.

16. Håkanson S. Trigeminal neuralgia treated by retrogasserian injection of glycerol (thesis). Stockholm, Tryckeri Balder AB, 1982.

17. Rengachary S, Watanabe IS, Singer P, Bopp WJ. Effect of glycerol on peripheral nerve: an experimental study. Neurosurgery 13:681–688, 1983.

18. Bennett MH, Lunsford LD. Percutaneous retrogasserian glycerol rhizotomy for tic douloureux. Part 2. Results and implications of trigeminal evoked potential studies. Neurosurgery 14:431–435, 1984.

19. Apfelbaum RI. Surgery for tic douloureux. Clin Neurosurg 31:667–683, 1984.

20. Burchiel KS. Percutaneous retrogasserian glycerol rhizolysis in the management of trigeminal neuralgia. J Neurosurg 69:361–366, 1988.

21. Lunsford LD. Treatment of tic douloureux by percutaneous retrogasserian glycerol injection. JAMA 248(4):449–453, 1982.

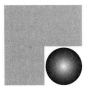

C H A P T E R   2 7

Trigeminal Neuralgia— Percutaneous Radiofrequency Rhizotomy

JAMAL M. TAHA, MD

Percutaneous radiofrequency (RF) rhizotomy is an effective surgical treatment for selected patients with trigeminal neuralgia. In this procedure, RF energy is delivered to selected trigeminal retrogasserian rootlets to inflict thermal injury to pain-mediating fibers. This is achieved using an electrode, which is introduced through a needle inserted percutaneously through the patient's face under fluoroscopic control.

HISTORICAL BACKGROUND

Sweet[1] introduced percutaneous RF rhizotomy for the treatment of trigeminal neuralgia 40 years ago when he refined the practice of diathermy coagulation of the trigeminal system. Sweet used short-acting anesthetic agents, which allowed surgeons to awaken patients during surgery for sensory testing; used electrical stimulation for precise localization; produced a reliable energy current for controlled destruction of neural tissue; and used temperature monitoring for precise lesion production. The technique was based on the physiologic findings of relative destruction of Aδ and C nociceptive fibers by graded temperature application to the trigeminal ganglion and rootlets.[2]

After its introduction, RF rhizotomy became widely practiced with good results; however, few subsequent reports of associated postoperative facial dysesthesia and anesthesia dolorosa encouraged investigators to explore other percutaneous destructive procedures.[3] Tew and Nugent are credited for refining the technique of RF rhizotomy to reduce the risk of dysesthesia. Tew[4] introduced a curved-tip electrode that allowed selective destruction of trigeminal rootlets, while Nugent[5] used a small cordotomy electrode to achieve a similar result. Both investigators independently created a milder thermal lesion that produced less facial numbness and less dysesthesia, reestablishing RF rhizotomy as the gold standard surgery to which other procedures compare.

PATIENT SELECTION

RF rhizotomy is indicated for patients with trigeminal neuralgia who no longer respond to medications or who suffer from side effects. Best candidates are the elderly or patients in poor medical condition with pain in the cranial nerve V3 or V2 trigeminal divisions. Young healthy patients and patients with pain involving cranial nerve V1 or all three trigeminal divisions can undergo RF rhizotomy, but may better be treated with other procedures that have less risk of corneal or facial numbness, such as microvascular decompression or balloon compression. Patients with trigeminal neuralgia associated with multiple sclerosis are good candidates for RF rhizotomy. RF rhizotomy has also been successfully used in patients with trigeminal neuralgia associated with tumor, aneurysm, arteriovenous malformation, or stroke.[6] Patients with vagoglossopharyngeal neuralgia related to head and neck cancer and selected patients with cluster headache can also benefit from percutaneous trigeminal RF rhizotomy.[6] Poor patient candidates for RF rhizotomy include most patients with trigeminal neuropathic pain presenting with continuous dysesthetic facial pain and most patients with atypical facial pain syndromes. These conditions can be associated with a high risk of postoperative severe dysesthesia after RF rhizotomy.[6]

SURGICAL TECHNIQUE

RF rhizotomy is performed in the operating room or radiology suite under intravenous sedation. The procedure involves image-guided cannulation of the foramen ovale, stimulation of the trigeminal system for physiologic localization, and creation of a thermal lesion using radiofrequency energy. The patient needs to be awakened for a brief period during surgery for proper localization of the electrode and for proper creation of the lesion.

227

Preoperative Preparation

Prior to surgery, the patient is fully informed of the options available for the treatment of trigeminal neuralgia and of the outcome. Anticoagulant medications must be stopped before surgery, but antiplatelet medications can be continued. The patient is brought to the hospital the same day of surgery and intravenous access is secured opposite to the patient's pain. The patient's oral intake is restricted 6 hours before the procedure and 0.4 mg of atropine is administered intramuscularly 30 minutes before surgery to reduce oral secretions and to prevent bradycardia during sedation. I do not administer prophylactic antibiotics; however, some surgeons recommend a single dose of intravenous antibiotics against normal oropharyngeal flora before needle insertion.

Surgical Positioning

The patient lies supine with the head in neutral position and the arms strapped at the sides to minimize movement during sedation. Three anatomic landmarks are marked on the patient's face: 3 cm anterior to the external auditory meatus along the inferior border of the zygomatic arch; 1 cm beneath the medial aspect of the pupil; and 2.5 cm lateral to the oral commissure (Fig. 27-1). A reference pad is used for patient grounding. The patient's face lateral to the oral commissure is prepared with antiseptic solution. Sterile towels cover the patient's neck and chest, but the patient's face is left exposed.

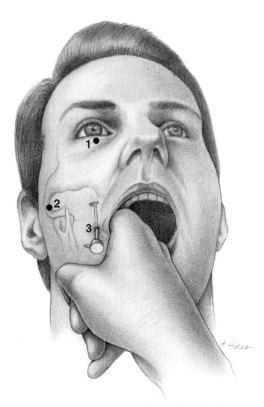

FIGURE 27-1 Electrode placement. External landmarks are as follows: (1) the medial aspect of the pupil; (2) 3 cm anterior to the external auditory meatus; and (3) site of needle penetration 2.5 cm to 3 cm lateral to oral commissure. (Printed with permission from Mayfield Clinic, Cincinnati, OH.)

The patient's blood pressure, heart rate, and oxygen saturation are continuously monitored during the procedure. An oral airway is placed between the patient's jaws to prevent involuntarily biting of the surgeon's index finger during placement of the needle. The patient is anesthetized with an intravenous injection of 30 to 50 mg methohexital (Brevital; Eli Lilly, Indianapolis, Indiana) before needle insertion.

Needle Placement

The surgeon places the index finger in the patient's mouth, inferior to the lateral pterygoid wing to prevent the needle from penetrating the oral mucosa and to guide it into the medial portion of the foramen ovale. A standard 100-mm length 20-gauge needle with a stylet penetrates the skin 2.5 cm lateral to the oral commissure but should not penetrate the buccal mucosa. The needle is aimed in the lateral-medial direction toward the skin mark inferior to the pupil and in the superior-inferior direction toward the skin mark 3 cm anterior to the external auditory meatus (see Fig. 27-1). The needle is advanced under intermittent lateral fluoroscopy toward the angle formed by the shadows of the petrous bone and the clivus, 5 to 10 mm below the sella floor along the clival line. Needle entrance into the foramen ovale is achieved at a depth of approximately 6 to 8 cm and is signaled by a facial wince and a brief contraction of the masseter muscle, indicating contact with the mandibular sensory and motor fibers.

Proper positioning of the needle within the trigeminal cistern allows free flow of cerebrospinal fluid as the stylet is removed in most patients. Cerebrospinal fluid may not be obtained in patients who had previous percutaneous ablative procedure. Egress of cerebrospinal fluid does not ensure the needle is properly positioned in the retrogasserian area. Cerebrospinal fluid can be obtained from the infratemporal subarachnoid space if the needle is too deep or from the region distal to the gasserian ganglion if the dural subarachnoid sleeve extends beyond the rootlets.

In positioning the needle, care must be taken to avoid injury to other vascular or neural structures by strictly adhering to the landmarks described previously and by frequently utilizing fluoroscopy during needle advancement. The internal carotid artery is vulnerable to injury at three sites: the foramen lacerum, where its cartilaginous covering can be penetrated if the needle is deviated posterior and medial; Meckel's cave, where the artery is frequently devoid of bony covering at its entrance into the petrous bone and which can be injured if the needle is deviated posterior and lateral; and the cavernous sinus, if the needle is advanced too far cephalad, anterior, and medial. If the carotid artery is penetrated, the needle should be withdrawn promptly and manual pressure applied over the posterior pharyngeal space. The procedure should be discontinued but can be repeated a few days later.

Foraminae that lie adjacent to the foramen ovale should not be cannulated, such as the superior orbital fissure, which lies anterior and superior, and the jugular foramen, which lies posterior and inferior. The abducens nerve may be injured if the needle is advanced more than 5 mm beyond the profile of the clivus on lateral fluoroscopy. The trochlear and oculomotor nerves can be injured if the needle is too cephalad close to the cavernous sinus.

Electrode Localization

The cannula is calibrated to permit extrusion of the electrode in 1-mm increments. The curved electrode tip is a coil spring that carries a thermocouple, stimulator, and lesion-generating probe. When the electrode is fully inserted into the cannula, the curved tip extends 5 mm beyond the end of the cannula and projects 3 mm perpendicular to the axis of the electrode. The cannula is Teflon insulated to the tip so that only the extruded portion of the electrode (0 to 5 mm) is conductive. The electrode can be rotated through a 360-degree axis for stimulation and lesion production.

After needle cannulation of the foramen ovale, the surgeon changes his or her gloves and the patient is allowed to wake up. The electrode is placed, initially guided by its anatomic location on lateral fluoroscopic projection. For cranial nerve V3 pain, the electrode tip lies within 5 mm proximal to the clivus profile and is directed caudal; for cranial nerve V2 pain, the electrode tip is placed at the clivus profile; and for cranial nerve V1 pain, the electrode tip lies within 5 mm distal to the clivus profile and is directed cephalad (Fig. 27-2).

Final placement of the electrode tip is determined by the patient's response to electrical stimulation. A square wave current of 0.2 to 0.5 V at 50 cycles/second and 0.1 msec duration produces paresthesias in the distribution of the involved nerve or trigger zone or reproduces the paroxysmal bouts of pain reminiscent of trigeminal neuralgia. It is important to distinguish patient's responses to stimulation from intraoperative spontaneous bouts of trigeminal neuralgia. Stimulation can also be achieved with mild heating (<40 °C). Stimulation at higher voltage (0.5 to 1 V) may be required in patients who had a previous percutaneous destructive procedure. Rotation of the curved electrode about its axis, depth of penetration, and angle of trajectory permit stimulation of different portions of the nerve. Medial rotation of the electrode tip provides better access to the fibers of the ophthalmic division while lateral rotation contacts the mandibular fibers. Advancement of the electrode within 5 mm beyond the clival line on lateral fluoroscopy provides better contact with the ophthalmic division while an electrode that lies within 5 mm short of the clival line provides better contact with the mandibular fibers. A cannula which is redirected more anteromedial bringing the tip closer to the posterior clinoid achieves better contact with the ophthalmic division. The motor root lies medial to the ganglion and can be avoided by rotating the curved electrode laterally if stimulation produces masseter contraction. If ocular movement occurs during stimulation, the cannula is too deep in the cavernous sinus or too near the brainstem. Stimulus evoked facial contractions indicate that the electrode is either too deep or is inclined too low on the clivus, or that the stimulation level is too high.

Lesion Production

The geometry of the lesions varies with the medium; reproducible lesions are $5 \times 5 \times 4$ mm and are eccentric with orientation toward the curve of the electrode. The electrode tip measures 0.5 mm in diameter. A thermocouple sensor is located at the electrode tip and provides calibration accuracy of ± 2 °C over the range of 30 °C to 100 °C.

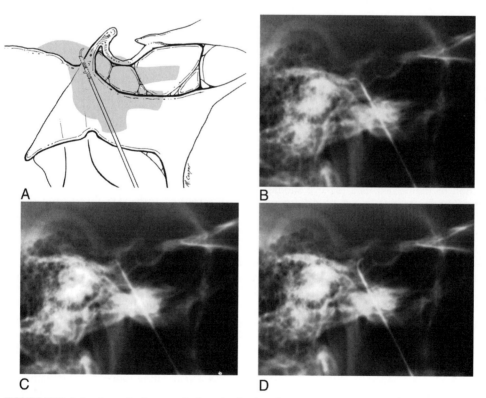

FIGURE 27-2 *A*, A schematic diagram of a lateral sella view demonstrating the relationship of the trigeminal rootlets to the clivus. Lateral radiographs demonstrate the location of the electrode for stimulation of *(B)* V3, *(C)* V2, and *(D)* V1 trigeminal divisions. (Printed with permission from Mayfield Clinic, Cincinnati, OH.)

Additional intravenous anesthetic is administered and a preliminary lesion is usually produced at 70 °C for 70 seconds. For pain along cranial nerve V1, the author starts with a lesion of 60 °C for 60 seconds. Facial flush (partly secondary to antidromic release of vasodilatory neuropeptides such as substance P and calcitonin gene–related peptide) usually appears and helps to localize the region of the nerve root undergoing thermal destruction.[7] When the patient is fully awake, facial sensations are carefully examined. Repeat lesions are produced until the desired effect is achieved. Generally, sequential lesions are made by increasing the temperature 5 °C to 10 °C and the duration of lesions by 5 to 10 seconds with each lesion. The lesion can be controlled by carefully altering the location of the electrode, controlling the temperature, and monitoring the location and severity of sensory deficits. After a partial lesion has been produced, it is frequently possible to complete lesion production without using additional anesthetics and with constant sensory testing to finely control denervation.

Surgery is completed when dense hypalgesia but not anesthesia develops in the primarily affected divisions, especially over the trigger zone and when the patient cannot reproduce trigeminal pain after touching the trigger point or after performing maneuvers known to induce pain. If the patient is cooperative and reliable, he or she is asked to compare the sensations in the treated division with that of the normal opposite side. Hypalgesia of 75% or more is a good end point. Another end point is loss of sensations to superficial light touch but not deep touch. In uncooperative patients, I have found it helpful to observe the patient's facial reactions as a needle testing sensations is advanced from hypalgesic to normal areas of the face.

Once the desired degree of sensory loss has been achieved, the patient is observed for an additional 15 minutes to determine if a fixed lesion has been produced. Masseter, pterygoid, facial, and ocular muscle functions are recorded. Patients return to their rooms and are observed for 4 hours. During this period, ice packs are applied to the jaw and cheek areas to reduce facial swelling. The patient is informed of the necessity for eye care, of avoiding jaw strain, and of the consequences of facial analgesia. If substantial loss of corneal sensation occurs, artificial tears are used on the cornea every 2 to 4 hours. The patient should inform the surgeon of blurring of vision or injection of the cornea, and the eye should be inspected. Diet should be restricted to soft food for 1 week postoperatively; jaw opening exercises are practiced for 2 weeks. The patient should avoid biting the lip, tongue, and buccal mucosa, as well as scratching or irritating the analgesic skin. If maceration occurs, the mouth is irrigated with warm saline solution every 4 hours. After surgery, patients receive half of the daily dose of anticonvulsant medications, which are thereafter slowly tapered before being discontinued.

RESULTS

Several series with large number of patients have reported the results of RF trigeminal rhizotomy in the treatment of trigeminal neuralgia.[8] In summary, pain is immediately relieved in 99% of patients. Occasionally, some patients suffer from bouts of tic pain for 1 day after surgery before it subsides. In our experience, rate of pain recurrence is similar to that of microvascular decompression—approximately 15% to 20% in 10 to 15 years.[9] All patients develop numbness in the face after a successful RF rhizotomy which, in the majority of patients, is tolerable. In a review of 500 patients who underwent percutaneous RF rhizotomy using the curved Tew electrode, 9% of patients described an intermittent crawling, burning, or itching sensation that did not require treatment; 2% complained of numbness that was disturbing and required treatment; and anesthesia dolorosa developed in 0.2%.[8] Drooling, loss of taste, and difficulty chewing as a result of diminution of sensory perception were infrequently objectionable. Ocular complications, including neurogenic keratitis or corneal abrasion, developed in less than 1% of patients, exclusively in patients who had tic pain involving the first or second trigeminal divisions. Weakness of the masseter, temporalis, and pterygoid muscles occurred in 10% of patients but was rarely permanent. Difficulty in hearing with tinnitus, random roaring, and popping sounds was reported by few patients. These symptoms are attributable to paresis of the small muscles around the eustachian tube (tensor veli palatini) and tympanic membrane (tensor tympani). Other complications, such as ocular nerve injury, seizures, meningitis, stroke, intracranial hemorrhage, and death have been reported but are rare. In a review of 1200 patients observed for 1 to 20 years (mean, 9 years), 93% reported excellent or good results, 4% reported fair results because of undesirable side effects, and 1% reported poor results because of severe denervation dysesthesias.[4]

DISCUSSION

There is no current surgical cure for trigeminal neuralgia; however, several surgical procedures offer high rates of postoperative long-term pain relief with low morbidity. Of the percutaneous procedures, I have found RF rhizotomy to be associated with the highest success rate and the lowest pain recurrence rate, similar to microvascular decompression. Complications of dysesthesia are markedly reduced by attention to the following details:

- Using a curved electrode which, compared to the straight electrode, has a distinct capability to closely contact the involved sensory fibers and enables the production of a selective lesion with minimal injury to adjacent noninvolved fibers.
- Testing sensations continuously during lesion making. The first lesion is performed using intravenous sedation at a temperature of 60 °C to 70 °C while the remaining lesions are usually performed with the patient fully awake.
- Asking the patient if facial numbness is tolerable during the procedure.
- Quantitating rather than qualitating numbness by asking the patient to compare the pinprick sensation on the treated side to that of the contralateral side.
- Restricting the final lesion to dense hypalgesia (i.e., pinprick sensation in the treated trigeminal dermatome

is less than one third of the normal side) in the primary affected trigeminal division and the trigger zone, and to mild hypalgesia (i.e., pinprick sensation in the treated trigeminal dermatome is greater than one third of the normal side) in the secondarily affected trigeminal divisions.

Smaller rates of dysesthesia are obtained if lighter sensory lesions in the primary trigeminal divisions are produced but with higher rates of pain recurrence.

With few exceptions, RF rhizotomy is the destructive procedure of choice. The ease by which the procedure can be repeated allows production of sensory lesions that best suit the patient as much as possible in the degree of numbness desired. Compared to glycerol rhizotomy, RF rhizotomy gangliolysis producing mild hypalgesia achieves the same results without the technical difficulties associated with glycerol rhizotomy when cerebrospinal fluid flow is not obtained. Temporary relief associated with mild sensory deprivation may provide a trial period for any apprehensive patient concerned about tolerating the effects. When pain recurs, patients frequently request a more analgesic lesion and occasionally request a duplication of the earlier procedure, noting that 2 or 3 years of relief was appreciated and that increased numbness would be tolerable. Most patients do not express concern about repeating the procedure to control recurrence of tic pain.

Compared to balloon compression, RF rhizotomy achieves longer pain relief without the risks of general anesthesia. One advantage of balloon compression, however, is that it destroys the larger myelinated fibers, relatively sparing small myelinated fibers that innervate the cornea. Therefore, elderly patients with pain around the eye may better be treated by balloon compression.

REFERENCES

1. White JC, Sweet WH. Pain and the Neurosurgeon. Springfield, Ill, Charles C Thomas, 1969.
2. Letcher FS, Goldring S. The effect of radiofrequency current and heat on peripheral nerve action potential in the cat. J Neurosurg 29:42, 1968.
3. Siegfried J. Percutaneous controlled thermocoagulation of gasserian ganglion in trigeminal neuralgia. Experience with 1000 cases. *In* Samii M, Jannetta P (eds). The Cranial Nerves. Berlin, Springer-Verlag, 1981, pp 322–330.
4. Tew JM Jr, Taha JM. Percutaneous rhizotomy in the treatment of intractable facial pain (trigeminal, glossopharyngeal, and vagal nerves). *In* Schmidek HH, Sweet WH (eds). Operative Neurosurgical Techniques. Philadelphia, WB Saunders, 1996, pp 3386–3403.
5. Nugent R. Radiofrequency treatment of trigeminal neuralgia using a cordotomy-type electrode. A method. Neurosurg Clin North Am 8:41–52, 1997.
6. Taha JM, Tew JM. Therapeutic decisions in facial pain. Clin Neurosurg 46:410–431, 2000.
7. Tran Dinh Y, Thurel C, Cunin G, Serrie A, Seylaz J. Cerebral vasodilation after the thermocoagulation of the trigeminal ganglion in humans. Neurosurgery 31:658–663, 1992.
8. Taha JM, Tew JM. Comparison of the surgical treatment of trigeminal neuralagia. Reevaluation of radiofrequency rhizotomy. Neurosurgery 38:865–871, 1996.
9. Taha JM, Tew JM Jr. A prospective 15-year follow up of 154 consecutive patients with trigeminal neuralgia treated by percutaneous stereotactic radiofrequency thermal rhizotomy. J Neurosurg 83:989–993, 1995.

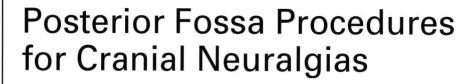

CHAPTER 28

Posterior Fossa Procedures for Cranial Neuralgias

AMIN KASSAM, MD AND MICHAEL HOROWITZ, MD

A number of pain syndromes involving the head and face take their origins from compression or dysfunction of the cranial nerves. These syndromes include trigeminal neuralgia, geniculate neuralgia, and glossopharyngeal neuralgia. The management of these cranial neuropathies through microvascular decompression (MVD) and neural sectioning will form the basis of this chapter.

TRIGEMINAL NEURALGIA

Trigeminal neuralgia (TN) is the term for a pain syndrome involving the face and at times oral cavity. Typical TN can be classified as a unilateral, lancinating, sudden, and intermittent facial pain that can be triggered by touch or facial movements. Patients typically describe a memorable onset of their discomfort and report pain relief/control with anticonvulsant medications such as carbamazepine or phenytoin. TN can be managed in a number of ways including medical therapy with anticonvulsant medications, balloon compression of the trigeminal ganglion, glycerol rhizotomy, radiofrequency rhizotomy, focused stereotactic radiosurgery, and microvascular decompression.

The goal of microvascular decompression is to treat the underlying cause of cranial neuropathy, which is compression of the nerve by arteries or veins from the root entry zone to the exit into Meckel's cave. This procedure is outlined in a stepwise manner below.

Step 1: The patient is placed under general anesthesia with appropriate monitoring of arterial pressure using an indwelling arterial catheter. Always be sure to identify the correct surgical side.

Step 2: Brainstem function and eighth cranial nerve function is monitored using brainstem auditory-evoked potentials (BSAEPs). Bilateral monitoring is conducted so that comparisons between the surgical and nonsurgical side can be made.

Step 3: The patient is placed into the lateral decubitus position with the head secured in a rigid pin type head holder. All pressure points are padded and an axillary roll is used. The patient is secured to the table with tape and the head is positioned laterally with the chin slightly tucked leaving two fingerbreadths between the chin and chest.

Step 4: The retromastoid region is shaved and cleaned.

Step 5: A straight or slightly curved 5- to 6-cm incision is made just behind the hairline.

Step 6: Using a monopolar cautery a subperiosteal dissection is carried out so that a window of bone is exposed that includes the mastoid's digastric groove. Self-retaining cerebellar retractors are placed.

Step 7: A half-dollar size craniotomy or craniectomy is fashioned with a drill and Kerrison and Leksell rongeurs. The bone removal is carried out until the inferior lateral edge of the transverse sinus and the medial edge of the sigmoid sinus are exposed. Overall, a region of dura 5 × 3 cm is uncovered.

Step 8: All mastoid air cells are waxed to avoid latent cerebrospinal fluid leaks.

Step 9: The dura is opened in a curvilinear fashion and reflected laterally using 4–0 suture. It is important to make the lateral bone removal along the sigmoid sinus as straight as possible so that when the dura is reflected laterally it can be retracted flush with the bone so that maximal lateral exposure of the cerebellum is possible. This will reduce the need for excessive cerebellar retraction.

Step 10: It is important at this point to obtain cerebellar relaxation. If a spinal drain was inserted at the start of the operation, it can be opened. If a drain was not used then either the 11th or 5th cranial nerve cisterns can be opened. It is often advantageous and safer to open the 11th cranial nerve cistern first because it is easier to access and there are fewer venous bridging veins in this area. In any event, opening of the cistern permits for cerebellar relaxation and visualization of the fifth nerve. In some cases, especially in young patients, the posterior fossa can be quite full despite mild hyperventilation and preoperative mannitol infusion. In these cases wide opening of the dura will often lead to cerebellar herniation from the wound and tissue injury. In such instances we often first open only a small caudal window of dura and then open the 11th cranial nerve cistern to obtain cerebellar relaxation before widely opening and retracting the dura. In the event of cerebellar herniaton it is important to keep the cerebellum in the head and below the dural edges so that the tissue is not strangulated. In these situations gentle counter pressure with cotton paddies will often keep the cerebellar herniation under control and permit the surgeon to minimize cerebellar trauma while he or she identifies the cisterns. Often, when the posterior fossa is tight, simple retraction on the cerebellar tonsil and movement toward the 11th cistern will lead to arachnoid disruption and spontaneous egress of spinal fluid.

Step 11: Once the cerebellum is relaxed, the surgeon can focus the microscope on the rostral aspect of the exposure and identify the junction between the tentorium cerebelli and the petrous bone. At times, sudden venous bleeding will occur when beginning to retract the corner of the cerebellum. This is generally a consequence of a torn bridging vein running from the tentorial surface of the cerebellum to the tentorium. Such bleeding can be quickly controlled with cotton tamponade and bipolar coagulation. Gentle retraction on the cerebellum will allow for visualization of the trigeminal cistern. Once opened, the petrosal venous complex (Dandy's veins) often comes into view. In most cases this complex or a portion of it needs to be cauterized and divided to allow for access to the underlying trigeminal nerve. Care should be taken when dividing these veins because they can easily be avulsed from the dural entry site or be incompletely cauterized before sectioning, thus leading to contamination of the subarachnoid space with venous blood.

Step 12: At this point the trigeminal nerve's motor and sensory components are visualized. To see the full extent of the nerve and its entry into the pons, the cerebellar ala must be sharply dissected free of the nerve. All arachnoid should be divided so that the nerve in its entirety is visualized from pons to Meckel's cave entry site. Arachnoid that is adherent to the eighth cranial nerve should also be sharply divided so that cerebellar retraction does not transmit stretch forces on the auditory nerve. These forces will be detected by increases in BSAEP wave latencies and decreases in wave amplitude. Often, if a bony protuberance makes distal visualization difficult, a 30- or 45-degree endoscope or microsurgical mirror can be used to view the distal portion of the nerve. We find the endoscope to be useful for both visualization and surgical manipulation of hidden vessels, thus minimizing our need for cerebellar or nerve manipulation.

Step 13: At this point the surgeon should look for arteries and veins that may be compressing the TN. The superior cerebellar artery (SCA) is the most common arterial culprit. Once arising from the basilar trunk it wanders along the inferior tentorial surface, but may be quite ectatic in its course. When decompressing the TN the surgeon must account for both the rostral and caudal SCA divisions because decompression of one and not the other can be a cause for procedure failure. The SCA is gently dissected free of the TN and its surrounding arachnoid bands and separated from the TN using Teflon padding that is rolled into different cigar-shaped sizes by the nurse. If Teflon is not available, another inert substance can be substituted. It is important to decompress the entire nerve from the SCA and be sure that in the process of doing so the vessel and its perforant branches are not permanently kinked so as to induce a stroke. It is also important to avoid manipulation of the fourth cranial nerve during the SCA manipulations to minimize the risks of postoperative diplopia.

Once the SCA has been dealt with the surgeon should look for other vascular compressions from smaller arteries and veins. We make a point of moving all arteries, even small arterioles, from the nerve and padding them. Veins are also treated. In the past we simply coagulated and divided these structures; however, we came to realize that recurrent TN often developed as a result of other veins dilating in response to previous venous interruption. For that reason, we have begun to decompress veins whenever possible using Teflon felt. Such decompression is technically more difficult than arterial decompression because the veins tend to be more closely adherent to the nerve. Nevertheless, using sharp microsurgical technique most veins can be atraumatically separated from the nerve. Those veins that cannot be surgically elevated from the nerve surface are divided without coagulation (unless they are large). Hemostasis is easily achieved with gentle tamponade using Teflon felt. By limiting our use of coagulation, we think we are able to minimize the risks of postoperative hypesthesia. If coagulation must be done near the nerve, the nerve is first covered with felt to insulate it from the bipolar current.

On occasion the basilar artery can compress the TN. This ectatic vessel can be difficult to decompress because of its size and turgor. Nevertheless, it can generally be achieved with persistence and care. Often its movement requires additional work more caudally so that the course of the vessel can be deflected.

While microvascular decompression has focused on the importance of compression at the root entry zone, its is known that the junction between central and peripheral myelin (the region of susceptibility) is variable. We have seen symptomatic compression all along the length of the TN and for that reason we are quite radical in our degree of decompression. At the conclusion of the case the nerve is essentially completely encased in felt rostrally, caudally, dorsally, and ventrally. Using this technique we have significantly reduced our recurrences and failures (Figs. 28-1 and 28-2).

Step14: The dura is closed in a watertight fashion. Muscle patches may be necessary to completely close the defect.

Step 15: The air cells are again waxed.

Step 16: A perforated titanium mesh is placed over the defect and secured with screws.

Step 17: The muscle, fascia, subcutaneous tissue, and skin are closed sequentially.

Step 18: The patient is extubated and transferred to the recovery room.

Special Notes and Considerations

1. We do not cut the trigeminal nerve as a part of our treatment because we have obtained excellent results with atraumatic decompression alone. We think that nerve sectioning leads to increased incidence of numbness and

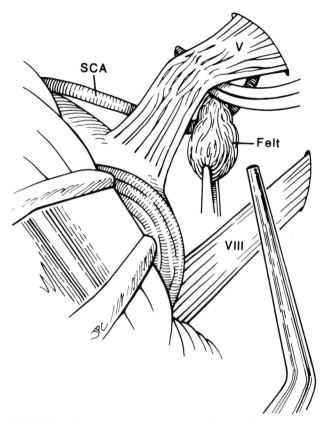

FIGURE 28-1 Sketch showing the right cranial nerve V being decompressed from the right superior cerebellar artery.

risk for anesthesia dolorosa. We have found that sectioning the nerve or a portion of it for atypical TN may result in temporary pain relief only with recurrence of symptoms within 6 to 12 months.

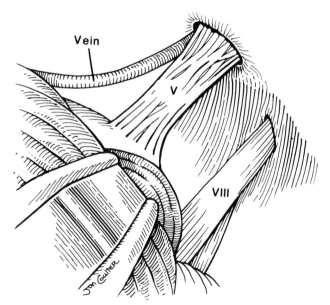

FIGURE 28-2 Sketch showing a vein compressing cranial nerve V as it exits toward Meckel's cave.

2. We treat atypical TN with MVD in those patients who have both typical and atypical components (transitional TN) and in those patients who respond partially to anticonvulsant therapy. Atypical pain is often the result of venous pathology located distal to the root entry zone and is often seen with motor root compression.

3. In our experience, the complication rate for MVD in TN is less than 5%. These include hematoma (0.1%), significant edema (0.4%), infarction (0.1%), hydrocephalus (0.1%), seventh cranial nerve paralysis (1.7%), eighth cranial nerve injury (1.4%), other cranial nerve palsy (4.6%), cerebrospinal fluid leak (1.6%), meningitis (0.2%), and death (0.2%).

4. Bradycardia or asystole is a common occurrence during fifth cranial nerve manipulation. Heart rate will generally recover when the manipulation stops. Use of thoracic Doppler can alert the surgeon to changes in heart rate during the dissection and decompression.

5. Our results with typical TN in over 2000 patients reveal complete immediate pain relief in 84% and partial relief (greater than 60% reduction in pain) in 13%. At 5 years, complete relief is maintained in approximately 75% of patients and partial relief in another 8% to 10%.

6. Our results with atypical TN in 672 cases reveal complete immediate pain relief in 45% to 55% and partial relief in 30% to 40%. At 5 years, complete relief is maintained in 35% to 45% and partial relief in another 10% to 15% of patients.

GENICULATE NEURALGIA

Geniculate neuralgia (Hunt's neuralgia) is a syndrome involving paroxysmal, lancinating deep ear pain that is often described by patients as a feeling of an ice pick in the ear. Occasionally the pain can also involve the auricle, eye, cheek, and deep nasal region. Cutaneous triggers can exist around the ear. Other triggers include swallowing, loud noise, and cold temperatures. Geniculate neuralgia (GeN) can be cryptogenic, although herpetic ganglionitis (Ramsay Hunt syndrome) must always be considered.

The surgical management of GeN centers around the innervation of the deep ear. General sensation from the external acoustic meatus and the external surface of the tympanic membrane is conducted along the auriculotemporal branch of cranial nerve V3. The inferior portion of the membrane and the meatus is innervated by the auricular branch of the 10th cranial nerve and by a branch of the facial nerve called the nervus intermedius (NI). This latter structure, located between the seventh and eighth cranial nerves, also carries sensation from the skin of the concha of the auricle, a small area of skin behind the ear and the wall of the acoustic meatus. General sensation from the internal surface of the eardrum is carried by the tympanic plexus of the ninth cranial nerve.

Surgical management of GeN involves MVD of cranial nerves V, IX, and X and sectioning of the NI. After completing the MVD of the fifth cranial nerve as described previously and MVD of cranial nerves IX and X as described subsequently, sectioning of the NI is carried out.

The NI is located between the eighth and seventh cranial nerves. It may consist of a single or more commonly as multiple filaments. From the retromastoid approach these filaments are generally not visible even with extreme microscopic angulation because of the overlying auditory and vestibular structures. Occasionally, however, they can be readily visualized and manipulated.

Manipulation, isolation, and sectioning of the NI can be achieved in a number of ways, some of which are more successful than others in individual cases. One method of isolating the nerve(s) is to blindly pass a micro-hook beneath cranial nerve VIII and slowly rotate it in an attempt to secure the NI. Once secured and pulled out from between cranial nerves VIII and VII, the filament(s) can be cut with a micro-scissors. Often the surgeon must blindly sweep from both the rostral and caudal side of cranial nerve VIII to deliver the fascicle(s). If this technique does not work, then an attempt can be made to visualize the space between cranial nerves VIII and VII using a micro-mirror. While this device is useful in some cases, it often provides poor visualization and proves less than desirable. We have stopped using the mirror and have begun to use the 30- and 45-degree endoscope to identify the NI when it cannot be delivered using the hook technique alone. The endoscope provides perfect visualization of the underside of cranial nerve VIII and the top side of cranial nerve VII, making identification and sectioning of NI simple and safe. The surgeon can perform this procedure alone by holding the endoscope in one hand and hook in the other. Once the NI is secured the endoscope is put down and the NI is cut using the microscope and scissors. Alternatively, if an endoscope holder or assistant is available the nerve can be identified, secured, and cut using the endoscopic image alone (Fig. 28-3).

Special Notes and Considerations

We perform GeN cases using neurophysiologic monitoring that includes BSAEPs, and cranial nerve VII, IX, and X electromyographs (EMGs), and are always prepared to do facial nerve stimulation in the advent that we are unsure whether or not we have isolated the NI or a portion of motor cranial nerve VII. Because EMG is being used, the patient cannot be paralyzed while under general anesthesia.

GLOSSOPHARYNGEAL NEURALGIA

Glossopharyngeal neuralgia (GPN) is a syndrome that presents with severe, lancinating, deep throat pain that is triggered by swallowing. GPN can result in significant morbidity due to inanition. Medical management has not been effective. Surgical therapy includes sectioning of the fascicles of cranial nerves IX and upper fascicles of X or MVD of the fascicles of cranial nerve IX and the upper fascicles of cranial nerve X. The latter procedure is discussed below.

The initial portion of the surgical procedure for treatment of GPN is discussed in steps 1 to 10 under TN. Once the exposure has been completed, the remainder of the steps are as follows:

> Step 11: The arachnoid over cranial nerves XI, X, and IX is opened sharply and these cranial nerves are sharply released from the cerebellum.
>
> Step 12: The flocculus is separated using sharp dissection from the 9th and 10th nerves and the nerves are dissected back until their origin from the brainstem can be clearly visualized. The choroid plexus and the foramen of Luschka should be clearly exposed.
>
> Step 13: Inspection of the fascicles of cranial nerves IX and X near the brainstem will reveal compressing vessels. These may consist of a large posterior inferior cerebellar artery (PICA), medullary branches from the PICA, or an ectatic vertebral artery (VA). Veins may also be found impinging upon the nerve fascicles. Decompression at the brainstem nerve junction is carried out using Teflon felt. Veins that can be decompressed are padded while those that cannot are either divided and tamponaded or cauterized and cut.
>
> Step 14: If a large PICA or VA cannot be adequately displaced where it impinges upon cranial nerve IX and X, it may be useful to first move the VA away from the medulla where it lies medial to cranial nerve XI. This more caudal deflection with felt can make it easier to deliver, manipulate, and move the more rostral vessel(s). Once again, the surgeon must be aware of avoiding permanent kinks in the diplaced vessels so as to avoid ischemic brainstem or cerebellar strokes (Figs. 28-4 and 28-5).
>
> Step 15: Closure is identical to that for TN and GeN.

Special Notes and Considerations:

1. All patients undergo cranial nerve IX and X EMG monitoring during these cases along with BSAEPs. Therefore, paralysis cannot be used as part of the anesthetic technique.
2. BSAEP changes during these cases are more commonly due to transmitted pressure to the cochlear nucleus rather than traction on the extramedullary portion of cranial nerve VIII. Nevertheless, removing the arachnoid bands that connect the cerebellum to cranial nerve VIII

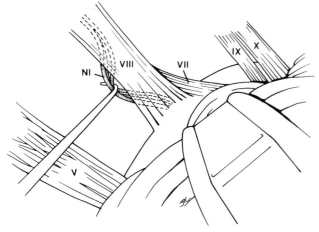

FIGURE 28-3 Sketch showing fascicles of the nervus intermedius being dissected and exposed so that they can be cut. These fascicles are located between cranial nerves VIII and VII.

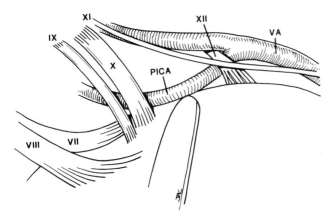

FIGURE 28-4 Sketch showing a posterior inferior cerebellar artery compressing cranial nerves IX and X near the root entry zones. Usually the fascicles of cranial nerve IX and the first one or two fascicles of cranial nerve X are compressed at the brainstem level.

can often be effective in improving BSAEP waveforms when they degrade during the case. If this fails to help with BSAEP recording then the retractor needs to be removed or moved so that compression of the cochlear nucleus can be diminished.

3. In a series of 217 cases of GPN treated at University of Pittsburgh Medical Center overall immediate complete pain relief was achieved in 65% of patients while an additional 25% had significant improvement in their symptoms (90% good to excellent results). Long-term complete relief was achieved in 58% of patients while another 18% had significant improvement in their symptoms (76% good to excellent results). Best results were seen in patients who presented with throat pain only. In this subgroup, long-term cure was achieved in greater than 95% of cases.

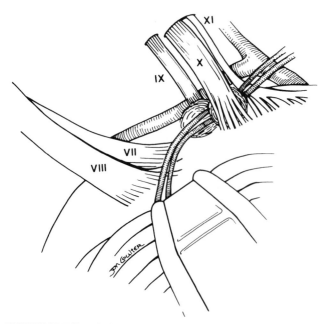

FIGURE 28-5 Sketch showing small arteries compressing fascicles of cranial nerves IX and X at the brainstem level. These vessels have been decompressed with Teflon pledgets.

4. Complications resulting from MVD for GPN occur in fewer than 5% of cases. These include cranial nerves IX and X palsy or paresis (3% to 4% since 1988), other cranial nerve injury (2% to 4% since 1988), and spinal fluid leak (1% to 2% since 1988). Since 1993, we have experienced no intracranial hematomas, brainstem infarctions, or deaths.

GENERAL CONSIDERATIONS AND POINTS TO REMEMBER FOR ALL PROCEDURES DISCUSSED

1. Try to minimize the use of brain retractors.
2. Arachnoid is your enemy.
3. Papaverine placed on cranial nerve VIII can often help it function when all other causes for BSAEP decline can be identified.
4. Be cognizant of reductions in patient blood pressure because this can adversely affect BSAEP recordings.
5. Sinus bleeding can generally be controlled with gentle tamponade and bone wax secured against a bony surface.
6. The nerves should be visualized from brainstem to dural exit sites to be sure no vessels remain in contact. Having said this, the brainstem/nerve junction remains the most critical site in most cases.

CONCLUSION

Pain syndromes related to posterior fossa neuropathies are varied but are based on known pathways of innervation. MVD and occasionally neural sectioning can help alleviate these syndromes in the majority of patients provided they are selected properly.

REFERENCES

Barker FG II, Janetta PJ, Bissonette DJ, et al. The long-term outcome of microvascular decompression for trigeminal neuralgia. N Engl J Med 334:1077–1086, 1996.

Brown JA, Coursaget C, Preul MC, et al. Mercury water and cauterizing stones: Nicolas Andre and tic douloureux. J Neurosurg 90:977–981, 1999.

Burchiel KJ, Slavin KV. On the natural history of trigeminal neuralgia. Neurosurgery 46:152–155, 2000.

Fothergill J. Of a painful affection of the face. *In* Society of Physicians in London: Medical Observations and Inquiries, vol 5. London, T Cadell, 1773, pp 129–142.

Hamlyn PJ, King TT. Neurovascular compression in trigeminal neuralgia: a clinical and anatomical study. J Neurosurg 76:948–954, 1992.

Janetta PJ, Rand RW. Transtentorial retrogasserian rhizotomy in trigeminal neuralgia by microneurosurgical technique. Bull LA Neurol Soc 31:93–99, 1966.

Klun B. Microvascular decompression and partial sensory rhizotomy in the treatment of trigeminal neuralgia: personal experience with 200 patients. Neurosurgery 30:49–52, 1992.

Pollack IF, Janetta PJ, Bissonnette DJ. Bilateral trigeminal neuralgia: a 14-year experience with microvascular decompression. J Neurosurg 68:559–565, 1988.

Schmidt JE. Medical Discoveries. Springfield, Ill, Charles C Thomas, 1959.

Sun T, Saito S, Nakai O, et al. long-term results of microvascular decompression for trigeminal neuralgia with reference to probability of recurrence. Acta Neurochir 126:144–148, 1994.

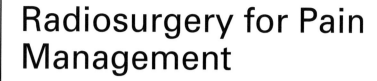

C H A P T E R 2 9

Radiosurgery for Pain Management

RONALD F. YOUNG, MD

In this chapter, the use of stereotactic radiosurgery, for the treatment of chronic pain as well as trigeminal neuralgia, will be reviewed. The early experiences of the pioneers of radiosurgery in the treatment of chronic pain and trigeminal neuralgia will be discussed and subsequently the criteria for patient selection will be described and a description of current radiosurgical techniques will be provided. The results of our recent experience and those of others in treating these two pain disorders will also be described. The treatment of these two conditions is covered in detail throughout this textbook; therefore, this chapter will not discuss the pathophysiology and alternative surgical methods available for the treatment of chronic pain or trigeminal neuralgia, except as they relate directly to radiosurgical management.

HISTORY

Leksell originally described the concept of "radiosurgery" in 1951 and in that paper described "therapeutic destruction of normal brain tissue with a narrow beam, as for example in thalamotomy."[1] It is clear that one of Leksell's main areas of emphasis in developing the concept of radiosurgery, was for the treatment of functional disorders of the brain.[2] In 1963, Larson and colleagues described a radiosurgical method using a proton beam generator, for the treatment of three patients with different types of functional disorders. One of the patients suffered from chronic pain due to a malignancy and a mesencephalic tractotomy was carried out using the proton beam method for treatment of this patient's pain. In 1960, before these early attempts to use radiosurgery to produce destructive lesions in the brain in attempts to treat functional disorders including chronic pain, Leksell and colleagues described the production of lesions in the goat brain by high-energy proton beams.[3] Radiosurgical doses between 200 and 380 Gy produced necrotic lesions surrounded by perivascular hemorrhage in postmortem examinations carried out 1 to 4 months after the procedure. In 1967, Mair and colleagues described a mesencephalic tractotomy created using the radiosurgical method in the midbrain of a 59-year-old man who suffered from intractable pain in the left scapula, arm,

and fingers related to a squamous cell carcinoma of the left lung.[4] This lesion was also made with a proton beam generator and a radiosurgical dose of 200 Gy. The patient was apparently relieved of his pain within 1 month of the treatment, but the pain subsequently recurred and gradually increased in severity until the patient's death 2 months following the treatment. Autopsy in this patient showed a lesion approximately 7 mm in diameter, appropriately located and demonstrating central necrosis and perivascular hemorrhages, virtually identical to those that had been previously described in the goat brain experiments.

In 1968, Leksell reported two patients with intractable pain who had been treated with a medial thalamotomy using the prototype gamma unit to treat pain related to a metastatic cancer of the bladder in one patient and metastatic carcinoma of the rectum in another patient.[5] In the first patient, there was significant improvement in the patient's pain, but he unfortunately died 10 weeks after the operation. In the second patient, staged bilateral thalamotomy was carried out in the centre' median nuclei 2 months apart. Radiosurgical doses of 200 and 250 Gy were used. Approximately 2 months after the second procedure, there was a slow improvement in the patient's pain and a marked decrease in analgesic medication usage. This patient died 20 weeks after the first procedure. Autopsy in both patients showed lesions virtually identical to those described in the previous experimental situations with central necrosis and surrounding perivascular changes. The target points for the lesions in both of these patients were located using pneumoencephalography. In 1970, Andersson and colleagues reported on the histopathology of lesions made in the goat brain with autopsies performed as late as 1453 days after the initial radiosurgical lesions were made.[6] The early lesions showed histologic changes similar to those previously described, but the later lesions showed small areas of glial scar consisting of astrocytic fibers and some macrophages. There was a fairly abrupt transition between these areas and the surrounding areas, which were essentially normal, with preserved neurons and normal myelinated nerve fibers. The vessels surrounding the lesions showed no evidence of any histologic changes with follow-up as long as 48 months. Kjellberg and colleagues described similar lesions created using the proton beam generator and the Bragg peak effect.[7] The first large series of patients treated using radiosurgical thalamotomy was reported by Forster and then by Steiner and colleagues.[8,9] A total of 52 patients with intractable pain due to cancer underwent medial thalamotomy using the cobalt-60 gamma unit at the Karolinska Institute in Stockholm, Sweden. Of the 52 patients described by Steiner and colleagues, 8 experienced good pain relief, 18 had moderate relief, and in 24 the operation did not significantly reduce the pain.[9] In two patients, the effect of the treatment was not reported. A second procedure when pain recurred after an initial thalamotomy was reported to be rarely of any value. Steiner and colleagues indicated that the procedures were more effective for the treatment of pain located in the face or the arm or shoulder, rather than pain in the lower body. Contralateral lesions seemed to be most effective, but ipsilateral lesions were described as also possibly providing some relief. The best results were obtained when the lesions were placed posteriorly in the thalamus, close to the wall of the third ventricle just anterior to the posterior commissure. Steiner and colleagues concluded that medial thalamotomy using the gamma knife could be tried as a last resort in the treatment of cancer pain in patients with a short life expectancy.[9]

In 1983, Leksell described 83 patients treated for intractable pain using the gamma knife.[10] No accounting of the outcomes in these patients was ever provided, although it is assumed that the 52 patients described by Steiner and colleagues were included in these latter 83 described by Leksell. In addition, there is no description as to whether any of the 83 patients were treated for non–cancer-related pain. Before our efforts, beginning in 1992, to use gamma knife thalamotomy to treat chronic pain, we are unaware of any other significant experience using radiosurgical methods to treat chronic pain of noncancer origin.[11–13]

PATIENT SELECTION

The selection of patients for gamma knife thalamotomy is identical to that which would be appropriate for patient selection for any type of ablative surgical intervention to treat chronic pain. Briefly, these procedures are reserved for situations in which other less invasive treatments have failed. A variety of other treatment methods may be explored prior to considering thalamotomy to treat chronic pain. These would include pharmacologic methods, physical therapy, psychological intervention, nerve blocks, and stimulation procedures, such as spinal cord stimulation or chronic spinal opiate infusion. Management in a multidisciplinary chronic pain treatment program before considering ablative surgical procedures is also desirable.

Despite the indications from the early reports of Steiner that a unilateral thalamotomy may be useful to treat bilateral pain, it has been our observation that thalamotomy is generally effective only for contralateral pain. Bilateral thalamotomy with the gamma knife is not safe because the location of the two isocenters is so close that dose interaction occurs raising the risk of radiation necrosis with serious permanent neurologic side effects. On the other hand, medial thalamotomy is useful for the treatment of both nociceptive and neuropathic

pain or for combinations of the two types of pain. The procedure is considerably more effective for nociceptive pain than for neuropathic pain. Patients with combinations of the two types of pain fall in between in terms of the effectiveness of the procedure.

RADIOSURGICAL TECHNIQUE

Our initial attempts to perform medial thalamotomy to treat chronic pain had as their intent the development of a lesion identical in size and location to that created using the radiofrequency technique.[11–14] In addition, the original radiosurgical thalamotomies made by Leksell and colleagues used a slotted or oval collimator helmet, which resulted in cylindrical lesions. Since the modern gamma knife used spherical isocenters, it was necessary to design a treatment plan that combined two or more spherical isocenters to create an oval lesion (Fig. 29-1). This technique has been previously published.[12] As a result of complications that occurred with the multi-isocenter technique, we then modified the technique to use only a single isocenter, which resulted in a smaller spherical lesion (Fig. 29-2).[15–19] While considerably safer than the multi-isocenter lesion, the single isocenter lesion has proven to be less effective in terms of pain treatment. The most common radiosurgical technique we have used is a single isocenter using the 4-mm secondary collimator helmet and maximum radiosurgical doses between 120 and 140 Gy. The stereotactic coordinates for the isocenter are determined from magnetic resonance images (MRIs) obtained in the axial and coronal planes. The intent is to place the lesion in the lateral portion of the mediodorsal nucleus, including the intralaminar nuclei and portions of the centre' median and parafascicular nuclei. In an average-sized brain with an intercommissural distance of approximately 26 mm and a normal-sized third ventricle, the stereotactic coordinates are in the "X" or mediolateral plane, 7 to 9 mm lateral to the midline of the third ventricle, 4 to 6 mm anterior to the posterior commissure in

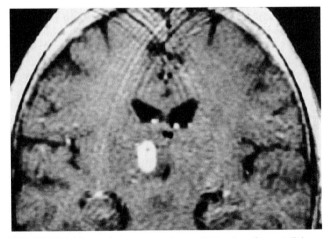

FIGURE 29-1 Magnetic resonance image 6 months after medial thalamotomy with the gamma knife using two adjacent isocenters. See text for details.

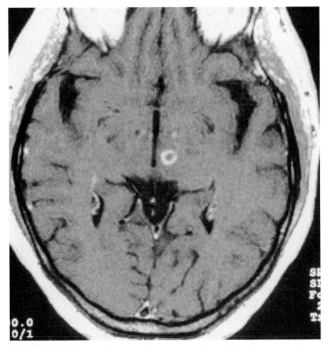

FIGURE 29-2 Magnetic resonance image 6 months after medial thalamotomy with the gamma knife using a single isocenter. See text for details.

the "Y" or anterior-posterior axis, and 3 to 4.5 mm superior to the intercommissural plane in the "Z" or vertical axis.

More recently, we have used a technique that involves two superimposed isocenters, one with the 4-mm collimator helmet and one with the 8-mm collimator helmet. The isocenters are weighted by altering the exposure times of the two isocenters so that the relative exposure of the 8- and 4-mm collimators is 0.5 to 1. This results in a calculated lesion volume at the 50% isodose line of approximately 180 mm³. This is considerably larger than the lesions made with a single 4-mm collimator (approximately 90 mm³), but is smaller than the double or triple isocenter lesions used previously.

RESULTS

Approximately 4 weeks after the radiosurgical procedure, MRIs demonstrate an area of decreased attenuation at the lesioning site.[15–19] At this time, the lesions do not enhance with intravenous gadolinium and patients do not normally notice any alteration in their pain. Over the next 2 to 4 months, the lesions become more distinct and begin to enhance rather intensely with gadolinium. The lesions measure approximately 6 to 8 mm in diameter when made with a single exposure using the 4-mm collimator helmet and contain a small central zone a few millimeters in diameter that does not enhance with intravenous contrast material and is surrounded by an area of low signal attenuation (see Fig. 29–2). The peripheral rim of the lesion enhances rather intensely. During this interval, which is 2 to 4 months after the procedure, patients begin to notice a gradual reduction in pain.

Over the ensuing 6 to 9 months, the lesions generally remain stable and then gradually begin to decrease in size in most patients. By 2 to 3 years following the radiosurgical procedure, the lesions usually do not enhance with contrast, although sometimes persistent contrast enhancement is seen as long as 3 to 5 years subsequent to the procedure. Using the single isocenter technique, unexpectedly large lesions are uncommon, but may rarely occur. In this situation, the lesions continue to enlarge over a period that may last as long as 9 to 36 months, reaching a maximum diameter as large as 15 mm. With the earlier technique, which used two or three adjacent isocenters, extremely large lesions, measuring as much as 3 to 5 cm in diameter were seen in as many as 25% of the patients and were often accompanied by significant neurologic deficits that in some cases were permanent. These deficits included contralateral sensory loss, paralysis, uncoordination, dysphasia, and balance difficulties. With the single isocenter technique, we have seen only one patient in whom a relatively mild permanent contralateral balance problem developed that was related to a lesion larger than expected.

Our experience now includes a total of 74 medial thalamic lesions performed in 71 patients for the treatment of a variety of pain complaints. In patients with nociceptive pain, usually due to unsuccessful spinal operations related to intervertebral disk disease, spinal stenosis, and so on, excellent or good pain relief was achieved in 86%. In those suffering from neuropathic pain related to conditions such as the thalamic syndrome, anesthesia dolorosa of the face, postherpetic neuralgia, and peripheral nerve injury, among others, excellent or good relief was achieved in only 45% of patients. In patients who suffered a combination of nociceptive and neuropathic pain, for instance, low back pain of a nociceptive nature and leg pain related to chronic radiculopathy, excellent or good pain relief was achieved in 60%. In patients who were treated with the older two- or three-isocenter technique, regardless of the type of pain they were treated for, excellent or good relief was achieved in 62.5% overall; whereas in patients who underwent medial thalamotomy using the single isocenter technique, excellent or good relief was achieved in only 44.1%. While these values are not statistically significantly different, based on the relatively small number of patients in each group, they do suggest that the single isocenter technique may be less effective and that is what led us to use the more recent double superimposed isocenter method. Currently, the follow-up with the latter method is too short and the number of patients too small to give an accurate assessment of the safety and effectiveness of this approach. The mean follow-up in our patient group is 42.6 months and a total of 2453 patient months of follow-up are encompassed in our overall experience.

From the standpoint of complications, in patients who were treated with the single isocenter technique using the 4-mm collimator helmet, only one (2.9%) experienced any permanent complication and another (2.9%) experienced temporary complications which eventually resolved completely. In patients who underwent the double isocenter thalamotomy technique, 4.2% experienced temporary complications and 21% experienced permanent complications. There was also one death due to radiation necrosis of the brainstem in a patient who underwent bilateral thalamotomy with a 3-month interval between the procedures.

CONCLUSIONS

Medial thalamic lesions may be made safely in the human brain using a single exposure with the 4-mm collimator and the Leksell gamma unit with maximum radiosurgical doses of 120 to 140 Gy. While there has been considerable discussion in the literature regarding the accuracy of lesion placement using only image guidance without electrophysiologic corroboration of the target, in no patient, in our experience, has a complication resulted from misplacement of a radiosurgical thalamic lesion. In fact, the maximum deviation in any coordinate direction with these lesions is 1.5 mm, and the usual deviation is 0.5 mm or less. All complications that we have experienced have been due to lesions that developed larger than expected, rather than to misplacement. With the single isocenter technique, lesions larger than expected occur approximately 5% of the time and permanent complications occur in only 2.9% of patients. The success rate for relieving chronic pain with gamma knife thalamotomy is approximately equal to that using the radiofrequency medial thalamic lesioning method, whether or not guided by electrophysiologic control. Medial thalamotomy with the gamma knife is an excellent method to treat chronic pain in patients who are not suitable candidates for open stereotactic procedures, such as those who take anticoagulants chronically, but the procedure is also attractive to many patients because of its noninvasive nature. My experience with radiofrequency thalamotomy for the treatment of chronic pain suggests that the complication rate of gamma thalamotomy using the single isocenter method is significantly lower.

TRIGEMINAL NEURALGIA

History

It appears that trigeminal neuralgia may have been the first entity treated with Leksell's original prototype version of a radio-surgical instrument.[20] This unit consisted of an orthovoltage x-ray tube attached to the arc of Leksell's standard stereotactic frame. The beam was collimated by a circular diaphragm in one patient to 6 mm and the other to 10 mm to treat trigeminal neuralgia. These treatments were described by Leksell in 1971, more than 18 years after the original treatments.[20] The original treatments were performed in April and June 1953 and both patients were described as free of trigeminal neuralgia at the time of their last follow-up.

Neither patient had experienced any facial numbness or loss of facial function or sensation. By 1983, Leksell reported that he had treated 63 patients with trigeminal neuralgia using the early versions of the gamma knife, but no description of either the results or the technique was provided.[10] In 1993, Alexander and Lindquist reported that 46 patients had been treated with the original gamma knife using a combination of bony landmarks and cisternography with the treatment target directed at the trigeminal ganglion.[21] Only 18% of these patients were pain free by 30 months after the treatment. Alexander and Lindquist also described more recent attempts to treat trigeminal neuralgia using the modern version of the gamma knife directed at the trigeminal sensory root adjacent to its entry into the pons using a 4-mm collimator and a radiosurgical dose maximum of 70 Gy. A total of 10 patients were treated and of those observed more than 6 months, all were described as having good pain control. One patient developed an increase in preexisting facial numbness and no other changes in facial sensation were described. In 1993, Rand and colleagues from Good Samaritan Hospital in Los Angeles, California, described gamma knife treatment of trigeminal neuralgia in a small series of patients in whom the treatment was directed at the trigeminal ganglion and the trigeminal nerve root in various combinations.[22] The results with treatments directed at the ganglion were disappointing, but the authors suggested that treating the trigeminal nerve root would be more effective. Based on this early experience, we used a consistent technique in the treatment of more than 400 patients with trigeminal neuralgia.

Patient Selection

Surgical treatment of trigeminal neuralgia is usually reserved for patients who fail extended attempts at pharmacologic treatment. Carbamazepine (Tegretol®) is the most effective pharmacologic agent for the treatment of trigeminal neuralgia. Successful treatment of facial pain with carbamazepine is an additional diagnostic feature that confirms the diagnosis of trigeminal neuralgia. Side effects, including allergic reactions, may necessitate the utilization of other drugs such as Neurontin®, Dilantin®, baclofen, mexiletine, or Lamictal®. These latter are generally not as successful as carbamazepine, but are sometimes effective. Because radiosurgical treatment with the gamma knife is equally effective to results with other forms of surgical intervention and because the only side effect of the procedure is the development of some degree of facial numbness on a delayed basis after the treatment in about 15% of patients, we thought that it may be more appropriate to treat patients early with the gamma knife, rather than requiring a prolonged period of pharmacologic treatment. Because all of the surgical methods to treat trigeminal neuralgia, including the gamma knife, are most successful in patients who exhibit the classical symptoms of trigeminal neuralgia, it is very important to establish the diagnosis clearly before any form of surgical intervention is undertaken. Unfortunately, there are no diagnostic imaging studies or laboratory studies that confirm the diagnosis. The diagnosis is made based on the typical clinical complaint of brief, severe, knifelike or electric shock–like pains limited to one or more of the major trigeminal divisions virtually always on one side of the face. Trigger zones from which innocuous mechanical stimuli, such as brushing the teeth, touching the lips, speaking, and chewing elicit the typical pain are characteristic as well. Trigeminal neuralgia is most common in patients in their fifties or sixties and increases in frequency into the seventies, eighties, and nineties. The disease may occasionally be seen in patients in their thirties or forties and rarely patients in their twenties or in the teenage period. The above features, coupled with a prompt and significant reduction in pain with pharmacologic treatment, confirm the diagnosis.

In addition to the classical presentation, there are a number of atypical presentations of trigeminal neuralgia. The most common atypical features are a constant background aching or pressure sensation or the absence of trigger zones. These latter two features place the trigeminal neuralgia in the category of atypical trigeminal neuralgia. In such patients, all forms of treatment, be they pharmacologic or surgical, are less successful. Some patients present with even more atypical symptoms, which include constant aching, pressing, or throbbing pain through the entire face, often extending beyond the trigeminal distribution into the occipital region or into the cervical area or across the midline. The pain usually is unresponsive to any form of pharmacologic treatment and many patients with these complaints have suffered from the pain for many years without effective treatment. Psychological profiles in such patients often include hypochondriasis, hysteria, somatization, and depression, among others. The latter group of patients, those with atypical facial pain, generally fares poorly with any form of surgical treatment, including radiosurgery.

The only significant features of trigeminal neuralgia that correlate with the success of radiosurgical treatment are the presence of the classical symptoms.[23] The more the symptoms deviate from the classical pattern described previously, the less successful will radiosurgical treatment be. Patients who have had unsuccessful treatment of classical trigeminal neuralgia by surgical methods, be that an initial failure or a recurrence after initial successful treatment, respond as well to radiosurgical treatment with the gamma knife, as do those who have never had a surgical intervention.

It has been our feeling that early surgical treatment of trigeminal neuralgia is probably more effective than delayed treatment.[23–26] Once the diagnosis has been established by the classical symptoms described previously and the response to appropriate pharmacologic agents, we recommend surgical treatment. It is our belief that radiosurgical treatment represents the best combination of safety and effectiveness of any of the available surgical procedures, and a comparison of the alternate surgical methods will be described subsequently. In the past, surgical treatment has been frequently delayed because of the concern about complications associated with these methods. Because the only complications of radiosurgical treatments so far described have been delayed alteration in facial sensation in approximately 10% to 15% of patients, we believe that there is no reason to delay radiosurgical treatment once the diagnosis has been clearly established. Many patients find that carbamazepine and the alternate pharmacologic treatments result in significant side effects, including lethargy, confusion, loss of short-term memory, and balance difficulties, which lead to impairment of the quality of life, and in many patients, the inability to function at all in activities of daily living or in an employment situation. These side effects as well as occasional other complications, which include allergic reactions, and alterations in liver and bone marrow function, among others, can be avoided by early successful radiosurgical treatment.

Radiosurgical Technique

Our approach has been directed exclusively at the trigeminal sensory root adjacent to the pons, as described earlier by Alexander and colleagues[21] and Kondziolka and colleagues.[27] The rationale for this target is that the putative cause of trigeminal neuralgia, namely vascular cross compression, occurs at this site.[24,28] Previous and more recent histologic studies, including electron microscopy, have demonstrated segmental demyelination at this location. It is presumably this segmental demyelination that results in ectopic signal generation, and as a consequence, the spontaneous and triggered pain of trigeminal neuralgia. Thus, it seems most logical to treat at this site, the site of the pathology of

the illness, rather than at some more distal site, such as the trigeminal ganglion, which was previously tried relatively unsuccessfully. We identified the trigeminal sensory root on axial, coronal, and reconstructed stereotactic MRIs, obtained with the Leksell model "G" stereotactic frame in place. The images were transferred by fiberoptic link to the gamma plan, computer dose planning system for the Leksell gamma unit. We used exclusively the 4-mm secondary collimator helmet of the gamma unit and simulated the treatment by placing the isocenter directly over the trigeminal posterior root so that the 50% isodose line is tangential to the surface of the pons (Figs. 29-3 and 29-4).[29] Despite prior concerns, our own and other recent studies have demonstrated that stereotactic MRI is sufficiently precise to allow for functional targeting.[16] This is particularly important in the treatment of trigeminal neuralgia where the target is extremely small and targeting errors of a few millimeters will lead to mistargeting and thus an insufficient radiosurgical dose being delivered to the trigeminal nerve root with corresponding poor results. There has been some evolution in the maximum radiosurgical dose recommended for treatment of trigeminal neuralgia. Based on our initial experience and that of others, a maximum radiosurgical dose of 76 Gy was initially used. In an attempt to increase the success rate, we gradually increased our radiosurgical dose maximum of 87 Gy and then to 98 Gy. Observation of patients treated at 98 Gy reveal that while there was a small increase in the success rate, there was a correspondingly much larger increase in the incidence of delayed facial numbness, and therefore we have recently used 87 Gy as our usual maximum radiosurgical dose. The treatment is accomplished under local anesthesia with minimum intravenous sedation normally used only for application of the stereotactic frame. The remainder of the procedure can usually be carried out without further sedation. Upon completion of the procedure, the stereotactic frame is removed and patients are subsequently observed. In some centers patients are discharged on the same day as the procedure, and in others, they are observed overnight

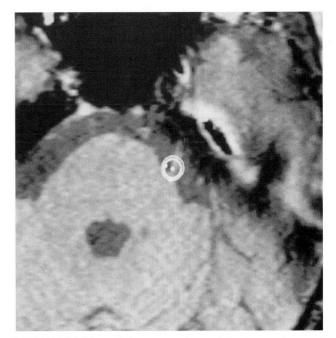

FIGURE 29-3 Axial magnetic resonance image demonstrates placement of the isocenter for gamma knife treatment of trigeminal neuralgia.

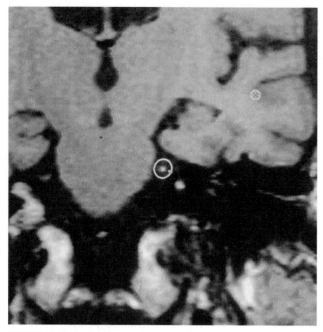

FIGURE 29-4 Coronal magnetic resonance image demonstrates placement of the isocenter for gamma knife treatment of trigeminal neuralgia.

and discharged the following morning. Because of the noninvasive nature of the procedure, immediate return to normal activities is possible. DeSalles recently described treatment of trigeminal neuralgia with a radiosurgical method using the linear accelerator.[30] Targeting was similar to that which we have described in this chapter. DeSalles used a 5-mm collimator and a radiosurgical maximum dose of 70 to 80 Gy. Results were variable in these patients who had both primary and secondary (caused by tumors) forms of trigeminal neuralgia. Overall, DeSalles described that 70% of patients were benefited from the treatment.

Patients in whom initial radiosurgical treatment fails, or in whom recurrent pain develops after an initial successful radiosurgical treatment, have recently been considered for retreatment with the gamma knife. Our experience with retreatment is limited to approximately 35 patients. In these cases, we have used the same general method of targeting and placement of the isocenter, except that we have reduced the maximum radiosurgical dose of the second treatment so that when added to the dose of the first treatment, the combined dosage for both treatments does not exceed 130 to 140 Gy. Approximately 435 treatments have been administered for trigeminal neuralgia with the gamma knife by our groups between 1991 and 1999.

Results

Successful relief of pain following radiosurgical treatment of classical trigeminal neuralgia has been achieved in slightly more than 90% of patients.[23–30,31] This is divided into approximately 60% of patients who achieve complete relief of pain and are able to discontinue all medications and approximately 30% of patients who have reductions in pain to the extent that they can be managed on a small, tolerable dose of medication without side effects. Pain relief after radiosurgical treatment of trigeminal neuralgia rarely occurs immediately. Approxi-

mately 10% to 15% of patients will achieve immediate relief of pain, but more usually, there is a latency period varying from a few days to as long as 6 months and averaging 2 to 4 months before the pain gradually subsides. Recurrent pain after initial successful treatment reduces the long-term success rate to approximately 77% for classical trigeminal neuralgia. For patients who exhibit atypical trigeminal neuralgia, the initial success rate is approximately 88% but recurrences reduce the long-term success to approximately 71%.

Retreatment of initial failures or subsequent pain recurrences is successful in approximately 80% of patients, although, as mentioned, the number of patients retreated is relatively small and the follow-up interval at this time is relatively short. Maximum follow-up interval for initial treatment of trigeminal neuralgia at this time is approximately 7 years, and average follow-up is more than 3 years. Maximum follow-up for patients retreated at this time is slightly over 2 years and an average follow-up after retreatment is less than 1 year.

Initial reports of the radiosurgical treatment of trigeminal neuralgia described alterations in facial sensation in approximately 5% of patients. Our detailed follow-up of a much larger number of patients followed over a longer time suggests that with a maximum treatment dose of 76 Gy, the incidence of facial sensory alterations is approximately 10%; for 87 Gy, approximately 15%; and for 98 Gy, approximately 25% to 30%. In our experience, alterations in facial sensation have occurred a minimum of 6 weeks and a maximum of 26 months following the procedures. The peak incidence of alterations in facial sensation is between 6 months and 1 year. The magnitude of sensory loss and the distribution of sensory loss following radiosurgical treatment are rather variable. Mild subjective paresthesias only, without any objective facial sensory loss, is the minimum alteration we have noted and the maximum is complete analgesia throughout all three trigeminal divisions, including the intraoral distribution with absence of the corneal reflex. The latter degree of sensory loss has been seen in approximately 2% of patients. Most patients have experienced alterations in facial sensation midway between these two extremes and virtually all patients have experienced a gradual decrease in the amount of facial sensory loss over 3 to 12 months following the initial treatment. Many patients who have experienced sensory loss of a significant degree have subsequently recovered completely normal facial sensory function. Painful dysesthesias have occurred in approximately 1% of patients, but no patients have experienced anesthesia dolorosa or neuroparalytic keratitis after such treatment. Unlike all of the other surgical treatments, we have seen no other complications of any kind following radiosurgical treatment of trigeminal neuralgia with the gamma knife.

Comparison to Other Surgical Methods

MVD should theoretically be the ideal treatment of trigeminal neuralgia since it treats the putative cause of trigeminal neuralgia, namely vascular cross compression of the trigeminal sensory root.[28] The initial success rate of MVD is similar to that of radiosurgical treatment, but is accompanied in the case of MVD by a mortality rate of approximately 1% and a significant proportion of other relatively serious complications, including hearing loss, facial sensory loss, facial paralysis, diplopia, brainstem infarction, and cerebellar infarction and/or hemorrhage requiring reoperation. In addition, less serious, but nevertheless bothersome and expensive complications, of MVD, such as cerebrospinal fluid leakage, meningitis, and prolonged pain at the operative site are also seen. Gradual recurrences of pain following microvascular decompression reduce the long-term success rate to approximately that of the gamma knife varying in different reports from approximately 75% to 80% success. The percutaneous treatments are equally successful, but the accompanying sensory loss with these procedures is problematic for many patients and even the percutaneous procedures have associated morbidity and rare mortality.[32] Inadvertent placement of a percutaneous treatment needle into the temporal lobe has resulted in hematoma and abscess requiring surgical treatment. Carotid cavernous fistulae from inadvertent puncture of the cavernous sinus and then the carotid artery, inadvertent placement of the needle through other foramina (e.g., jugular foramen, superior orbital fissure) among others, also reduce the attractiveness of the percutaneous procedures. In addition, recurrence of pain after the percutaneous procedures is high. In our experience, following radiofrequency rhizolysis, the recurrence rate is 3% to 5% per year, resulting in a 10-year recurrence rate of approximately 30% to 50%. The recurrence rate after glycerol rhizolysis is even higher. Even prolonged pharmacologic treatment of trigeminal neuralgia is not without morbidity and, very rarely, mortality. We believe that there is sufficient evidence to say that on balance, radiosurgery with the gamma knife offers the best current treatment of trigeminal neuralgia. In the event of a radiosurgical treatment failure, or of recurrence of pain following successful treatment, retreatment with the gamma knife, at a reduced dose, is an option. Initial radiosurgical treatment also does not exclude later treatment with microvascular decompression, one of the percutaneous procedures, or pharmacologic treatment.

The safety and effectiveness of radiosurgery with the gamma knife in treating trigeminal neuralgia has been documented by recent reports from a number of centers around the world. Gamma knife treatment of so-called secondary trigeminal neuralgia due to structural lesions, such as tumors, multiple sclerosis, and vascular lesions, may also be effective.[23,33] Our general approach to the treatment of trigeminal neuralgia due to tumors or vascular lesions has been to treat these lesions directly using standard radiosurgical doses. This approach has resulted in relief of secondary trigeminal neuralgia in approximately 85% of patients. In two patients in whom recurrence of secondary trigeminal neuralgia developed after initial successful treatment, we subsequently treated with the trigeminal nerve root using the methods described in this report for classical trigeminal neuralgia. In many patients with secondary trigeminal neuralgia, the structural lesion causing the trigeminal neuralgia obliterates the trigeminal nerve root and it cannot be identified as a separate structure on imaging studies. In these cases, if radiosurgical treatment of the underlying structural lesion is unsuccessful, then we have recommended percutaneous treatment of the persistent trigeminal neuralgia. The effectiveness of gamma knife treatment of secondary trigeminal neuralgia is approximately equal to that of open surgical treatment in the form of craniotomy to remove the underlying structural lesion or reduce its bulk. The mortality and morbidity of gamma knife treatment, however, is lower and the cost is also lower.

Two other forms of craniofacial pain have also been recently treated by gamma knife radiosurgery. Pollack and Kondziolka recently reported radiosurgical treatment of a patient with sphenopalatine neuralgia using the gamma knife.[34] The treatment was directed at the sphenopalatine ganglion, located in the pterygopalatine fossa and identified on stereotactic imaging studies. A maximum radiosurgical dose of 98 Gy was delivered using a single 8-mm collimator. This patient initially experienced a significant decrease in pain so that by 8 months after the treatment, she was virtually pain free. By 17 months after the treatment, her pain had increased to approximately 50% of the original intensity and a second radiosurgical treatment was performed, again with a single 8-mm collimator and a maximum dose 87 Gy. Seven months after the second procedure and 24 months after the first procedure, the patient was described as free of pain with no associated neurologic deficits.

Ford and colleagues recently described the radiosurgical treatment of six patients with refractory cluster headache using the gamma knife.[35] In this report, the treatment was directed at the trigeminal sensory nerve root using a 4-mm secondary collimator helmet at a maximum radiosurgical dose of 76 Gy, identical to the treatment method we have described in this report for the treatment of trigeminal neuralgia. Four of the six patients were reported as having had excellent relief of pain and of the other two patients, one had good relief and one had fair relief. Neither postradiation complications nor facial sensory loss were seen in any of the patients during a follow-up period, which varied from 8 to 14 months. Ford and colleagues concluded that radiosurgical treatment of the trigeminal nerve root with the gamma knife afforded great promise in the management of chronic and refractory cluster headache. Our experience in treating cluster headache is extremely small, but our results are similar to those described by Ford. Of the four patients we have treated, one had excellent relief with follow-up over 2 years, whereas in two others, there has been greater than a 50% reduction, with concomitant marked reduction in medication and ability to resume a reasonably normal life. In the fourth patient, follow-up is too short to make definitive conclusion.

Conclusions

Radiosurgical treatment of trigeminal neuralgia is recommended as an early form of treatment, once the diagnosis has been clearly established based on the clinical symptoms and response to pharmacologic treatment. The effectiveness of the radiosurgical treatment of trigeminal neuralgia seems well enough established that it can be recommended enthusiastically. The success rate is approximately equal to the other forms of surgical treatment and the overall morbidity is significantly lower. A limited experience suggests that radiosurgical treatment of trigeminal neuralgia with linear accelerator-based radiosurgery may be as successful as that with the gamma knife, although the number of patients treated by that modality is, so far, rather small.

OTHER RADIOSURGICAL PAIN TREATMENTS

Several other forms of radiosurgical treatment have been described for chronic pain. We have limited experience with two of these, namely hypophysectomy and bilateral cingulotomy.

Surgical hypophysectomy or stereotactic cryohypophysectomy for the treatment of intractable pain in patients who suffer cancer with widespread bone metastases has been used in metastatic carcinoma of the breast and prostate gland with some success. Radiosurgical hypophysectomy may be utilized as an alternate to either transsphenoidal or stereotactic cryohypophysectomy or radiofrequency hypophysectomy. Because the life expectancy of most patients with diffuse metastatic carcinoma with bone metastases is relatively short, an early response to the treatment is desirable. To accomplish the hypophysectomy with the gamma knife in a short time, a high radiosurgical dose is recommended, 140 to 200 Gy. Multiple 4-mm isocenters directed at the pituitary gland, as identified on stereotactic MRIs, may be used for this method. Appropriate blocking of the secondary collimator helmet of the gamma knife will flatten the radiosurgical dose curve to keep the dose to the optic chiasm within acceptable limits. Stereotactic radiofrequency cingulotomy has been used for many years for the treatment of intractable pain. Recent metabolic studies have identified the cingulate cortex as an important termination point of pain-generated activity within the nervous system. Radiofrequency lesioning of the cingulum bundle has been demonstrated to produce significant reductions in pain that may be diffusely located through the body. Similar lesions may be created using radiosurgical methods, although experience with the technique is limited. We have utilized a single exposure with either the 4- or 8-mm collimator helmet and a maximum radiosurgical dose of 141 Gy centered on the cingulum bundle bilaterally at a point 25-mm posterior to the tips of the frontal horns of the lateral ventricles.

Our experience at this point is too small to permit a definitive recommendation about the specifics of the technique, but all treated patients appeared to benefit from the treatment with reduced pain complaints and decreased medication usage.

REFERENCES

1. Leksell L. The stereotaxic method and radiosurgery of the brain. Acta Chir Scand 102:316–319, 1951.
2. Larsson B, Leksell L, Rexed B. The use of high energy protons for cerebral surgery in man. Acta Chir Scand 125:1–7, 1963.
3. Leksell L, Larsson B, Andersson B, Rexed B, Sourander P, Mair W. Lesions in the depth of the brain produced by a beam of high energy protons. Acta Radiol 54:251–264, 1960.
4. Mair W, Rexed B, Sourander P. Histology of the surgical radiolesion in the human brain as produced by high-energy protons. Radiat Res 7(Suppl):384–389, 1967.
5. Leksell L. Cerebral radiosurgery: gamma thalamotomy in two cases of intractable pain. Acta Chir Scand 134:585–595, 1968.
6. Andersson B, Larsson B, Leksell L, Mair W, Rexed B, Sourander P, Wennerstrand J. Histopathology of late local radiolesions in the goat brain Acta Radiol Ther Phys Biol 9:385–394, 1970.
7. Kjellberg RN, Koehler AM, Preston WM, Sweet WH. Intracranial lesions made by the Bragg peak of a proton beam. In Haley TJ, Snider RS (eds). Response of the Nervous System to Ionizing Radiation. Boston, Little, Brown, 1964, p 36.
8. Forster DMC, Meyerson BA, Leksell L, Steiner L. Stereotactic Radiosurgery in Intractable pain. In Janzen R (ed). Pain. London, Thieme, 1972, pp 194–198.
9. Steiner L, Forster D, Leksell L, Meyerson BA, Boethius J. Gamma thalamotomy in intractable pain. Acta Neurochir 52:173–184, 1980.
10. Leksell L. Stereotactic radiosurgery. J Neurol Neurosurg Psychiatry 46:797–803, 1983.
11. Young RF, Jacques DB, Rand RW, Copcutt BC, Vermeulen SS, Posewitz AE. Medial thalamotomy with the leksell gamma knife for treatment of chronic pain. Adv Radiosurg Acta Neurochir 62(Suppl Wien):105–110, 1994.
12. Young RF, Jacques B, Rand RW, Copcutt BC, Vermeulen SS, Posewitz, AE. Technique of stereotactic medial thalamotomy with the leksell gamma knife for treatment of chronic pain. Neurol Res 17(1):59–65, 1995.
13. Young RF, Jacques DB, Rand RW, Copcutt BC, Vermeulen SS, Posewitz AE. Gamma knife thalamotomy for the treatment of persistent pain. Stereotact Funct Neurosurg 64(Suppl 1):172–181, 1995.
14. Young RF, Rinaldi P. Stereotactic ablative procedures for pain relief. In Wilkins RH, Rengachary SS (eds). Neurosurgery (2nd ed). New York, McGraw-Hill, 1996, pp 4061–4065.
15. Young RF, Posewitz A. Noninvasive lesioning: functional radiosurgery. In Alexander EB III, Maciunas RM (eds). Advanced Neurosurgical Navigation, vol. 41. New York, Thieme, 1998, pp 1–11.
16. Young RF, Vermeulen SS, Grimm P, Posewitz A. Electrophysiological target localization is not required for the treatment of functional disorders. Stereotact Funct Neurosurg 66(Suppl 1):309–319, 1996.
17. Young RF, Vermeulen SS, Posewitz A, et al. Functional neurosurgery with the leksell gamma knife. Radiosurgery 1:218–228, 1996.
18. Young RF. Functional disease of the brain: treatment by gamma knife radiosurgery. In DeSalles A, Lufkin R (eds). Minimally Invasive Therapy of the Brain. New York, Thieme, 1997, pp 225–234.
19. Young RF. Functional neurosurgery with the leksell gamma knife. Stereotact Funct Neurosurg 66(1–3):19–23, 1996.
20. Leksell L. Stereotaxic radiosurgery in trigeminal neuralgia. Acta Chir Scand 137:311–314, 1971.
21. Alexander EB III, Lindquist C. Special indications: radiosurgery for functional neurosurgery and epilepsy. In Alexander EB III, Loeffler JS, Lunsford LD (eds). Stereotactic Radiosurgery. New York, McGraw-Hill, 1993, pp 221–225.
22. Rand RW, Jacques DB, Melbye RW, Copcutt BG, Levenick MN, Fisher MR. Leksell gamma knife treatment of tic douloureux. Stereotact Funct Neurosurg 6:93–102, 1993.
23. Young RF, Vermeulen SS, Grimm P, Blasko J, Posewitz A. Gamma knife radiosurgery for treatment of trigeminal neuralgia: idiopathic and tumor related. Neurology 48(3):608–614, 1997.
24. Young RF. Radiosurgery versus microsurgery for trigeminal neuralgia. In Salcman M (ed). Current Techniques in Neurosurgery. New York, Springer, Current Medicine, 1998, pp 35–43.
25. Young RF, Vermeulen SS, Posewitz A. Gamma knife radiosurgery for the treatment of trigeminal neuralgia. Stereotact Funct Neurosurg 70(Suppl 1):192–199, 1998.
26. Young RF. Treatment of trigeminal neuralgia by radiosurgery with the gamma knife. In Fisher WS (ed). Perspectives in Neurological Surgery. New York, Thieme, 1999, pp 1–16.
27. Kondziolka D, Lundsford LD, Flickinger JC, et al. Stereotactic radiosurgery for trigeminal neuralgia: a multi-institution study using the gamma unit. J Neurosurg 84(6):940–945, 1996.
28. McLaughlin MR, Jannetta PJ, Clyde BL, Subach BR, Comey CH, Resnick DK. Microvascular decompression of cranial nerves: lessons learned after 4400 operations. J Neurosurg 90:1–8, 1999.
29. Young RF. Stereotactic radiosurgery for the trigeminal nerve root for treatment of trigeminal neuralgia. In Rengachary SS, Wilkins R (eds). Neurosurgical Operative Atlas Volume. Chicago, American Association of Neurological Surgeons, 1997, pp 87–91.
30. DeSalles AF, Buxton W, Solberg T, et al. Linear accelerator radiosurgery for trigeminal neuralgia. In Kondziolka D (ed). Radiosurgery, vol. 2. Basel, Karger, 1998, pp 173–182.
31. Kondziolka D, Lunsford LD, Flickinger JC. Gamma knife radiosurgery as the first surgery for trigeminal neuralgia. Stereotact Funct Neurosurg 70(Suppl 1):187–191, 1998.
32. Young RF. Stereotactic procedures for facial pain. In Apuzzo M (ed). Brain Surgery: Complication, Avoidance & Management. New York, Churchill Livingstone, 1993, pp 2097–2114.
33. Regis J, Metellus P, Lazorthes Y, Porcheron D, Peragut JC. Effect of gamma knife on secondary trigeminal neuralgia. Stereotact Funct Neurosurg 70(Suppl 1):210–217, 1998.
34. Pollock BE, Kondziolka D. Stereotactic radiosurgical treatment of sphenopalatine neuralgia. Case report. J Neurosurg 87:450–453, 1997.
35. Ford RG, Ford KT, Swaid S, Young P, Jennelle R. Gamma knife treatment of refractory cluster headache. Headache 38(1):3–9, 1998.

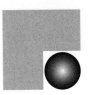

Miscellaneous Topics

Physical Medicine and Rehabilitation in Pain Management

MARC Y. WASSERMAN, MD AND SRIDHAR V. VASUDEVAN, MD

Physical methods of pain control are used in patients with both acute and chronic pain, but take on an especially critical role in those patients who have chronic pain. Victims of chronic pain have often been in the medical system for a long period of time, shifting from physician to physician in the hopes of a cure. Their charts are often quite convoluted, and both the physician and the patient can be confused and irritated by these long histories and no apparent relief.

The scope of the problem is tremendous: 75 million Americans suffer from chronic debilitating pain and 80% of all physician visits involve pain, costing $70 billion a year in medical claims, disability payments, and lost productivity. An additional factor is that many patients with chronic pain do not just have problems stemming directly from the physical suffering. The toil they have experienced by the time they finally arrive at a pain clinic often involves depression, anxiety, fear, estrangement from family members and friends, and despair.[1,2]

Pain rehabilitation programs were established, beginning in the early 1960s, to treat these patients. The programs were and remain comprehensive interventions designed especially to help patients increase their functioning, both physical and emotional, despite the presence of pain.[3] Their goals are to maximize the ability of the patient to function despite pain; reduce medications to the minimum level required to maintain this function; help the patient self-manage his or her own pain complaints and flare-ups without excessive inappropriate use of healthcare resources or falling back into a cascade of physicians and referrals; reduce depression, anxiety, anger, and other emotional states that can actually worsen the pain; help with disability or compensation issues, if these are present; and finally, to reduce pain intensity.

Not all patients are candidates for pain rehabilitation programs. Luckily, most patients can be treated on an outpatient or intermittent basis, as the majority of pain is acute and resolves fairly quickly. A major differentiation should be made here between acute pain and chronic pain. Acute pain is "useful" pain. It is a warning signal from the body that something is wrong—this can include infection, injury, hemorrhage,

tumor, and endocrinologic problems. This pain resolves when the problem is treated. In some patients, however, the pain does not resolve after medical or surgical treatment; when pain lasts for more than 3 to 6 months past the expected healing period of an injury or illness, then the pain is considered chronic, or intractable, pain. This intractable pain is not a warning signal—it is pain that is present but is no longer "useful." The intensity, frequency, and quality of this pain vary considerably between people and may bear no resemblance in character to the original injury.

Even at this point, however, some patients function well. Unfortunately, other patients become virtual slaves to their chronic pain, developing several problems that significantly affect their ability to function in society and to lead a normal family, social, and vocational life. These difficulties can be summarized with the mnemonic "The Ds"[4]:

1. *Disuse.* The patient tends not to use the part of the body that is causing them pain. As a result, that part of the body tends to contract and become stiff. This causes the patient to use the part even less, causing further stiffness in a repeating cycle.
2. *Deconditioning.* The gradual loss of muscle strength and stamina.
3. *Drug misuse.* Patients are often prescribed medications to help them deal with the pain. A patient who feels that they are always in pain can easily misuse some of these medications. These are not only narcotic medications, which tend to be the first medications that come to mind for possible abuse and misuse; patients can easily use doses of aspirin and nonsteroidal anti-inflammatory medications that lead to anticoagulation and gastrointestinal bleeding problems, or enough acetaminophen to cause permanent liver damage.
4. *Dependence.* This does not so much refer to drugs as a certain dependence on the family and healthcare system. Many patients with chronic pain have withdrawn from society, feeling that they are unable to accomplish anything at all due to their chronic pain. Complaints of

doing nothing but sitting and staring at the television set are, unfortunately, not uncommon. This allows the patient to concentrate fully and only on their pain. Worse, many individuals with chronic pain receive reinforcing gains for their "pain behaviors." Family members often allow the individual to become inactive and cater to the patient's requests and needs,[5] thus inadvertently increasing and reinforcing the patient's dependence.

5. *Depression*. This can be manifested by feeling hopeless and crying frequently, sleep disturbances, weight gain, and a lack of control that can lead to a risk of suicide.

6. *Disability*. Patients often have a significant dependence on social and financial assistance, particularly if they are not working due to their pain. Disability is defined as an inability or limitation in performing socially defined activities and roles of the individuals within a social and physical environment.[6] Over 75% of chronic pain patients display difficulties with job or housework, leisure activities, sexual function, or vocational endeavors.[5]

REHABILITATION PROGRAMS

Early rehabilitation programs were mostly inpatient. Unfortunately, with the rise of cost-cutting measures throughout hospitals and insurance plans, these are seen more rarely today. There were several advantages to inpatient programs, particularly the ability to supervise medication use, and the ability of patients to see other patients with chronic pain and share their experiences. In addition, transportation to and from the facility, often an issue in the outpatient setting, is not a difficulty in the inpatient programs.

However, the outpatient programs seen more commonly now also have unique advantages. More flexible scheduling is possible, the programs can occur over a much longer time (often an issue for chronic pain patients), and the cost to the patients is less. Outpatient programs also remove the potential stress of taking the patient out of their home environment; however, as mentioned previously, this can also be a disadvantage if that home environment is reinforcing their pain behaviors and pain complaints.

Due to the increased focus on outpatient facilities, it is important to ensure follow-up as well as to try and remove the potential for family reinforcement regarding their pain complaints. It should be emphasized to the patient's family and significant others that they are to be an active support system for helping the patient recover, not just offering passive sympathy. They have an important role in maintaining treatment gains—their support can be a powerful positive reinforcing stimulus for the patient to continue to improve. In addition, with every visit, a planned follow-up must be arranged, as well as who to call if a problem develops. This helps reassure the patient that they will not be abandoned by the healthcare system.

Pain rehabilitation programs may seek voluntary accreditation by the Commission on Accreditation of Rehabilitation Facilities, which analyzes organizational quality, structure, and management. Such accreditation ensures that facilities provide "coordinated, goal oriented, interdisciplinary team

services to improve functioning and decrease the dependence on health care systems by persons with pain."[7]

Most pain rehabilitation programs are led by a physician who is involved in education of the patient in the medical aspects of pain, particularly acute versus chronic pain. It is the physician who prescribes medications as needed, explains the results of tests to the patient and his or her family, and provides medical interventions such as injections. A physician is generally also the medical director of the rehabilitation clinic, board certified within his or her specialty, with at least 2 years of experience, membership in at least one national or regional pain society, and who receives continuing medical education in pain management or physical rehabilitation.

Psychologists also play a major role in the pain rehabilitation setting. They assist the patient in evaluating their behaviors and how these behaviors affect their pain. It should be emphasized to the patient that being referred to a psychologist does not in any way mean that the pain is "all in their head." In fact, it is not; pain is an intensely personal experience and can lead to depression, anxiety, fear, and many other psychological components. These can be best addressed through counseling, not through medications or other intervention alone. Psychologists are also able to help the patient rely more on positive thinking rather than focusing on their pain. They can teach stress management skills and relaxation techniques such as progressive muscle relaxation, deep breathing, imagery, and meditation. Psychologists also are particularly adept at helping the patient determine what role pain plays in their belief systems and views of self. The more the patient views the pain as a signal demanding a reduction in activity and thus increasing disability, the more difficult it becomes for the patient to achieve compliance with rehabilitation.[5] A psychologist can address these views and help the patient address the pain in a more constructive manner.

Group therapy encourages patients to actively discuss their behaviors, feelings, and thoughts about their pain, the way it affects their lives, and whether the program is helping them. Patients who are being helped by the program are often a source of encouragement for those patients just entering the program, leading to increased self-esteem, reduced isolation, and reduced feelings of worthlessness. Support groups need not stop at the end of therapy; patients can establish friendships and long-term support groups that can help reinforce coping.

Physical therapists perform and teach exercises designed to increase strength and range of motion as well as remove contractures caused by long disuse of muscles. They teach proper posture as body awareness, as well as start exercises that have been shown to help stimulate endorphin release, increase circulation, and escalate activity level. Patients should be instructed in the difference between "hurt" and "harm." Many patients are afraid to use their painful muscles because of the fear of harm. They should be told that the exercises may in fact "hurt" (that is, they may cause pain) but they will not "harm" (that is, they will not cause physical damage). The difference is critical—although the muscles will hurt for a time, they will improve their function, not get worse or become harmful to them; allowing the patient not to use the muscles and to remain at bed rest all day is, in fact, far more harmful. Physical therapists also often perform heat and cold therapy, massage, and other physical modalities discussed subsequently.

Vocational counselors aid in helping the patient return to work in some capacity. This is critical, as it gives the patient a goal to achieve as they gain control over their pain, a financial support, and the self-esteem of accomplishment. It should be noted that many patients have a pain complaint from a work injury, so it is important to pair this with psychology to keep a patient's anxiety about returning to work and potentially causing another injury from becoming a factor. Vocational counselors look at the patient's education and work history, often perform functional capacity evaluations, and evaluate the patient's motivation and ability to work. They often coordinate activities with prospective employers and case managers to help the patient find work suitable for them.

Other members of a pain rehabilitation team often include nurses that provide assistance and education, occupational therapists to improve function and endurance and provide assistive devices, nutritionists, social workers, pharmacologists, and recreational therapists.

Most multidisciplinary pain clinics use the Fordyce Model, which uses the general principles of interruption of the pain behavior reinforcement cycle, rewards for healthy behavior, appropriate goals, measurement of improvement by pain level, and psychosocial adjustment.[2] Pain management programs are designed to reduce, not necessarily eliminate, pain while increasing the patient's functional capabilities. Exercise is emphasized but is focused on what the patient can perform, with progressive increases. Pain complaints and behaviors are essentially ignored; the patient has to understand that the goal of the program is not to eliminate the pain—that may be impossible. The focus is instead on improved management of the pain.

The patient should understand and recognize that the program can increase function (physical, psychosocial, and vocational), but the patient must take an active role by attending treatment regularly and complying with treatment recommendations. The patient can and should discuss goals and treatments, and most major decisions are made with the patient's active input. Pain programs should have a weekly team conference to coordinate treatment, with the patient present at the conference, and the perception of progress from both the team and the patient should be discussed. Physical rehabilitation approaches are useful for both acute and chronic pain, and should become an integral part of aggressive, nonsurgical conservative treatment in patients with acute as well as chronic pain from musculoskeletal and neurologic disorders.[8]

REFERRAL OF PATIENTS TO PHYSICAL REHABILITATION PROGRAMS

It is often not enough for the physician simply to refer his or her patient to physical therapy and assume that all sessions are the same. Physical therapists are able to modulate the patient's perception of pain, instruct the patient about their pain syndrome and how to treat it, assist the patient in relaxation, improve the patient's physical fitness, and help patients learn back and joint mechanics that prevent reinjury. Patients' abilities, however, are improved when they fully understand exactly why the physician has referred the patient to physical therapy.[9] A helpful physical therapy prescription includes the patients' name, diagnosis, precautions, expected duration of treatment, goals, and the date of the next follow-up with the physician.

Referral diagnosis often tends to be "chronic pain," which is not very specific nor helpful; it tends to be more useful to state exactly where this chronic pain is located, its duration, exacerbating and alleviating factors, and radiation. Areas of contracture, weakness, or poor mobility can be diagnosed with musculoskeletal examination and listed as specific "target areas" to be addressed during treatment. The physician should also carefully note the patient's past medical history, particularly conditions that could potentially interact with therapy, such as hypertension, seizure disorder, diabetes, coronary artery disease, chronic obstructive pulmonary disease, or a history of spinal fusion, fracture, or total hip replacement. In addition, the physician should list specific goals of the therapy—which impairments are most critical to address, and what result is expected or reasonable to achieve in a given time.[9]

Referral should also not be delayed for too long with patients with chronic pain. In the United Kingdom, the Clinical Standard Advisory Group Committee on Back Pain notes the utility of active rehabilitation within the first 6 weeks of onset of pain to prevent long-term disability.[10] Studies in the United States confirm that individuals who have been removed from the labor market due to pain for less than 6 months have a 90% chance of returning to full employment, but those removed from the labor force due to pain for more than 1 year have less than a 10% chance of ever returning.[5] Patients with low back pain referred to physical therapy earlier (within 1 month of injury) also tended to return to work earlier (less than 60 days absence) than those patients referred later.[11]

Referral methods vary by state; access to physical therapy in many states requires a prescription by a physician.[12] A few states, such as Maryland and Massachusetts, have now enacted direct access legislation that allows patients to enter physical therapy without referral.

PHYSICAL REHABILITATION MODALITIES

Physical rehabilitation focuses on the use of physical modalities such as heat, cold, and electricity, as well as hands-on manual techniques such as manipulation, mobilization, massage, and traction. It also involves balancing rest to the injured part with exercises, as well as prevention of reinjury through appropriate orthotic devices such as braces and splints, with an exercise program and active movement.[8]

There are six major methods for managing pain: surgical, anesthesiologic, pharmacologic, physical rehabilitative, psychological, and alternative. Surgical and anesthesiologic techniques are covered well in other chapters of this book. A full investigation of complementary medicine is beyond the scope of this chapter; however, it should be noted that alternative treatments are frequently used by chronic pain patients, particularly those frustrated by the lack of success of traditional medical or surgical interventions. These range from chiropractors to faith healers to Rolfers to herbs. Many patients will not discuss these alternative treatments unless specifically asked; therefore, it is important to ask the patient what treatments they have tried—both traditional and alternative—because this can be important both to treatment as well as to assess their psychological state and their views on pain and pain control.

Traditional western medicine has tended to deemphasize alternative practices in favor of surgical and pharmacologic treatments. Interestingly, western medicine has also tended to deemphasize physical methods for the control of pain. This is partially because of wide advances in technology that have vastly improved the technique, success, and recovery time involved in surgical and anesthesiologic interventions. The same technology has allowed greater understanding of the neurochemical basis of pain, and has enabled us to pinpoint pain receptors and design pharmacologic agents to directly block those receptors (as evidenced by the recent COX-2 inhibitors), vastly improving our arsenal of powerful anti-inflammatory and anesthetic drugs. In addition, in the past 20 years there has been a great amount of focus on the psychological dimensions of pain and the need to incorporate psychological principles in the treatment of patients with both acute and chronic pain.

In recent years, however, there has been increased interest in physical agents to treat pain. Most information regarding the rationale for the use of physical agents in pain management is based on tradition, data extrapolated from basic science research, and randomized (albeit not always controlled) clinical trials.[13] Physical methods, however, unlike traditional surgical and pharmacologic treatments, involve the active participation of the patient, and patients tend to report better subjective pain recovery when they are actively involved in their own care.[3]

Physical modalities include superficial heat, deep heat (also called diathermy), cold (cryotherapy), and electrical current (electrotherapy).

Therapeutic Heat

Heat has been used extensively as an effective agent to relieve pain. Superficial heat can be provided by means of hot packs, hot water bottles, moist compresses, heating pads, or chemical and gel packs. It can also be provided through immersion in water (hydrotherapy) via whirlpool. All of these convey heat by conduction (directly) or by convection (indirectly, through a current). The greatest effect is at approximately 0.5 cm from the surface of the skin.[8]

Diathermy (deep heat) converts energy into heat. Short-wave diathermy uses high-frequency electrical current, and microwave diathermy uses electromagnetic radiation, but these are rarely used today; both are contraindicated in the presence of pacemakers, and microwave diathermy in particular is contraindicated in the presence of metal because the metal can be rapidly heated by the microwave radiation. Much safer and more frequently used is ultrasound diathermy. In ultrasound, acoustic vibrations of high frequency are converted into heat. These deep-heating modalities increase the temperature at depths far greater than superficial heat, up to 5 cm into the skin. This is particularly useful in the treatment of painful disorders of the deep soft tissues and tendons, as the structures are heated with ultrasound without increasing the temperature of the overlying skin.[14]

The physiologic effects of heat include pain relief, an increase in extensibility of tissues, and the reduction of muscle spasm. The increased muscle temperature decreases the muscle spindle sensitivity and relaxes the muscle.[15] Thus, superficial heating devices are indicated when muscles are in spasm. Heat also causes the vessels in the skin to dilate, bringing more blood flow to the area. This increased blood flow and availability of oxygen may also play a role in producing pain relief in the muscle.

By increasing the extensibility of the muscle, heat is an important adjunct in the stretching exercises of physical therapy. Deep-heating modalities such as ultrasound are very useful in the treatment of tight tissues such as those seen in frozen shoulder. Tight hamstrings, heelcords, or postsurgical scarring can also be softened with the use of deep heat and stretching.[8,9,14]

An additional advantage of heat therapy is that the patient can easily use these methods at home. A Hydrocollator pack, which uses conductive heating, is frequently used in heat therapy. It is applied to the painful area under varying thicknesses of terry cloth towels. The use of paraffin wax is another option for specific areas such as the hands, fingers, or feet; it is not indicated for other areas of the body.

Fluidotherapy is sometimes seen in physical therapy offices as well. It is a machine that contains a bed of very finely divided ground corn or cellulose particles. These particles can be heated and blown around rapidly. The patient then dips his or her hand, foot, or other affected part into the particles. The effect is something like heated sand—patients report that it is very soothing, and a major advantage is the prevention of edema, because fluidotherapy avoids the dependency position that is assumed with hydrotherapy. Disadvantages are that it cannot be used at home, and is difficult to apply to any part of the body except the extremities.

Hydrotherapy is the most common heating modality used in physical therapy departments. It is usually provided in the form of a whirlpool. Its major advantage is that any part of the body, or the entire body, can be submerged. In addition, the whirlpool provides buoyancy, minimizing stress to the joints during exercises and eliminating the gravitational pull on the lower extremities and spine.

In summary, superficial heating is useful before exercise, provides pain relief and muscle relaxation, and can easily be used at home. Deep heating is more useful when the intention is to treat deep structures such as joints and ligaments. Ultrasound is the method of choice, as it can treat deep structures, trigger points, tight tendons, can be used under water, and the presence of metal is not a contraindication. Diathermy of any type, however, is contraindicated in the presence of active malignancy.[14]

Cold Therapy

Cold therapy involves the use of ice and gel packs, vapocoolant sprays, and cold baths. Like heat therapy, cold therapy affects the muscle spindle and may also modulate neurotransmitters.[16] Cold packs are applied for approximately 15 minutes, and are also wrapped in terry cloth. Cold therapy has the advantage of providing longer pain relief than does heat. It is contraindicated, however, in any condition in which vasoconstriction of arteries produces symptoms, such as in Raynaud's phenomenon. In general, patients report that cold therapy produces first a subjective coolness for 1 to 2 minutes, then a burning sensation for 1 to 2 minutes, and then finally numbness.[14] Cold is particularly useful for trigger points, tendons, and can be used before stretching, just like heat therapy.

Cold is the treatment of choice in acute injuries because of its effect of decreasing the initial inflammatory response and its accompanying edema. Heat, in contrast, would actually make this process worse. Cold reduces the metabolism of the underlying tissues, reduces nerve conduction velocity (including pain nerves), and directly cools the muscle spindle, reducing spasm. Ice packs can also be conveniently used by the patient at home.

Manual Therapy

The most "hands-on" part of physical therapy, manual therapy involves direct massage, mobilization, and manipulation of tissues, and is usually preceded by heat or cold therapy described above so that the tissues are more accommodating to the stretch.

Massage generally involves stroking, friction, and kneading of the tissues.[17] Stroking involves pushing the tissues from periphery toward the center. It decreases edema. Friction and kneading is a more aggressive handling of the tissues, and breaks down intramuscular adhesions, reducing stiffness and pain and allowing the tissues to be stretched more easily.

Mobilization is a technique in which a trained physical therapist directly mobilizes specific soft tissues, particularly fascia; this is sometimes referred to as a "myofascial release." Normally, the fascia covering muscles is slightly mobile, but pain can cause it to shorten and tighten around the muscle. These fascial restrictions can generate enormous pressure, as evidenced by such pathologic conditions as compartment syndrome. Also, fascia is richly innervated by nerves, but unfortunately are not very well vascularized; thus, irritation of the fascial tissues leads to a great deal of pain and slow healing.[18] Myofascial release stretches the fascia back into its normal position, stretching it until the soft tissue below it is felt to relax, or "release."[19]

Manipulation is a skilled passive movement to a spinal segment, most often associated with chiropractic medicine. It is also an accepted technique among osteopaths, many medical doctors, and physical therapists as well, although all of them approach the technique differently. It is possible that manipulative therapy helps release tissue trapped between collapsed facet joints, but unfortunately, manipulative therapy can be overused and create a patient dependency, and its general efficacy remains uncertain.[20]

Another physical modality that is sometimes used is traction, in which tissues and vertebral bodies (generally cervical) are mechanically distracted. Overhead intermittent cervical traction of approximately 10 to 25 lbs can be useful in cervical radiculopathy, because it widens the intervertebral foramina and reduces pressure on the nerves. However, it is impractical for lumbar disk diseases, as the force required to widen the foramina between the lumbar vertebral bodies is far too high for most patients to tolerate.[17]

Electrical Stimulation

Transcutaneous electrical nerve stimulation (TENS) is considered a relatively new therapy, but, in fact, it is one of the earliest; historical notes from the Roman Empire included descriptions of patients using electric "torpedo" fish to treat gout and headaches.

TENS uses electrical energy transmitted from the surface of the skin to the nervous system. The rationale is based on the gate control theory of pain proposed in 1965 by Melzack and Wall,[21] which suggests that the larger myelinated fibers that transmit non-noxious somatosensory impulses can shut down the "gate" that allows the smaller unmyelinated C fibers that transmit pain to function. TENS stimulates the larger fibers, causing the smaller pain fibers to be suppressed.

TENS seems to work best at high frequency and low intensity, frequently called "conventional TENS."[22] However, high-intensity, low-frequency TENS ("acupuncture TENS") also can produce pain relief. This may occur through stimulation of endogenous opioids, as the effect of TENS can be reversed with the opiate antagonist naloxone.[23] TENS has been studied for both acute and chronic back pain. Some find no difference between placebo and TENS for the relief of chronic low back pain[24]; others find utility for TENS, particularly in phantom pain, complex regional pain syndrome,[8] postoperatively,[25] and in arthritic conditions.[26]

Despite the controversy, TENS has a sound physiologic rationale for its use, it is noninvasive, can be taught to the patient, and can be used as part of a broader approach to pain management. Therefore, it is accepted as a major intervention for pain syndromes.

Acupuncture

Acupuncture is an ancient Chinese therapy in which thin metal needles are inserted into specific body sites and slowly twisted. The Chinese believe acupuncture restores the balance between spirit and blood, which flow in 14 channels, or "meridians" with a total of 361 acupuncture sites. Research shows that acupuncture may stimulate large sensory afferent fibers and suppress pain perception through gate control, much like TENS. The fact that some acupuncture needles are not simply twisted but stimulated electrically in acupuncture lends support to this possibility.

In addition, there is a significant overlap between traditional acupuncture sites and muscular trigger points.[5] The insertion of the needle into these areas is similar to the experience of the insertion of a needle into a trigger point, regardless of the substance injected. Therefore, acupuncture may be a form of neuromodulation, encouraging the production of endogenous opiate-like substances.[27]

Therapeutic Exercises

The natural reaction for the individual who has pain is to restrict that body part. This is reasonable in acute pain, as to move the part could cause further harm; hence, splinting and rest are appropriate interventions. However, in chronic pain, quite the opposite is the case; restricting that body part will inhibit normal functioning of that body part, and that disuse can result in further declines in function as well as deconditioning.[28] In fact, strict rest can result in up to a 20% loss in strength, as well as rapid muscle atrophy, cardiopulmonary deconditioning, bone mineral loss, and increased risk for thromboembolism.[29]

Worse, returning the patient to work after this disuse and loss of strength occurs is a risk factor for additional injury due to the weakened state. Bed rest of 2 to 3 days may be reasonable for some acutely injured patients, but prolonged bed rest, more than 2 weeks, is inadvisable. To break the cycle of pain leading to stiffness leading to weakness leading to pain, exercises should be reinstituted, albeit at a pace agreed upon by physician and patient.[30]

Once a patient has stopped exercising due to pain, it is often difficult to get them to start again. Many factors are involved in the overall decrease of activity levels of patients with pain. Patients who are not fully informed about the differences between "hurt" and "harm" try and avoid the initial hurt that exercise can produce.[31] It is also difficult to convince patients that rest will not help the healing process in chronic pain, unlike acute pain.

Exercise programs are focused, much like physical rehabilitation in general, on improving the patient's physical and functional capacity and his or her quality of life; the main focus is not on relieving the pain specifically, although with strengthening and stretching of the muscles, that is often the result. Therapeutic exercises include range of motion, stretching, strengthening, general conditioning, and relaxation.

Range-of-motion exercises are those done to maintain and increase the motion of joints and the flexibility of muscles. These exercises can be done passively by physical therapists, actively by the patient, or through a combination in which the patient's active range of motion is supplemented by the therapist's passive increase in mobility. Range-of-motion exercises increase and maintain the elasticity of connective tissue around joints.

Stretching exercises should be done slowly and steadily, and the stretch should be sustained. The stretch brings the contracted and atrophied muscle back to its normal length (remembered by the adage "a long muscle is a strong muscle"). The stretch should be smooth and controlled; jerking or bouncing movement can cause further injury to tissues. Pretreatment with heat or ice is reasonable to facilitate the stretch. Both range-of-motion and stretching exercises can be carried over to the home without equipment.

Strengthening exercises are done against resistance, and fall into three categories: isometric (static strengthening), isokinetic (constant speed with maximum torque), and isotonic (active movement and movement against resistance, as with free weights). Isometric exercises are generally not helpful for chronic pain. Isokinetic exercises of the back are particularly useful for the erector spinae muscles, and can decrease low back pain.[32] Isotonic exercises are very good for general strengthening, and a gradual increase in weights and repetitions tends to produce the best result. Isotonic exercises have the additional advantage of being able to target specific weak muscles; also, free weights can be used by the patient at home. Randomized clinical trials support the usefulness of stretching and strengthening exercises in the treatment of chronic low back pain.[24,33]

Aerobic exercises improve the general physical capability of the patient. These exercises include rhythmic and repetitive activities such as running, cycling, and swimming, and involve large muscle groups. Patients with chronic pain, whether from low back pain, fibromyalgia, or other causes, are very deconditioned; aerobic exercise provides a rapid and useful way to address this problem, particularly when coupled with muscle strengthening. Aerobic exercise may increase

endogenous opioids, increases pain threshold, boosts confidence, can be done independently, is inexpensive, and improves cardiovascular endurance. When accompanied by appropriate warm-up and cool-down exercises, aerobic exercise appears to offer long-lasting relief from low back pain.[29] In addition, individuals who perform aerobic exercises seem to have less pain during activities of daily living and a greater endurance for activities.[34,35]

Patients should, of course, have a say in how much exercise is instituted into their recovery. An exercise "quota system" can be established by physician and patient that provides an achievable increase in both exercises and expectancy while simultaneously decreasing concern regarding overexercising. It is often beneficial to make the early goals in the quota system below what the patient can already currently achieve so that progress appears to be made immediately and early success is provided. Goals are set for all forms of exercise, and increasing quotas are provided as signs of achievement.

Aerobic exercises, particularly walking and gentle running, can be done with other patients. This is often beneficial; the flexibility, coordination, general conditioning, strengthening, endurance building, peer pressure, competition, and mutual support all work together, and some of the more advanced patients can be role models for new patients.

OUTCOME MEASURES

Feine and Lund,[36] in a major analysis of review articles for chronic musculoskeletal pain techniques, show strong evidence that symptoms improve during treatment with most forms of physical therapy, including placebo. They note, however, that many studies have had difficulty measuring outcomes. The reasons for this are multiple, but often have to do with the fact that pain is subjective, and measuring it is difficult. The sample populations and locations of pain tend to be very heterogenous, and small sample sizes in many of the studies also make drawing definitive conclusions risky. In addition, most studies compare different forms of treatment regimens, and most regimens included several forms of therapy. Research into the management of chronic pain is also complicated by the fact that many patients with chronic pain have complex symptoms treated over many years by multiple modalities that are difficult to disentangle as individual components.[37]

That said, Feine and Lund agree that physical rehabilitation programs do help patients; the reason for this, they propose, is that physical therapy and even placebo allowed the patients to concentrate less on the pain as they worked on increasing range of motion; the patients were given the ability to take an active role in decreasing their pain, helping them cope. Malone and Strobe[38] concur, stating that physical rehabilitation's effectiveness, as well as other methods, seems to be attributable to something that the treatments all have in common: the identification of psychological factors that affect pain, contact with empathetic team members, and hope.

Other outcome measures have been more definitive. Flor, Fydrich, and Turk's large meta-analytic reviews of pain centers show that the mean cost of a multidisciplinary pain program is approximately $8100, versus about $15,000 for just one typical lumbar laminectomy surgery. Patients also reported a reduction in subjective pain intensity of about 25% following rehabilitation, maintained at 5 years; 65% discontinued narcotic medications, and 50% returned to work. In addition, even at long-term follow-up, patients treated in multidisciplinary pain clinics were functioning better than 75% of a sample either untreated or treated by conventional unimodal approaches. Patients treated in these pain clinics are almost twice as likely to return to work as the unimodally treated patients, with 43% more patients working after as compared to before treatment, potentially saving billions of dollars annually.[39]

The need for psychologists to be a part of pain rehabilitation programs is emphasized by studies that show 60% to 80% improvement in patients with chronic pain without psychosocial components and 30% to 50% in patients with chronic pain who also have significant psychosocial components.[40] In addition, in a study of 94 chronic pain patients enrolled in a multidisciplinary chronic pain program with cognitive-behavioral components, decreases in pain helplessness were linked to pain severity reduction at 6 months of follow-up, even after controlling for effects of a decrease in depression, suggesting that cognitive and physical capacity changes that occur during pain treatment contribute favorably to long-term outcome.[41]

The cost of pain programs has been a concern, particularly to third-party payors who think that the initial costs are not worth the investments. However, the outcomes ensure that patients use fewer healthcare resources; patients with chronic pain are more than five times more likely than patients without chronic pain to use healthcare resources, and frequently experience anxiety and depression that must also be evaluated and treated.[42] A retrospective study of 53 chronic pain patients demonstrated, using a model to project costs, an average cost benefit of $238,515 per patient.[43]

CONCLUSIONS

In the normal course of events, pain signals the need for attention to a pathologic condition that can be diagnosed and appropriately treated; this is acute pain, and serves a useful function. Chronic pain, on the other hand, persists after the pathologic condition has been treated, or occurs in the absence of any pathologic condition. This pain does not serve any useful biologic function. However, that does not mean that it is not real or that it is "all in the patient's head." The chronic pain is quite real to the patient, and leads to tremendous costs in terms of depression, pain, and anxiety, as well as significant emotional, physical, vocational, economic, and social alterations that affect not just the patient but also their family and friends and society as a whole.

Programs that focus on rehabilitation approaches that use specific treatment goals reduce patient pain in a cost-effective manner.[1] The incorporation of physical rehabilitation in a pain management program is crucial for any patient with pain. Primary care physicians and specialists should both be knowledgeable about the rationale, physiology, and appropriate use of physical agents in pain control. Physical rehabilitation should certainly be used along with appropriate pharmacologic, surgical, anesthesiologic, and psychological approaches for the management of pain.

REFERENCES

1. Vasudevan SV. Rehabilitation of the patient with chronic pain: is it cost effective? Pain Digest 2:99–101, 1992.
2. Fordyce WE. Behavioral Methods For Chronic Pain And Illness. St. Louis, CV Mosby, 1976.
3. Chapman S. Pain rehabilitation programs. *In* Abram S, Haddox J (eds). The Pain Clinic Manual. Philadelphia, Lippincott Williams and Wilkins, 2000.
4. Vasudevan SV. Pain: a Four Letter Word You Can Live With (2nd ed). Milwaukee, P.A.I.N. LLC, 1995.
5. Walsh NE, Dumitru D, Ramamurthy S, Schoenfield LS. Treatment of the patient with chronic pain. *In* DeLisa J (ed). Rehabilitation Medicine: Principles and Practice. Philadelphia, JB Lipincott, 1988.
6. Vasudevan SV. Role of functional capacity assessment in disability evaluation. J Back Musculoskel Rehabil 6:237–248, 1996.
7. Commission on Accreditation of Rehabilitation Facilities (CARP). 1996 Standards Manual and Interpretive Guidelines for Medical Rehabilitation, Tucson, 1996.
8. Vasudevan SV, Hegmann, K, Moore A, et al. Physical methods of pain management. *In* Raj PP (ed). Practical Management of Pain (2nd ed). Chicago: YearBook Medical, 1992, pp 669–679.
9. Bloodworth-Schramm DM. Physical therapy in the pain clinic setting. *In* Abram S, Haddox J (eds). The Pain Clinic Manual. Philadelphia, Lippincott Williams and Wilkins, 2000.
10. Clinical Standard Advisory Group. Back Pain. London: HMSO, 1994.
11. Ehrmann-Feldman D, Rossignol M, Abenhaim L, Gobeille D. Physician referral to physical therapy in a cohort of workers compensated for low back pain. Phys Ther 76(2):150–156, 1996.
12. Mitchell JM, deLissovoy G. A comparison of resource use and cost in direct access versus physician referral episodes of physical therapy. Phys Ther 77(1):8–10, 1997.
13. Fedorczyk J. The role of physical agents in modulating pain. J Hand Ther 10(2):110–121, 1997.
14. Michlovitz S. Thermal Agents in Rehabilitation. Philadelphia, FA Davis, 1986.
15. Lehmann JF, ed. Therapeutic Heat and Cold (3rd ed). Baltimore, Williams and Wilkins, 1982.
16. Fields HL, Basbaum AL. Brain stem control of spinal pain–transmission neurons. Annu Rev Physiol 40:217–248, 1978.
17. Bonica JJ, ed. The Management of Pain (2nd ed, vol. 2). Philadelphia, Lea & Febiger, 1990.
18. Calliet R. Soft Tissue Pain and Disability. Philadelphia, FA Davis, 1997.
19. Manheim CJ, Lavett DK, eds. The Myofascial Release Manual. Thorofare, New Jersey, Slack, 1989.
20. McKenzie RA. A perspective on manipulative therapy. Physiotherapy 8:440–444, 1975.
21. Melzack R, Wall PD. Pain mechanisms: a new theory. Science 150:971–979, 1965.
22. Soric R, Devlin M. Transcutaneous electrical nerve stimulation: practical aspects and applications. Postgrad Med 78:101–107, 1985.
23. Sjolund BH, Eriksson MB. The influence of naloxone on analgesia produced by peripheral conditioning stimulation. Brain Res 173:295–301, 1979.
24. Deyo RA, Walsh N, Martin D, et al. A controlled trial of transcutaneous electrical nerve stimulation and exercise for low back pain. N Engl J Med 322:1627–1634, 1990.
25. Manheimer JS. TENS: uses and effectiveness. *In* Michel TH (ed). Pain. New York, Churchill Livingstone, 1985, pp 73–121.
26. Minor MA, Sanford, MK. The role of physical therapy and physical modalities in pain management. Rheum Dis Clin North Am 25(1):233–248, 1999.
27. Melzack R. Acupuncture and related forms of folk medicine. *In* Wall PD, Melzack R (eds). Textbook of Pain. New York, Churchill Livingstone, 1984, pp 691–700.
28. King JC, Dumitru D, Walsh NE. Rehabilitation of the pain patient: a U.S. perspective. Pain Digest 2:106–126, 1992.
29. Muller EA. Influence of training and inactivity on muscle strength. Arch Phys Med Rehabil 51:449–463, 1970.
30. Deyo RA, Diehl AK, Rosenthal, M. How many days of bed rest for acute low back pain: a randomized clinical trial. N Engl J Med 315:1064–1070, 1986.
31. Soric R, Devlimn M. Role of physical medicine. *In* Tollison CD (ed). Handbook of Chronic Pain Management. Baltimore, Williams & Wilkins, 1989.

32. Timm K. Case studies: use of Cybex trunk extension/flexion unit in the rehabilitation of back patients. J Sports Orthop Ther 8:578–581, 1987.

33. Nachemson AL. Advances in low back pain. Clin Orthop 200:266–278, 1985.

34. Jackson C, Brown M. Analysis of current approaches and a practical guide to prescription exercise. Clin Orthop 179:46–53, 1983.

35. Jackson C, Brown M. Is there a role for exercise in the treatment of patients with low back pain? Clin Orthop 179:39–43, 1983.

36. Feine J, Lund J. An assessment of the efficacy of physical therapy and physical modalities for the control of chronic musculoskeletal pain. Pain 71:5–23, 1997.

37. Justins DM. Management strategies for chronic pain. Ann Rheum Dis 55:588–596, 1996.

38. Malone MD, Strobe MJ. Meta-analysis of nonmedical treatments for chronic pain. Pain 34:231–244, 1988.

39. Flor H, Fydrich T, Turk DC. Efficacy of multidisciplinary pain centers: a meta-analytic review. Pain 49:221–230, 1992.

40. Chapman SL, Brena SF, Brandford LA. Treatment outcome in a chronic pain rehabilitation program. Pain 11:255–268, 1981.

41. Burns JW, Johnson BJ, Mahoney N, Devine J, Pawl R. Cognitive and physical capacity process variables predict long-term outcome after treatment of chronic pain. J Consult Clin Psychol 66(20):434–439, 1998.

42. Marcus D. Treatment of nonmalignant chronic pain. Am Fam Phys 61(5):1331–1338, 2000.

43. Stieg RL, Williams RC, Timmermann-Williams G, et al. Cost benefits of interdisciplinary chronic pain treatment. Clin J Pain 1:189–193, 1986.

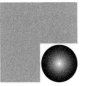

CHAPTER 31

The Multidisciplinary Pain Treatment Program

RONALD P. PAWL, MD

FUNDAMENTAL CONCEPTS

Collaboration among medical therapists in the treatment of chronic disorders has occurred somewhat more or less throughout the history of medicine. However, pain has been historically usually viewed as a symptom that is a primary nociceptive process related to some sort of tissue injury, caused by a process threatening bodily integrity. The diagnosis of the source of a given patient's pain was the domain of any and, to some extent, every medical expert, and the focus of treatment of pain was determined by the nature of the practitioner's expertise. That was the situation until the formation of the interdisciplinary medically integrated International Association for the Study of Pain by the late Dr. John Bonica in 1972. Thereafter, for the first time in history, pain was addressed as a medical problem generally, and collaboration among numerous types of medical experts, ranging from basic scientists to the various categories of clinical specialists, nurses, physical and occupational therapists, and psychologists occurred in a formal scholarly manner. Pain, it came to be realized through interdisciplinary investigation, is not purely a strictly sensory process. Pain is a perception that depends to some more or less extent on sensory nociception, in many instances, but it also depends on the integration of central nervous system function that includes cognition and motor activities and with psychological functioning and personality. It came to be realized also that this is the case with both acute and chronic pain. Further, chronic diseases that produce more or less nociception by disruption of tissue through metastatic invasion, inflammation, or infectious destruction came to be distinguished from chronic pain syndromes in which personality, other psychological factors, and cognition play the greater role.

Distinction between Chronic Disease and Chronic Pain

Diseases such as cancer and arthritis, and degenerative spinal disorders can and do produce acute pain that is primary nociception, through damage to tissue. Often in these diseases, acute pain is recurrent and intermittent, and in that sense the associated pain disorder, often in the past, was called chronic.

Those diseases and the pain associated with them are now what have now come to be called chronic pain syndromes (CPSs), although at times these completely different types of painful disorders may coexist. Typically, CPSs are divided into two categories, although at times there may be an overlap between them. Myofascial pain syndromes are characterized by tight muscles, tender spots at the region of the musculotendinous border in the muscles involved or trigger points, and a tendency toward diffuse pain. CPSs may be regional, as in low back, cervical, or temporomandibular syndromes, or more diffuse, as in fibromyalgia. Vascular CPSs are characterized by alteration in blood flow to the part involved, such as in classic migraine headaches or reflex sympathetic dystrophy syndromes. Myofascial syndromes may have some associated changes in blood flow, but it is the myofascial component that is dominant. Similarly, vascular syndromes may be accompanied by myofascial tightness, but the vascular component is dominant. Clinically, a CPS starts acutely. This means that a patient's pain complaint does not have to be present for a specific number of weeks or months to be a CPS.

Clinical Characteristics of Chronic Pain Syndrome

It is particularly important for neurosurgeons and other spinal surgeons to be able to distinguish between a patient's pain complaints that can be improved or relieved by surgical intervention and those that will not. It is equally important to be able to distinguish which pain problems will benefit from coordinated therapy in a multidisciplinary pain treatment program (MPTP).

The descriptions of pain by the patient with CPS are couched in affective as opposed to descriptive terms.[1] "Excruciating, throbbing, stabbing, like a red-hot poker running down my leg (or arm), hurting, like someone kicked me, a fist in the back (or shoulder blade, or neck), a knife sticking through me" are typical examples. In CPSs in the cervical or lumbar region, the pain complaint is mainly in the spinal region, or at least the pain there is coequal with the extremity complaint. On the other hand, patients with radicular syndromes in the neck or low back describe "electric-like, tingling, or pins and needle" paresthesias that follow a distal distribution in the upper or lower extremity, consistent with the

255

dermatome of the root involved. In those instances, the pain in the spinal area is little or none. In a patient with a radiculopathy, the pain described radiates to or is located in the myotome, that is, the specific muscular elements supplied by the nerve root. The patient with chronic pain, on the other hand, describes a more diffuse and often anatomically impossible radiation that involves more of the upper or lower extremity than would be accounted for by a root syndrome. Paresthesias do not follow a neurologic pattern in a CPS, and are diffuse, overlapping several dermatomes, and often involve the entire limb. The paresthesias are often equated with the pain by patients with CPSs, and not distinguished from it as by patients with radiculopathy.

The manner in which a patient behaves during the examination is important and often quite characteristic for a CPS. Verbal or bodily expression of emotional states, particularly anger or depression, are frequently demonstrated by patients who have CPSs. On the other hand, some patients with CPSs describe the pain problem in horrific terms, but appear almost happy and laughing inappropriately. Patients with CPSs often demonstrate pain behaviors, such as grimacing, sighing, or grunting during the description of the problem or the physical examination. The patient may hold the afflicted part, such as the head, neck, or low back stiffly. Camptocormia may be demonstrated. Camptocormia is a bent forward and sometimes sidewise posturing at the waist, mostly seen in low back syndromes. However, a similar posturing of the head and neck may be demonstrated by patients with cervical syndromes. Waddell's signs[2,3] and other nonorganic signs such as complaints of increased low back or neck pain when walking on heels or toes and reports of pain when the subcutaneous tissues are palpated frequently occur.

Psychological and Socioeconomic Components

Psychological, personality, and socioeconomic factors play the major underlying role in CPSs. When formal psychological tests are performed on patients with a CPS, somatization is the most consistent finding.[4] An example is the score on the Minnesota Multiphasic Personality Inventory (MMPI), which is perhaps the best-documented and validated psychometric test in the English language. The score on the test is printed out on a graphic scale that has three validity scales, 10 primary clinical scales, and a number of other secondary scales. In patients with CPSs, elevations are commonly seen on the 1 and 3 scales, the hysteria and hypochondriasis scales, the combination of which is now called somatization. Somatization is a psychological process in which emotional distress is converted into bodily or somatic complaints. Patients with somatization are also intently focused on their bodies, to the point that innocuous bodily functions or non-painful stimuli are interpreted as uncomfortable. The Waddell signs have been shown to correlate well with elevations on the 1 and 3 scales, particularly in males.[5] Elevations on the 1 and 3 scales also correlate with a personality that is passive and fearful of moving the painful part.[6] Frequently, an elevation occurs on the 8 scale. The 8 scale is called the schizophrenia scale, but is not, of itself, diagnostic of schizophrenia. When the 8 scale is elevated in female CPS patients, it has been shown to correlate with Waddell's signs. Catastrophizing is

characteristic of patients with chronic pain and along with rumination, correlates with pain and disability. The correlation is independent of anxiety and depression.[7,8]

Childhood psychological traumas, such as physical and sexual abuse, emotional neglect or abuse, abandonment by parent(s), or chemically dependent parent(s) correlate highly with chronic pain syndromes.[9,10] Of particular note to the surgeon is the negative correlation between the outcome of lumbar spinal surgery and the number of such traumatic childhood psychological events. That negative correlation is stronger than the positive correlation between the outcome of surgery and the surgical selection criteria.[11] When a patient who is being considered for surgical intervention for pain relief is found with a significant number of the foregoing characteristics, evaluation in a multidisciplinary pain treatment center is warranted.

ORGANIZATION OF THE MULTIDISCIPLINARY PAIN TREATMENT PROGRAM

The medical therapists essential to a MPTP are a physician, a psychologist, physical and/or occupational therapy (PT), and in many centers, including the one at Lake Forest, Illinois, nurses who also act as case managers.

Physician

The physician in an MPTP may come from any specialty, but usually is a physiatrist, neurosurgeon, neurologist, psychiatrist, or anesthesiologist. The MPTP physician must be thoroughly familiar with the biopsychosocial medical model, critical to the understanding and treatment of pain. The American Board of Pain Medicine provides a certification examination for physicians in pain medicine, which is based on that model. The American Board of Anesthesiology also provides a special certification in pain management. Although the exam does cover a broad scope of pain diagnosis and treatment, there is a greater stress on invasive therapy, such as injection treatment, placement of pumps to deliver medications, and spinal cord stimulation.

The medical director of an MPTP is usually a physician, but that is not always the case. Some well-qualified centers have psychologists, nurses, or therapists acting as directors, but physicians are a necessary part of the therapeutic team. The MPTP physician must be knowledgeable about musculoskeletal problems because spinal and extremity pains make up the majority of patients with CPS. It is ideal if the MPTP physician is capable of interpreting radiologic studies. Patients with CPS often feel that something has been missed diagnostically in the case, and another view of the radiographic investigations is welcomed. If the physician is not able to interpret radiographic diagnostic studies, readily available radiologic consultation is necessary, for the same reason, and to assure that any other diagnosis has been ruled out. This is important not only diagnostically, but also therapeutically, since outcome of treatment requires patient acceptance of the diagnosis.

Nursing

Nurses play a major role in the care of patients with chronic pain. The nurse should have training in case management, and be knowledgeable about medication use and drug interactions. The nurse will often bear the brunt of the patient's expression of anger. Anger is a characteristic psychological component of many patients with CPS. The nurse's role in coordinating patient care requires regular and frequent contact with the patient. Therefore, the nurse for an MPTP requires the fortitude and skill to handle such expressions of anger as well as patients' attempts to manipulate the secondary gains, which are also characteristic of the CPS.

Therapy

Physical therapy, occupational therapy, and ergonomic therapy and education are all significant components of chronic pain treatment. These components will be addressed under the heading of PT. The role of PT is not confined, however, to therapeutic maneuvers of and education about the musculoskeletal system. The therapist must know the theory and methods of behavioral modification and participate actively in that process. In the usual course of events, a physical therapist ordinarily will stop treatment when a patient no longer demonstrates improvement in physical functioning. When treating patients with a CPS, therapy does not necessarily stop when there is a plateau in a patient's progress. The decision to stop treatment is a team action, which is often dependent on multiple factors—physical, cognitive, and psychological.

Psychology

Psychologists are critical to the MPTP. Even more critical is that the psychologist be knowledgeable about the psychological foundation of the CPS. Psychologists who have not been exposed to diagnosis and treatment in chronic pain disorders are often confounded by some or all of the psychological distress found in patients with CPS. In such a circumstance, the psychological distress of a patient may be interpreted as a reaction to a primarily nociceptive process. Personality and psychological factors are part and parcel of the matrix and origin of chronic pain. Psychological therapy differs considerably between a circumstance where the psychological problem is reactive to an organic disorder, or is the substance of the basis of the problem. The approach of the psychologist in treatment is critical to a successful outcome.

Also, some psychologists are not trained in biofeedback, which is a key therapeutic component, particularly for patients with a myofascial CPS. Biofeedback is used to reduce muscular tension. The therapeutic effect of biofeedback is really twofold. The technique of treatment is such that the patient sees the tension of muscles measured graphically on a television screen. When the patient learns the relaxation technique, the muscular nature of the pain becomes apparent to the patient. That point is important to establish firmly the diagnosis, which often is suspect by the patient, as noted earlier. Thus, the biofeedback treatment directly helps reduce abnormal muscular tension and also gives the psychologist a better position from which to begin therapy that directly addresses psychological issues. Biofeedback can also be useful in chronic pain disorders associated with vascular changes, such as chronic migraine or reflex sympathetic dystrophy.

Biofeedback as the sole form of treatment for a CPS is not successful. It is only when biofeedback is used as a component of the cognitive-behavioral therapeutic approach that successful treatment emerges. The cognitive-behavioral approach includes traditional counseling, altering a patient's pain behavior, changing coping techniques, educating the patient about CPS, and addressing the issues of secondary gain. The psychologist must also educate and guide the nurses, physical therapists, and physician in cognitive-behavioral techniques, generally, and in specific reference to each individual patient.

Alternative and Complementary Techniques

Alternative and complementary medical therapies have gained in popularity in the last decade. For instance, some 40% of American patients seek chiropractic care for low back pain.[12] Because chronic low back pain accounts for 50% or more of the patients treated in an MPTP, many programs have added chiropractic manipulation to the therapeutic regimen.[13,14] Although there are now a good number of prospective studies on the usefulness of chiropractic in certain acute myofascial conditions, the science-based data on acupuncture is not yet as secure. Acupuncture is often offered in pain management, but lacks adequate scientific documentation in the treatment of CPS. The National Institutes of Health have formed a center for complementary and alternative medicine, the National Center for Alternative and Complementary Medicine. That center is currently funding studies that include prospective studies of acupuncture effectiveness in the treatment of pain.

WHEN TO REFER A PATIENT TO A MULTIDISCIPLINARY PAIN TREATMENT PROGRAM

The CPS starts acutely. When a patient's history is couched in affective terminology; the patient demonstrates pain behaviors or emotions of anger, anxiety, or depression; or the intensity of the voiced pain is excessive for the underlying pathology, early referral to an MPTP should be made. Even when the clinical circumstance is acute, referral should occur as soon as the diagnosis of a CPS is suspected, because of the manner in which the patient presents. Delay in referral costs average more than $25,000 per patient who is on workman's compensation, which is enough to pay for the treatment of three patients.[15] It is also clear that the longer a patient with CPS is away from work, the less likely that there will be a successful outcome of therapy,[8] consequently early referral to an MPTP is clinically imperative as well.

Since psychological and behavioral phenomena play such a major role in the patient with a CPS, psychological testing is of value in helping to establish that a patient has a CPS.[16] It is not necessary to have every patient a neurosurgeon sees with a pain problem carry out testing as extensive as the MMPI. The pain drawing has been found to be a reliable method of determining when psychological or motivational factors may be playing a significant role in a patient's complaint of pain.[17] The pain drawing does not consume as much time and effort as does filling out and charting the MMPI and many other psychological tests, thus it is valuable as a screening device. The decision whether or not to operate should not be made solely on the pain drawing, however.

Most patients with CPS complain of cervical, thoracic, or low back symptoms. Other syndromes best treated in an MPTP setting include chronic pelvic pain in women,[18] chronic genital pain in men,[19] temporomandibular disorders without primary joint disease,[20,21] atypical facial pain, reflex sympathetic dystrophy also referred to as chronic regional pain syndrome,[22,23] and patients with rheumatoid arthritis.[24] The biopsychosocial model of patient care is spreading into many aspects of general medicine, particularly where the disease process is chronic.

When a patient requires heavy or persistent use of narcotic medications, it should be a signal to the surgeon that there may be a CPS. One important study found that physicians prescribe narcotic medications primarily on the basis of observed pain behavior demonstrated by the patient, rather than the voiced complaint of the patient or the ongoing disease process.[25] Pain behaviors that are associated with patient requests for narcotic medication should lead to referral to an MPTP.

Although persistent pain that occurs in patients with cancer is often recurrent acute nociceptive pain related to infiltration of the tumor, the psychological distress of the patient may also be expressed with behavior similar to that found in CPSs. In those circumstances, referral to an MPTP is quite in order.[26]

EVALUATION IN A MULTIDISCIPLINARY PAIN TREATMENT PROGRAM

Initial Evaluation in a Multidisciplinary Pain Treatment Program

During the initial evaluation of a patient in an MPTP, a history is taken by each of the core team members, nurse, physician, psychologist, and PT. The physical examination of the physician and the therapist focus on the main area of pain complaint, and also includes a general examination, appropriate to the patient's disorder. The PT also determines the patient's cardiopulmonary conditioning. Often, patients with CPS become deconditioned because of reduced activity levels associated with the CPS. Treatment of the CPS patient requires reconditioning as part of the process, so the level at which the patient is functioning during the evaluation phase is important. Stance and posture are also important aspects of the musculoskeletal examination because of the role these functions play in muscular tension. Many CPSs are related to work activities. Therefore, the PT, as well as the physician, must become informed about the patient's job and the ergonomics involved.

The examination by the psychologist is not only focused on the immediate pain problem. The psychological examination also includes a structured formal general psychological interview, which includes inquiry as far back as childhood and the dynamics of family interactions then as well as in the present. Secondary gain issues need to be probed. An interview with the patient's spouse or other significant person(s) in the patient's life is also important. The significant other interview provides another and often quite different perspective on the patient's condition as well as information about current interpersonal actions. Psychometric testing is carried out. The MMPI is the most commonly used test, but other tests that measure personality traits, levels of depression and anxiety, or feelings of dysfunction or disability may also be used.

The Initial Staffing Session

The staffing session is essentially the dynamic that broadens the view of the patient's problem for the staff of the MPTP. Objectivity requires the initial staffing session be carried out without the patient present. The history obtained from each professional is compared, as are physical findings and observations of behavior. In the current environment, most PTs and nurses are female, and the physician and psychologist often are males, although in many countries such may not be the case, and that situation, in North America at least, is rapidly changing. Gender differences between the health providers play a role in how the patient relates the history and the type of information offered. Furthermore, the patient's perception of the place the individual health professional occupies on the ladder of medical importance plays a significant role. Consequently, the information obtained historically from the patient by each of the core team members may differ considerably. These differences are critiqued in the staffing session, and add a perspective concerning the patient's attitude toward gender and medical professionals. That kind of knowledge will play an important role in planning the manner in which the patient's treatment is carried out, because modification of the patients' pain behavior is such an important part of the treatment.

Radiographic studies and pertinent past medical records are reviewed; the psychological testing is analyzed. Psychological testing has proven to be of considerable value in determining outcome of treatment as well as analyzing the patient's personality. For instance, it is recognized that inconsistency of scores on psychometric testing and two or more positive Waddell signs are predictors of patients anticipating financial compensation as part of their motivation,[27] and such a secondary gain must be taken into account when planning treatment. Dealing with the secondary gains is incorporated into the therapeutic approach and must not be ignored or left to others outside the team. The importance of the secondary gain from the patient's reported pain determines to a significant extent the outcome of treatment. If the secondary gain is very important to the patient and cannot be addressed therapeutically because of personality factors or motivation of the patient, therapy is unlikely to succeed. However, disability exaggeration, of itself, should not exclude a patient from therapeutic consideration because the outcome of therapy has been shown to be the same, whether or not the patient exaggerates disability.[28]

Patients who come from controlling and disorganized families and who are high on negative thinking require special attention to those components in the therapy program.[29] The team therefore needs insight into the family relations to plan appropriate therapy.

Outside information may play a significant part when the team is planning therapy. Often, this information is provided by a nurse, hired as a case manager by an insurance company, especially in workman's compensation and litigation-related cases. When any outside source is present at staffing sessions, the prior approval of the patient must be obtained, barring any medical or legal requirement to the contrary. For instance, in some regions an independent medical examination by an MPTP may be obtained by the insurance carrier or the legal representative of an insurance carrier, who can be at the staffing session without the approval of the patient being examined.

After analysis of all the information, the team decides whether or not treatment is needed and appropriate, and specifically what therapeutic program to recommend.

Intensive versus Customized Program

Patients whose chronic pain problem is associated with regular significant dysfunction in daily activities of living require an intensive approach therapeutically. Patients who are by and large housebound, or spend significant daily time at rest, or persistently seeking alternative diagnostic studies or treatments for the problem, or taking prescription and over-the-counter medications regularly throughout the day for the problem all qualify for an intensive treatment regimen. Patients who are addicted to medications may not require an intensive program, but those whose behavioral and verbal requests, especially for narcotics, are excessive will require intensive treatment. The intensive regimen is a daily program, lasting up to 8 hours per day, 5 days a week for 3 to 4 weeks.

Patients who are functioning fairly regularly at home or on the job, but who have a chronic pain problem that distresses them or their family enough to seek medical attention, will benefit from less intense therapy. Such programs consist of treatment sessions of from 2 to 3 hours, twice a week or so, for 6 to 8 weeks.

MULTIDISCIPLINARY TREATMENT

Techniques and Methods

The main course of therapy includes education, teaching behavioral and cognitive skills, stretch and exercise programs, medication reduction, goal setting and pacing, and relaxation training.[30] Education of the patient occurs in one-on-one therapy with PT and the psychologist, and in formal educational sessions by the nurse and physician. The myofascial and vascular components of chronic pain are discussed, as well as more generalized health concerns, such as the endocrine and adrenal effects of chronic anger that is so often a significant component of chronic pain.

The nurse-case manager coordinates the demographics of dealing with insurance carriers and outside rehabilitation workers assigned to the case, and also supervises the withdrawal of drugs on a scheduled basis.

Behavioral Methods

Interactions between the healthcare professionals and the patient are key in the appropriate functioning of a MPTP.[16] Therapy should be aimed at changing beliefs and altering cognitive coping strategies because this is correlated with good outcome.[31,32] The PT has the most lasting contact with the patient in day-to-day therapy, and conveys information regarding myofascial concepts through teaching and training, and contributes to alteration of patient behavior by supervising the patient response to pain during the diurnal fluctuation of discomfort. The psychologist teaches relaxation techniques, using electromyographic or skin temperature biofeedback, but this is intertwined with therapeutic counseling and practical goal-setting that must include dealing with secondary gain issues.

Dealing with Secondary Gain and Motivation

Patients applying for disability, and, by inference, those seeking financial compensation through litigation, respond poorly to an MPTP, unless those issues are dealt with as part of the therapeutic process.[33–37] The attitude and motivation of the patient with a CPS and that patient's support system determines whether the pain reported is allowed to be totally disabling,[37] and these factors must be confronted in a manner that supports altering such behavior. Anger is a significant component of the CPS. Dealing with the way a patient manages anger is therefore also an important part of an MPTP.[38] For instance, in males anger expression correlates negatively with outcome of increasing lifting capacity, whereas anger suppression correlates negatively with improvement in depression and general activities.

CPS patients have a less clear understanding of the diagnosis[39] and a belief that they have a different or more serious physiologic disorder than has been diagnosed.[8] But, beliefs about pain and attributes of pain control can be changed by therapy in an MPTP.[40] Education is thus an important component to an MPTP. Education of the patient improves outcome for the patient and reduces patient dissatisfaction with physician attempts to treat the condition.[39] Reduction of a patient's subjective feelings of disability is the most important predictor of success in pain rehabilitation, including eventual return to work.[41] Although all members of the core team participate in the behavioral aspect of an MPTP, the direct input of the psychologist is most useful for patients found to have perceived helplessness.[42]

Staffing Sessions and Coordination of Therapies

Two types of staffing sessions are held at least once per week. The working session is held without the patient present so that frank and open discussion regarding patient progress and motivation can be discussed, and alterations in the therapeutic plan can be made when needed. The second session is with the team and patient present together so that interaction with the entire team and the patient occurs. Any problems, including lack of motivation by the patient, are confronted in the session. Such confrontation is carried out in a manner planned according to the needs and personality of the patient. The psychologist plays a key role in such an interaction.

The goal is to produce a positive alteration of behavior on the part of the patient or, if needed, on the part of the staff.

OUTCOME OF TREATMENT USING A MULTIDISCIPLINARY PAIN TREATMENT PROGRAM

Prospective studies have demonstrated the value of MPTP in return to work and recreational activities, reduction of pain behavior and use of pain medication, as well as improved psychological well being and quality of life.[30,34,43–52] Intensive programs produce better results than less intense programs or those that offer physical therapy restoration techniques alone.[32,44,53] Long-term follow-up indicates that the good outcome persists in 50% of all patients selected for treatment.[54,55] Reduction of pain intensity and unpleasantness ranging from 33%[50] to 70%[56] have been reported, concurrent with reduction of pain medication by 72%, and elimination of all narcotics.[50,57]

Changes in the patient's behavior, that is, in cognitive-behavioral and physical capacity processes predict outcome of MPTP. The pretreatment medical history, physical impairment, and general physical variables have little predictive value in determining whether or not a patient will return to work after an MPTP.[8] Likewise, findings on diagnostic studies, such as computerized tomographic scanning, whether normal or demonstrating degenerative changes including bulges, protrusions, or stenosis, do not predict outcome of MPTP treatment.[13] Interestingly, positive responses to therapy are unrelated to a change in depression.[58]

Because the therapeutic approach of MPTP is focused on functional restoration,[53] and somatization complaints are managed in a consistent manner by all personnel on the therapy team, the presence of Waddell signs in chronic low back patients does not predict, by itself, a poor outcome to such therapy.[34] Factors that do predict poor outcome with MPTP are a high predominance of psychological factors,[53] a high degree of pain complaint, personality disorders, secondary gain, divorced marital status, unemployment, diffuse complaints, and postsurgery status.[4,59] As might be expected, working patients improve the most with MPTP. However, permanently unemployed patients on disability pension do as well with MPTP. Patients applying for disability, on the other hand, have the poorest response to MPTP.[33,35] Likewise, patients on workmen's compensation report more depression, pain, and disability than those that are not on compensation, both before and after rehabilitation.[36] The length of time a patient has been off of work correlates negatively with treatment outcome.[44] Smokers and patients with exposure to vibrations on the job are more likely to end up with a disability pension.[44] Patients who improve in isometric back muscle endurance are less likely to end up on a disability pension, and experience reduction of back pain level even at a 1-year follow-up after an MPTP.[44] The age of the patient correlates with outcome with regard to return to work.[60] Younger patients are more likely to return to work, whereas older patients tend to end up on disability pensions.[44] When patients undergoing MPTP are compared to a control group without therapy, 64% return to work, as opposed to 29% in the control group.[47] Long-term follow-up results of 1.5 to 2 years show stabilization of the outcome with 49% good job outcome, correlating with a 53% good feeling of well being. However,

38% persisted with a poor job outcome and 47% had the same or worse well being.[55] One report notes an 80% return to work at 4 years follow-up.[52] Treated patients have fewer sick days, less disability, less contact with healthcare professionals, and less intensity of pain.[47] In a prospective study, at 6-month follow-up improvement was significant in patients compared to controls in a quality-of-life questionnaire, anxiety, pain related to movements, psychosomatic symptoms, and need for pain-related medicines.[49]

Preinjury perceptions of the job, particularly job satisfaction, excessive physical demands, employee conflicts, job liking, job dangerousness, supervisory conflicts, job stress, and a voiced intent not to return to work are significant negative predictors of return to work after MPTP.[41,60,61] A pessimistic belief that the patient cannot return to the former occupation is a significant negative predictor of outcome.[59] Women are twice as likely to return to work as men.[44]

MPTPs have changed the clinical response to patient complaints of chronic pain. Clearly, patients who are somaticizing, and those with significant psychological distress and personality disorders, are not candidates for surgical interventions that are primarily aimed at relieving pain. The alternative treatment of rehabilitation is certainly more effective than surgical intervention in such instances, and far less destructive, but rehabilitation does not solve all patients' problems. Research resulting from the application of MPTP to chronic pain syndromes has enlarged the medical view of pain and pain treatment. The biopsychosocial model developed as a result has had application for medicine at large. The learning process is far from complete. Neuroimaging with functional magnetic resonance imaging is beginning to shed light on the cerebral experience in pain. Studies on the now recognized psychological matrix in chronic pain syndromes are more frequent and more scientifically oriented, providing insight into better methods of successful therapies. The multidisciplinary approach to evaluation and treatment remains at this time the best method for achieving good therapeutic results.

REFERENCES

1. Adler RH, Zamboni P, Hofer T, et al. How not to miss a somatic needle in the haystack of chronic pain. J Psychosomatic Research 42(5):499–505, 1997.
2. Gaines WG Jr, Hegmann KT. Effectiveness of Waddell's nonorganic signs in predicting a delayed return to regular work in patients experiencing acute occupational low back pain. Spine 24(4):396–400; discussion 401; 1999.
3. Novy DM, Collins HS, Nelson DV, et al. Waddell signs: distributional properties and correlates. Arch Phys Med Rehabil 79(7):820–822, 1998.
4. Elkayam O, Ben Itzhak S, Avrahami E, et al. Multidisciplinary approach to chronic back pain: prognostic elements of the outcome. Clin Exp Rheumatol 14:281–288, 1996.
5. Maruta T, Goldman S, Chan CW, et al. Waddell's nonorganic signs and Minnesota Multiphasic Personality Inventory profiles in patients with chronic low back pain. Spine 22(1):72–75, 1997.
6. Vendrig AA, de Mey HR, Derksen JJ, van Akkerveeken PF. Assessment of chronic back pain patient characteristics using factor analysis of the MMPI-2: which dimensions are actually assessed? Pain 76(1–2):179–188, 1998.
7. Sullivan MJ, Stanish W, Waite H, Sullivan M, Tripp DA. Catastrophizing, pain, and disability in patients with soft tissue injuries. Pain 77(3):253–260, 1998.
8. Pfingsten M, Hildebrandt J, Leibing E, Franz C, Saur P. Effectiveness of a multimodal treatment program for chronic low-back pain. Pain 73(1): 77–85, 1997.
9. Schofferman J, Anderson D, Hines R, Smith G, Keane G. Childhood psychological trauma and chronic refractory low-back pain. Clin J Pain 9(4):260–265, 1993.

10. Sherry DD, Weisman R. Psychologic aspects of childhood reflex neurovascular dystrophy. Pediatrics 81(4):572–578, 1988.

11. Schofferman J, Anderson D, Hines R, Smith G, White A. Childhood psychological trauma correlates with unsuccessful lumbar spine surgery. Spine 17(Suppl 6):S138–S144, 1992.

12. Waddell G. Low back pain: a twentieth century health care enigma. Pain 21(24):2820–2825, 1996.

13. Elkayam O, Avrahami E, Yaron M. The lack of prognostic value of computerized tomography imaging examinations in patients with chronic non-progressive back pain. Rheumatol Int 16:19–21, 1996.

14. Elkayam O, Ben Itzhak S, Avrahami E, et al. Multidisciplinary approach to chronic back pain: prognostic elements of the outcome. Clin Exp Rheumatol 14:281–288, 1996.

15. Gallagher RM, Myers P. Referral delay in back pain patients on worker's compensation. Psychosomatics 37(3):270–284, 1996.

16. Boureau F, Luu M, Doubere JF. Principles of organization of a center for pain evaluation and treatment. Rev Med Interne 16(9):696–704, 1995.

17. Chan CW, Goldman S, Ilstrup DM, Kunselman AR, O'Neill PI. The pain drawing and Waddell's nonorganic physical signs in chronic low-back pain. Spine 18(13):1717–1722, 1993.

18. Reiter RC. Evidence-based management of chronic pelvic pain. Clin Obstet Gynecol 41(2):422–435, 1998.

19. Costabile RA, Hahn M, McLeod DG. Chronic orchialgia in the pain prone patient: the clinical perspective. J Urol 146(6):1571–1574, 1991.

20. Foreman PA. The changing focus of chronic temporomandibular disorders: management within a hospital-based, multidisciplinary centre. NZ Dent J 94(415):23–31, 1998.

21. Cooper BC, Cooper DL. Multidisciplinary approach to the differential diagnosis of facial, head and neck pain. J Prosthet Dent 66(1):72–78, 1991.

22. Wilder RT, Berde CB, Wolohan M, Vieyra MA, Masek BJ, Micheli LJ. Reflex sympathetic dystrophy in children. Clinical characteristics and follow-up of seventy patients. J Bone Joint Surg (Am) 74(6):910–919, 1992.

23. Geertzen JH, de Bruijn H, de Bruijn-Kofman AT, Arendzen JH. Reflex sympathetic dystrophy: early treatment and psychological aspects. Arch Phys Med Rehabil 75(4):442–446, 1994.

24. Vliet Vlieland TP, Breedvold FC, Hazes JM. The two-year follow-up of a randomized comparison of in-patient multidisciplinary team care and routine out-patient care for active rheumatoid arthritis. Br J Rheumatol 36(1):82–85, 1997.

25. Turk DC, Okifuji A. What factors affect physicians' decisions to prescribe opioids for chronic noncancer pain patients? Clin J Pain 13(4):330–336, 1997.

26. Gaston-Johansson F, Ohly KV, Fall-Dickson JM, Nanda JP, Kennedy MJ. Pain, psychological distress, health status, and coping in patients with breast cancer scheduled for autotransplantation. Oncol Nurs Forum 26(8):1337–1345, 1999.

27. Hayes B, Soloym CA, Wing PC, Berkowitz J. Use of psychometric measures and nonorganic signs in detecting nomogenic disorders in low back patients. Spine 18(10):1254–1259, 1993.

28. Hazard RG, Bendix A, Fenwick JW. Disability exaggeration as a predictor of functional restoration outcomes for patients with chronic low-back pain. Spine 16(9):1062–1067, 1991.

29. Tota-Faucette ME, Gil KM, Williams DA, Keefe FJ, Goli V. Predictor of response to pain management treatment. The role of family environment and changes in cognitive processes. Clin J Pain 9(2):115–123, 1993.

30. Williams AC, Nicholas MK, Richardson PH, et al. Evaluation of a cognitive behavioural programme for rehabilitating patients with chronic pain. Br J Gen Pract 43(377):513–518, 1993.

31. Jensen MP, Turner JA, Romano JM. Correlates of improvement in multidisciplinary treatment of chronic pain. J Consult Clin Psychol 62(1):172–179, 1994.

32. Pither CE, Nicholas MK. Psychological approaches in chronic pain management. Br Med Bull 47(3):743–761, 1991.

33. Becker N, Hojsted J, Sjogren P, Eriksen J. Sociodemographic predictors of treatment outcome in chronic non-malignant pain patients. Do patients receiving or applying for Disability Pension benefit from multidisciplinary pain treatment? Pain 77:279–287, 1998.

34. Polatin PB, Cox B, Gatchel RJ, et al. A prospective study of Waddell signs in patients with chronic low back pain. When they may not be predictive. Spine 22(14):1618–1621, 1997.

35. Ciccone DS, Just N, Bandilla EB. A comparison of economic and social reward in patients with chronic nonmalignant back pain. Psychosom Med 61(4):552–563, 1999.

36. Rainville J, Sobel JB, Hatrigan C, et al. The effects of compensation involvement on the reporting of pain and disability by patients referred for rehabilitation on chronic low back pain. Spine 22(17):2016–2024, 1997.

37. Aronoff GM, McAlary PW, Witkower A, et al. Pain treatment programs: do they return workers to the workplace? Occupational Medicine: State of the Art Reviews 3(1):123–136, 1988.

38. Burns JW, Johnson BJ, Devine J, et al. Anger management style and the prediction of treatment outcome among male and female chronic pain patients. Behav Res Ther 36(11):1051–1062, 1998.

39. Roth RS, Horowitz K, Bachman JE. Chronic myofascial pain: knowledge of diagnosis and satisfaction with treatment. Arch Phys Med Rehabil 79(8):966–970, 1998.

40. Lipchik GL, Milles K, Covington EC. The effects of multidisciplinary pain management treatment on locus of control and pain beliefs in chronic non-terminal pain. Clin J Pain 9(1):49–57, 1993.

41. Hildebrandt J, Pfingsten M, Saur P, et al. Prediction of success from a multidisciplinary treatment program for chronic low back pain. Spine 22(9):990–1001, 1997.

42. Jensen I, Nygren A, Gamberale F, et al. The role of the psychologist in multidisciplinary treatments for chronic neck and shoulder pain: a controlled cost-effectiveness study. Scand J Rehabil Med 27(1):19–26, 1995.

43. Johansson C, Dahl J, Jannert M, et al. Effects of a cognitive-behavioral pain-management program. Behav Res Ther 36(10):915–930, 1998.

44. Bendix AF, Bendix T, Haestrup C. Can it be predicted which patients with chronic low back pain should be offered tertiary rehabilitation in a functional restoration program? Spine 23(16):1775–1783, 1998.

45. Bendix AF, Bendix T, Labriola M, et al. Functional restoration for chronic low back pain. Two-year follow-up of two randomized clinical trials. Spine 23(6):717–725, 1998.

46. Bendix AF, Bendix T, Lund C, et al. Comparison of three intensive programs for chronic low back pain patients: a prospective, randomized, observer-blinded study with one-year follow-up. Scand J Rehabil Med 29(2):81–89, 1997.

47. Bendix AF, Bendix T, Vaegter K, et al. Multidisciplinary intensive treatment for chronic low back pain: a randomized, prospective study. Cleve Clin J Med 63(1):62–69, 1996.

48. Bendix AF, Bendix T, Ostenfeld S, et al. Active treatment programs for patients with chronic low back pain: a prospective, randomized, observer-blinded study. Eur Spine J 4(3):148–152, 1995.

49. Grahn B, Ekdahl C, Borquist L. Effects of a multidisciplinary rehabilitation programme on health-related quality of life in patients with prolonged musculoskeletal disorders: a six month follow-up of a prospective controlled study. Disabil Rehabil 8:285–297, 1998.

50. Hubbard JE, Tracy J, Morgan SF, et al. Outcome measures of a chronic pain program: a prospective statistical study. Clin J Pain, 12(4): 330–337, 1996.

51. Mengshoel AM, Forseth KO, Haugen M, et al. Multidisciplinary approach to fibromyalgia. A pilot study. Clin Rheumatol 14(2):165–170, 1995.

52. Tyre TE, Walworth DE, Tyre EM. The outcome status of chronic pain patients 4 years after multidisciplinary care. Wisc Med J 93(1):9–12, 1994.

53. Rosomoff HL, Rosomoff RS. Comprehensive multidisciplinary pain center approach to the treatment of low back pain. Neurosurg Clin North Am 2(4):877–890, 1991.

54. Maruta T, Swanson DW, McHardy MJ. Three year follow-up of patients with chronic pain who were treated in a multidisciplinary pain management center. Pain 41(1):47–53, 1990.

55. Lanes TC, Gauron EF, Spratt KF, et al. Long-term follow-up of patients with chronic back pain treated in a multidisciplinary rehabilitation program. Spine 20(7):801–806, 1995.

56. Gil IA, Barbosa CM, Pedro VM, et al. Multidisciplinary approach to chronic pain from myofascial pain dysfunction syndrome: a four-year experience at a Brazilian center. Cranio 16(1):17–25, 1998.

57. Deardorff WW, Rubin HS, Scott DW. Comprehensive multidisciplinary treatment of chronic pain: a follow-up study of treated and non-treated groups. Pain 45(1):35–43, 1991.

58. Burns JW, Johnson BJ, Mahoney N, et al. Cognitive and physical capacity process variables predict long-term outcome after treatment of chronic pain. J Consult Clin Psychol 66(2):434–439, 1998.

59. Burns JW, Sherman ML, Devine J, et al. Association between workers' compensation and outcome following multidisciplinary treatment for chronic pain: roles of mediators and moderators. Clin J Pain 11(2):94–102, 1995.

60. Fishbain DA, Rosomoff HL, Cutler RB, et al. I. Do chronic pain patients' perceptions about their preinjury jobs determine their intent to return to the same type of job post-pain facility treatment? Clin J Pain 11(4):267–278, 1995.

61. Fishbain DA, Cutler RB, Rosomoff HL, et al. Impact of chronic pain patients' job perception variables on actual return to work. Clin J Pain 13(3):197–206, 1997.

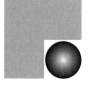

C H A P T E R 3 2

Disability and Impairment in the Patient with Pain

RICHARD L. STIEG, MD, MHS

There is evidence that the number of persons assigned to disability status is growing at an alarming rate in many countries. The factors related to pain and disability have been extensively studied but, it seems, these are largely ignored within medical entitlement systems and by most practicing physicians.[1,2] This is not surprising, given the multifactorial nature of disability. Physical, psychological, and social issues all play a role in the development of disability. These multiple variables make scientific study of disability exceptionally difficult.

The purpose of this chapter is to briefly outline some of the issues, to discuss attempts at measuring disability, and, most importantly, to discourage practicing physicians from engaging in formal disability assessment procedures on their patients.

ON THE NATURE OF IMPAIRMENT AND DISABILITY

Although the concept of disability dates back hundreds of years, disability benefit programs are a phenomenon of the modern era.[3] Such programs were developed to provide injured or sick individuals with resources to help regain access to competitive opportunities in society. In this century, the concept of disability in modern countries has broadened considerably as a result of several interactive factors:

1. Improved societal resources for those unable to resume fully productive roles
2. The decreasing role of the family as an agency of social welfare
3. An increasing awareness and expanding body of knowledge about mind/body inseparability
4. Improved resources for remediating the disabled[1]

There are significant distinctions and considerable confusion between impairment and disability. Impairment has been defined by the World Health Organization as "any loss or abnormality of psychological, physiological, or anatomic structure or function." The AMA Guides to the Evaluation of Impairment, 4th Edition, defines impairment as "an alteration

of an individual's health status." Permanent impairment occurs when that status "has become static or stabilized during a period of time sufficient to allow optimal tissue repair and one that is unlikely to change in spite of further medical or surgical therapy." Under most definitions it is implied that impairment must be assessed by medical means and is a medical issue.

In contrast, the World Health Organization defines disability as "any restriction or lack (resulting from an impairment) of ability to perform an activity in the manner or within the range considered normal for a human being." The AMA Guides define it as "an alteration of an individual's capacity to meet personal, social, or occupational demands or statutory or regulatory requirements because of an impairment." The Social Security Act defines disability as "the inability to work at any substantial gainful activity because of a medically determinable physical or mental impairment expected to result in death or to last for at least 12 months."

In contrasting impairment and disability, a few further distinctions are notable:

1. Impairment is generally determined medically, while disability is generally determined legally and is variably defined under different entitlement systems.
2. Either impairment or disability can exist in the absence of the other. As an example, an individual who is a violinist may, under a workman's compensation law, be unimpaired because of a fall that has resulted in malfunctioning of a small finger. Yet that same injury can be exceedingly disabling if it significantly affects the individual's ability to continue earning a living at his or her customary job.
3. Although determined medically, impairment is still significantly modified by regulatory requirements, especially in the workman's compensation arena. For example, in Colorado under the Workman's Compensation Act, all impairment ratings must be based on the Third Edition (Revised) of the AMA Guides and "a physician cannot rate chronic pain without anatomical or physiological correlation."

These definitions clearly indicate the multifactorial nature of impairment and disability and the influence of entitlement systems on those definitions. Issues about the relationship of pain and disability (as, for example, noted in the definition of disability under Social Security) include, but are certainly not limited to:

1. Poor correlation among pain, pathologic and anatomic findings, functional performance, and the probability that various medical interventions will restore normal functioning
2. A reductionistic and pervasive medical logic that symptoms can be explained on the basis of anatomic or physiologic findings while ignoring or discounting psychosocial confounding issues[4–6]
3. Great variability in definitions and benefits among various disability entitlement programs in which the physician may be asked to participate in decisions about his or her patient that can have far-reaching physical and psychosocial consequences
4. Ethical problems for treating physicians such as: a) attending to system/societal needs, which might be in conflict with the needs of their individual patients; b) taking on medical and social roles for which one may be poorly trained; or c) potentially harming one's own patients by participation in the process of impairment and disability determinations

PHYSICIAN PARTICIPATION IN IMPAIRMENT RATINGS

Impairment determinations should be made by physicians who are not, and do not plan to be, involved in the treatment of the patient in question. These physicians should have special training, insight, and interest in evaluating impaired individuals for the purpose of helping to arrive at legal/regulatory determination of disability. Knowledge of the medical problems being evaluated is essential, as is recognition of the psychosocial issues that may be confounding factors. Numerous studies indicate that psychosocial factors are often paramount in the eventual production of disability.[1] In the workman's compensation arena, an individual's work status, job performance, employer benefit package, satisfaction with work, family support system, preexisting or concurrent psychological issues, and/or preexisting personality profile may all play a significant role in an individual's perception of impairment and disability. Impairment, therefore, cannot be measured simply in physical terms. In an earlier publication, I attempted to make that point very clear.[5] In that publication, I pointed out that the most appropriate way of evaluating impairment in patients with chronic pain was either directly or indirectly through the use of multidisciplinary services. It is beyond the scope of most practicing physicians to be able to fully evaluate and comprehend all of the medical, physical, and psychosocial issues during the course of an impairment evaluation. Special training for physicians in this emerging field of medicine is readily available (see Appendix).

For physicians who may be developing an interest in doing impairment ratings, a good place to start would be the American Medical Association Guides to the Evaluation of Permanent Impairment. There are several editions of this document. The 4th edition is the one most commonly used at present. I would recommend beginning by studying the index on page 354 of the 4th edition of the Guides. Think anatomically. The Guides are arranged from caudad to cephalad in Chapters 3 and 4 (the musculoskeletal and nervous systems). Learn about the confusing areas and where to obtain additional help. For Pain Medicine physicians, a study of Chapter 15 of the 4th edition is particularly important. This chapter calls for transcending the usual biomedical model in the evaluation of impairment for patients in pain (as just discussed above). At the same time, it acknowledges problems relating to evaluating pain, pointing out that many of them cannot be solved. Ambiguities and areas of confusion exist. Additionally, the guidelines may be altered or changed by regulatory demands in different entitlement venues. As one reads further about how to deal with pain and impairment, the "general measurement principles" on page 112 are also important. Here it states that "pain, fear of injury or neuromuscular inhibition may limit mobility by diminishing the patient's effort, leading to inaccurately low readings in the absence of any objective evidence of significant disease." It goes on to say that an impairment is valid "only if there is medical evidence of a documented injury or illness with a physiological residual." Impairment, however, may be valid and not involve anatomic or physiologic changes if there is documented bonafide psychiatric illness related to an injury or medical problem. Further problems in the use of the Guides for patients in pain, including those suffering with complex regional pain syndrome (formerly called RSD) have been discussed elsewhere and underscore the ambiguities in the use of the widely accepted "standard" for measuring impairment as published in the AMA Guides, 4th edition.[7]

THE PRACTICING PHYSICIAN AND THE PRODUCTION OF IATROGENIC DISABILITY

Failure to understand the multifactorial nature of impairment and disability can lead to a perpetuation of the biomedical approach to treatment. It is not uncommon in my practice to see patients who have had dozens of physical tests and treatment interventions, many of which are of unproven utility, only to suffer inexorable and progressive loss of functionality, physical and emotional health, and loss of spirit. While there is little "scientific" data to prove my point, I find it impossible not to intuit that such prolonged lack of success, coupled with overdependency on physicians practicing in that manner, significantly contribute to the perception of disability in these individuals. Physicians alone, however, should not have to bear the brunt of the responsibility for creating iatrogenic disability. A task force on back pain convened in 1992 and 1993 boldly challenged and called for sweeping systems changes in a controversial monograph to which I have referred several times in this chapter.[1] This work, like that from many other pain medicine visionaries, points out the enormous responsibility of society in general, and physicians in particular, in properly evaluating and caring for the disabled among us.

PROBLEMS IN RATING PAIN AS AN IMPAIRMENT

Pain is subjective and must be correlated in most impairment rating systems with objective evidence of anatomic abnormalities and/or physiologic disturbance and/or pertinent psychosocial issues. The examiner must rely on his or her skill and experience in applying this biopsychosocial (as opposed to biomedical) model to the rating. Working within a skilled team structure, when available, can be very helpful in this regard. The examiner should acknowledge and deal with the ethical issues he or she will confront in this arena. The relationship of pain to anatomic, physiologic, or psychosocial factors is often unclear and requires time, patience, and insightful thinking. Additionally, the examiner must understand the rules he or she is working under. Indeed, the 4th edition to the AMA Guides, Chapter 15, points out that "the physician's judgment about pain must be characterized not so much by scientific accuracy as by procedural regularity and should be evaluated by physicians who are conversant with this disorder."[8] The examiner should be a rating expert and should not be the treating physician.

Tools for rating impairment are inadequate. The AMA Guides, the most widely used tool, have widespread use and availability within training courses. They allow for some consistency in reporting from patient to patient. However, it has been demonstrated that there is very poor inter-rater reliability in the use of the guides.[7] The AMA Guides may not be the required guideline within a given entitlement system. As already discussed, when applied to patients with pain, the AMA Guides may be ambiguous and difficult to use.

Physicians often try to determine functionality through functional capacity testing. It is my belief, because of the multifactorial nature of impairment (particularly in the patient with chronic pain), that reliance on this kind of data alone is futile and should never be the only source of information used by an impairment rating physician.[5]

There are numerous psychological tests that have been normed on populations of patients with pain. The contribution of psychosocial factors in impairment is best determined by an experienced mental health professional who has knowledge of these test batteries.[2,4,5] Ideally, he or she has also interviewed the patient and fully examined all pertinent psychosocial issues.

CONCLUSIONS

This chapter has been written to introduce the concepts of impairment and disability. It is especially addressed to pain medicine physicians who should have an interest in the rela-

tionship of impairment and disability to pain. We have pointed out how physicians may, iatrogenically, help to produce a situation of disability. I believe treating physicians should not be involved in the formal process of evaluating impairment and disability. For those who choose to take on this responsibility as part of clinical practice, there are sources of information and formal training programs available. Many physicians, myself included, do this sort of specialty work in selected patients who are not under their care. I believe more pain medicine physicians should take on this additional responsibility in an effort to solve some of the social issues that have become a part of the growing disability problem in modern countries.[1]

REFERENCES

1. Fordyce WE (ed). Back Pain in the Workplace: Management of Disability in Nonspecific Conditions. Seattle, IASP Press, 1995.
2. Turk D, Rudi TE, Stieg RL. The disability determination dilemma: toward a multi-axial solution. PAIN 34:217–229, 1988.
3. Mendelson G. Psychiatric Aspects of Personal Injury Claims. Springfield, Ill, Charles C Thomas, 1988.
4. Kinsman R, Durks JF, Wunder J, Carbaugh R, Stieg R. Multidimensional analysis of peak pain symptoms and experiences. Psychother Psychosom 51:101–112, 1989.
5. Stieg RL. The futility of physical testing in the assessment of disability. APS J 3(3):187–190, 1994.
6. Stieg RL. Disability evaluations: medical/legal evaluations. In Wallace M, Staats P (eds). Just the Facts: Pain Medicine. Dubuque, Iowq, McGraw-Hill, 2003.
7. Stieg RL. Pain and the AMA guides to the evaluation of permanent impairment (4th ed). Disability 4(1):1–8, 1995.
8. AMA Guides to the Evaluation of Permanent Impairment (4th ed). Chicago, AMA, 1993, p. 304.

APPENDIX

Resources for Medical/Legal Training and Information

1. SEAK Incorporated Legal and Medical Information Systems: PO Box 729, Falmouth, MA 02541. www.seak.com
2. American Academy of Disability Evaluating Physicians. www.aadep.org
3. American Academy of Pain Medicine. www.painmed.org
4. American Medical Association. www.ama-assn.org
5. The Comprehensive Forensic Services Manual: *The Essential Resources for all Experts by Steven Babitsky, JD, James J. Mangraviti, Jr.* JD and Christopher J. Todd, JD, published SEAK Incorporated Legal and Medical Information Systems, 2000.

Outcome Assessment

NORMAN MARCUS, MD AND AMY BLEYER, MD

While the field of pain medicine is replete with disagreement, it is generally agreed that the modern practice of pain medicine/management is linked to the work of John Bonica, MD. Bonica recognized the multidetermined aspects of pain and encouraged assessment and treatment appropriate to the specific needs of each patient. In the preface to his second edition, he describes the purpose of his tome as "a reference source in helping to make or to confirm the correct diagnosis of complex pain problems and to deduce what therapy or combination of therapies should be carried out and what treatments should *not* be done . . . By providing appropriate guidelines, it is hoped that patients will be spared the risk of iatrogenic complications such as the development of chronic pain syndromes, drug toxicity, useless operations, and other ineffective therapies."[1]

Despite Bonica's cogent proposition made over a decade ago, the field of pain medicine has evolved in the absence of evidence-based guidelines. Treatment guidelines do exist for pain medicine practitioners,[2–7] but they are recommendations based on small studies, which lack the scientific rigor of the gold standard double-blinded randomized controlled trial (RCT). Even the guidelines produced by the Agency for Healthcare Policy and Research (AHCPR) in their 1994 clinical practice guideline for acute low back problems in adults lacked the support of any large scale RCTs.[2]

Although pain is the most common reason for visits to the physician's office,[8] there is little cross-specialty, and often times little intra-specialty agreement among physicians as to how to approach the patient who has pain.[9–13] There is no algorithm that physicians have agreed on to utilize in their approach to the patient with pain because there is a relative dearth of data proving that any approach actually achieves distinctly superior outcomes. In contrast to objective outcome measurement in patients who undergo angioplasty or antibiotic treatment for infectious disease, pain treatment outcome is more difficult to codify.[14,15] The variables that should be assessed include pain intensity, functional capacity, medication use, return to work, mood, and satisfaction with treatment.

In the attempt to determine how to best approach the patient with pain, the field of pain medicine, therefore, turned to the outcomes movement[16] and has attempted to collect data that is universal to all practitioners of pain medicine. If all practitioners could actually compare their patients before and after any intervention(s), we could begin to establish evidence-based guidelines that are based on meaningful data. It would be ideal if there was a single instrument, such as a self-report questionnaire, that patients could complete before and after treatment that would reflect whether or not the intervention achieved its stated outcomes. By using the knowledge and tools of the outcomes movement, and with the assistance of public health organizations (i.e., the AHCPR) the field of pain medicine has begun to define for itself what are reasonable and meaningful outcomes to measure and how to accomplish such measurements in a reasonable and meaningful way.[17,18]

The Uniform Outcome Measures (UOM) project of the American Academy of Pain Medicine (AAPM) has demonstrated the potential for multisite data collection using uniform, standardized tools while reconfirming the complexity of administering such a project. There were major problems encountered in the UOM project, such as the significant respondent burden placed on physician practices that participated in the structured data gathering and the inability to provide validated reports that could be used in clinical practice for quality assurance, quality improvement, and presentation to insurance companies. If there is to be more universal data collection from individual clinicians, a user-friendly instrument is needed.

The AAPM's UOM project is working on such an instrument, but it is important for individual pain treatment practices to begin to measure their outcomes today. Although there are disagreements as to what constitutes proper outcome measures for pain treatment assessment, our suggestion, based on a review of the literature,[15] is to collect the data along the following six axes:

I. Demographics
II. Symptom presentation
III. Putative diagnosis
IV. Comorbid conditions
V. Quality of life
VI. Immediate and long-term costs

One of the goals of this chapter is to provide the tools necessary to assess the utility of any protocol for the treatment of pain. It has become critical that all practitioners ascertain the validity of any treatment approach for the specific condition being treated that is distinct from the technical success of the procedure itself. The reliance on technical proficiency in performing a procedure is no longer sufficient to satisfy the demands of data collection for the establishment of evidence-based treatment guidelines and proof of effectiveness of the intervention. The imperative to offer valid proof for the effectiveness of what we do has been exaggerated by the potential withholding of authorization and payment for a variety of treatments and procedures. Cost containment pressures have made evidence-based medicine a necessity rather than a wish.[19] More detailed data collection on clinical outcomes will allow physicians to provide their services to their patients with less interference from insurance carriers. Focused data collection is important in setting appropriate levels of expectation for treatment outcome. The awareness of comorbid states, such as depression and anxiety, family and work dysfunction, and physical deconditioning, will allow the physician to address these issues explicitly to enhance successful outcome and to understand why less than optimal outcomes are achieved with patients perceived as "excellent candidates for treatment."

Our collective experience as physicians has shown us that many interventions that we have used and many that we continue to implement, while having been perfected in their execution, are not the most reasonable treatments for the disease or symptoms being treated. Examples include gastrectomies for ulcer disease, implantation of the internal mammary artery for angina, chymopapain injection for intervertebral disk herniation,[20,21] and laminectomies, diskectomies, foraminotomies, and fusions for a variety of putative diagnoses of low back pain.[22–24] No doubt that some patients have done well with all of the above procedures as measured by some criteria; however, each of the above interventions has been challenged as being the best approach for their intended outcome and a few are no longer used. Some of our colleagues knew that the particular procedure they performed was not achieving success at acceptable levels before the official reevaluation by the organized medical community. Our goal is to provide the tools to each physician such that he or she is able to assess the appropriateness of their chosen procedures.[25]

Clinical research is difficult. The demands of the busy practice are frequently at odds with collecting data that appears to be extraneous to the immediate clinical problem. Given these constraints, we will present two different models: section A will present and discuss a wide range of possible data collection instruments for those readers who wish to consider a more detailed clinical research paradigm, and section B will present the authors' suggestions for a streamlined approach via a basic data collection module.

SECTION A

Each additional item of data we collect potentially increases the sensitivity and specificity of our outcomes. Unfortunately, each additional item of data collected increases the burden of data analysis as well as respondent burden. If we do not plan to use the data collected, and we are not engaged in a study where someone else plans to use the data, there is no good reason to collect more information than is absolutely necessary.

Assuming you will be performing your own data analysis, you must first devise a strategy to use all of the data collected

so that you have enough data to yield significant results yet aren't faced with extraneous, time-consuming data. Use of previously validated instruments is suggested wherever possible. This eases the burden of analysis and provides measures that will be understood by colleagues who will be familiar with the parameters assessed by a commonly used instrument.

Demographics

Important demographic variables are age, gender, marital status, work status, payer type, income, and educational level. All of these factors will contribute to defining distinct cohorts with unique characteristics surrounding their particular pain presentation.

Symptom Presentation

We like to employ the PQRST mnemonic, which is as follows:

P is for any *p*alliative or *p*rovocative factors (what exacerbates or alleviates the pain).
Q is for the *q*uality of pain (is the pain burning, shooting, stabbing, aching, etc.).
R is for *r*adiation of pain (yes or no).
S is for the *s*patial distribution (where is the pain).
T is for the *t*emporal aspect (is the pain constant or intermittent).

Once you have collected the above data with respect to the patient's symptoms, you will need to define how to address common presentations of pain. For example, low back pain is one of the most common complaints and is, in fact, a rather generic catchphrase for a plethora of diagnoses. With respect to low back pain, the UOM committee created subcategorized cohorts in their beta testing that were based on radiation and spatial distribution of low back pain. The three subcategories that were beta tested were (1) predominantly back pain without radiation, (2) back pain with radiation to the lower extremity, and (3) lower extremity pain. Just beware—the more subcategories to which to assign your data, the more difficult it will be for any given data collector to amass the numbers needed to produce reliable statistics.[18]

Putative Diagnoses

It is important to realize that imaging studies by themselves are not adequate to provide a reliable cause of back pain. It has been shown repeatedly that magnetic resonance imaging is frequently read as abnormal in asymptomatic individuals[26–28]; therefore, an abnormal study is not diagnostic merely because it is coexistent with a specific pain syndrome. Imaging studies should confirm your putative diagnosis and *not* be used as a means by which to make a diagnosis.[29] The authors suggest that even in any case where radiographic evidence appears to be explicit as a diagnostic criteria, you also delineate the associated clinical factors that support the putative diagnosis. For example, spinal stenosis and disk herniation are common diagnoses often assigned to patients who report low back pain and are based solely on the chief complaint and imaging studies. We suggest that you further define these diagnoses using explicit diagnostic criteria such as follows:

- *Spinal stenosis*: low back pain associated with one out of three of the following: pseudoclaudication, stooped posture when weight bearing, and inability to stand erect.
- *Disk herniation*: patients must present with three of the following six additional criteria: radicular sensory loss, radicular weakness, radicular pain, decreased reflexes, sphincter incontinence, and progression of any or all symptoms over days or weeks.

These descriptors were chosen as examples of what could be used to more specifically define a patient cohort. You may, however, choose different descriptors. What is important to realize is that any explicit definitions of how a diagnosis is derived, which are then consistently applied to your diagnostic data, will elevate your data above the norm and increase the power of your outcomes measurement.

Comorbid Conditions

Conditions that are commonly accepted as exacerbating a pain state or making treatment more difficult should be considered. Diabetes mellitus with its frequent neuropathies and less frequent soft tissue problems would be an important cohort modifier, i.e., _____ pain with diabetes mellitus type 1 or 2. Collecting such data will allow you to have more discrete outcome groups and less confounded analyses.

Psychological comorbidity is particularly important in our patients with pain. Depression, coexisting with persistent pain, has been shown in a number of studies to be associated with diminished physical and emotional functioning.[30,31]

Depression and anxiety scales are almost universally collected in large back pain outcome studies because psychological disturbance systematically affects patients' pain experience.[32,33] Two of the most commonly used instruments to assess depression are the Beck[34] and the Hamilton[35] inventories. Two commonly used scales to assess anxiety are the Zung[36] and the Spielberger.[37–39] It is crucial to document psychological comorbidity because it may be the cause of or the result of the pain syndrome. Depression may be associated with lower levels of serotonin, which can diminish the effectiveness of endogenous opiates. Anxiety may increase the perception of pain and result in pain through its expression as muscle tension.

Quality of Life Measures

Quality of life (QOL) is probably the most useful and important measure of outcome that is generally collected. QOL measures reflect the physical and emotional function of the individual and are considered as a true test of clinical effectiveness for an intervention. The standard QOL measure has been the SF-36.[40–43] The SF-36 was normalized on a chronic illness population and, therefore, is not specific for a chronic pain population.[44] Adding pain-specific items to the SF-36 created enhanced pain-specific QOL measures (TOPS; SF-61).[45] These instruments are more sensitive to small pain-related functional changes that may be missed on the SF-36. Those wishing to use an abbreviated, albeit less sensitive, measure could use the SF-12, which is an abbreviated, validated version of the SF-36.[46,47]

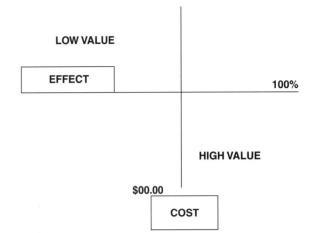

FIGURE 33-1 Cost vs. effect. Because "value" in healthcare is defined as the amount of effect per unit of cost, one can determine whether an intervention is of low value or high value.

Cost

Cost for a treatment is a relative factor. You may have an inexpensive procedure with poor results or an expensive procedure with excellent results. Therefore, it is useful to discuss the *value* of an intervention where *value* is defined as the effect of the intervention divided by its cost[48] (Fig. 33-1).

Various outcomes researchers have published quite different results of similar or equivalent interventions. For example, two studies of the success of spinal fusion surgeries for chronic low back pain had diametrically opposite results based on the different postoperative patient queries that were used to determine the success of the procedure.[49,50] Before determining an intervention's ultimate value, you must first define what are your desired, or ideal, results. These "ideal" results equal 100% effectiveness. Once you have defined your ideal results, you will then be able to quantify the effect of your intervention by comparing its effect, or results, with your predetermined ideal. Once the effect of your intervention is established, your cost data will become meaningful via its *value* analysis. Based on Figure 33-1, the clinician should aim for *value* outcomes in the lower right quadrant and avoid outcomes in the left upper quadrant.

Cost may be misleading. Early, successful, costly intervention may, in the long term, be cost-effective based on reduced post-treatment cost. Included in any cost analysis needs to be a consideration of the cost of care before and after treatment. The cost of treatment is factored into the post-treatment cost to compare the *value* of the treatment provided. If the post-treatment cost is not less or the functional capacity of the individual is not more over time, then the intervention was not of great value (Fig. 33-2).

SECTION B

It is important for even the most overextended clinician to have a useful data collection system that will allow quality assurance and improvement of their practice. When we present our

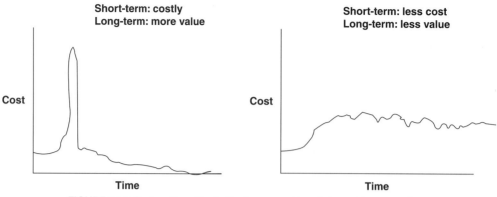

FIGURE 33-2 Cost vs time: Cost-effectiveness of two interventions over time.

"positive" treatment results to our colleagues or insurance carriers, we are frequently asked "where is your data?" If pain is an important indexed symptom, we should at least record measures of pain intensity, pain relief, and mood alteration as they relate to our various interventions. The Memorial Pain Assessment Card (MPAC) is an easy to administer test that assesses these fundamental parameters. The MPAC is a simple instrument that was designed to provide rapid evaluation of pain intensity, pain relief, and psychological distress in patients with pain related to cancer.[51] Because the important parameters concerning pain treatment success (pain intensity, pain relief, and mood alteration) are constant across disease states and only vary with respect to the relative importance of each variable, the MPAC can be used as a simple measure of outcome for **any** pain treatment. The four indices measured are pain intensity via a visual analogue scale *and* a categorical rating; pain relief via a visual analogue scale; and mood also via a visual analogue scale. The MPAC is merely a single card that is folded in half and presents these four scales for the patient to complete (Fig. 33-3).

Although the instrument was normalized on a cancer population, it does provide global measures of pain intensity, relief, and psychological distress that can be distinctively assessed. Because of the problems with respondent burden that are replete in using any of the validated instruments described previously, it is our belief that use of the MPAC along with a demographic analysis and cohort definition based on the six factors noted previously will suffice to allow the practicing clinician to systematically assess their interventions for effectiveness.

The MPAC or any other pain assessment instrument should be administered at each patient visit and before and after any procedures that may decrease or increase the patient's pain. The data can be recorded on the progress note itself or on a separate pain assessment sheet. Below is an example of how to incorporate the MPAC data into the medical record (Fig. 33-4).

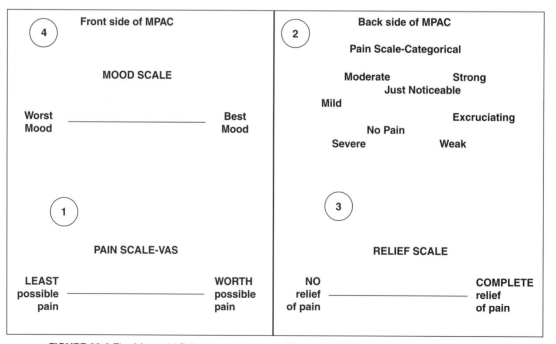

FIGURE 33-3 The Memorial Pain assessment card. The card is folded in half and each scale is presented to the patient individually.

Date	3/10/01	3/24/01
Pain-VAS	6	7
Pain-Categorical	Moderate	Strong
Mood-VAS	4	3
Analgesic Orders: Med-Analgesic	MSIR po	MSIR po
Dose	30/4h; 8/1 h prn	45/4h; 15/1h prn
Adjuvant Analgesic	APAP 650 qid po	same

FIGURE 33-4 Incorporation of the MPAC data into the medical record.

"Opinion breeds ignorance, while facts produce wisdom." (Hippocrates)

Let us all join together to accumulate facts to improve our collective wisdom, improve our patient care, and reestablish physicians and allied clinicians as the proper stewards of our beloved profession.

REFERENCES

1. Bonica JJ. The Management of Pain (2nd ed). Philadelphia, Lea & Febiger, 1990, p vii.
2. Bigos S, Bowyer O, Braen G, et al. Acute Low Back Problems in Adults. Clinical Practice Guideline No. 14. AHCPR Publication no. 95–0642. Rockville, MD: Agency for Health Care Policy and Research, Public Health Service, U.S. Department of Health and Human Services, December 1994.
3. Stanton-Hicks M, Baron R, Boas R, et al. Complex regional pain syndromes: guidelines for therapy. Clinical Journal of Pain 14(2):155–166, 1998.
4. Rose VL. Guidelines from the American Geriatric Society target management of chronic pain in older persons. Am Fam Phys 58(5):1213–1214, 1217, 1998.
5. McGrath PA. Development of the World Health Organization guidelines on cancer pain relief and palliative care in children. J Pain Symptom Management 12(2):87–92, 1996.
6. Finley RS. Clinical practice guidelines for the management of cancer pain. Cancer Pract 2(3):236–238, 1994.
7. Jacox A, Carr DB, Payne R. New clinical-practice guidelines for the management of pain in patients with cancer. N Engl J Med 330(9):651–655, 1994.
8. Nelson C, Woodwell D. National Ambulatory Medical Care Survey: 1993 summary. Vital & Health Statistics, series 13: Data from the National Health Survey. U.S. Department of Health and Human Services, 136:iii–vi, 1–99, 1998 April.
9. Cherkin DC, Deyo RA, Wheeler K, Ciol MA. Physician variation in diagnostic testing for low back pain: who you see is what you get. Arthr Rheum 37:15–22, 1994.
10. Cherkin DC, Deyo RA, Loeser JD, Bush T, Waddell G. An international comparison of back surgery rates. Spine 19:1201–1206, 1994.
11. Carey TS, Garrett J, North Carolina Back Pain Project. Patterns of ordering diagnostic tests for patients with acute low back pain. Ann Intern Med 125:807–814, 1996.
12. Osterweis M, Kleinman A, Mechanic D, eds. Pain and Disability: Clinical, Behavioral, and Public Policy Perspectives. Washington, DC, National Academy Press, 1987.
13. Swedlow A, Johnson G, Smithline N, Milstein A. Increased costs and rates of use in the California workers' compensation system as a result of self-referral by physicians. N Engl J Med 327:1502–1506, 1992.
14. Farrar JT, Portenoy RK, Berlin JA, Kinman JL, Strom BL. Defining the clinically important difference in pain outcome measures. Pain 88:287–294, 2000.
15. Turk DC, Rudy TE, Sorkin BA. Neglected topics in chronic pain treatment outcome studies: determination of success. Pain 57(2):253–254, 1994.
16. Benjamin K. Outcomes research and the allied health professional. J All Health 24(1):3–12, 1995.
17. Marcus NJ. Establishing uniform outcome measures for pain treatment centers: the need and an effort. J Back Musculosk Rehabil 8(2):89–93, 1997.
18. Farrar JT. What is clinically meaningful: outcome measures in pain clinical trials. Clin J Pain 16:S106–S112, 2000.
19. Larson EB. Evidence-based medicine: is translating evidence into practice a solution to the cost-quality challenges facing medicine? Joint Commission Journal on Quality Improvement 25(9):480–485, 1999.
20. Javid MJ, Nordby EJ. Lumbar chymopapain nucleolysis. Neurosurg Clin North Am 7(1):17–27, 1996.
21. Nordby EJ, Wright PH. Efficacy of chymopapain in chemonucleolysis. A review. Spine 19(22):2578–2583, 1994.
22. Porchet F, Vader JP, Larequi-Lauber T, Costanza MC, Burnand B, Dubois RW. The assessment of appropriate indications for laminectomy. J Bone Jt Surg 81B(2):234–239, 1999.
23. Mayer T, McMahon MJ, Gatchel RJ, Sparks B, Wright A, Pegues P. Socioeconomic outcomes of combined spine surgery and functional restoration in workers' compensation spinal disorders with matched controls. Spine 23(5):598–605, 1998.
24. Woertgen C, Rothoerl RD, Henkel J, Brawanski A. Long term outcome after cervical foraminotomy. J Clin Neurosci 7(4):312–315, 2000.
25. Phelps CE. The methodologic foundations of studies of the appropriateness of medical care. N Engl J Med 329(17):1241–1245, 1993.
26. Boden SD, Davis DO, Dina TS, Patronas NJ, Wiesel SW. Abnormal magnetic-resonance scans of the lumbar spine in asymptomatic subjects: a prospective investigation. J Bone Jt Surg Am 72:403–408, 1990.
27. Jensen MC, Brant-Zawadzki MN, Obuchowski N, Modic MT, Malkasian D, Ross JS. Magnetic resonance imaging of the lumbar spine in people without back pain. N Engl J Med 331:69–73, 1994.
28. Weishaupt D, Zanetti M, Hodler J, Bood N. MR imaging of the lumbar spine: prevalence of intervertebral disk extrusion and sequestration, nerve root compression, end plate abnormalities, and osteoarthritis of the facet joints in asymptomatic volunteers. Radiology 209:661–666, 1998.
29. Zimmerman RD. A review of utilization of diagnostic imaging in the evaluation of patients with back pain: the when and what of back pain imaging. J Back Musculosk Rehabil 8:125–133, 1997.
30. Gallagher RM, Mossey JM, Moree C, Lynch C. Impact of comorbid depression on self-reported pain and physical and emotional functioning in low back patients. Presented at the AAPM 17th annual meeting. February 2001, Miami Beach.
31. Mossey JM, Gallagher RM. Evaluation of the effects of pain and depression on the physical functioning of continuing care retirement residents: implications for the treatment of pain in older individuals. Presented at the AAPM 17th annual meeting. February 2001, Miami Beach.
32. Prieto EJ, Hopson L, Bradley LA, et al. The language of low back pain: factor structure of the McGill pain questionnaire. Pain 8(1):11–19, 1980.
33. McCreary C, Turner J, Dawson E. Principal dimensions of the pain experience and psychological disturbance in chronic low back pain patients. Pain 11(1):85–92, 1981.
34. Beck AT. Beamesderfer A. Assessment of depression: the depression inventory. Modern Probl Pharmacopsychiatry 7:151–169, 1974.
35. Hamilton M. Development of a rating scale for primary depressive illness. Br J Social Clin Psychol 6(4):278–296, 1967.
36. Zung WW. A rating instrument for anxiety disorders. Psychosomatics 12(6):371–379, 1971.
37. Spielberger CD, Gorusch RL, Lushene RE. Manual for the State-Trait Anxiety Inventory. Palo Alto, CA, Consulting Psychologists Press, 1970.
38. Spielberger CD. State-Trait Anxiety Inventory for Adults. Palo Alto, Calif, Mind Gardens, 1983.
39. Spielberger CD. State-Trait Anxiety Inventory: A Comprehensive Bibliography (2nd ed). Palo Alto, CA, Consulting Psychologists Press, 1989.
40. Ware JE Jr, Sherbourne CD. The MOS 36-item short-form health survey (SF-36). I. Conceptual framework and item selection. Med Care. 30(6):473–483, 1992.
41. McHorney CA, Ware JE Jr, Raczek AE. The MOS 36-Item Short-Form Health Survey (SF-36): II. Psychometric and clinical tests of validity in measuring physical and mental health constructs. Med Care 31(3):247–263, 1993.
42. McHorney CA, Ware JE Jr, Lu JF, Sherbourne CD. The MOS 36-item Short-Form Health Survey (SF-36): III. Tests of data quality, scaling assumptions, and reliability across diverse patient groups. Med Care 32(1):40–66, 1994.
43. Hays RD. Sherbourne CD. Mazel RM. The RAND 36-Item Health Survey 1.0 [see comments]. Health Econ 2(3):217–27, 1993.

44. Wagner A, Sukienik A, Kulich R, et al. Outcome assessment in chronic pain treatment: the need to supplement SF-36. Int Assoc Pain Newslett 8:2, 1996.

45. Rogers WH, Wittik H, Wagner A, Cynn D, Carr DB. Assessing individual outcomes during outpatient multidisciplinary chronic pain treatment by means of an augmented SF-36. Pain Med 1:44–54, 2000.

46. Ware J, Jr., Kosinski M, Keller SD. SF-12: A 12-item short-form health survey: Construction of scales and preliminary tests of reliability and validity. Med Care 34(3):220–233, 1996.

47. Ware J Jr, Kosinski M, Keller SD. SF-12: How to Score the SF-12 Physical and Mental Health Summary Scales (2nd ed). Boston, Health Institute, New England Medical Center, 1995.

48. Nelson EC, Mohr JJ, Batalden PB, Plume SK. Improving health care, Part 1: The clinical value compass. Joint Commission Journal on Quality Improvement 22(4):243–258, 1996.

49. Deyo RA, Ciol MA, Cherkin DC, Loeser JD, Bigos SJ. Lumbar spinal fusion. A cohort study of complications, reoperations, and resource use in the Medicare population. Spine 18(11):1463–1470, 1993.

50. Franklin GM. Haug J. Heyer NJ. McKeefrey SP. Picciano JF. Outcome of lumbar fusion in Washington State workers' compensation. Spine 19(17):1897–1903; discussion 1904; 1994.

51. Fishman B, Pasternak S, Wallenstein SL, Houde RW, Holland JC, Foley KM. The Memorial Pain Assessment Card: a valid instrument for the evaluation of cancer pain. Cancer 60:1151–1158, 1987.

C H A P T E R   3 4

Building (and Surviving) a Neurosurgical Pain Practice

ROBERT M. LEVY, MD, PhD

Surgical therapy for medically intractable pain represents a significant area of growth in neurosurgical practice. Nowhere is the issue of cross specialty practice competition more evident than in the setting of interventional pain management. Historically, the sole territory of neurosurgeons, surgical pain therapy has been largely assumed by other specialties, most notably anesthesia, over the past three decades.

Neurosurgeons have recently demonstrated a renewed interest in surgical pain management, due both to their inherent interest in the pathologic mechanisms of pain transmission and modulation as well as their desire to maintain and grow their clinical practice. As neurosurgeons increase their visibility to the community of pain management physicians and patients with chronic pain, they have almost universally rapidly recognized a busy practice in interventional pain management. With this growth in practice come many significant benefits, responsibilities, and challenges.

Surgical management of chronic pain problems can be particularly satisfying to the neurosurgeon. Patients with chronic pain represent complex clinical challenges for the neurosurgeon. These patients usually present with complex nervous system pathology, and understanding the underlying physiology of their problems can be challenging and intriguing. No other pain practitioners have the degree of experience and training in the fields of neurophysiology, neuroanatomy, neuropharmacology, and neuropathology, and this renders neurosurgeons as uniquely able to evaluate and treat these difficult clinical problems. Furthermore, no other specialty allows its practitioners the breadth of approaches available to treat these chronic pain syndromes. Medical management; neuroaugmentative procedures such as deep brain stimulation, spinal cord stimulation, and intraspinal drug administration; and neuroablative procedures such as cordotomy and dorsal root entry zone lesioning are all within the spectrum of neurosurgical practice. The neurosurgeon can offer the full breadth of therapeutic approaches to bear on chronic pain problems. Furthermore, interventional pain management can be uniquely satisfying. Most patients with chronic pain presenting to the neurosurgeon have failed aggressive medical therapy and are desperate for help. When successful, our therapies can provide profound and lasting relief.

The practice of surgical pain therapy is complicated, however, by the biopsychosocial problems related to chronic pain and the problems that patients with chronic pain bring to bear on a clinical practice. Patients with chronic pain can be uniquely demanding of practitioner's time and attention; they can be physically and emotionally draining to the neurosurgeon, nurses, and support staff. Patients with chronic pain, almost universally, have significant issues that are not common to the general neurosurgical patient. These issues include drug overuse and abuse problems, overuse and overdependency on the healthcare system, employment and vocational problems, and financial stresses and difficulties with interpersonal and family relationships. Associated with these issues are the resulting depression, anxiety, anger, and frustration that require therapeutic consideration if surgical pain therapies are to be successful.

The most significant strategy required to successfully initiate a practice that includes surgical pain management is to ally with or develop a multidisciplinary pain management team. Multidisciplinary pain management has been demonstrated to be superior to unimodality pain therapy in both patient satisfaction and objective outcomes; this difference is so significant that many third-party payers refuse reimbursement for unimodality pain therapy. The reason for the greater success of multidisciplinary pain management is the multifaceted nature of chronic pain problems. Patients with chronic pain demonstrate not only evidence of dysfunction or dysregulation of the pain transmission pathways, but also have the complex biopsychosocial issues noted previously. It is only using a multifaceted, "holistic" approach that all of these issues can be addressed and outcomes can be optimized. Modern multidisciplinary pain clinics include input from neurosurgery, anesthesia, physical therapy, nursing, oncology, physiatry, social work, psychology, and psychiatry. Consultation is often obtained from orthopedics, neurology, and general medicine. Having such a comprehensive team up to date on all aspects of pain management can only help to improve the quality and coordination of patient care.

The neurosurgeon's role in the comprehensive pain management team is clear. The neurosurgeon has the comprehensive knowledge of the neuroanatomy and neurophysiology underlying chronic pain problems. Second, the neurosurgeon is the only member of the pain management team with the expertise and ability to perform the full spectrum of interventional pain procedures, whether they are augmentative or ablative. Furthermore, the neurosurgeon, by virtue of neurosurgery training, has the ability to synthesize diverse pieces of information and establish a definitive plan. By virtue of the experience as neurosurgical chief resident, the neurosurgeon has experience with interpersonal organization and management.

The psychologist is critically important to the success of a neurosurgical pain practice. Medicare and Medicaid require psychological evaluation and clearance as a prerequisite for reimbursement for neuromodulation procedures. The psychologist, using a structured interview and psychological test instruments such as the Minnesota Multiphasic Personality Inventory, the Beck Depression Inventory, the McGill Pain Questionnaire, and others, can determine the presence of significant psychological issues that might prevent the success of pain-relieving procedures. In some cases, underlying psychiatric illness can be revealed. More often, patients with significant untreated depression are identified; after successful psychological therapy and possible pharmacologic therapy, these patients might become suitable candidates for pain surgery. Also, such evaluation often reveals patient's unrealistic expectations or poor understanding of the pain procedures to be performed; the psychologist can serve a significant support and education function as well. Furthermore, many patients suffering from chronic pain require ongoing short-term and long-term psychological therapy; the psychologist can either provide this therapy or refer to colleagues able to provide these critical patient care services. In addition to therapy, there are a number of psychological approaches to pain management, such as biofeedback, hypnosis, relaxation training, and stress management, which can be provided to patients with chronic pain by the pain clinic psychologist.

While the clinical psychologist has been the most often used mental health professional in the multidisciplinary pain setting, it is our experience that the psychiatrist can play an equally significant role. Within psychiatry is an active area of addiction medicine, and the psychiatrist is uniquely suited to address issues of chemical dependence that frequently affect the patient with chronic pain. In this regard, psychiatry frequently supervises drug detoxification programs in the pain clinic setting. Finally, the psychiatrist can best perform the administration and monitoring of medicines for the treatment of depression and other psychiatric issues.

The anesthesiologist plays both a critical diagnostic and therapeutic role in a comprehensive pain practice. In the hands of a skilled regional anesthesia specialist, diagnostic blocks of many kinds can be performed to help elucidate the nature and distribution of chronic pain disorders. These can be uniquely helpful in determining the neurosurgical procedures that may or may not be effective in ameliorating the patient's chronic pain complaints. Furthermore, therapeutic nerve blocks, trigger point injections for myofascial pain syndrome, and epidural steroid injections are the mainstay of many nonsurgical pain programs.

Over the past few decades, physiatry has played an increasingly important role in chronic pain therapy. There has been considerable work in the areas of exercise physiology as it applies to many chronic pain syndromes and the physiatrist is uniquely suited to apply rehabilitation techniques for chronic pain management. Because workman's compensation claims often complicate the treatment of patients with chronic pain

complaints, the physiatrist can also assist by supervising functional capacity evaluations and work hardening programs as indicated. Finally, once results of other therapies have been optimized, functional restoration programs as designed by physiatry can help to improve the functional outcomes for patients with chronic pain.

It may be argued that the most important member of the comprehensive pain management team is the pain clinical nurse specialist. Certainly, from the perspective of the neurosurgeon, the clinical nurse specialist is the key to a successful pain practice. The nurse serves those critical needs that allow the neurosurgeon to function effectively while minimizing the stress and other emotional and logistic burdens that can doom a neurosurgical pain practice. The nurse first serves as the patient liaison; by having good communication skills combined with empathy and knowledge of pain medicine, the nurse can supplement the therapeutic approaches of the clinical pain practitioners. The nurse provides critical pharmacologic documentation, including refill and compliance data. In most neurosurgical pain settings, the nurse provides monitoring of interventional pain therapy trials, provides intraoperative assistance in neuromodulation procedures, and performs outpatient pump refills and reprogramming of pumps and stimulators. These clinical functions, when properly reimbursed, can more than cover the cost of such skilled nurse practitioners.

The multidisciplinary approach to chronic pain management can seem daunting to the neurosurgeon new to chronic pain practice. It is critically important, however, that such an approach be initiated. Not only does such an approach optimize outcomes, but also with a team of practitioners with expertise in pain medicine, the tremendous needs of the chronic pain patient can be shared and the burden on the neurosurgical pain specialist can be limited to a manageable degree.

For such a multidisciplinary pain management team to succeed, each of the members must have a dedicated, but not necessarily exclusive, interest in chronic pain management. Each team member must maintain an up to date knowledge of the pain management principles, techniques, and pharmacology appropriate to their specialty. To function effectively, such a multidisciplinary pain management team must meet regularly, either in real or virtual space, to discuss patient care issues and to outline treatment plans. Such staffing allows for multidisciplinary assessment prior to interventional pain procedures. Another critical function of this multidisciplinary staffing is to delegate the clinical tasks appropriate to each specialty; such delegation of responsibility not only optimizes patient care but also decreases the significant burden that chronic pain patients can have on the individual practitioner. Finally, an adequate support staff is required to ensure that the administrative and logistic needs of the clinic are met.

What might be optimal in certain environments, but is not at all necessary, is a formal or fiducial relationship among the members of the multidisciplinary pain management team. What is required is the common knowledge, interest, and commitment to pain medicine. While certain marketing, billing, and reimbursement issues might be more easily accomplished by having a single clinic entity, they can be effectively addressed regardless of the affiliation of the team members.

Once the value, nature, and requirements of a multidisciplinary pain management team are recognized, the neurosurgeon is then faced with the potentially difficult reality of trying to accomplish this goal. In evaluating comprehensive pain treatment centers around the country, it appears that there are three major approaches to multidisciplinary pain management available to the neurosurgeon establishing a new chronic pain practice.

The first approach is to establish a comprehensive, multidisciplinary team *de novo*. The major benefit of such an approach is the significant degree of control that the neurosurgeon can exercise. By selecting individuals with a comprehensive, modern knowledge of pain medicine and a dedication to pain management, the neurosurgeon can create a high-quality, cohesive team. Not only does this approach allow for quality control, but also it can provide for optimal patient flow, access, and coordination of care. These logistic issues cannot be overemphasized. Also, such a cohesive, formal association between practitioners tends to provide for optimum billing and collection procedures. The real drawback of this approach, however, is the significant time and labor commitment required of the neurosurgeon to establish such a program. This may become overwhelming and detract from the neurosurgeon's non-pain-related practice.

The second approach is to ally with a preexisting interdisciplinary team. This is often the easiest approach and requires little input on the part of the neurosurgeon. Problems with this approach include the relative rarity of preexisting interdisciplinary pain management teams, especially within the private practice environment. Second, such a preexisting clinic may have well-established patterns of referral that tend to exclude the neurosurgeon and may foster competition rather than collegiality between the neurosurgeon and interventional pain therapists in anesthesia or physiatry. The neurosurgeon must first establish a niche in this already established referral pattern, such as in the area of ablative neurosurgery, and then expand this niche to other pain management procedures as they become better established within the practice environment. Third, the quality of treatment in such programs may not be satisfactory and the ability to control or direct the quality of therapy may be outside the purview of such a consulting neurosurgeon.

The third approach to multidisciplinary pain management involves a casual affiliation of pain practitioners. While this is the easiest and the most common practice about the country, it is the most likely to frustrate and overwhelm the neurosurgeon. Problems with inadequate communication among practitioners, poorly articulated objectives and treatment plans, and poorly coordinated patient care ultimately lead to poor outcomes and patient dissatisfaction. These loosely affiliated, casual "pain clinics" are the most likely to fail.

In addition to establishing or allying with a preexisting multidisciplinary pain clinic, there are a number of strategies that can be used in a neurosurgical practice to protect the neurosurgeon and the support staff from those burdens and stresses which so often lead to frustration and burn out. To make a more rewarding and long-term interventional pain practice, the neurosurgeon might well benefit from incorporating the following recommendations into their neurosurgical practice.

OFFICE MANAGEMENT

Patients with chronic pain tend to be somewhat different than the usual neurosurgical patient. They require more time in the office to address their medical and social issues. They have multiple medical, psychological, social, financial, and legal issues that need to be addressed. Unfortunately, there is seldom time available to address all of their needs. The office front-end staff needs to be aware of and understand these increased needs. They must further be made aware of the importance of workman's compensation, insurance, and litigation issues, which are so common to this patient population. By being aware of these issues, and maintaining adequate documentation, the office staff can optimize both patient care and reimbursement.

It is important that office staff members are aware of the importance of prompt and courteous responses to patient, insurance, and referring physician contacts. One key to survival in a pain practice is ensuring that payer preapproval be obtained for all neurosurgical pain procedures. Vendors of neuromodulation hardware have considerable expertise in the field of optimizing reimbursement; the practitioner should learn to make appropriate use of these resources.

The neurosurgeon should further be mindful of the critical role that the hospital plays in neurosurgical pain management. The equipment and patient care costs associated with neuromodulation in particular can be quite expensive. Unless reasonable reimbursement can be arranged for the hospital, they may be unwilling to allow practitioners the option of performing these procedures at their facility. There are a number of complex issues related to hospital reimbursement for implantable devices; it behooves the neurosurgeon to investigate these issues, with the help of support staff from the equipment manufacturers to ensure that the procedures are performed in compliance with the requirements of third-party payers and that they are billed in the manner that ensures proper reimbursement.

CLINICAL NURSE SPECIALIST

In our practice, the skills of a clinical nurse are absolutely necessary for the success of the neurosurgical pain practice. Dedicated to and knowledgeable about all facts of pain medicine, the clinical nurse provides services that are critical to maintaining a chronic pain practice while limiting the potentially overwhelming demands on the neurosurgeon. Excellent education and training for clinical nurse specialists is available either directly or indirectly from a number of sources including the American Pain Society, the International Association for the Study of Pain, the American Association of Neuroscience Nurses, and through the manufacturers of equipment used in neurosurgical pain procedures.

PRACTICE MANAGEMENT

The uninterrupted stream of patients with chronic pain, with their significant medical and emotional needs, can become overwhelming for the neurosurgeon and lead to early burn out. The most successful neurosurgical pain practitioners have found that alternating patients with chronic pain with general neurosurgical patients leads to less stress and frustration. By spreading out the pain patient load, either by scheduling pain clinic patients on alternating or dedicated clinic days, the neurosurgeon can remain fresher and limit the stresses on the clinic support staff.

There are specific issues that must be addressed in the clinic management of patients with chronic pain. On the provider's side, patient visits must include a significant element of empathy and understanding. The usual neurosurgical diagnostic and therapeutic encounter is insufficient for most patients with chronic pain. The office visit must include clearly articulated diagnostic information and outline a specific treatment plan. Many have found that providing a copy of the office note describing the assessment and plan is useful for patients with chronic pain complaints.

The schedule must allow for ample office time for these often complex and challenging clinical problems. The average chronic pain clinical encounter requires as much as 100% more time as compared to the general neurosurgical patient. With appropriate documentation and coding, these encounters are billed and reimbursed at an accordingly higher level.

On the patient's side, there are certain requirements that must be clearly articulated to maintain an orderly and safe clinical practice. With such overwhelming needs, the patient with chronic pain often demands levels of attention and support that are unreasonable and impossible in a clinical practice setting. Thus, it is often necessary and appropriate to set limits with these patients. These limits may include defining a maximum number of nonemergency clinic contacts per unit time, limits on the length of patient encounters, and limits on the times and amounts of medication refills. We frequently provide patients with informal "contracts" that define the length and purpose of initial patient evaluations and follow-up visits, the number of nonemergent calls that will be returned in a given week, and the days of the week and the hours of the day when medication refill calls will be accepted. When using chronic opioid therapy, we articulate very clearly a number of limits, which must be respected if we are to continue prescribing opioids and if we are to continue seeing a patient in our practice.

SUMMARY

From the previous discussion, it is clear that there is an overwhelming demand for neurosurgical pain management. In a time when there is significant constriction and competition for patients, pain management provides a subspecialty area with almost unlimited growth potential. Chronic pain problems are often clinically complex and intellectually stimulating and as such their solution can be extremely satisfying for the neurosurgeon. Patients who have significant and diverse needs manifest these problems, however, and their care can be very labor and energy intensive. These patients, and the neurosurgical pain specialist, are best served by a multidisciplinary approach to pain management. By using such a comprehensive approach, and by being mindful of the particular issues that patients with chronic pain bring to bear on a clinical practice, the neurosurgical pain specialist can develop a practice that is extremely personally rewarding and that provides a critical service to their patients and the community.

Index

Note: Page numbers followed by f refer to figures; those followed by t refer to tables.

A

Aβ fibers, 18, 20, 21f
  in neuropathic pain, 35
Aδ fibers, 18, 20, 21f
A5 cell group, in descending pain pathway, 26, 26f
A7 cell group, in descending pain pathway, 26, 26f
AAPM (American Academy of Pain Medicine), Uniform Outcome Measures project of, 265
Abuse, and surgical outcome, 44
Acetaminophen (APAP, paracetamol), 47
Acetylsalicylic acid (ASA), 47–48
Activities of daily living, with myofascial pain syndromes, 69
Acupuncture, 249
  in multidisciplinary pain treatment program, 257
Acute pain, 5–7
  chronic vs., 4, 64
  recurring, 5
  spinal mechanisms of, 21, 22f
Addiction
  and surgical outcome, 41
  defined, 50
  to opioids, 50
    pseudo-, 50
AEDs (antiepileptic drugs). See Anticonvulsant drugs.
Aerobic exercises, 250
Affective-motivational pathways, 24–25, 24f
Afferent fibers
  cutaneous, 17
  muscle and joint, 18
  nociceptive
    deep somatic, 18
    neurochemistry of, 19
  primary, 17–18
  sensory, 18
    efferent function of, 19
  silent, 18
  visceral, 18–19
AFP (atypical facial pain), 84, 96, 103–104, 103t
Alcohol, and cluster headache, 94
Allodynia, 18f, 30
  functional reorganization in, 34
Alpha-amino-3-hydroxy-5-methyl-4-isoxazolepropionic acid (AMPA) receptors
  in central sensitization, 34
  in change from acute to inflammatory pain, 21, 22, 22f
  in hyperalgesia, 27
Alterative and complementary techniques, in multidisciplinary pain treatment program, 257
American Academy of Pain Medicine (AAPM), Uniform Outcome Measures project of, 265
American Medical Association Guides to the Evaluation of Permanent Impairment, 263, 264
Amitriptyline, 48
Analgesia
  patient-controlled, 51f
    oral, 52f
  pre-emptive, 23
  stress-induced, 63
Analgesics. See Pharmacologic therapies.
Anesthesia dolorosa, 103t
  motor cortex stimulation for, 161

Anesthesiologist, in neurosurgical pain practice, 272
Animal models, of neuropathic pain, 31, 31t
Antiarrhythmics, for neuropathic pain, 32–33
Anticonvulsant drugs
  for failed back surgery syndrome, 80
  for glossopharyngeal neuralgia, 85
  for neuropathic pain, 32–33, 52
  for occipital neuralgia, 88
  for pain, 49
  for post-stroke pain, 112
  for spinal cord injury pain, 112
  for trigeminal neuralgia, 104–106, 105t
  in balanced analgesic regimen, 53
Antidepressant agents
  for failed back surgery syndrome, 80–81
  for insomnia, 53
  for neuropathic pain, 52
  for occipital neuralgia, 88
  for pain, 48–49
  for post-stroke pain, 112
  for spinal cord injury pain, 112
Antiepileptic drugs (AEDs). See Anticonvulsant drugs.
Anxiety
  and surgical outcome, 39, 41
  assessment of, 267
  with failed back surgery syndrome, 79
  with myofascial pain syndromes, 70
APAP (acetaminophen), 47
Arachidonic acid, in tissue injury, 47
Arachnoiditis, failed back surgery syndrome due to, 75
Array, 132
ASA (acetylsalicylic acid), 47–48
Ascending pain pathways, 23–25, 24f
Aseptic meningitis, with NSAIDs, 47
Aspirin, 47–48
Aspirin triad, 48
ATN (atypical trigeminal neuralgia), 103–104, 240–241
Attitude issues, in failed pain syndrome, 10
Atypical facial pain (AFP), 84, 96, 103–104, 103t
Atypical trigeminal neuralgia (ATN), 103–104, 240–241
Autonomic disturbance, in complex regional pain syndrome, 120
Autotraction, for myofascial pain syndromes, 68

B

Back pain, lower
  facet rhizotomy for, 206–208
  "functional" vs. "organic," 39
  management of, 61–66, 69f
  "Back schools," 80
Baclofen (Lioresal), for trigeminal neuralgia, 104, 105t, 106–107
Balanced analgesic regimen, 52–53
Balloon compression, for trigeminal neuralgia, 107, 214–218
  anesthesia for, 214–215
  background of, 214
  bilateral, 217
  equipment placement and draping for, 215, 215f
  indications for, 214
  intraoperative imaging for, 215
  operative techniques for, 214
  positioning for, 215

Balloon compression, for trigeminal neuralgia, (*Continued*)
  preoperative preparation for, 214
  pressure monitoring technique for, 215–216, 216f
  recurrence after, 217
  results of, 108t, 216–218
  volume-controlled approach for, 216
Basilar artery, compression of trigeminal nerve by, 233
Battered root syndrome, 74
Beck Depression Inventory, for spine surgery, 40, 42
Behavioral management
  in multidisciplinary pain treatment program, 259
  of myofascial pain syndromes, 70–71
Benadryl (diphenhydramine), for spinal cord injury pain, 112
Biceps brachii syndromes, 60, 68f
Biofeedback
  for myofascial pain syndromes, 71
  in multidisciplinary pain treatment program, 257
Bonica, John, 265
Brachial plexus avulsion, DREZotomy for, 179, 181f, 183, 184t
Brachialis syndromes, 60, 68f
Brainstem ablative procedures, 189–192
Buprenorphine, 49
Butorphanol, 49

C

C fibers
  cutaneous afferent, 18
  in chronic pain, 23
  in dorsal horn, 20, 21f
C1/C2 fusion, 100
C1/C3 posterior rhizotomy, 100
C2 decompression, 100
C2 ganglionectomy, 99–100
C2-3–mediated pain, 99
Calcitonin, for phantom limb pain, 115
Calcitonin gene–related peptide (CGRP), in nociceptive afferent fibers, 19
Calcium (Ca^{2+})
  in change from acute to inflammatory pain, 23
  in chronic pain, 23
Camptocormia, 256
Cancer pain
  dorsal rhizotomy for, 205
  DREZ lesions for, 183
  intracranial ablative procedures for, 195, 196, 197
  midbrain tractotomy for, 189–190
Carbamazepine (Tegretol), 49
  for trigeminal neuralgia, 104, 105–106, 105t, 219, 240
Carisoprodol, 50
Carotidynia, 90
Catastrophizing, in chronic pain syndromes, 256
Cauda equina lesions, DREZ lesions for, 183, 185t
Caudalis DREZ lesions
  for facial pain due to malignancy, 92–93
  for postherpetic neuralgia, 96
Causalgia. *See* Complex regional pain syndrome (CRPS).
Ceiling effect, of NSAIDs, 46, 47
Celecoxib, 48
Central lateral nucleus, in post-stroke pain, 111
Central myelotomy, 172
Central pain syndromes, 110–115
  classification of, 110
  defined, 110
  intracranial ablative procedures for, 196–197
  medical strategies for, 112–113
  pathophysiology of, 110–112
  surgical strategies for, 113–114
  treatment outcomes for, 114–115
Central sensitization, 17, 21–23, 22f
  in neuropathic pain, 34–35
  pathologic, 34–35
Cerebral blood flow, with motor cortex stimulation, 161–162
Cervical facet(s), innervation of, 207
Cervical facet block, 208

Cervical medial branch block, 208
Cervicogenic pain, 99
CGRP (calcitonin gene–related peptide), in nociceptive afferent fibers, 19
Channel, 132
Chaotic reinnervation, 112
Chemotherapy, for head and neck cancer, 91
Chest wall pain, dorsal root ganglionectomy for, 206
Chiropractic, in multidisciplinary pain treatment program, 257
Chronic disease, *vs.* chronic pain, 255
Chronic pain, 7
  acute *vs.*, 4, 64
  chronic disease *vs.*, 255
  defined, 131
  depression with, 65
  difficulties of, 247–248
  drug abuse with, 64–65
  epidemiology of, 247
  intractable benign, 66
  obligations in care for, 4–5
  spinal mechanisms of, 23
Chronic pain syndromes (CPSs), 255
  clinical characteristics of, 255–256
  multidisciplinary pain treatment program for, 256–260
  psychological and socioeconomic components of, 256
Chronic paroxysmal hemicrania (CPH), 94
Cingulate cortex, pain-related, 194
Cingulotomy, 197
  radiosurgical, 246
Clinical nurse specialist, in neurosurgical pain practice, 272, 273
Clonazepam (Klonopin), for trigeminal neuralgia, 105t
Cluster headache (CH), 93–95
  nucleus caudalis DREZ for, 190–192
  radiosurgery for, 243
Cluster-tic syndrome, 94
Codeine, 49
Cold therapy, 250–255
Commissural myelotomy, 172–173, 173f, 174f
Commissurotomy, midline, for spinal cord injury pain, 113
Comorbid conditions
  in outcome assessment, 267
  with pain, 53
Compensation factors, in failed pain syndrome, 8
Complex regional pain syndrome (CRPS), 119–127
  clinical features of, 120–121, 126–127
  diagnosis and evaluation of, 121–123, 122t–124t, 126–127
  differential diagnosis of, 121, 122t
  epidemiology of, 119–120
  pathophysiology of, 121, 122f
  peripheral nerve stimulation for, 145–146
  psychological factors in, 123–124
  sympathectomy for, 202, 204–205
  taxonomy of, 119, 120t
  treatment regimens for, 124–125
Computed tomography (CT), of failed back surgery syndrome, 77t, 78
Conditioned nociception, 43
Constipation, due to opioids, 52
Contact, 132
Controlled substances, 50, 53
Conus medullaris lesions, DREZ lesions for, 185t
Cordectomy, for spinal cord injury pain, 113
Cordotomy, 165–170
  alternatives to, 166–167, 167t
  bilateral, 168, 169
  complications of, 168–169, 169f
  for phantom limb pain, 115
  for post-stroke pain, 114
  for spinal cord injury pain, 113, 114
  history of, 165
  indications for, 165–166, 166t
  mechanism of, 165
  operative technique for, 167–168, 167f
  results of, 168
Cortex, in neuropathic pain, 35
Corticalization, of pain, 43

Cost, in outcome assessment, 267, 267f, 268f
COX (cyclo-oxygenase) inhibitors, 47–48
COX-1 (cyclo-oxygenase-1), 20
COX-2 (cyclo-oxygenase-2), 20
CPH (chronic paroxysmal hemicrania), 94
CPSs. *See* Chronic pain syndromes (CPSs).
Cranial neuralgia(s), 102–108
    clinical presentation of, 102, 103t
    diagnosis of, 103t
    differential diagnosis of, 103–104
    epidemiology of, 102
    etiology of, 102, 103t
    evaluation of, 104
    medical management of, 104–107, 105t
    pathophysiology of, 102
    posterior fossa procedures for, 232–236, 234f–236f
    surgical treatment of, 107–108, 108t
    treatment algorithm for, 107–108
Craniofacial pain, 84–96
    approach to, 84
    atypical, 84, 96, 103–104, 103t
    aural, 85t
    common causes of, 84, 85t, 102, 103t
    dental and periodontal, 85t
    due to carotidynia, 90
    due to geniculate or intermedius neuralgia, 86–87
    due to glossopharyngeal neuralgia, 84–86
    due to headache, 85t
        cluster, 93–95
    due to malignancy, 90–93
    due to occipital neuralgia, 87–89, 88t
    due to postherpetic neuralgia, 95–96
    due to sphenopalatine neuralgia, 89
    due to superior laryngeal neuralgia, 90
    due to trigeminal neuralgia, 84
    due to vidian neuralgia, 89–90
    neuropathic, 84, 85t
    nontrigeminal, 84–96
    ocular and periocular, 85t
    of midface, 85t
Craniovertebral junction (CVJ), imaging of, 88
Crossed afterdischarge, in neuropathic pain, 34
Cross-excitation, in neuropathic pain, 34
CRPS. *See* Complex regional pain syndrome (CRPS).
Cryoablative facet joint denervation, 208
CT (computed tomography), of failed back surgery syndrome, 77t, 78
Cutaneous afferent fibers, 18
CVJ (craniovertebral junction), imaging of, 88
Cyclo-oxygenase (COX) inhibitors, 47–48
Cyclo-oxygenase-1 (COX-1), 20
Cyclo-oxygenase-2 (COX-2), 20
Cystitis, interstitial, peripheral nerve stimulation for, 141
Cytochrome P-450 (CYP 450) system, acetaminophen effect on, 47

D
DBS. *See* Deep-brain stimulation (DBS).
Deafferentation pain syndromes, 110–115
    classification of, 110
    defined, 110
    medical strategies for, 112–113
    motor cortex stimulation for, 161
    pathophysiology of, 110–112
    surgical strategies for, 113–114
    treatment outcomes for, 114–115
Deconditioning, with chronic pain, 245, 258
Deep heat, 248
Deep somatic nociceptive afferent fibers, 18
Deep-brain stimulation (DBS), 156–159
    chronic, 158–159
    complications and side effects of, 157–158, 159
    for phantom limb pain, 115
    for postherpetic neuralgia, 95–96
    for post-stroke pain, 114, 115

for spinal cord injury pain, 114
    indications for, 156
    long-term effectiveness of, 159
    physiology of, 156
    postoperative, 158
    preoperative preparation for, 157
    surgical technique for, 157
    target selection for, 157–158, 157f, 158f
Demographics, in outcome assessment, 266
Depakote (sodium valproate), for trigeminal neuralgia, 105t
Dependence, with chronic pain, 245–246
Depression
    and spine surgery, 39, 40–41, 43
    assessment of, 267
    with chronic pain, 65, 246
    with failed back surgery syndrome, 79
    with myofascial pain syndromes, 70
Descending fibers, 21f
Descending modulation, of pain, 25–26, 26f
    inflammatory, 27
Descending pain pathways, 25–26, 26f
Diagnosis(es), putative, in outcome assessment, 266–267
Diathermy, 248
Diclofenac, 48
Dilantin (phenytoin), 49
    for trigeminal neuralgia, 105t, 106
Diphenhydramine (Benadryl), for spinal cord injury pain, 112
Diphenylhydantoin (phenytoin), 49
    for trigeminal neuralgia, 105t, 106
Disability
    impairment *vs.*, 262
    in patient with pain, 262–264
    nature of, 262–263
    pain and, 263
    production of iatrogenic, 263
    with chronic pain, 246
Disk herniation, root syndrome or radiculopathy due to, 57
Diskogenic pain, 7
Diskography, of failed back surgery syndrome, 77t, 78
Disuse, with chronic pain, 245
DLF (dorsolateral funiculus), in descending pain pathway, 25, 26f
DLPT (dorsolateral pontine tegmentum), in descending pain pathway, 26, 26f
Domestic issues, in failed pain syndrome, 8–9
Dorsal column(s), in ascending pain pathway, 24, 24f
Dorsal column medial lemniscal system, in post-stroke pain, 111
Dorsal horn, of spinal cord, 20–27, 21f
Dorsal horn neurons, in central sensitization, 34
Dorsal interscapular approach, for upper thoracic sympathectomy, 203
Dorsal rhizotomy, 205, 206
Dorsal root entry zone (DREZ), 176, 177f
Dorsal root entry zone (DREZ) lesion(s), 176–187
    anatomic-physiologic rationale for, 176
    at lumbosacral level, 179–180, 182f
    for brachial plexus avulsion, 179, 181f, 183, 184t
    for cancer pain, 183
    for cauda equina lesions, 183, 185t
    for facial pain due to malignancy, 92–93
    for hyperspastic states with pain, 184–187
    for laterocervical pain, 184
    for occipital neuralgia, 184
    for Pancoast syndrome, 179f
    for peripheral nerve lesions, 183–184
    for phantom limb pain, 115, 184
    for postherpetic neuralgia, 96, 184
    for spinal cord injury pain, 113, 114, 183, 185t, 186f
    for stump pain, 184
    history of, 176
    indications for, 187, 187f
    laser, 181
    microsurgical, 176–180, 178f–182f
    nucleus caudalis, 190–192
        for facial pain due to malignancy, 92–93
        for postherpetic neuralgia, 96

Dorsal root entry zone (DREZ) lesion(s) (*Continued*)
    radiofrequency thermocoagulation, 180–181
    somatosensory evoked potentials with, 179–180, 182f
    ultrasonic, 181
Dorsal root ganglion (DRG) neurons, in neuropathic pain, 33
Dorsal root ganglionectomy, 205–206
Dorsolateral funiculus (DLF), in descending pain pathway, 25, 26f
Dorsolateral pontine tegmentum (DLPT), in descending pain
        pathway, 26, 26f
DREZ. *See* Dorsal root entry zone (DREZ).
Drug(s)
    efficacy of, 46
    half-life of, 46
    potency of, 46
    steady state of, 46
Drug abuse
    and surgical outcome, 41
    with chronic pain, 64–65
Drug misuse, with chronic pain, 247
Drug therapy. *See* Pharmacologic therapies.
Dynorphins, 26
Dysesthesias, 29
    due to cordotomy, 169

E

Ectopic activity
    in chronic pain, 23
    in neuropathic pain, 32–33, 32f
EESG (evoked electrospinogram), with DREZ lesions, 182f
Efficacy, of drug, 46
Electrical stimulation, 251
    for postherpetic neuralgia, 95–96
    of peripheral nervous system. *See* Peripheral nerve
        stimulation (PNS).
    of spinal cord. *See* Spinal cord stimulation (SCS).
Electrode(s)
    defined, 132
    for spinal cord stimulation, 136, 136f
        placement of, 138–139, 138f, 139f
Electromyography, of failed back surgery syndrome, 78
Electrophysiologic studies, of failed back surgery syndrome, 78
Elimination half-life, 46
El-Naggar/Nashold electrode, 191, 192
"Enabling behaviors," in failed pain syndrome, 8–9
Endomorphins, 26
β-Endorphin, 26
Ephaptic connections, 201
Epidural fibrosis, failed back surgery syndrome due to, 75
Epidural spinal cord stimulation
    for phantom limb pain, 115
    for spinal cord injury pain, 113
Epidural steroid injections, for failed back surgery syndrome, 81
EPSPs (excitatory postsynaptic potentials), in acute pain, 21
Equianalgesic dose, 46
Ergonomics, for myofascial pain syndromes, 71
Evoked electrospinogram (EESG), with DREZ lesions, 182f
Excitatory amino acids, as neurotransmitters for nociceptive afferent
        fibers, 19
Excitatory interneurons, 20, 21f
Excitatory postsynaptic potentials (EPSPs), in acute pain, 21
Exercises
    for failed back surgery syndrome, 80
    for myofascial pain syndromes, 68
    therapeutic, 251–252
Expectations, of patient, 5, 6f, 10, 12, 14
    and patient satisfaction with spine surgery, 39
Extralemniscal myelotomy, 172
    stereotactic, 173

F

Facet joint denervation, 208
    for failed back surgery syndrome, 81

Facet joint syndrome
    clinical diagnosis of, 207–208
    facet rhizotomy for, 206–208
Facet rhizotomy, 206–208
Facial pain. *See* Craniofacial pain.
Failed back surgery syndrome (FBSS), 73–82
    characteristics of, 65
    cingulotomy for, 197
    defined, 65, 73
    due to arachnoiditis, 75
    due to battered root syndrome, 74
    due to epidural fibrosis, 75
    due to improper patient selection, 74, 75
    due to operative complications, 74, 75
    due to pseudoarthrosis, 76
    due to technical difficulty, 74
    early, 75, 75t
    electrophysiologic studies for, 78
    etiology of, 73–76, 74t–76t
    evaluation of, 76–79, 77t
    hematologic analysis for, 79
    immediate, 73–74, 74t
    incidence of, 65, 73
    intermediate, 75–76, 75t
    late, 76, 76t
    myofascial pain syndromes in, 76, 80
    onset of symptoms of, 73–74, 74t–76t
    patient education for, 80
    patient history in, 76
    physical examination for, 76–77
    physical therapy for, 80
    psychological evaluation for, 79
    psychological factors in, 74, 80
    radiographic evaluation for, 77–78, 77t
    reoperation for, 65, 79
    treatment for, 79–82
Failed pain syndrome, 7–11
Family dynamics, in failed pain syndrome, 8–9
Family groups, for myofascial pain syndromes, 70
FBSS. *See* Failed back surgery syndrome (FBSS).
Fentanyl, 49
Fifth cranial nerve, pain from tumor involving, nucleus caudalis
        DREZ for, 190–192
Fluidotherapy, 248
Fordyce Model, in pain rehabilitation, 247

G

GABA (gamma-aminobutyric acid), in neuropathic
        pain, 35
Gabapentin, 49
Gain, secondary, 258, 259
Gamma knife cingulotomy, 246
Gamma knife hypophysectomy, 246
Gamma knife radiosurgery
    for cluster headache, 245
    for sphenopalatine neuralgia, 245
    for trigeminal neuralgia, 242–245, 243f, 244f
Gamma knife thalamotomy, 239–241, 240f, 241f
Gamma-aminobutyric acid (GABA), in neuropathic pain, 35
Ganglionectomy
    dorsal root, 205–206
    for occipital neuralgia, 89
Genetic factors, in failed pain syndrome, 8
Geniculate neuralgia (GeN), 86–87
    anatomy and pathophysiology of, 86
    clinical features and diagnosis of, 86–87, 104
    posterior fossa procedures for, 234–235, 235f
    surgical treatments for, 87
Glossopharyngeal neuralgia (GPN), 84–86
    clinical features of, 84–85, 103t, 104
    etiology and pathogenesis of, 85
    posterior fossa procedures for, 235–236, 236f
    treatment for, 85–86

Glutamate
in central sensitization, 34, 35
in change from acute to inflammatory pain, 21, 22, 22f
Gluteal muscle syndromes, 58, 61f
Glycerol, mechanism of action of, 220–221
Glycerol injection, for cluster headache, 95
Glycerol rhizolysis, for trigeminal neuralgia, 107, 108t
Glycerol rhizotomy, for trigeminal neuralgia, 219–225
anesthesia for, 221–222
complications of, 223–225
contraindications to, 225
history of, 220
indications and patient selection for, 220
landmarks, trajectory, and imaging during, 222–223, 222f–224f
mechanism of action of, 220–221
positioning for, 221
preoperative evaluation for, 221
reported success with, 225
GPN. *See* Glossopharyngeal neuralgia (GPN).
G-protein–coupled receptors, 20, 20f
in change from acute to inflammatory pain, 21, 22, 22f
Greater occipital nerve (GON), 87, 88
peripheral neurectomy of, 89
Group therapy, in pain rehabilitation, 248
Growth factors, in nociceptor sensitization, 20

H
Half-life, 46
Head and neck, cancer pain of, 90–93
Headache(s)
cluster, 93–95
nucleus caudalis DREZ for, 190–192
radiosurgery for, 245
craniofacial pain due to, 85t
lower-half, 89
occipital. *See* Occipital neuralgia.
posterior region, 99–101
transformed migraine, 99
Heat therapy, 248
Hematologic analysis, of failed back surgery syndrome, 79
Hemicrania, chronic paroxysmal, 94
Hemiparesis, due to cordotomy, 169
Hepatotoxicity, of acetaminophen, 47
Herniated disk, root syndrome or radiculopathy due to, 57
Herpes simplex virus (HSV), reactivation of, due to trigeminal nerve irritation, 224–225
Herpes zoster, neuralgia after. *See* Postherpetic neuralgia (PHN).
Hippocampus, abuse effect on, 44
5-HT (serotonin), in descending pain pathway, 25–26, 26f
Human herpesvirus-3, postherpetic neuralgia due to, 95–96
Hunt's neuralgia. *See* Geniculate neuralgia (GeN).
Hydrocodone, 49
Hydrocollator pack, 250
Hydromorphone, 49
Hydrotherapy, 250
Hyperalgesia
defined, 30
neuroanatomic and neurophysiologic basis of, 22f, 23
primary *vs.* secondary, 17, 27
stimulus intensity and, 18f
Hyperesthesias, 29
Hyperhidrosis, sympathectomy for, 202
Hyperpathia, 30
Hyperspastic states with pain, DREZ lesions for, 184–187
Hypophysectomy, 195, 198
radiosurgical, 244
Hypothalamus, in cluster headache, 93

I
IASP (International Association for the Study of Pain), 30
diagnostic criteria for complex regional pain syndrome by, 122, 126
Ibuprofen, 48

Ice application, for myofascial pain syndromes, 67
Iliopsoas syndrome, 58, 60f
Immediate early genes (IEGs), 22f
Immobilization, 58, 63
Impairment
disability *vs.*, 262
in patient with pain, 262–264
nature of, 262–263
problems in rating pain as, 264
Impairment ratings, physician participation in, 263
Implantable pulse generator (IPG), 132, 136, 137f
Improvement, response to, 11
Incident pain, 51
Indomethacin, 48
Inflammation, 19–20
Inflammatory pain
attenuation of, 20
descending modulation of, 27
neuropathic *vs.*, 29
spinal mechanisms of, 21–23
Infraorbital nerve, peripheral denervation of, 211f, 212, 212f, 213
Infraspinatus syndrome, 59–60, 67f
Inhibitory interneurons, 20, 21f
Innocuous stimuli, 18f
Insomnia, due to pain, 53
Interleukin 1β, in neuropathic pain, 33
Intermedius neuralgia. *See* Geniculate neuralgia (GeN).
Internal capsule, deep-brain stimulation of, 158, 159
International Association for the Study of Pain (IASP), 30
diagnostic criteria for complex regional pain syndrome by, 122, 126
Interneurons
excitatory, 20, 21f
inhibitory, 20, 21f
Interstitial cystitis, peripheral nerve stimulation for, 141
Intracranial ablative procedure(s), 194–198
anatomic and physiologic considerations for, 194–195
cingulumotomy as, 197
hypophysectomy as, 195, 198
indications for, 195–196
medial thalamotomy as, 196–197, 197t
radiothalamotomy as, 197
Intracranial rhizotomy, for glossopharyngeal neuralgia, 86
Intraoperative management, 12
Intraspinal analgesic infusion therapy, for failed back surgery syndrome, 81
Intrathecal (IT) analgesic administration, 150–155
advantages of, 150
complications of, 155
for failed back surgery syndrome, 81
for post-stroke pain, 114
for spinal cord injury pain, 113
implantation technique for, 151–153, 152f
indications for, 150–151
outcomes of, 153–155, 154t
preimplant considerations for, 151
trials for, 150, 151
types of pumps and catheter placements for, 153
Intraventricular opiates (IVOs), for head and neck cancer, 91–92
IPG (implantable pulse generator), 132, 136, 137f
Isokinetic exercises, 252
Isometric exercises, 252
Isotonic exercises, 252
IT analgesic administration. *See* Intrathecal (IT) analgesic administration.
IVOs (intraventricular opiates), for head and neck cancer, 91–92

J
Job satisfaction, and surgical outcome, 41
Job simulation, for myofascial pain syndromes, 69
Joint afferent fibers, 18

K
Ketamine, for phantom limb pain, 115
Ketoprofen, 48

Kinesophobia, 43
Klonopin (clonazepam), for trigeminal neuralgia, 105t

L

Laminae, of spinal cord, 20, 21f
Laminotomy electrodes, for spinal cord stimulation, 139–140, 140f
Laser DREZ lesions, 181
Lateral medullary infarction, motor cortex stimulation for, 161
Laterocervical pain, DREZ lesions for, 184
LBP (lower back pain)
    facet rhizotomy for, 206–208
    "functional" vs. "organic," 39
    management of, 61–66, 69f
Lead(s)
    defined, 132
    for spinal cord stimulation, 136, 136f
        implant techniques for, 137–140, 137f–139f
Legal information, resources on, 264
Legal issues, with opioids, 50, 53
Lesser occipital nerve, 87–88
Leuenkephalin, 26
Leukotrienes, inflammation due to, 57
Levator scapulae syndromes, 59, 64f
Lidocaine, for post-stroke pain, 115
Ligand-gated channels, in nociceptor sensitization, 19–20, 20f
Limbocortical–diencephalic–
        mesopontomedullary–spinal cord circuit, 25, 26f
Limited midline myelotomy, 173, 173f, 174, 174f
Lioresal (baclofen), for trigeminal neuralgia, 104, 105t, 106–107
Locus coeruleus, in descending pain pathway, 26, 26f
Low threshold cells, 20
Lower back pain (LBP)
    facet rhizotomy for, 206–208
    "functional" vs. "organic," 39
    management of, 61–66, 69f
Lower-half headache, 89
Lumbar facet block, 208
Lumbar facet joint, anatomy of, 206–207
Lumbar facet syndrome
    clinical diagnosis of, 207–208
    facet rhizotomy for, 206–208
Lumbar medial branch block, 208
Lumbar pain
    facet rhizotomy for, 206–208
    "functional" vs. "organic," 39
    management of, 61–66, 69f
Lumbar puncture, for intrathecal morphine trials, 151
Lumbar spine surgery, psychological considerations in, 38–44
Lumbar sympathectomy, 204

M

Macrophages, in neuropathic pain, 33
Magnesium (Mg^{2+}) block, of NMDA receptor, 21, 22, 22f
Magnetic resonance imaging (MRI), of failed back surgery
        syndrome, 77t, 78
Malignancy, facial pain due to, 90–93, 103t
Mandibular nerve, peripheral denervation of, 211f, 212, 212f, 213
Manipulation, 251
Manual therapy, 251
Massage therapy, 251
MBT (midbrain tractotomy), 93, 189–190
MCX. See Motor cortex stimulation (MCX).
MDT. See Microsurgical dorsal root entry zone– otomy
        (micro-DREZotomy, MDT).
MEAC (minimum effective analgesic concentration), 50–51, 51f
Medial lemniscus, in ascending pain pathway, 24, 24f
Medial thalamotomy, 196–197, 197t
    radiosurgery for, 239–241, 240f, 241f
Medical therapy. See Pharmacologic therapies.
Medical/legal training and information, resources for, 264
Melatonin, in cluster headache, 93
Memorial Pain Assessment Card (MPAC), 268–269, 268f, 269f

Meningitis, aseptic, with NSAIDs, 47
Mental nerve, peripheral denervation of, 211f, 212, 212f, 213
Meperidine, 49
Mesencephalotomy, 93
Metenkephalin, 26
Methadone, 49
Mexiletine, for post-stroke pain, 112, 115
Mg^{2+} (magnesium) block, of NMDA receptor, 21, 22, 22f
Microsurgical dorsal root entry zone–otomy (micro-DREZotomy, MDT),
        176–180, 178f–182f
    for brachial plexus avulsion, 179, 181f, 183, 184t
    for cancer pain, 183
    for cauda equina lesions, 183, 185t
    for hyperspastic states with pain, 184–187
    for laterocervical pain, 184
    for occipital neuralgia, 184
    for peripheral nerve lesions, 183–184
    for phantom limb pain, 184
    for postherpetic neuralgia, 184
    for spinal cord injury pain, 183, 185t, 186f
    for stump pain, 184
Microvascular decompression (MVD)
    for geniculate neuralgia, 87, 234–235, 235f
    for glossopharyngeal neuralgia, 85–86, 235–236, 236f
    for trigeminal neuralgia, 107, 108t, 232–234, 234f, 244–245
Micturition, cordotomy effect on, 169
Midbrain tractotomy (MBT), 93, 189–190
Midline commissurotomy, for spinal cord injury pain, 113
Midline myelotomy
    limited, 173, 173f, 174, 174f
    punctate, 173–174, 174f
Migraine headache(s), transformed, 99
Minimum effective analgesic concentration (MEAC), 50–51, 51f
Minnesota Multiphasic Personality Inventory (MMPI)
    for spine surgery, 39, 41–42
    in chronic pain syndromes, 256
Mobilization, 251
Mood disorders, and surgical outcome, 39, 40–41
Morphine, 49, 50
    intrathecal administration of. See Intrathecal (IT) analgesic
        administration.
    side effects of, 155
Motivational issues
    in failed pain syndrome, 8
    in multidisciplinary pain treatment program, 259
Motor cortex stimulation (MCX)
    and cerebral blood flow, 161–162
    for anesthesia dolorosa, 161
    for neuropathic pain syndromes, 160–163
    for postherpetic neuralgia, 96, 161
    for post-stroke pain, 114, 115
    for trigeminal neuropathy, 161
    history of, 160–162
    indications for, 162
    mechanism of, 161–162
    operative technique for, 162–163, 162f, 163f
    preoperative evaluation for, 162
    therapeutic parameters for, 163
Motor disturbance, in complex regional pain syndrome, 121
Movement therapy, for myofascial pain syndromes, 68
MPAC (Memorial Pain Assessment Card), 268–269, 268f, 269f
MRI (magnetic resonance imaging), of failed back surgery
        syndrome, 77t, 78
MS. See Multiple sclerosis (MS).
Multidisciplinary pain treatment program (MPTP), 255–260
    dealing with secondary gain and motivation in, 259
    effectiveness of, 70f, 71
    for myofascial pain syndromes, 64, 66–71
    fundamental concepts of, 255–256
    initial evaluation in, 258
    initial staffing session in, 258–259
    intensive vs. customized, 259
    maximizing outcomes with, 13–14
    neurosurgeon in, 271–273

organization of, 256–257
outcome of using, 260
referral to, 257–258
staffing sessions and coordination of therapies in, 259–260
treatment techniques and methods in, 259
Multiple sclerosis (MS)
    nucleus caudalis DREZ for, 190–192
    percutaneous trigeminal nerve compression for, 217
    trigeminal neuralgia in, 219
Multisynaptic ascending system, 25
Muscle afferent fibers, 18
Muscle contraction, in myofascial pain syndromes, 57–58
MVD. *See* Microvascular decompression (MVD).
Myelography, of failed back surgery syndrome, 77t, 78
Myelotomy, 172–175
    central, 172
    commissural, 172–173, 173f, 174f
    extralemniscal, 172
        stereotactic, 173
    history of, 172
    indications for, 172, 174–175
    mechanism of, 173
    midline
        limited, 173, 173f, 174, 174f
        punctate, 173–174, 174f
Myofascial pain syndromes, 57–71
    behavioral management for, 70–71
    clinical presentation of, 57, 255
    ergonomics for, 71
    in failed back surgery syndrome, 76, 80
    multidisciplinary team for, 64, 66–71
        effectiveness of, 70f, 71
    of lower quadrants, 58–59, 59f–63f
    of upper quadrants, 59–60, 64f–68f
    pathophysiology of, 57
    physical examination for, 58
    physical medicine and rehabilitation for, 67–69
    secondary effects of, 57–58, 60–61
    spray and stretch for, 80
    treatment overview for, 61–66, 69f
    vocational rehabilitation for, 69–70
Myofascial release, 249

N
Na+ (sodium) channels
    in chronic pain, 23
    in ectopic activity, 32
Nalbuphine, 49
Naproxen, 48
NCD. *See* Nucleus caudalis DREZ (NCD).
NE (norepinephrine)
    in descending pain pathway, 26, 26f
    in neuropathic pain, 33
Neck pain, due to cancer, 90–93
Negative phenomena, 29
Negative symptoms, 29
Neo-spinothalamic pathway, 194
Nerve conduction studies, of failed back surgery syndrome, 78
Nerve damage
    clinical symptoms following, 30
    pain due to. *See* Neuropathic pain.
Nerve fiber interactions, pathologic, in neuropathic pain, 33–34
Nerve growth factor (NGF), in nociceptor sensitization, 20
Nerve inflammation, in neuropathic pain, 33
Nerve injury, anatomic reorganization after, 34, 34f
Nervus intermedius (NI), 234, 235
Neural excitotoxicity, 23
Neuralgia(s). *See under* specific neuralgia, e.g., Occipital neuralgia.
    sphenopalatine, radiosurgery for, 245
Neuraxial analgesic administration, 150–155
    advantages of, 150
    complications of, 155

implantation technique for, 151–153, 152f
    indications for, 150–151
    outcomes of, 153–155, 154t
    preimplant considerations for, 151
    trials for, 150, 151
    types of pumps and catheter placements for, 153
Neurectomy, peripheral. *See* Peripheral neurectomy.
Neurokinin-1 (NK-1) receptors
    in central sensitization, 35
    in change from acute to inflammatory pain, 22, 22f
    in pre-emptive analgesia, 23
Neuromas
    experimental, 32, 32f
    pathophysiology of, 201
    prevention of, 201
Neuropathic pain
    algorithm for, 187, 187f
    anatomic reorganization following injury in, 34, 34f
    animal models of, 31, 31t
    central sensitization in, 34–35
    characteristics of, 162
    classification of, 30–31, 30t
    defined, 7, 17, 30
    diagnosis of, 30
    DRG neurons in, 33
    ectopic activity in, 32–33, 32f
    etiology and anatomic distribution of, 30, 30t
    intracranial ablative procedures for, 196–197, 197t
    loss of endogenous pain inhibitory controls in, 35
    motor cortex stimulation for, 160–163, 162f, 163f
    nerve inflammation in, 33
    pathologic fiber interactions in, 33–34
    pathophysiology of, 29–36
    peripheral mechanisms of, 31–34, 32f
    physiologic *vs.*, 29, 30f
    scope of, 29
    spinal mechanisms of, 34–35, 34f
    supraspinal mechanisms of, 35
    sympathetic nervous system in, 33
    thalamus and cortex in, 35
    treatment of, 17, 36, 52
    trigeminal, 84, 103t, 104
Neuropeptide(s), in nociceptive afferent fibers, 19
Neuropeptide Y (NPY), in neuropathic pain, 33
Neurosurgeon, consultation with, 4
Neurosurgical pain practice, building (and surviving) a, 271–274
Neurotransmitters, for nociceptive afferent fibers, 19
Neurotrophins, in nociceptor sensitization, 20
NGF (nerve growth factor), in nociceptor sensitization, 20
NI (nervus intermedius), 234, 235
Nitric oxide (NO) synthase, in change from acute to inflammatory pain, 23
NK-1 receptors. *See* Neurokinin-1 (NK-1) receptors.
N-methyl-*D*-aspartate (NMDA) receptors
    in central sensitization, 34, 35
    in change from acute to inflammatory pain, 21, 22, 22f
    in pre-emptive analgesia, 23
    in secondary hyperalgesia, 27
NO (nitric oxide) synthase, in change from acute to inflammatory pain, 23
Nociception, conditioned, 43
Nociceptive afferent fibers
    deep somatic, 18
    neurochemistry of, 19
Nociceptive pain, 7, 29
    intracranial ablative procedures for, 195–196, 197t
Nociceptive specific (NS) neurons, 20
Nociceptor sensitization, 19–20, 20f
Nociceptors
    defined, 17–18
    silent (sleeping), 18
non-NMDA receptors
    in change from acute to inflammatory pain, 21, 22, 22f
    in hyperalgesia, 27

Nonsteroidal anti-inflammatory drugs (NSAIDs), 47–48
    efficacy of, 46
    for failed back surgery syndrome, 80
    for inflammatory pain, 20
    in balanced analgesic regimen, 53
Norepinephrine (NE)
    in descending pain pathway, 26, 26f
    in neuropathic pain, 33
Normal pain, 29
Nortriptyline, 49
Noxious stimuli, 17, 18f
NPY (neuropeptide Y), in neuropathic pain, 33
NRG (nucleus reticularis gigantocellularis), in descending pain pathway, 26f
NS (nociceptive specific) neurons, 20
NSAIDs. See Nonsteroidal anti-inflammatory drugs (NSAIDs).
Nuclear medicine, of failed back surgery syndrome, 77t, 78
Nucleus caudalis DREZ (NCD), 190–192
    for facial pain due to malignancy, 92–93
    for postherpetic neuralgia, 96
Nucleus cuneiformis, in descending pain pathway, 26, 26f
Nucleus raphe magnus, in descending pain pathway, 25, 26f
Nucleus reticularis gigantocellularis (NRG), in descending pain pathway, 26f
Nucleus reticularis magnocellularis, in descending pain pathway, 25, 26f
Nucleus reticularis paragigantocellularis, in descending pain pathway, 25, 26f
Nucleus submedius, in post-stroke pain, 111
Nurses, in multidisciplinary pain treatment program, 257

O
Occipital nerve
    greater, 87, 88
    lesser, 87–88
Occipital nerve block, for occipital neuralgia, 89
Occipital nerve neurectomy, 99
Occipital nerve neurolysis, 99
Occipital nerve stimulation, for occipital neuralgia, 89, 100–101
Occipital neuralgia, 87–89, 99–101
    anatomy and pathophysiology of, 87–88
    clinical presentation of, 99
    diagnosis of, 88
    dorsal root ganglionectomy for, 206
    DREZ lesions for, 184
    etiology of, 88, 88t, 99
    peripheral nerve stimulation for, 141
    treatment for, 88–89, 99–101
Occupational therapy, for myofascial pain syndromes, 68–69
OFF cells, 26
    in opioid analgesia, 27, 27f
Office management, for neurosurgical pain practice, 273
ON cells, 26
    in opioid analgesia, 27, 27f
Opiates, intraventricular, for head and neck cancer, 91–92
Opioid(s), 49–53
    addiction to, 50
    around-the-clock use of, 51, 51f
    as peripheral analgesics, 20
    different responses to, 51–52, 51f, 52f
    efficacy of, 46, 49
    endogenous, 26, 27f
    for failed back surgery syndrome, 81
    for neuropathic pain, 36, 52
    for postherpetic neuralgia, 95
    in balanced analgesic regimen, 52–53
    legal issues with, 50, 53
    long-acting, 52f
    minimum effective analgesic concentration of, 50–51, 51f
    mixed agonist-antagonist, 49
    naturally occurring, 49
    partial agonist, 49
    pharmacology of, 26–27, 27f
    physical dependence on, 50
    pseudoaddiction to, 50
    pure μ-agonist, 49
    refilling prescriptions for, 50, 53
    semisynthetic, 49
    side effects of, 52
    synthetic, 49
Opioid receptors, 26
Orthoses, for failed back surgery syndrome, 81
Oscillopsia, due to deep-brain stimulation, 157–158
Otalgic geniculate neuralgia, 87
Outcome(s)
    maximizing, 13–14
    patients expectations about, 5, 6f, 10, 12
    psychological factors related to surgical, 39–40
Outcome assessment, 265–269, 267f–269f
Oxcarbazepine (Trileptal), for trigeminal neuralgia, 105t, 107
Oxycodone, 49

P
Paddle electrode, 132
PAG. See Periaqueductal gray (PAG).
Pain
    acute, 5–7
        chronic vs., 4, 64
        recurring, 5
        spinal mechanisms of, 21, 22f
    and disability, 263
    and impairment, 264
    approach to patient with, 3–15
    chronic, 7
        acute vs., 4, 64
        chronic disease vs., 255
        defined, 131
        depression with, 65
        difficulties of, 247–248
        drug abuse with, 64–65
        epidemiology of, 247
        intractable benign, 66
        obligations in care for, 4–5
        spinal mechanisms of, 23
    classification of, 5–7, 7f
    comorbidities with, 53
    corticalization of, 43
    incident, 51
    inflammatory
        attenuation of, 20
        descending modulation of, 27
        neuropathic vs., 29
        spinal mechanisms of, 21–23
    neuroanatomic and neurophysiologic basis of, 17–27
    neuropathic. See Neuropathic pain.
    nociceptive, 7, 29
    normal, 29
    pathologic, 29, 30f
    perception of, 17, 18f
    physiologic, 29, 30f
    protective functions of, 17
    psychogenic, 70
    reflexive, 29
    somatic, 17–20, 20f
    subacute, 5–7
    transient, 29
    types of, 5–7, 7f
"Pain generator," 7, 40
    in cluster headache, 93
    in failed back surgery syndrome, 79–80
Pain inhibitory controls, loss of endogenous, 35
Pain management, failures of, 3–4, 5
Pain pathways
    ascending, 23–25, 24f
    descending, 25–26, 26f
Pain rehabilitation, 245–251
    modalities of, 247–250
    outcome measures for, 250–251

programs for, 246–247
referral for, 247
Pain threshold, 8
Paleospinothalamic pathway, 194
Pancoast syndrome, DREZotomy for, 179f, 183
Paraffin wax, for heat therapy, 248
Paresthesias, 29
   due to deep-brain stimulation, 158
Pathologic pain, 29, 30f
Patient, expectations of, 5, 6f, 10, 12, 14
   and patient satisfaction with spine surgery, 39
Patient "contracts," 274
Patient education, for failed back surgery syndrome, 80
Patient satisfaction, with spine surgery, 39
Patient selection, 12
Patient-controlled analgesia (PCA), 51f, 150
   oral, 52f
Patrick's test, 58, 62f
Pentazocine, 49
Percutaneous balloon compression, for trigeminal neuralgia, 214–218
   anesthesia for, 214–215
   background of, 214
   bilateral, 217
   equipment placement and draping for, 215, 215f
   indications for, 214
   intraoperative imaging for, 215
   operative techniques for, 214
   positioning for, 215
   preoperative preparation for, 214
   pressure monitoring technique for, 215–216, 216f
   recurrence after, 217
   results of, 216–218
   volume-controlled approach for, 216
Percutaneous cordotomy, 165–170
   alternatives to, 166–167, 167t
   complications of, 168–169, 169f
   for spinal cord injury pain, 113
   history of, 165
   indications for, 165–166, 166t
   mechanism of, 165
   operative technique for, 167–168, 167f
   results of, 168
Percutaneous glossopharyngeal rhizotomy, 86
Percutaneous leads, for spinal cord stimulation, 138–139, 138f, 139f
Percutaneous neurostimulation, for occipital neuralgia, 100–101
Percutaneous radiofrequency (RF) rhizotomy, for trigeminal neuralgia, 227–231
   electrode localization for, 228f, 229, 229f
   historical background of, 227
   lesion production in, 229–230
   needle placement for, 228
   patient selection for, 227
   positioning for, 228
   preoperative preparation for, 228
   reducing complications of, 230–231
   results of, 230
   surgical technique of, 227–230
Percutaneous radiofrequency (RF) sympathectomy, 203
Percutaneous retrogasserian glycerol rhizotomy (PRGR), for trigeminal neuralgia, 219–225
   anesthesia for, 221–222
   complications of, 223–225
   contraindications to, 225
   history of, 220
   indications and patient selection for, 220
   landmarks, trajectory, and imaging during, 222–223, 222f–224f
   mechanism of action of, 220–221
   positioning for, 221
   preoperative evaluation for, 221
   reported success with, 225
Percutaneous trigeminal nerve compression, 214–218
   anesthesia for, 214–215

background of, 214
bilateral, 217
equipment placement and draping for, 215, 215f
indications for, 214
intraoperative imaging for, 215
operative techniques for, 214
positioning for, 215
preoperative preparation for, 214
pressure monitoring technique for, 215–216, 216f
recurrence after, 217
results of, 216–218
volume-controlled approach for, 216
Percutaneous trigeminal tractotomy and nucleotomy, 92
Periaqueductal gray (PAG)
   deep brain stimulation of, for postherpetic neuralgia, 95
   in descending pain pathway, 25, 26, 26f
   in opioid analgesia, 27, 27f
Perineal pain, dorsal root ganglionectomy for, 206
Peripheral ablative technique(s), 200–209
   advantages and disadvantages of, 200
   dorsal rhizotomy as, 205, 206
   dorsal root ganglionectomy as, 205–206
   facet rhizotomy as, 206–208
   peripheral neurectomy as, 200–202
   splanchnicectomy as, 204
   sympathectomy as, 202–205
Peripheral mechanisms
   of neuropathic pain, 31–34, 32f
   of somatic pain, 17–20, 20f
Peripheral nerve injury, spinal mechanisms of chronic pain due to, 23
Peripheral nerve lesions, DREZ lesions for, 183–184
Peripheral nerve pain, pathophysiology of, 200–201
Peripheral nerve stimulation (PNS), 144–148
   for occipital neuralgia, 89, 100–101
   for postherpetic neuralgia, 95
   history of, 144
   indications for, 146
   mechanism of, 144
   outcome studies of, 145–146, 148f
   spinal cord stimulation vs., 147
   technique of, 144–145, 145f–148f
   uses and future of, 147
Peripheral nerve terminals, sensitization of, 200–201
Peripheral nervous system, electrical stimulation of, 141
Peripheral neurectomy, 200–202
   for trigeminal neuralgia, 210–213
      indications and patient selection for, 210–211
      needle techniques for, 211–212, 211f
      open surgical techniques for, 212–213, 212f
      outcomes of, 213
      rationale for, 210
   of greater occipital nerve, 89
Peripheral sensitization, 17, 22f, 200–201
Peripheral trigeminal denervation, 210–213
   indications and patient selection for, 210–211
   needle techniques for, 211–212, 211f
   open surgical techniques for, 212–213, 212f
   outcomes of, 213
   rationale for, 210
Periventricular gray (PVG), deep brain stimulation of, 157–159, 157f
   for postherpetic neuralgia, 95
Personality disorders, and surgical outcome, 41
Personality factors, in failed pain syndrome, 8
Personality testing, for spine surgery, 39, 41–42
PGH$_2$ (prostaglandin H$_2$), effect of NSAIDs and acetaminophen on, 47
Phantom limb pain
   DREZ lesions for, 115, 184
   medical strategies for, 113
   pathophysiology of, 112
   surgical strategies for, 114
   treatment outcomes for, 115

Pharmacologic therapies, 46–54
  for failed back surgery syndrome, 80–81
  general principles of, 46
  with acetaminophen, 47
  with anticonvulsant drugs, 49
  with antidepressant agents, 48–49
  with aspirin, 47–48
  with COX inhibitors, 48
  with NSAIDs, 47–48
  with opioids, 49–53, 51f, 52f
Phenytoin (Dilantin, diphenylhydantoin), 49
  for trigeminal neuralgia, 105t, 106
PHN. See Postherpetic neuralgia (PHN).
Physiatry, in neurosurgical pain practice, 272
Physical dependence, on opioids, 50
Physical rehabilitation, 247–253
  for myofascial pain syndromes, 67–69
  modalities of, 249–252
  outcome measures for, 252–254
  programs for, 248–249
  referral for, 249
Physical therapy (PT)
  for failed back surgery syndrome, 80
  in multidisciplinary pain treatment program, 257, 258
  in pain rehabilitation, 246
Physician, in multidisciplinary pain treatment program, 256
Physiologic pain, 29, 30f
Piriformis syndrome, 58, 62f
Piroxicam, 48
Placebo response, in spine surgery, 43
Plate electrode, 132
PNS. See Peripheral nerve stimulation (PNS).
Positive phenomena, 29
Positive symptoms, 29
Postcentral gyrectomy, 160
Postcentral gyrus stimulation, 160
Posterior complex, of thalamus, in ascending pain pathway, 24, 24f
Posterior fossa procedures, 232–236
  for geniculate neuralgia, 234–235, 235f
  for glossopharyngeal neuralgia, 235–236, 236f
  for trigeminal neuralgia, 232–234, 234f
  general considerations for, 236
Postganglionic sympathectomy, 202
Postherpetic neuralgia (PHN), 95–96
  clinical features of, 103t, 104
  deep brain stimulation for, 95–96
  DREZ lesions for, 96, 184
  epidemiology of, 95
  motor cortex stimulation for, 96, 161
  nucleus caudalis DREZ for, 96, 190–192
  pathophysiology of, 95
  pharmacologic treatment of, 95
  surgical treatment of, 95–96
Post-laminectomy syndrome. See Failed back surgery syndrome (FBSS).
Postlaparotomy pain, dorsal root ganglionectomy for, 206
Postoperative issues, 12
Post-stroke pain
  medical strategies for, 112–113
  nucleus caudalis DREZ for, 190–192
  pathophysiology of, 111–112
  surgical strategies for, 114
  treatment outcomes for, 115
Postsynaptic dorsal column (PSDC) neurons, 24, 24f
Post-thoracotomy pain, dorsal root ganglionectomy for, 206
Post-traumatic pain, nucleus caudalis DREZ for, 190–192
Potassium bromide, for trigeminal neuralgia, 104
Potency, of drug, 46
PQRST mnemonic, 266
Practice management, for neurosurgical pain practice, 273–274
Precentral gyrus stimulation, 160
Pre-emptive analgesia, 23
Preganglionic sympathectomy, 202
Preoperative evaluation, 12
Pressure monitoring technique, for percutaneous trigeminal nerve
  compression, 215–216, 216f

Presynaptic inhibition, loss of, 35
PRGR. See Percutaneous retrogasserian glycerol rhizotomy (PRGR).
Primary afferent fibers, 17–18
Primary hyperalgesia, 17
Projection neurons, 20, 21f
Prostaglandin(s), vasodilatation due to, 57
Prostaglandin H₂ (PGH₂), effect of NSAIDs and acetaminophen on, 47
PSDC (postsynaptic dorsal column) neurons, 24, 24f
Pseudoaddiction, to opioids, 50
Pseudoarthrosis, failed back surgery syndrome due to, 76
Psychiatrist, in neurosurgical pain practice, 272
Psychological assessment
  for failed back surgery syndrome, 79
  for spinal cord stimulation, 135
  for spine surgery, 41–42, 42f
Psychological comorbidity, in outcome assessment, 267
Psychological consultation, for spine surgery, 42–43, 43t
Psychological counseling, for myofascial pain syndromes, 70
Psychological factors
  in complex regional pain syndrome, 123–124
  in failed back surgery syndrome, 74, 80
  in spine surgery, 38–44
  related to surgical outcomes, 39–40
Psychological "risk factors," for poor surgical outcome, 40–41, 40t, 44
Psychologists
  consultation with, 4
  in multidisciplinary pain treatment program, 13–14, 257, 258
  in neurosurgical pain practice, 272
  in pain rehabilitation programs, 248, 253
Psychosocial factors, in chronic pain, 11
PT. See Physical therapy (PT).
Pulvinotomy, for post-stroke pain, 114
Punctate midline myelotomy, 173–174, 174f
Putative diagnoses, in outcome assessment, 266–267
PVG (periventricular gray), deep brain stimulation of, 157–159, 157f
  for postherpetic neuralgia, 95

Q
Quadratus lumborum syndrome, 58, 59f
Quality of life (QOL) measures, in outcome assessment, 267

R
Radiation surgery. See Radiosurgery.
Radiation therapy, for head and neck cancer, 91
Radiculopathy, due to herniated disk, 57
Radiofrequency (RF) facet joint denervation, 208
Radiofrequency (RF) rhizolysis, for trigeminal neuralgia, 107, 108t
Radiofrequency (RF) rhizotomy
  for cluster headache, 94–95
  for trigeminal neuralgia, 227–231
    electrode localization for, 228f, 229, 229f
    historical background of, 227
    lesion production in, 229–230
    needle placement for, 228
    patient selection for, 227
    positioning for, 228
    preoperative preparation for, 228
    reducing complications of, 230–231
    results of, 230
    surgical technique of, 227–230
Radiofrequency (RF) stimulation system, 136, 137f
Radiofrequency (RF) sympathectomy, 203
Radiofrequency (RF) thermocoagulation DREZ lesions, 180–181
Radiographic evaluation
  of failed back surgery syndrome, 77–78, 77t
  of occipital neuralgia, 88
Radionuclide scans, of failed back surgery syndrome, 77t, 78
Radiosurgery, 239–246
  for cingulotomy, 246
  for cluster headache, 245
  for hypophysectomy, 246
  for medial thalamotomy, 197, 239–241, 240f, 241f

for sphenopalatine neuralgia, 243
for trigeminal neuralgia, 107, 108t, 240–243, 241f, 242f
Radiothalamotomy, 197, 239–241, 240f, 241f
Ramsay-Hunt syndrome, geniculate neuralgia in, 87
Range-of-motion exercises, 250
for myofascial pain syndromes, 68
Receiver, 132
Receptive field, of primary afferent fibers, 18
Rectus abdominis syndrome, 59, 63f
Recurring acute pain, 5
Referral
to multidisciplinary pain treatment program, 257–258
to physical rehabilitation program, 249
Reflex sympathetic dystrophy (RSD). See Complex regional pain syndrome (CRPS).
Reflexive pain, 29
Regression, response to, 11
Rehabilitation, 245–251
for myofascial pain syndromes, 67–69
modalities of, 247–250
outcome measures for, 250–251
programs for, 246–247
referral for, 247
Reinnervation, chaotic, 112
Relaxation training, for myofascial pain syndromes, 70
Reorganization, after nerve injury, 34, 34f
Respiratory compromise, due to cordotomy, 169
Respiratory depression, due to opioids, 52
Reticular formation, in descending pain pathway, 25, 26f
Retrogasserian glycerol injection, for cluster headache, 95
Retrogasserian RF rhizotomy, for cluster headache, 94–95
RF. See Radiofrequency (RF).
Rhizotomy
dorsal, 205, 206
facet, 206–208
for glossopharyngeal neuralgia, 86
percutaneous radiofrequency (RF), for trigeminal neuralgia, 227–231
electrode localization for, 228f, 229, 229f
historical background of, 227
lesion production in, 229–230
needle placement for, 228
patient selection for, 227
positioning for, 228
preoperative preparation for, 228
reducing complications of, 230–231
results of, 230
surgical technique of, 227–230
percutaneous retrogasserian glycerol, for trigeminal neuralgia, 219–225
anesthesia for, 221–222
complications of, 223–225
contraindications to, 225
history of, 220
indications and patient selection for, 220
landmarks, trajectory, and imaging during, 222–223, 222f–224f
mechanism of action of, 220–221
positioning for, 221
preoperative evaluation for, 221
reported success with, 225
Rhomboid syndrome, 59, 65f
"Risk factors," for poor surgical outcome, 39, 40–41, 40t
Rofecoxib, 48
Root syndrome, due to herniated disk, 57
Rostroventral medulla (RVM)
in descending pain pathway, 25–26, 26f
in neuropathic pain, 35
in opioid analgesia, 27, 27f
RSD (reflex sympathetic dystrophy). See Complex regional pain syndrome (CRPS).

S
SCA (superior cerebellar artery), compression of trigeminal nerve by, 233
Screening trial, for spinal cord stimulation, 135, 136t

SCS. See Spinal cord stimulation (SCS).
Secondary effects, of myofascial pain syndromes, 57–58, 60–61
Secondary gain, 258, 259
Secondary hyperalgesia, 17, 27
Selective serotonin reuptake inhibitors (SSRIs), 48, 49
Seniority issues, in failed pain syndrome, 9–10
Sensitization
central, 17, 21–23, 22f
in neuropathic pain, 34–35
pathologic, 34–35
nociceptor, 19–20, 20f
peripheral, 17, 22f, 200–201
Sensory afferent fibers, 18
efferent function of, 19
Sensory neurons, stimulus-independent activity of, 32
Sensory-discriminative pathways, 24, 24f
Sensory-sympathetic coupling, in neuropathic pain, 33
Serotonin (5-HT), in descending pain pathway, 25–26, 26f
Sexual abuse, and surgical outcome, 44
SF-36, 267
SG (substantia gelatinosa), 176, 177f
Shingles, postherpetic neuralgia after, 95–96
Silent nociceptors, 18
Silent synapses, in acute pain, 21
SIP (sympathetically independent pain). See Complex regional pain syndrome (CRPS).
Sleeping nociceptors, 18
Sluder's syndrome, 89
SMP (sympathetically maintained pain). See Complex regional pain syndrome (CRPS).
SMT (spinomesencephalic tract), 24f, 25
in spinal cord pain, 111
Sodium (Na+) channels
in chronic pain, 23
in ectopic activity, 32
Sodium valproate (Depakote), for trigeminal neuralgia, 105t
Somatic anxiety, and surgical outcome, 39, 41
Somatic pain, 17–20, 20f
Somatization
and surgical outcome, 41
in chronic pain syndromes, 256, 260
Somatosensory evoked potentials (SSEPs), with DREZ lesions, 179–180, 182f
SP. See Substance P (SP).
Sphenopalatine neuralgia, 89
radiosurgery for, 245
Spinal cord
dorsal horn of, 20–27, 21f
synaptic organization of, 21, 21f
Spinal cord inhibitory neurotransmission, loss of, 35
Spinal cord injury pain
DREZ lesions for, 113, 114, 183, 185t, 186f
medical strategies for, 112
pathophysiology of, 110–111
surgical strategies for, 113
treatment outcomes for, 114
Spinal cord stimulation (SCS), 131–141
complications of, 140–141
epidural
for phantom limb pain, 115
for spinal cord injury pain, 113
equipment for, 136–137, 136f, 137f
experience and training in, 133, 134t
for complex regional pain syndrome, 125
for failed back surgery syndrome, 81
historical background of, 131–132
indications for and efficacy of, 132–133
lead implant techniques for, 137–140, 138f–140f
patient selection criteria for, 133–134, 135t
peripheral nerve stimulation vs., 147
psychological screening for, 135
screening trial for, 135, 136t
terminology for, 132
Spinal fusions, failure of, 75

Spinal mechanisms
  of acute pain, 21, 22f
  of chronic pain, 23
  of inflammatory pain, 21–23
  of neuropathic pain, 34–35, 34f
Spine surgery
  psychological assessment for, 41–42, 42t
  psychological considerations in, 38–44
  psychological consultation for, 42–43, 43t
  psychological factors related to outcomes of, 39–40
  psychological "risk factors" for, 40–41, 40t
  return to work after, 39
Spinocervical tract, in post-stroke pain, 111–112
Spinomesencephalic tract (SMT), 24f, 25
  in spinal cord pain, 111
Spinoparabrachial system, in spinal cord pain, 111
Spinopontoamygdaloid pathway, in spinal cord pain, 111
Spinoreticular tract (SRT), 24–25, 24f
  in spinal cord pain, 111
Spinothalamic tract (STT), 24, 24f
  ventral, 25
Splanchnicectomy, 204
Spondylolisthesis, postoperative, 77–78
Spondylolysis, postoperative, 77–78
Spray and stretch, for myofascial pain syndromes, 80
SRT (spinoreticular tract), 24–25, 24f
  in spinal cord pain, 111
SSEPs (somatosensory evoked potentials), with DREZ lesions,
    179–180, 182f
SSRIs (selective serotonin reuptake inhibitors), 48, 49
Steady state, of drug, 46
Stereotactic extralemniscal myelotomy, 173
Stereotactic radiosurgery, 239–246
  for cingulotomy, 246
  for cluster headache, 245
  for hypophysectomy, 246
  for medial thalamotomy, 239–241, 240f, 241f
  for sphenopalatine neuralgia, 245
  for trigeminal neuralgia, 107, 108t, 242–245, 243f, 244f
Stereotactic thalamotomy, for spinal cord injury pain, 114
Stimulus intensity, and pain sensation, 18f
Strengthening exercises, 252
Stress-induced analgesia, 63
Stretching exercises, 252
Stroke, pain after
  medical strategies for, 112–113
  nucleus caudalis DREZ for, 190–192
  pathophysiology of, 111–112
  surgical strategies for, 114
  treatment outcomes for, 115
STT (spinothalamic tract), 24, 24f
  ventral, 25
Stump pain, 112
  DREZ lesions for, 184
Subacute pain, 5–7
Substance abuse
  and surgical outcome, 41
  with chronic pain, 64–65
Substance P (SP)
  in change from acute to inflammatory pain, 21, 22f
  in neuropathic pain, 33, 35
  in nociceptive afferent fibers, 19
Substantia gelatinosa (SG), 176, 177f
Subthreshold synapses, in acute pain, 21
SUNCT syndrome, 94
Superior cerebellar artery (SCA), compression of trigeminal nerve by, 233
Superior laryngeal neuralgia, 90
Supraclavicular approach, for upper thoracic sympathectomy, 203
Supraorbital nerve, peripheral denervation of, 211–212, 211f, 212f, 213
Supraspinal mechanisms, in neuropathic pain, 35
Supraspinatus syndrome, 59, 66f
Surgeon, in multidisciplinary approach, 13
Surgical outcomes, psychological factors related to, 39–40
Sweet, William, 5

Sympathectomy, 202–205
  indications for, 202
  lumbar, 204
  percutaneous radiofrequency, 203
  preganglionic vs. postganglionic, 202
  results of, 204–205
  upper thoracic, 202–203
  video-assisted thoracoscopic, 203–204
Sympathetic ganglion block, selective, 202
Sympathetic nervous system, in neuropathic pain, 33
Sympathetically independent pain (SIP). See Complex regional pain
    syndrome (CRPS).
Sympathetically maintained pain (SMP). See Complex regional pain
    syndrome (CRPS).
Sympatholysis, for complex regional pain syndrome, 125
Symptom presentation, in outcome assessment, 266
Synapses, subthreshold (silent), in acute pain, 21
Synaptic organization, of spinal cord, 21, 21f

T
TCAs (tricyclic antidepressants), 48–49
  for occipital neuralgia, 88
Technology issues, in failed pain syndrome, 10
Tegretol (carbamazepine), 49
  for trigeminal neuralgia, 104, 105–106, 105t, 219, 242
Tender points, 57
TENS (transcutaneous electrical nerve stimulation), 251
  for myofascial pain syndromes, 68, 80
Thalamic burst activity, motor cortex stimulation and, 160
Thalamic deep brain stimulation
  for phantom limb pain, 115
  for spinal cord injury pain, 114
Thalamic sensory nuclei, deep-brain stimulation of, 158, 158f, 159
Thalamotomy
  for phantom limb pain, 115
  for post-stroke pain, 114, 115
  for spinal cord injury pain, 114
  medial, 196–197, 197t
    radiosurgery for, 197, 239–241, 240f, 241f
Thalamus
  in neuropathic pain, 35
  posterior complex of, in ascending pain pathway, 24, 24f
Thebaine, 49
Therapeutic exercises, 251–252
Therapeutic heat, 250
Therapeutic range, 50, 51f
Therapeutic window, 50, 51f
Thoracic apex syndrome, DREZ lesions for, 183
Thromboxane, vasoconstriction due to, 57
Thromboxane A_2 (TxA_2), in tissue injury, 47
Tinel's sign, 32
TN. See Trigeminal neuralgia (TN).
TNF-α (tumor necrosis factor-α), in neuropathic pain, 33
TNP (trigeminal neuropathic pain), 84, 103t, 104
Tobacco, and cluster headache, 94
"Topectomy," for post-stroke pain, 114
Tract of Lissauer (TL), 176, 177f
Traction, 249
  for myofascial pain syndromes, 68
Tractotomy, midbrain, 93, 189–190
Transaxillary approach, for upper thoracic sympathectomy, 203
Transcutaneous electrical nerve stimulation (TENS), 251
  for myofascial pain syndromes, 68, 80
Transient pain, 29
Trazodone, 49
  for insomnia, 53
Treatment failure, 8
Tricyclic antidepressants (TCAs), 48–49
  for occipital neuralgia, 88
Trigeminal neuralgia (TN), 84, 102–108
  atypical, 103–104, 240–241
  classification of, 232
  clinical presentation of, 102, 103t

defined, 219, 232
diagnosis of, 103t
differential diagnosis of, 103–104
epidemiology of, 102, 219
etiology of, 102, 103t, 219
evaluation of, 104
glossopharyngeal vs., 84–85
medical management of, 104–107, 105t, 219
microvascular decompression for, 107t, 108t, 232–234, 234f, 244–245
natural history of, 219
nucleus caudalis DREZ for, 190–192
pathophysiology of, 102
percutaneous balloon compression for, 214–218
    anesthesia for, 214–215
    background of, 214
    bilateral, 217
    equipment placement and draping for, 215, 215f
    indications for, 214
    intraoperative imaging for, 215
    operative techniques for, 214
    positioning for, 215
    preoperative preparation for, 214
    pressure monitoring technique for, 215–216, 216f
    recurrence after, 217
    results of, 216–218
    volume-controlled approach for, 216
percutaneous glycerol rhizotomy for, 219–225
    anesthesia for, 221–222
    complications of, 223–225
    contraindications to, 225
    history of, 220
    indications and patient selection for, 220
    landmarks, trajectory, and imaging during, 222–223, 222f–224f
    mechanism of action of, 220–221
    positioning for, 221
    preoperative evaluation for, 221
    reported success with, 225
percutaneous radiofrequency rhizotomy for, 227–231
    electrode localization for, 228f, 229, 229f
    historical background of, 227
    lesion production in, 229–230
    needle placement for, 228
    patient selection for, 227
    positioning for, 228
    preoperative preparation for, 228
    reducing complications of, 230–231
    results of, 230
    surgical technique of, 227–230
peripheral neurectomy for, 210–213
    indications and patient selection for, 210–211
    needle techniques for, 211–212, 211f
    open surgical techniques for, 212–213, 212f
    outcomes of, 213
    rationale for, 210
posterior fossa procedures for, 232–234, 234f
radiosurgery for, 107, 108t, 242–245, 243f, 244f
secondary, 245
surgical treatment of, 107–108, 108t, 219–220
treatment algorithm for, 107–108
typical, 103
Trigeminal neuropathic pain (TNP), 84, 103t, 104
Trigeminal neuropathy, motor cortex stimulation for, 161
Trigeminal nucleotomy, percutaneous, 92
Trigeminal tractotomy
    open, 92
    percutaneous, 92

Trigger point(s), 57
Trigger point desensitization, for myofascial pain syndromes, 68
Trileptal (oxcarbazepine), for trigeminal neuralgia, 105t, 107
Trophic disturbance, in complex regional pain syndrome, 121
L-Tryptophan, with deep-brain stimulation, 158–159
Tumor necrosis factor-α (TNF-α), in neuropathic pain, 33
TxA$_2$ (thromboxane A$_2$), in tissue injury, 47
Typical trigeminal neuralgia (TTN), 103

U
Ultrasonic DREZ lesions, 181
Uniform Outcome Measures (UOM) project, 265
Upper thoracic sympathectomy, 202–203

V
Vail's syndrome, 89–90
Valdecoxib, 48
Value, in outcome assessment, 267, 267f
Varicella-zoster virus, postherpetic neuralgia due to. See Postherpetic neuralgia (PHN).
Vascular chronic pain syndromes, 255
VATS (video-assisted thoracoscopic sympathectomy), 203–204
Ventral posterior lateralis (VPL)
    deep-brain stimulation of, 157, 158
    in ascending pain pathway, 24, 24f
Ventral posterior medialis (VPM), 157, 158
Ventral spinothalamic tract, 25f
Ventrobasal complex, in post-stroke pain, 111
Video-assisted thoracoscopic sympathectomy (VATS), 203–204
Vidian neuralgia, 89–90
Visceral afferent fibers, 18–19
Vocational adjustment, 12
Vocational counselors, in pain rehabilitation programs, 247
Vocational rehabilitation, for myofascial pain syndromes, 69–70
Volume-controlled approach, for percutaneous trigeminal nerve compression, 216
VPL (ventral posterior lateralis)
    deep-brain stimulation of, 157, 158
    in ascending pain pathway, 24, 24f
VPM (ventral posterior medialis), 157, 158

W
Waddell signs
    in chronic pain syndromes, 256, 258, 260
    in failed back surgery syndrome, 76
Wage replacement ratio, 9
Wide dynamic range (WDR) neurons, 20
Work, return to, 8, 9–10
    after spine surgery, 39
Work conditioning, for myofascial pain syndromes, 69
Work hardening programs, for failed back surgery syndrome, 80
Workers' compensation
    and surgical outcome, 41
    in failed pain syndrome, 8
Workplace environmental problems, in failed pain syndrome, 9–10

Z
Zung Depression Inventory, 40